# TRANSLATIONAL AND EXPERIMENTAL CLINICAL RESEARCH

**Daniel P. Schuster, MD**
Professor of Medicine and Radiology
Associate Dean for Clinical Research
Director, Program in Translational and Experimental Medicine
Washington University School of Medicine
St. Louis, Missouri

**William J. Powers, MD**
Professor of Neurology, Neurological Surgery, and Radiology
Head, Cerebrovascular Diseases and Neuroimaging Sections
Washington University School of Medicine
St. Louis, Missouri

LIPPINCOTT WILLIAMS & WILKINS
A **Wolters Kluwer** Company

Philadelphia • Baltimore • New York • London
Buenos Aires • Hong Kong • Sydney • Tokyo

*Acquisitions Editor:* Sonya Seigafuse
*Developmental Editor:* Fran Murphy
*Project Manager:* David Murphy
*Senior Manufacturing Manager:* Ben Rivera
*Marketing Manager:* Kathy Neely
*Designer:* Doug Smock
*Production Services:* Schawk, Inc.
*Printer:* Edward Brothers

**Library of Congress Cataloging-in-Publication Data**
Translational and experimental clinical research / [edited by] Daniel P Schuster,
William J. Powers.
    p. ; cm.
  Includes bibliographical references and index.
  ISBN 0-7817-5565-4 (alk. paper)
  1. Medicine—Research—Methodology. 2. Medicine—Research—Statistical
methods. 3. Clinical trials—Methodology. I. Schuster, Daniel P. II. Powers,
Willliam J.
  [DNLM: 1. Biomedical Research—methods. 2. Clinical Trials—methods.
  3. Data Interpretation, Statistical. 4. Research Design. W 20.5 T772 2005]
  R850.T73 2005
  610'.72'4—dc22

                                            2005011068

# Preface

There are many fine textbooks about statistics in clinical research, about epidemiology and public health, even about the design and conduct of clinical trials. But, in our view, no introductory textbook has been available for the entry-level investigator interested in employing the tools of modern biology to answer a scientific question about human disease. Addressing this deficiency, in a nutshell, is the purpose and goal of this book.

In the Introduction, we address, in a more formal way, the definitions of "translational" and "experimental" clinical research. No question, however, that these buzzwords are "hot"; they are popular in the lay press as well as in scientific journals. Why now?

Well, "time" is certainly a major reason. Physicians and physician-scientists have been "translating" basic discoveries into clinical practice, in both formal and informal ways, for at least the last century. But there is a sense that the pace should (must?) now be accelerated. A decade or two interval between discovery and best practice is no longer acceptable. The public, the press, and Congress all want to see a quicker return on the research investment. Accordingly, funding agencies like the National Institutes of Health (NIH) are working to reengineer the clinical research enterprise and are putting their funding muscle behind such efforts. The interested reader can learn more about the NIH's Roadmap to transform how clinical research is conducted at its website (http://nihroadmap.nih.gov/overview.asp).

For these efforts to be fully realized, there is a general consensus that a new generation of clinical investigators must be trained, and that these new scientists must not only understand the need for rigor in research in general, the challenges of clinical research in particular, but they must also be familiar if not facile with the techniques of modern biology and its potential application to research in humans. It is our hope and intent that this book will begin to meet the didactic needs of this new generation.

Thus, the beginning and middle portions of the book focus on the mechanics of designing, conducting, and analyzing a translational or experimental clinical research study. In Section I, Chapters 1–4 contain material relevant to generating a testable hypothesis. Chapters 5–9 are about how to design a study to test that hypothesis. Chapters 10–13 consider practical implementation of that study.

Chapters 14 and 15 of Section II address ethical and regulatory issues that every investigator needs to understand. Chapters 16 and 17 concern the funding and financing of clinical research. The remaining chapters of Section II discuss a variety of subjects of more specialized interest.

Section III of the book focuses on how results should be analyzed, interpreted, and reported. Although this book does not purport to be a formal textbook on statistics, it is our view that a well-designed study must anticipate the statistical strategies that will be used to analyze the data it generates. Every clinical investigator needs to have an appreciation of the statistical approaches that are available to analyze most translational or experimental clinical research studies, their intended use, and their limitations. It is also important for the investigator to communicate these results to others. There is no point in making a discovery if no one but the discoverer knows about it. The goal of every scientist should be to communicate valuable new information to his or her colleagues. In the context of clinical research, it can also be argued that a failure to do so is a breach of ethical conduct, for an appeal to benefit others (through the dissemination of new knowledge) is often used as a powerful argument to elicit the participation of potential research participants. Imparting such information is the overall goal of Section III.

Finally, Section IV includes a review of some of the most commonly employed tools of modern biology that can be used in translational clinical research. In developing these chapters, our goal was to have the techniques briefly described, to include some cautionary comments about the obstacles that can be encountered when trying to implement these methods in a translational research study, and to end with some examples of where these techniques have been (and will be!) used to successfully answer interesting and important questions related to human health and disease.

As in any new writing endeavor, we anticipate finding out (and being told) that we have missed some important material or overemphasized some other. We look forward to the feedback. But if we have imparted even a small portion of the excitement we feel about the promise and value of performing our studies, we will certainly feel that the effort has been completely worthwhile.

## ACKNOWLEDGMENTS

It is always a Herculean effort to put a multi-authored textbook together, requiring enormous patience and persistence. In helping us meet these challenges, the editors are especially grateful to Karen Dodson, Julie Follman, and Claire Kramer of Academic Publishing Services, and Marcy Harstein and Vicki Friedman of MedPIC, all at Washington University.

The editors obviously wish to give special thanks to all of the authors for their contributions. In academic medicine, writing a chapter for someone else's textbook often feels about as close to a thankless task as any of us are likely to encounter. But in this case, the effort is fully acknowledged and totally appreciated.

This book began with a conversation with Richard Winters, evolved to a concrete proposal with Danette Knopp, and was brought to fruition through the efforts of Sonya Seigafuse and Fran Murphy at Lippincott Williams & Wilkins, and Jean Lou Hess at Schawk, Inc. (and undoubtedly, countless others unknown to us). We are very indebted to them all.

Daniel P. Schuster, MD

# Foreword

From 2000–2004, the Institute of Medicine chartered a national Clinical Research Roundtable to deliberate the plight of clinical research in the United States. Constituted of stakeholders from government, academia, consumers, patients, payers, providers, and business, this interdisciplinary group identified at least two obstacles to translating new science into everyday treatments. The first of these "translational blocks," as they became known, involves the transfer of new basic research findings into the human. The second involves dissemination of therapies already proven in large-scale clinical trials into everyday practice. This textbook, aimed as it is at the first of these two blocks, provides a relatively unique contribution to the medical literature.

While the intellectual disciplines underlying the second translational block—clinical trials, epidemiology, statistics, and outcomes research—do change over time, they exhibit sufficient stability to generate reliable textbooks in which the underlying principles evolve more at their margins than at their center. In contrast, first studies in humans—exemplifying strategies addressing the first translational block—generally utilize a somewhat different and more rapidly evolving spectrum of disciplines of medical science. They usually involve more intensive measurements in smaller numbers of patients; are more intimately tied to the pathophysiology of disease states; use diseases as 'models' of pathophysiology; and are more frequently conducted in National Institutes of Health-Funded General Clinical Research Centers in academic medical centers. The ever-changing spectrum and pace of change in the scientific disciplines in which they are embedded are thus usually determined by parallel rapid evolutions in basic research. Hence, these studies typically require intimate partnerships between clinical and basic investigators to a much greater degree than do later and larger-scale trials and outcomes research. Since these venues of the basic science/human investigation interface are as dynamic as the rapidly evolving basic science platforms that empower them, the education agenda of translational investigators has proven somewhat elusive and challenging for textbook authors.

Drs. Schuster and Powers and their excellent set of collaborators have gone a long way toward addressing this gap in the field. They have undertaken the important challenge of determining the general approaches, disciplines, and organizational principles that translational investigators require while meeting these needs in a concise fashion. As such, this textbook is long overdue and a welcome contribution for young clinical investigators seeking to work at this challenging but rewarding interface between basic and clinical science.

William F. Crowley, Jr., MD
Professor of Medicine, Harvard Medical School
Director of Clinical Research, Massachusetts General Hospital

# List of Contributors

## Editors

Daniel P. Schuster, MD
Professor of Medicine and Radiology
Associate Dean for Clinical Research
Director, Program in Translational and
Experimental Medicine
Washington University School of Medicine
St. Louis, Missouri

William J. Powers, MD
Professor of Neurology, Neurological Surgery,
and Radiology
Head, Cerebrovascular Diseases and Neuroimaging
Sections
Washington University School of Medicine
St. Louis, Missouri

## Associate Editors

Mario Castro, MD, MPH
Associate Professor of Medicine and Pediatrics
Washington University School of Medicine
St. Louis, Missouri

Jeffrey E. Saffitz, MD, PhD
Professor of Pathology
Washington University School of Medicine
St. Louis, Missouri

William Shannon, PhD
Assistant Professor of Biostatistics in Medicine
Washington University School of Medicine
St. Louis, Missouri

## Contributors

Dana R. Abendschein, PhD
Assistant Vice Chancellor/Dean for Animal Affairs
Associate Professor of Medicine and Cell Biology
and Physiology
Washington University School of Medicine
St. Louis, Missouri

Gerhard Bauer, PhD
Laboratory Director, GMP Facility
Siteman Cancer Center
Washington University School of Medicine
St. Louis, Missouri

Amanda Blackford, ScM
Department of Oncology
Johns Hopkins School of Medicine
Baltimore, Maryland

W. Richard Burack, MD, PhD
Assistant Professor of Pathology and Immunology
Washington University School of Medicine
St. Louis, Missouri

Denise A. Canfield, RN
Center for Clinical Studies
Washington University School of Medicine
St. Louis, Missouri

Theodore J. Cicero, PhD
Vice Chancellor for Research
Professor of Psychiatry and Neurobiology
Washington University School of Medicine
St. Louis, Missouri

Mickey Clarke
Human Subject Research QA Program Manager
Washington University School of Medicine
St. Louis, Missouri

Diane K. Clemens, DC
HIPAA Compliance Manager
Washington University School of Medicine
St. Louis, Missouri

Andrew R. Coggan, PhD
Research Associate in Medicine
Washington University School of Medicine
St. Louis, Missouri

Thomas G. Cole, PhD
Vice President/Laboratory Director
Clinical Trials Services
Linco Diagnostic Services
St. Charles, Missouri

Sharon Cresci, MD
Assistant Professor Medicine
Washington University School of Medicine
St. Louis, Missouri

Robert C. Culverhouse, PhD
Instructor in Medicine
Washington University School of Medicine
St. Louis, Missouri

Victor G. Davila-Roman, MD
Associate Professor of Medicine, Anesthesiology,
and Radiology
Washington University School of Medicine
St. Louis, Missouri

Michael DeBaun, MD, MPH
Associate Professor of Pediatrics and
Biostatistics
Washington University School of Medicine
St. Louis, Missouri

Lisa de las Fuentes, MD
Instructor in Medicine
Washington University School of Medicine
St. Louis, Missouri

Karen L. Dodson, BS
Director and Managing Editor
Academic Publishing Services
Managing Editor, American Journal of
Physiology: Endocrinology and Metabolism
Washington University School of Medicine
St. Louis, Missouri

Bradley Evanoff, MD, MPH
Associate Professor of Medicine
Washington University School of Medicine
St. Louis, Missouri

Thomas Ferkol, MD
Associate Professor of Pediatrics
Washington University School of Medicine
St. Louis, Missouri

Vicki M. Friedman
Director, MedPIC
Washington University School of Medicine
St. Louis, Missouri

Brian F. Gage, MD, MSc
Associate Professor of Medicine
Washington University School of Medicine
St. Louis, Missouri

David W. Gibson, BS
Department of Medicine
Washington University School of Medicine
St. Louis, Missouri

Steven Goodman, MD, MHS, PhD
Associate Professor of Oncology, Pediatrics,
Biostatistics, and Epidemiology
Johns Hopkins Schools of Medicine and Public
Health
Baltimore, Maryland

Patricia J. Gregory, PhD
Senior Director of Corporate and Foundation
Relations
Washington University School of Medicine
St. Louis, Missouri

Karen L. Hardinger, PharmD, BCPS
Clinical Professor of Pharmacy Practice
University of Missouri–Kansas City
Kansas City, Missouri

Marcy H. Hartstein
Art Manager, MedPIC
Washington University School of Medicine
St. Louis, Missouri

Janet T. Holbrook, PhD, MPH
Center for Clinical Trials
Johns Hopkins University
Baltimore, Maryland

Carlton A. Hornung, PhD, MPH
Professor of Epidemiology
Chair, Epidemiology and Clinical Investigation
Sciences
University of Louisville
Louisville, Kentucky

Janice Huss, PhD
Research Instructor in Medicine
Washington University School of Medicine
St. Louis, Missouri

Suzanne T. Ildstad, MD
Professor of Surgery
Director, Institute for Cellular Therapeutics
University of Louisville
Louisville, Kentucky

Elliot Israel, MD
Associate Professor of Medicine
Brigham & Women's Hospital
Harvard Medical School
Boston, Massachusetts

Allison King, MD, MPH
Instructor of Pediatrics
Washington University School of Medicine
St. Louis, Missouri

Samuel Klein, MD
Professor of Medicine and Nutritional Science
Director, Center for Human Nutrition
Chief, Division of Geriatric and Nutritional
Science
Washington University School of Medicine
St. Louis, Missouri

Judith E. C. Lieu, MD
Assistant Professor of Otolaryngology
Washington University School of Medicine
St. Louis, Missouri

Benjamin Littenberg, MD
Professor of Medicine
Director, General Internal Medicine
University of Vermont
Burlington, Vermont

Philip A. Ludbrook, MD
Professor of Medicine and Radiology
Associate Dean and Chair, Human Studies
Committee
Washington University School of Medicine
St. Louis, Missouri

Denise A. McCartney
Associate Vice Chancellor for Research
Administration
Washington University School of Medicine
St. Louis, Missouri

Janet B. McGill, MD
Associate Professor of Medicine
Director, Volunteer for Health
Washington University School of Medicine
St. Louis, Missouri

Curtis L. Meinert, PhD
Department of Epidemiology
Bloomberg School of Public Health
Johns Hopkins University
Baltimore, Maryland

J. Philip Miller
Professor of Biostatistics
Director, Biostatistics Core
Siteman Cancer Center
Washington University School of Medicine
St. Louis, Missouri

Bettina Mittendorfer, PhD
Research Assistant Professor of Medicine
Washington University School of Medicine
St. Louis, Missouri

David A. Mulvihill, BS, MCSD, MT(ASCP)
Department of Medicine
Washington University School of Medicine
St. Louis, Missouri

Ronald Munson, PhD
Professor of Philosophy of Science and Medicine
University of Missouri—St. Louis
St. Louis, Missouri

Andrea J. Myles
Senior Graphic Designer, MedPIC
Washington University School of Medicine
St. Louis, Missouri

Jan A. Nolta, PhD
Associate Professor of Medicine
Washington University School of Medicine
St. Louis, Missouri

Arie Perry, MD
Associate Professor of Pathology and Immunology
Washington University School of Medicine
St. Louis, Missouri

John D. Pfeifer, MD, PhD
Associate Professor of Pathology and
Immunology
Washington University School of Medicine
St. Louis, Missouri

Jay F. Piccirillo, MD, MPH
Associate Professor of Otolaryngology
Washington University School of Medicine
St. Louis, Missouri

William J. Powers, MD
Professor of Neurology, Neurological Surgery,
and Radiology
Head, Cerebrovascular Diseases and
Neuroimaging Sections
Washington University School of Medicine
St. Louis, Missouri

Neville Prendergast, BS, DipED, MLS
Senior Librarian and Associate Director for
Communication & Outreach
Becker Medical Library
Washington University School of Medicine
St. Louis, Missouri

Michael A. Province, PhD
Professor of Biostatistics and Genetics
Washington University School of Medicine
St. Louis, Missouri

Lauren M. Rohde
Supervisor, Computer Graphics, MedPIC
Washington University School of Medicine
St. Louis, Missouri

Kevin A. Roth, MD, PhD
Professor of Pathology
University of Alabama at Birmingham
Birmingham, Alabama

Nancy L. Saccone, PhD
Assistant Professor of Genetics
Washington University School of Medicine
St. Louis, Missouri

Jeffrey E. Saffitz, MD, PhD
Professor of Pathology
Washington University School of Medicine
St. Louis, Missouri

Mark S. Sands, PhD
Associate Professor of Medicine
Washington University School of Medicine
St. Louis, Missouri

Patricia M. Scannell, BA, CIP
Director Human Studies Committee
Washington University School of Medicine
St. Louis, Missouri

Kenneth B. Schechtman, PhD
Associate Professor of Biostatistics
Director, Biostatistics Core
Pepper Center
Washington University School of Medicine
St. Louis, Missouri

Mary Ellen Scheipeter, RN, BSN
Department of Medicine
Washington University School of Medicine
St. Louis, Missouri

Daniel P. Schuster, MD
Professor of Medicine and Radiology
Associate Dean for Clinical Research
Director, Program in Translational and
Experimental Medicine
Washington University School of Medicine
St. Louis, Missouri

David M. Shade, JD
Research Associate in Medicine
Johns Hopkins School of Medicine
Baltimore, Maryland

William D. Shannon, PhD
Assistant Professor of Biostatistics in Medicine
Washington University School of Medicine
St. Louis, Missouri

Barry A. Siegel, MD
Professor of Radiology and Medicine
Washington University School of Medicine
St. Louis, Missouri

Christina Sullivan, MLS, MSW
Librarian
Becker Medical Library
Washington University School of Medicine
St. Louis, Missouri

Paul A. Thompson, PhD
Research Associate Professor of Biostatistics
Washington University School of Medicine
St. Louis, Missouri

David J. Tollerud, MD, MPH
Professor and Chair, Department of Environmental
and Occupational Health Sciences
University of Louisville
Louisville, Kentucky

R. Reid Townsend, MD, PhD
Associate Professor of Medicine
Washington University School of Medicine
St. Louis, Missouri

Tom Videen, PhD
Research Associate Professor of Neurology
Washington University School of Medicine
St. Louis, Missouri

Janet Voorhees, APRN, BC, FNP, CCRC
Family Nurse Practitioner, Neurology
Washington University School of Medicine
St. Louis, Missouri

Mark A. Watson, MD, PhD
Assistant Professor of Pathology and
Immunology
Washington University School of Medicine
St. Louis, Missouri

Michael Wechsler, MD, MMSc
Instructor in Medicine
Brigham & Women's Hospital
Harvard Medical School
Boston, Massachusetts

Martin C. Weinrich, PhD
Professor of Nursing & Biostatistics
Medical College of Georgia
Augusta, Georgia

Robert A. Wise, MD
Professor of Medicine
Johns Hopkins University School of Medicine
Baltimore, Maryland

John Yang, MD
Instructor of Medicine
Washington University School of Medicine
St. Louis, Missouri

Xiao Yang, PhD
Genomics Technologies
Monsanto Company
St. Louis, Missouri

Roger D. Yusen, MD, MPH
Assistant Professor of Medicine
Washington University School of Medicine
St. Louis, Missouri

# Contents

SECTION III
# Analyzing and Reporting Results                                        247

SECTION IV
# Modern Techniques of Translational Clinical Research         331

# The Value of Translational and Experimental Clinical Research

Daniel P. Schuster

*"Clinical research will transform health care: will academic medicine step up to the task?"*

—Ralph Snyderman, MD, Chancellor for Health Affairs, Duke University, 1999 (1)

The purpose of biomedical research is to improve human health. Since World War II, a multibillion dollar biomedical enterprise has developed with the goal of reducing disease-related suffering and death. To do so, the enterprise supports a vast and complex array of research activity, including clinical research (2). Yet, if the aim of all biomedical research is ultimately to understand the physiology and pathophysiology of *human* illness (either as a fundamental process or for the purpose of treating disease), then clinical research is the *only* way to validate hypotheses related to human disease, regardless of how these hypotheses were originally generated. Furthermore, clinical research in most cases is required before new discoveries can be *applied* to the treatment of disease. Thus, it is imperative that clinical research be conducted with great care and integrity but quickly and efficiently so as to shorten the time required to bring the benefits of the research investment to fruition.

The impact of clinical research, however, goes beyond its critical role in establishing mechanisms of disease in humans or the benefits of new treatment. By offering laboratory-oriented, patient-oriented, and population-oriented scientists opportunities for collaboration, clinical research also helps integrate such disparate activities as scientific investigation, medical education, and patient care. Clinical research and medical education distinguish our medical schools from patient care clinics on the one hand and dedicated research institutes on the other (Figure I–1). At centers where clinical research is a major activity, a rich web of interactions and interrelationships can be found among clinical research, basic research, and clinical practice activities (Figure I–2).

The paradigm that drove such great support for biomedical research during the latter half of the 20th century is that knowledge in biology and biomedicine must first be advanced at a fundamental ("basic") level before new treatments that will eventually improve human health can be developed. Indeed, it is this very framework for success that is often used to justify the enormous amounts of funding that the federal government and national foundations spend each year for in vitro and animal science. However, the links between discovery and treatment are actually not as unidirectional as the paradigm implies nor are they even connected by a straight line from one to the other. Less well appreciated is how often important new insights into the origins of disease are first the result of novel *clinical* observations (3). Examples include the role of hypercholesterolemia in premature atherosclerosis, the role of smoking in lung cancer, the role of inhibiting angiotensin-converting enzyme inhibitor to improve survival independent of its effects on blood pressure, and the role of the bacterium *Helicobacter pylori* in duodenal ulcers. In each case, the first hypothetical statements of potential cause and effect were based on the results of *clinical* studies; later, additional confirmatory clinical investigations and other types of research studies were performed to determine the underlying mechanisms.

## DEFINITION OF CLINICAL RESEARCH

An exact definition of what constitutes clinical research has been surprisingly difficult to develop. At

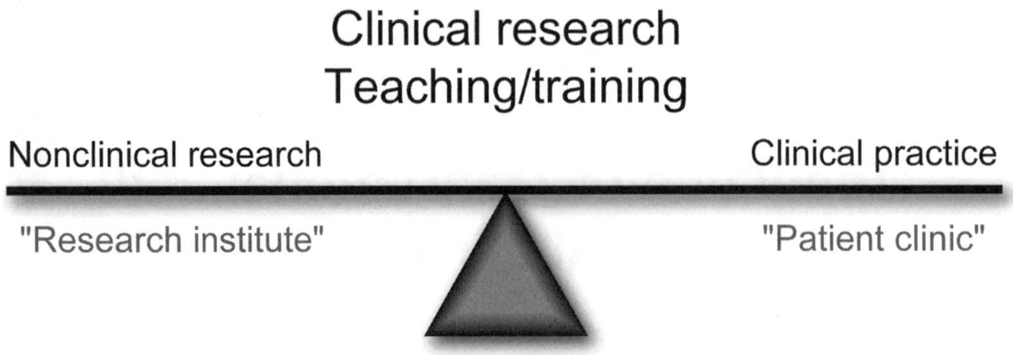

# Clinical research
# Teaching/training

Nonclinical research                                    Clinical practice

"Research institute"                                    "Patient clinic"

**FIGURE I–1** ● Clinical research exists at the intersection between nonclinical science and clinical practice. Along with traditional teaching and training functions, clinical research distinguishes a medical school from a research institute on the one hand and a highly specialized patient clinic on the other.

least five authoritative reports, from both individuals and institutions such as the Institute of Medicine and the Association of American Medical Colleges, include working definitions of clinical research (1–5). Among the most influential is the definition adopted by the National Institutes of Health (NIH) (6) (if for no other reason than the impact NIH has on research funding). According to this definition, clinical research includes the following areas of inquiry:

1. Patient-oriented research
2. Epidemiologic and behavioral studies
3. Outcomes and health services research

Patient-oriented research is defined as "research conducted with human subjects (or on material of human origin such as tissues, specimens, and cognitive phenomena) for which an investigator (or colleague) directly interacts with human subjects" (7). Accordingly, patient-oriented research specifically includes the following types of studies:

1. Research on mechanisms of human disease
2. Therapeutic interventions
3. Clinical trials
4. Development of new technologies

The NIH excludes from its definition of patient-oriented research in vitro studies in which human tissue samples are used but direct interactions with patients are absent. Thus, a study is considered to be clinical or patient-oriented research only when information

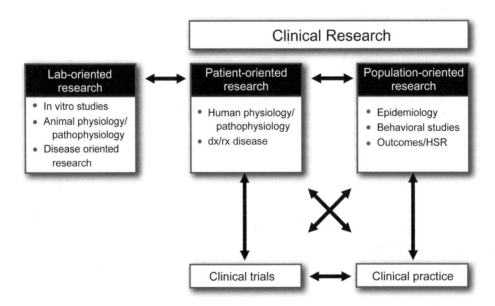

**FIGURE I–2** ● Interactions and interrelationships among clinical research, basic research, and clinical practice activities. *dx,* diagnostic studies; *rx,* therapeutic studies; *HSR,* health services research.

about the sources (i.e., the research participants) from which the tissues were obtained is available to properly interpret the research findings (7).

Other descriptive terms are sometimes used to define clinical research, including *basic patient-oriented research* (mechanistic studies), *applied patient-oriented research* (studies of disease management), and importantly (for the purposes of this textbook), *translational research* (a type of patient-oriented research, see following section).

Over and above the confusion raised by these various attempts to define clinical research, a problem with them all is that they provide virtually no *operational* guidance (i.e., no practical test) to determine whether a particular study should be classified as clinical research or not. Characterizing patient-oriented research as a type of investigation in which the physician and patient interact directly has led some to offer the "handshake test" as one rather tongue-in-cheek criterion. Another option is to depend on institutional review board approval as a requirement. However, this criterion would clearly allow some studies to be misclassified as clinical research by the NIH definition in that in vitro studies should be excluded if they use human tissues but do not involve patients directly (6).

As an alternative, in this textbook, we have adopted a very simple standard:

> *Clinical research includes any scientific investigation in which the unit of analysis is the person.*

This simple standard is consistent with the NIH recommendation that studies employing cell lines or tissues of human origin constitute clinical research only if the results can be related to the individuals from whom these materials were obtained. Similarly, studies that depend on databases of information about humans represent clinical research only if the analyzed information is about the individuals and not about some other convenient aggregate (e.g., hospitals or managed care groups).

According to this standard, a study that was limited to reporting changes in gene expression in human bronchial epithelial cells before and after stimulation with inflammatory cytokines would not be considered clinical research. However, a similar study comparing responses in cells harvested from five individuals with asthma with responses in cells from five healthy control volunteers *would* be characterized as clinical research.

Likewise, a study about the effectiveness of hand washing in reducing the spread of infection that compares practices at hospitals by geographic region would not be clinical research, but a similar study comparing the number of infections per patient-days *would* qualify.

Obviously, a published report about hand washing from such studies could easily contain *both* types of analyses, so scientific articles may contain elements of both clinical and nonclinical research. The nature of the studies, as well as the manner in which they are analyzed, determines how "clinical" the research is. Thus, to determine whether a study includes clinical research, the investigator need only determine what *n* represents in the data analysis. If *n* is the number of human beings from which the information is derived, the study can legitimately be characterized as clinical research. This standard is simple, practical, and unambiguous.

## TRANSLATIONAL AND EXPERIMENTAL MEDICINE

However, this textbook is not titled *Clinical Research*. Such a textbook, given the NIH definition, would include material related to patient-oriented research, epidemiology, behavioral studies, outcomes, and health services research—a vast compendium of research strategies and techniques. Rather, this book focuses on two subsets of clinical research: translational research and experimental medicine.

Both types of research activity constitute patient-oriented research according to the NIH definition, and the two terms are not mutually exclusive; their meanings, however, are distinct. *Translational research* connotes an attempt to bring information that has been confined to the laboratory into the realm of clinical medicine. As an example, suppose a gene recently discovered in mice appears to have important functions in regulating a cell's life cycle. Is a similar gene present in humans? Is the function of the gene product similar? Is its regulation the same as in mice? And, most importantly, what role does the gene play in disease? To the extent that clinical studies could be designed to answer such questions, they would each represent types of *translational* clinical research.

The term *translational research* has also come to convey a certain immediacy, suggesting an attempt to translate relatively recent information (at least within the last few years), obtained from nonhuman systems, to people. This emphasis on "cutting edge" research, too, is maintained within this book.

*Experimental medicine* is different. *Translational research* is about a *type* of inquiry. Experimental medicine is about a *method* of inquiry. Accept for the moment that all clinical research can be divided simply into two types: experimental and observational research. The distinctive feature of *experimental medicine* is that it is:

> *a method by which measurements are specifically obtained after an intervention controlled by the investigator.*

All other studies are observational; that is, regardless whether or not measurements are made after an intervention, the scientist is simply an observer if the intervention is *not* under his or her control (assuming one exists at all).

## THE VALUE OF CLINICAL EXPERIMENTS

Why is this distinction so important? The answer lies in the goals of research. Just as all research can be neatly (if not necessarily fairly) divided into two categories (experimental and observational), the goals of research can also be divided into two categories: explanatory and descriptive. In other words, in some cases, the goals of a study are to accurately *describe* phenomena or relationships; in other cases, research is performed to *explain* the causes of biomedical phenomena and to make predictive statements about them. Thus, although the overall goal of biomedical research may be to improve human health, the *means* by which this objective is achieved can vary. When physicians and other health care workers are armed with robust explanatory information, they can plan treatments with the greatest probability of a beneficial effect. Causal statements are the link between simple descriptions of what we believe to be real and predictive statements that allow us to affect that reality (7).

The most simple and straightforward causal statement takes the form of "A causes B" (Figure I–3). When such a declaration is made, a simple, linear "connection" is posited between A (the cause or mechanism) and B (the effect). For this reason, experimental studies are sometimes characterized as mechanistic research. Note that a cultural bias underlies the notion that A *causes* B. Other cultures may well reject such simple linear thinking; scientific reasoning, however, as it is practiced in Western cultures and societies, fully embraces this logic of linear causation (8).

As appealing as the "A causes B" concept may be, *proving* it to be so can be quite challenging. For instance, A may cause B by its effects on some intermediary (e.g., X) (Figure I–3). Alternatively, other factors (e.g., C) may also cause B (either directly or by affecting the same intermediary). The practical problem in such cases is that an investigator may not be able to show that A causes B unless he or she can account for (or eliminate) the effects of C. In the language of clinical research, C can "confound" efforts to show that A causes B.

From these considerations, three cardinal rules of causation can be identified:

1. The putative cause must precede the designated effect in time.
2. The effect must be related to the putative cause.
3. There must be no plausible alternative explanations, that is, no confounders.

Observational studies can provide evidence for the first two criteria, but ultimately such studies can only show association, not causation, because they cannot eliminate the potential effects of confounding. In contrast, experimental studies can provide proof of causation by imposing an intervention that is meant to either mimic or inhibit a putative mechanism while ensuring (by study design) that the subjects are otherwise treated identically.

It is important to note here that although control of the intervention is the critical event that distinguishes an experimental study from an observational one, the simple act of imposing an intervention by itself does not eliminate the problem of confounding. Other aspects of a *properly conducted* experiment (e.g., randomization, masking) are elements crucial to achieving this goal. However, without control of the intervention, these opportunities to eliminate confounding would not be available to the investigator.

Inferences about causation *can*, of course, be made from observational studies, but not with the same level of confidence that occurs as a result of a properly conducted experimental study, simply because the effects of confounders, especially unknown confounders, cannot be eliminated with the same degree of certainty. This distinction can

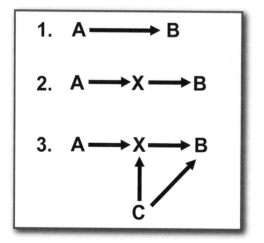

**FIGURE I–3** ● Identifying causation. (1) The cause A precedes the effect B (*arrow* indicates time). (2) In other cases, A causes B by means of some intermediary X. (3) If C can affect B directly or indirectly, then identifying A as a cause of B requires eliminating the confounding effects of C. This is best accomplished with an experimental study design.

be stated as a kind of the "central dogma" of experimental medicine:

> *Many study designs can answer whether two or more groups* differ *with respect to a particular variable, but only the randomized experiment can determine whether they differed* because *of that variable.*

Although this view has been disputed (9, 10), our position remains that a properly conducted experimental study provides the strongest evidence for causation (11).

## THE VALUE OF OBSERVATIONAL RESEARCH

If an experimental design is ultimately the most powerful way to generate data that can be used to make causal statements, why bother with any other type of research? There are several answers. Observational studies are often easier (and more practical) to perform. They are generally less costly and time consuming. They often provide the hypotheses to be tested by later, interventional (experimental) studies. In some instances, they may be more ethical, in that a particular intervention might require unacceptable safety risks to the research participant. For instance, an investigator would hardly want to prove that endotoxin causes shock in humans by intravenously administering enough of this material to demonstrate the point. (On the other hand, a highly specific inhibitor of endotoxin administered to patients with septic shock would provide proof for just such a hypothesis.) These factors alone mean that important information must often be obtained through properly conducted observational studies that would never, in any practical sense, be possible from experiments.

However, the most significant disadvantage of clinical experiments may be the very act itself of imposing an intervention on humans. By its very nature, this action is an artifice. By reducing study design to just one variable that is different between an experimental and a control group (the single intervention controlled by the investigator), the results of an experiment rarely present an accurate picture of reality. Often, they apply only to the peculiarities of that specific study—that is, the results may not extrapolate as well to the human population of interest.

This predicament continually bedevils clinical research: observational studies describe the real world because the investigator does nothing to interfere with that world (ignoring for the moment the deeper philosophical question of whether the act of observation itself disturbs the real world). On the other hand, observational studies are always confounded, sometimes by known and often by unknown variables, making it difficult to declare causation based on their results.

Experimental studies have the opposite problem: the ability to link events causally is what makes clinical experiments so powerful. Yet, for investigators to take advantage of this attribute, the studies may have to be so tightly controlled and narrowly defined as to be irrelevant to meaningful questions about human health.

What is the answer to this dilemma? Simply put, both types of studies have their value and place in the total clinical research portfolio (Table I–1).

---

**TABLE I–1**

### Some Goals of Experimental Versus Observational Studies

| Experimental studies | Observational studies |
| --- | --- |
| Mechanisms of disease | Impact of disease on the patient |
| Efficacy | Effectiveness |
| Effect of biochemistry and physiologic factors on biophysical outcomes | Effect of socioeconomic factors on patient-centered outcomes |
| Tests of drugs/devices | Tests of processes and delivery of care |
| Disease-centered | Patient- and community-centered |
| Inventing technology | Assessing technology |

Adapted from Rubenfeld G, Angus D, Pinsky M. Curtis J, Connors AJ, Bernard G. Outcomes research in critical care. Am J Respir Crit Care Med 1999:160:358–367, with permission.

## AN IDEALIZED SEQUENCE OF BIOMEDICAL RESEARCH

The value of clinical experiments comes from their ability to establish mechanisms responsible for disease. However, as already noted, they are only one part of the entire spectrum of biomedical research. Consider, for instance, the following hypothetical sequence of discovery, observation, experiment, and application (Figure I–4).

Assume that a fundamental new observation has been made in some isolated biologic system (for example, a new "Factor Q" is found to affect an in vitro cell function). Another scientist, reading about this discovery, designs a study to determine whether Factor Q affects cell function in an animal model of disease. A clinical investigator, after performing a literature review, reads this scientist's report. He decides to determine whether Factor Q is found at increased levels in tissues from patients with the human form of the disease in question. (This study might represent the first *translation* of the basic discovery into the clinical arena.) An additional observational study is designed and implemented to determine if Factor Q levels are a risk factor for disease severity. Then, having heard that Factor Q is expressed in higher concentrations in patients with the disease at a scientific meeting, another scientist works with a team to produce a Factor Q inhibitor directed against the Factor Q target that will be suitable for use in humans. Later, clinical experiments are designed in which the inhibitor is used as the intervention under the control of the investigator, to determine whether inhibiting Factor Q reestablishes normal cell function, providing evidence, in humans, that Factor Q is a potential pathogenetic mechanism for the disease. Another clinical experiment (a *clinical trial*) is conducted to determine whether Factor Q inhibitor reduces the morbidity associated with the disease. Eventually, outcome (observational) studies are performed to determine how the lives of patients using Factor Q inhibitor are affected. Making all of

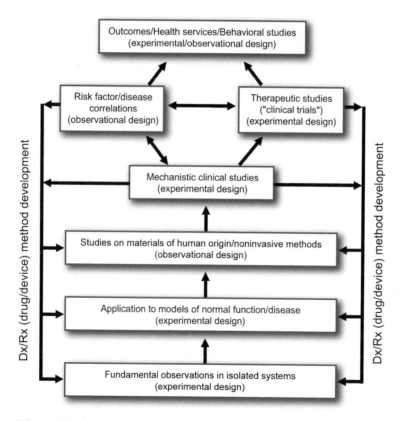

**FIGURE I–4** ● An idealized sequence of research in which a basic discovery is eventually translated into a clinical investigation, followed by clinical trials and other studies to establish efficacy and effectiveness of new treatments. Commonly employed research designs are shown at each step. These are not meant to be exclusive of other designs, however, at these points. Also shown are some pathways by which clinical observations provide incentives for basic laboratory investigations.

these studies possible is a series of new techniques developed to allow levels of Factor Q, or of the inhibitor, or of cell functions affected by Factor Q, to be determined in humans, including associated studies of measurement accuracy and precision.

The sequence of research events just described, in which studies moved steadily from a new basic science discovery to its application in human disease, its treatment, and its impact, is rarely so unidirectional. Instead, information usually flows in multiple directions (Figure I–4), often simultaneously. For instance, a *clinical* study rather than a bench study could just as easily generate the first clues that a specific pathway is important in a particular disease, providing incentive for bench scientists to learn more about the underlying molecular and cellular mechanisms. Nevertheless, the idealized sequence shown in Figure I–4 provides context for the topics of this book, specifically those studies that seek to provide the first *translation* of new laboratory discoveries to human biology and those studies that seek to establish, by the experimental method, mechanisms of physiology or pathophysiology in humans.

## THE VALUE OF CLINICAL RESEARCH

Given the importance of clinical research to improving human health, it is surprising that questions about its value still arise. For instance, a common perception is that clinical investigators in many academic centers have more difficulty in obtaining promotions and gaining the prestige commonly accorded to successful bench or laboratory scientists. While actual documentation that such practices exist is hard to come by, we can still ask why such a perception should even exist. One perspective is that basic science, by its very nature, provides a foundation (i.e., a basis) for studies yet to come. In this sense, an important basic discovery can have an impact on science that goes far beyond the specific study itself. Here we should keep in mind, of course, that it is not where the discovery is made (the "bench" or the "clinic") that is critical to its importance, but the nature of the discovery itself. Was not Harvey's discovery of the circulation *basic* science? Even so, most clinical investigation is more narrowly construed: the data in the majority of clinical studies admittedly only apply to a particular subset of the human population. In general, the results of such studies will not influence other fields as surely as an important basic discovery. Accordingly, they seem, to some, less important.

The discoveries of nonclinical science, on the other hand, can never have any *direct* impact on human health, even if the studies in which they are made were carried out in animal models of human disease. Only properly conducted clinical investigations can achieve this goal. Thus, although the impact of basic science may be broad, the impact of most clinical science is more focused and immediate. If the purpose of biomedical research is to improve human health, then both clinical and nonclinical science must be equally valued. In this context, it seems particularly fitting to recall the sage words of A. R. Feinstein (12):

> *The "basic scientist" often forgets the intellectual debts he owes the clinician for demonstrating what to explore . . . . The clinicians who treat patients, the clinicians who do clinical research or laboratory research, and the MDs and PhDs who do purely laboratory research all need each other. They destroy their opportunities for mutual progress if laboratory workers scorn clinical activities as unscientific art, or if clinicians reject laboratory research as impractical abstraction. Every scientist owes full allegiance and respect to the whole that is his own domain, but he forgets, at his peril, that his domain is a mere part of the whole of natural science and human life.*

## REFERENCES

1. AAMC. For the health of the public: ensuring the future of clinical research. Washington, DC: AAMC: Author 1999.
2. Sung N, Crowley W, Genel M et al. Central challenges facing the national clinical research enterprise. JAMA 2003;289:1278–1287.
3. Comroe JH. Bedside research. Am Rev Respir Dis 1978;118:941–945.
4. Shulman L. Clinical research 1996: stirrings from the academic medical centers. Acad Med 1996;71:362–363,398.
5. Kelly W, Randolph M. Careers in clinical research: obstacles and opportunities. Washington DC: National Academy Press; 1994.
6. Nathan D. Clinical research: perceptions, reality, and proposed solutions. NIH Director's Panel on Clinical Research. JAMA 1998;280:1427–1431.
7. Hill A. The environment and disease: association or causation? Proc Royal Soc Med 1965;58:295–300.
8. Gliner J, Morgan G, Harmon R. A tale of two paradigms. J Am Acad Child Adolesc Psych 1999;38:342–343.
9. Benson K, Hartz A. A comparison of observational studies and randomized, controlled trials. N Engl J Med 2000;342:1878–1886.
10. Concato J, Shah N, Horwitz R. Randomized, controlled trials, observational studies, and the hierarchy of research designs. N Engl J Med 2000;342:1887–1892.
11. Pocock S, Elbourne D. Randomized trials or observational tribulations? N Engl J Med 2000;342:1907–1909.
12. Feinstein AR. The scientific domain of the investigative clinician. In: Feinstein AR, ed. Clinical Judgement. Baltimore: Williams & Wilkins; 1967:381–390.

# Planning and Designing Clinical Research

# CHAPTER 1

# Defining the Research Question

## Daniel P. Schuster

In scientific investigations, various circumstances may serve as starting points for research; I will reduce all these varieties, however, to two chief types:

1. where the starting point for experimental research is an observation;
2. where the starting point for experimental research is an hypothesis or theory.

—Claude Bernard (1)

Many research studies begin with a question in the mind of the investigator. Clinical research studies are no exception.

Questions, of course, can be profound or trivial, difficult or straightforward, general or specific. In formulating a question for a research study, the investigator must invariably make decisions that affect the conduct, potential success, and value of the investigation that is designed to answer that question. A carefully constructed question will point the investigator down a very specific path—hopefully, but not necessarily, a path of discovery. Studies conducted to answer a vague or ill-defined question can be a waste of time and money. So, the first step on this path—defining the research question—is a crucial but often difficult one, especially for young investigators. Although a journey of a thousand miles [may] begin with a single step, it still hurts to stumble.

## FINDING QUESTIONS

Many junior investigators find that the most difficult part of formulating a research question is articulating a worthy question of any sort. Perhaps it is cold comfort to learn that virtually all scientists at some point confront this equivalent of writer's block. Not only fear of the unknown but fear of failure and fear of inadequacy are emotional barriers to be overcome. Although all scientists hope to make great and important discoveries, most know that a trip to Stockholm to accept a Nobel Prize is not likely to be part of their career paths. Nevertheless, almost anyone can make real and valuable contributions, especially if desire is coupled with a conscientious and methodical plan.

A curious mind is a great gift, and many of the most famous discoveries began when both curiosity and preparation converged in response to a seemingly mundane observation. (Louis Pasteur said that "in the field of observation, chance only favors the prepared mind"[2].) In reality, "Eureka!" moments are rare, and most investigators must resort to less spectacular, and admittedly more pedestrian, approaches to generating questions. Although the advances generated by studies that answer these questions may be smaller, they are no less real, and cumulatively, no less important. New investigators should avoid becoming discouraged because they are not yet able to generate questions from their own novel observations.

Thankfully, there are numerous sources for identifying questions (Table 1–1). Questions may develop naturally from attempts to verify the predictions of existing theories. Many literature reports end with questions that the authors suggest are appropriate for additional investigation. Conflicting results from different studies also frequently produce questions, the answers to which might help resolve the conflict.

Advances in technology are another common starting point to generate a study question. Sometimes there is a need to develop new technology; at other times, the need is to carefully characterize the performance of existing technology. Applying a new technology to a new field of inquiry and applying improved technology to validate and replicate results from a previous study are also frequent sources for study questions.

3

For those new to scientific investigation, an experienced mentor is an invaluable resource for study questions. Eventually, however, a successful career in research cannot be based on the ideas of others; each investigator needs to make the effort to develop his or her own ideas. The advice and direction of a thoughtful mentor, however, can certainly help less experienced investigators avoid naive mistakes.

## TYPES OF QUESTIONS

Content is not the only important factor to be considered when a research question is formulated. How the question is framed also affects how the study should be designed. For instance, some questions simply ask for descriptions of a particular phenomenon, a group, or a test of interest. An example might be the following question.

*Q1  "How much saturated fat do Americans consume in their diet each day?"*

The answer to this question describes the Americans' average saturated fat intake.

Other questions are meant to determine whether a relationship exists between two (or more) variables or whether a difference exists between two (or more) groups. For instance, one might ask,

*Q2  "Is the intake of saturated fat associated with atherosclerosis?"*

Or, alternatively,

*Q3  "Is the intake of saturated fat by patients with atherosclerosis different from that of individuals without evidence for atherosclerosis?"*

Thus, apparently similar questions can be asked in different ways (Table 1–2). Descriptive questions are about one variable in one group (in the case of Q1, the saturated fat intake of Americans). Questions about relationships involve more than one variable in a single group. In Q2, the relationship between a diet containing saturated fat and the presence of atherosclerosis is considered. However, the focus is still on one group (Americans). Comparative questions are answered by studies that measure differences in two or more variables among two or more groups. The variable (sometimes also referred to as a *factor*) that defines the difference among the groups is called the *independent* variable, and each value for this variable represents a different level (more on this topic in Chapter 3). The variable that is being compared is the *dependent* or *outcome* variable. In the case of Q3, the dependent variable is the intake of saturated fat and the independent variable is the presence or absence of atherosclerosis (representing two different levels). When the independent variable that defines differences among groups is not under the control of the investigator, it is often referred to as an *attribute*. In contrast, independent variables that are under the control of the investigator represent *interventions*, the defining characteristic of an *experiment*. As discussed in Chapters 7 and 8, how the question is framed (descriptive, relational, comparative) has a powerful effect on the type of research design used to answer it (3).

A simple feature distinguishes the descriptive question from relational and comparative questions: the latter two (but not the descriptive question) can always be reformulated so that the answer (at least theoretically) can be a simple "yes" or "no." For instance, instead of Q2, the investigator could have asked, "What is the relationship between the intake of saturated fat and the development of atherosclerosis?" But this question can be restated as Q2 (answer: possibly yes,

**TABLE 1–2**

### Basic Types of Research Questions

| Type of Question | Variables | Groups |
|---|---|---|
| Descriptive | One | One |
| Relational | Two (or more) | One |
| Comparative | Two (or more) | Two (or more) |

possibly no). In contrast, the investigator cannot restate Q1 in a yes/no format.

This simple distinction is actually quite important, because yes/no questions are really declarative statements in a question format, and declarative statements are (potentially) testable hypotheses. The transition from a research question to a testable hypothesis is a necessary step in planning studies in experimental medicine (Figure 1–1).

## THE IMPACT OF OBSERVATION ON FORMULATING A RESEARCH QUESTION

Although research questions can be developed from a number of sources (Table 1–1), some of the most interesting questions start with a simple (and hopefully novel) observation. For purposes of illustration, the problem that has already been posed, the relationship between diet and atherosclerosis, will be considered. (Actually, the story behind the "lipid hypothesis" of atherosclerosis is a dramatic example of the successes provided by interactions between basic and clinical science—that is, translational medicine, in the latter half of the 20th century [4].)

Suppose a physician notices that some patients with hypercholesterolemia have more frequent complications from atherosclerosis (e.g., myocardial infarction) than other patients in the clinic. Because cholesterol is a lipid, the following questions occur to the physician:

*Q4 Is the saturated fat intake of persons with hypercholesterolemia different from persons with normal cholesterol levels?*

And,

*Q5 Is the likelihood of having a myocardial infarction associated with the amount of saturated fat intake?*

It is interesting to ask *why*, in the first place, the physician made the potentially interesting observation that patients with hypercholesterolemia have a high rate of myocardial infarction. The key element

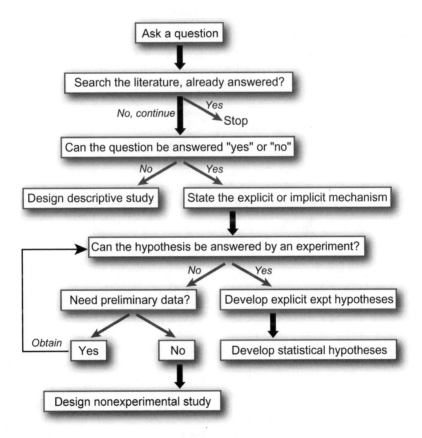

***FIGURE 1–1*** ● The iterative process of defining, and refining, a research question into a testable experimental hypothesis.

it seems is that the observation was *unexpected* (5). The events themselves (hypercholesterolemia, myocardial infarction) may not be unusual or uncommon, but it is their potential *association* with one another that may be strange or exceptional, especially if the observation is to be considered worthy of additional time, effort, and inquiry. This reaction is reasonable enough: everyone wants to control the world by understanding it; so, naturally, we take note of those things or events that do not "fit" our preconceptions. The potential *relatedness*, in this case of hypercholesterolemia to myocardial infarction, can cause a researcher to pause and ask, "Are they *really* related?"—or more provocatively— "Are they *causally* related"?

Of course, what strikes one person as unexpected may strike someone else as obvious, uninteresting, or even, boring. A legitimate concern is whether an individual's "novel" observation is actually quite well known in the world. Clearly, there is little reason to study a problem that has already been solved, and many seemingly important observations have turned out to be unimportant, once the investigator discovered others had already reported the same observation. Fortunately, the tools for searching the universe of scientific knowledge have improved dramatically in the last decade. An efficient and effective search of the available literature is the next step in refining the research question for study (Figure 1–1). This topic is addressed in detail in Chapter 2.

Although the unexpected nature of an observation is an important stimulus for *generating* a research question, observations made while attempting to *answer* the question are another matter entirely. These latter observations (in effect, measurements) are made to either confirm or refute the original impression that two variables are related or that two groups are different. For instance, to *confirm* that hypercholesterolemia is frequently present in patients with myocardial infarction, an investigator might measure the frequency of myocardial infarction in patients both with and without hypercholesterolemia. The investigator might find that the frequency of myocardial infarction is much higher in subjects with hypercholesterolemia; but now, these observations no longer *surprise* the investigator; rather, they *confirm* a relationship he or she suspected was present, a relationship that was the motivation for making the measurements in the first place.

This transformation in the nature of scientific observation was elegantly described by Claude Bernard, the 19th-century physician and physiologist who introduced the concept of homeostasis. Bernard distinguished two types of observations—

those that are passive and those that are active (1). Passive observations were made without any preconceived idea. It was only *because* the observations were unexpected that they caught the observer's attention. Active observations, on the other hand, were made specifically with a *preconceived* idea in mind; the *purpose* of these observations was an attempt to verify that idea.

Bernard felt strongly that an "anticipative idea or a hypothesis [must be the] necessary starting point for all experimental reasoning" (4) *because passive observations are vulnerable to bias*. Because uncommon events occur commonly (i.e., they are uncommon in any one instance but common in the aggregate), some uncommon events, by chance, will appear to be related. This unexpected but apparent connection between events may appear as both novel and interesting because the investigator's knowledge of the world is always incomplete. Investigators must filter the observations that constantly bombard them, discarding the ones that neither interest them nor strike them as unexpected. If an investigator verifies that an improbable co-occurrence has not previously been noted by someone else, he or she naturally believes that it is likely to be significant; the mere fact that these events occur together suggests in some fashion that they may be related, perhaps even causally related. However, recognizing that some apparent relationship may simply be the result of a filtering bias, it is essential to validate what appears to be novel and important by making the transition from passive to active observation. Formulating a question is often the result of a passive observation; transforming that question into a hypothesis that can be tested by making active observations is the next step and is at the heart of the scientific method.

Until recently, the passive, unexpected observation that led to a hypothesis and an experimental study was the province of the individual scientist. The "case report" in the medical literature is a classic example of the importance traditionally afforded such observations. However, in the modern era, it is no longer necessary to limit the unexpected to what is observed by the human mind alone. Enormous amounts of information can now be retrieved with the use of computers and the search for unexpected associations can be systematized. Using this strategy to generate hypotheses is sometimes referred to as *data dredging* (characterized more pejoratively as a *fishing expedition*). The concept is quite seductive because the seemingly unbiased computer should free the process of human prejudice and flawed logic (6). Using such methods to analyze genomic information is just one recent example of how computer searches for information are being used to generate hypotheses. Ultimately, however, the risks are the same: associations that appear to be interesting *because* they are unexpected are the result of a filtering process that can never, in and of itself, eliminate the possibility that they are merely associated by chance. The goal of clinical experimentation is to reduce this chance to an acceptable minimum level, one that investigators can live with as they go about the task of making decisions, the outcomes of which may depend on the truth of a causal relationship.

## FROM QUESTIONS TO HYPOTHESES

Relational questions can often be turned into comparative questions (and vice versa). Consider this question:

**Q6** *"Is the concentration of blood cholesterol associated with the intake of saturated fat in Americans?"*

The answer to this question seeks to relate the values for two variables (the amount of saturated fat in the diet and blood cholesterol concentrations) in one group (Americans). However, the same question can be asked differently (as in Q4):

**Q4** *Is the saturated fat intake of persons with hypercholesterolemia different from persons with normal cholesterol levels?*

In this case, one variable (dietary saturated fat intake) is compared in two groups (Americans with and without high blood cholesterol concentrations). Comparison questions are somewhat more complex than relational questions because operative criteria are needed to identify the different groups (in this case, a definition for what constitutes hypercholesterolemia and what constitutes a normal cholesterol concentration).

Changing a relational question to a comparative one can be valuable but risky. Defining groups can put measurements into a meaningful context (at least to the investigators). After all, the association between dietary fat and blood cholesterol (if it exists) would not be very meaningful if no association existed between some clinical disorder (such as myocardial infarction) and values for blood cholesterol at one extreme or the other. These extremes, then, may become part of the criteria by which research participants are designated as having "hypercholesterolemia" or "normal" cholesterol levels.

The risk in adopting this strategy is that by changing the concentration of blood cholesterol from a continuous to an ordinal variable (levels of blood cholesterol), statistical power is lost and a weak association may be missed (see Chapter 3). The exact operative choice for defining the levels may influence the results. For instance, groups might simply be defined on the basis of arbitrary blood cholesterol concentrations or by dividing the patients into arbitrary numbers of equal-sized groups. On the other hand, groups could be defined by levels of blood cholesterol chosen on the basis of their clinical relevance, such as a level associated with coronary artery disease as a clinical syndrome and another level designated as *borderline*. These groups, then, are no longer defined simply by virtue of their blood cholesterol levels but by other attributes as well, and these other attributes may or may not be relevant to the purported association with dietary fat.

A related risk can occur after the data have already been collected. Consider the following example: An investigator collects data about saturated fat and blood cholesterol concentrations in a group of patients in an effort to address Q6 but fails to identify a strong association. However, a further analysis of the data reveals that the saturated fat intake of the top third of patients with high cholesterol levels is statistically greater than that of the lower third of patients. Perhaps there is no statistically significant difference if the top half is compared with the lower half (possibly because there is too much variation among measurements) and there is no difference when the top quarter is compared with the lowest quarter (too few patients).

Publishing that the top and bottom tertiles of data were statistically different as an answer to Q4 (comparing cholesterol concentrations in two groups of patients) would be misleading. Unfortunately, this method of using post hoc data analyses to "answer" a research question is quite common. Of course, it is perfectly appropriate to perform such analyses. The misleading aspect of the practice is to imply that the question being answered was generated *before* the data were gathered or analyzed. Issues related to post hoc data analysis are addressed in more detail in Chapter 24.

All of these questions about the relationship between saturated fat intake and cholesterol levels are actually, in a sense, "second-level" questions. For instance, Q3 ("Is the intake of saturated fat by patients with atherosclerosis different from that of individuals without evidence for atherosclerosis?") is really a question about whether a high intake of dietary fat somehow *causes* atherosclerosis. Recognizing this implied *mechanistic* question is important because such questions are *best* answered by studies with an *experimental* design (see the Introduction). When groups are compared in *nonexperimental* studies, a specific attribute (e.g., the level of dietary fat or the level of blood cholesterol) distinguishes one group from the other. Experimental studies, however, are a special case of comparison in which the *intervention* becomes the criterion used to define the groups to be compared (Table 1–3). Comparison questions, as noted earlier, are simply declarative statements in a question format, and declarative statements are hypotheses that can be tested—in this case, with the intervention that is the basis for the experiment.

A desire to identify a mechanism (i.e., a cause-effect relationship) underlies many research questions. Because formal experiments are the best method of establishing cause and effect, it is sensible to determine whether a research question, restated as a hypothesis, could be answered by a study with an experimental design. If not, are additional preliminary data required before an acceptable experiment can be designed? Or is an experiment not feasible (e.g., too costly or too time consuming) or desirable (e.g., unethical)?

In summary, a research question for a study can be defined—and then refined—in a logical and deliberate manner (Figure 1–1). Once a research question is posed, an investigator should determine whether the question can be restated so that it could be answered theoretically with a "yes" or "no" (Figure 1–1). If it can, the question should be restated as a declarative hypothesis. Although this step may seem trivial, it is necessary because statistical analyses are performed on hypotheses, not questions.

The question or hypothesis should, then, be evaluated for an implied mechanism. If a mechanism can be identified, the question or hypothesis should be restated to address the potential mechanism.

Next, the investigator should determine whether the hypothesis can be tested in a study with an experimental design (i.e., in which an intervention is imposed on the research participants). If not, additional preliminary data may be required (in studies designed to answer other relevant descriptive, relational, or comparative questions). If an experiment cannot be performed, the original question may still be addressed in a nonexperimental relational or comparative study.

## OBJECTIVES, SPECIFIC AIMS, QUESTIONS, AND HYPOTHESES: PROGRESSIVE SPECIFICITY

Clinical research costs money. In many instances, this money is provided by the National Institutes of Health or a charitable foundation such as the American Heart Association or the American Cancer Society. Why should these institutions and organizations decide to fund a particular project? After all, funding is always finite and there are always more studies to fund than there are dollars to fund them.

A major criterion is the perceived importance of the proposed work. For the purpose of assessing importance, the proposed work must fit into some bigger picture—its *clinical* significance must be made clear. It is useful—and in the context of requesting funding, often mandatory—for an investigator to think about the overall *objectives* of a research project after he or she first conceives of a specific research question to be evaluated.

Beyond the overall objectives, most applications for research funding require the investigator to also define the *specific aims* of the research program. These statements are meant to convey a focused approach to meeting the overall objectives of the research. If each specific aim is clearly articulated, a testable hypothesis (or more often, *hypotheses*) should follow naturally.

For instance, recall the fictional example given in the Introduction. A clinical investigator reads in a medical journal that a newly discovered molecule (Factor Q) affects the function (F) of cells derived in

---

### TABLE 1–3

**Clinical Studies as a Type of Research Question**

| Type of Question | Purpose | Variables | Groups | Analytic Approach (Examples) |
|---|---|---|---|---|
| Descriptive | Describe | One | One | Mean, SD, etc. |
| Relational | Find associations | Two (or more) | One | Regression |
| Comparative | Compare; determine cause; make predictions | Two (or more) | Two (or more) Attribute Intervention | ANOVA |

cell culture (from an organ in which he or she is interested). After reading this paper, the investigator asks the question, "Might Factor Q cause Disease D in humans?"

As the investigator thinks about the study that would be performed to answer that question, he or she quickly realizes that funds will be needed to pay for technical help, supplies, and equipment. In preparing an application to request funding, the investigator makes the following statements about the proposal:

> *The overall objective of this research project is to understand the mechanisms responsible for Disease D. Our specific aim is to determine the role of Factor Q in Disease D. We hypothesize that Factor Q causes Disease D by interfering with cell Function F.*

Although this is a good start, the "devil is in the details," and the details are certainly missing from these statements. Therefore, the next step is to move from a general (study) hypothesis—a general predictive statement about the relationship between two variables or the difference between two or more groups—to an explicit (experimental) hypothesis, which specifies *exactly* how the variables identified in the hypothesis are to be related or compared. This step has been described as stating the "who," "what," "how much," "which," and "when" of an experimental hypothesis (7). The specific questions are as follows: *Who* will constitute the target population and how will that population be sampled for purposes of the study? *What* intervention and *how much* of it will be imposed on the participants? *Which* outcome variable(s) will be measured and *when* (and under what conditions)? The topic of choosing and sampling from a target population is considered in greater detail in Chapter 4. Issues related to choosing and making measurements of an outcome variable are addressed in Chapter 3.

In the fictional example, the investigator is fortunate enough to have access to a new drug, called Factor Q Inhibitor. This drug has been shown to alter cell Function F and is now ready for use in humans. Accordingly, the investigator realizes that the administration of Factor Q Inhibitor would allow him or her to test the hypothesis that Factor Q causes Disease D by affecting cell Function F. But to do so, the investigator needs to make some important decisions. Which human patients will get the drug (i.e., how will Disease D be defined for the purposes of this study)? What dose of the drug will be administered ("how much")? For how long will the drug be administered ("when")? And which variables will be used to determine whether Factor Q inhibitor affects Disease D? Ultimately, the explicit hypothesis might take the following form:

*H1 Factor Q Inhibitor, given in Dose S for W Weeks in P Patients with Disease D, improves Function F by Percent %.*

The study, which is designed to test this hypothesis, is obviously very specific. For the creation of this hypothesis, a great deal of information (preliminary data) must be available to make the experimental hypothesis explicit (and possible). Yet, if the results of the study fail to support the hypothesis, the investigator is left to wonder whether it is because the definition used to choose patients with Disease D was imprecise, because the dose was wrong, or because the duration of treatment was wrong. The *study* hypothesis (that Factor Q causes Disease D by interfering with Function F) may still be true even though a test of the *explicit* hypothesis fails to provide supporting evidence.

Alternatively, it might have been tempting to hypothesize that:

*H2 Factor Q Inhibitor, given in Dose S for W Weeks in P Patients with Disease D, improves Disease D.*

This hypothesis, although perhaps more clinically relevant that hypothesis H1, is also more problematic. It has all the risks associated with testing H1 (e.g., risks associated with choosing specific dosing schedules, duration of treatment), but may be even more difficult to interpret if the study results fail to generate evidence to support the hypothesis. If the study design includes some measurement of Function F that is affected by Factor Q Inhibitor, then the investigator may reasonably conclude that improvements in Function F and relief of symptoms associated with Disease D are related. However, the hypothesis in H2 doesn't mandate measurements of Function F, and it is common for studies to be designed that simply assume that the intervention (in this case, Factor Q Inhibitor) will affect the putative mechanism (in this case, Function F). In the event of a negative study, the investigator will wonder whether the definition of disease improvement was inadequate, and also whether Function F was *actually* affected.

A third variation on the hypothesis raises still other issues.

*H3 Factor Q Inhibitor, given in Dose S for W Weeks in P Patients with Disease D, improves Disease by improving Function F by Percent %.*

Superficially, this hypothesis seems to address the issues just raised with hypotheses H1 and H2. It is specific, clinically relevant, and links outcome to putative mechanism. However, the problem now is that compound, multiple response variables (improvements in Disease D and improvements in Function F) have been chosen. Thus, if only one of the two outcome measures changes in response to the intervention, does the evidence support or refute the hypothesis?

It is indeed common for an investigative team to make more than one "outcome" measurement (of dependent variables) when performing a clinical study. Often, some measurements are made as part of quality control (sometimes referred to as *validation measurements*); other measurements may be made that are also relevant to the hypothesis being tested. For instance, although measuring changes in Function F may be one way to test the effects of Factor Q Inhibitor, there may be several others. These alternatives may require additional data to be obtained, or they may simply be alternative methods of analyzing the data already obtained (e.g., rather than percentage change in Function F, a comparison of mean values before and after the administration of Factor Q Inhibitor). As a result, it quickly becomes possible to test the general hypothesis with multiple explicit "experimental" hypotheses, each one differing only by the measurement used to assess effect. In so doing, the investigator increases the risk of making a false conclusion about the efficacy of the intervention (i.e., if enough measurements are made, sooner or later, one of them will seem to "change" after the intervention; see Chapter 24).

The best solution to avoid this dilemma is to choose a single *primary* outcome measure and to then design a study to maximize the likelihood that the results can be correctly interpreted to either support or refute the appropriate experimental hypothesis. The other measurements should be considered as secondary outcomes. A study that only shows changes in the secondary outcomes, and not in the primary outcome variable, should be interpreted with considerable caution.

Thus, in the fictional example, hypotheses H1 and H2 could be combined, with one chosen as a primary outcome test, the other as a test for the secondary outcome. A study to test Hypothesis H1 would be an excellent example of translational clinical research; a study to test Hypothesis H2, on the other hand, would be more typical of a therapeutic clinical trial.

Eventually, each experimental hypothesis must be converted into an explicit *statistical* hypothesis. A statistical hypothesis is basically a mathematical expression of the experimental hypothesis. Statistical hypotheses come in two forms: a *null hypothesis*, which posits that there is no statistically significant difference between the two (or more)

groups being tested (or no statistically significant relation between the variables measured in one group), and an *alternative hypothesis*, which posits that a difference (or a relation) does exist. The rationale for putting statistical hypotheses in these forms is given in Chapter 23.

Although this discussion about a study that seeks to determine whether a Factor Q Inhibitor is effective in treating Disease D may seem fanciful, it is in reality a very general and common approach to testing hypotheses in humans. For example, by the 1960s, investigators knew both the absorption of cholesterol from food and the de novo hepatic synthesis of cholesterol affected concentrations of blood cholesterol. Investigators also knew high levels of blood cholesterol were associated with the development of atherosclerosis. These observations led to the general hypothesis that high levels of blood cholesterol, regardless of source, contribute to ("cause") atherosclerosis. The logical derivative hypothesis was that lowering blood cholesterol levels by any means (not just by dietary restriction) should reduce the consequences of atherosclerosis. When investigators discovered that hepatic synthesis of cholesterol is regulated by the enzyme 3-hydroxy-3-methylglutaryl coenzyme A (HMG-CoA) reductase, the search was on for a drug that would inhibit this enzyme. With the development of the statin class of HMG-CoA reductase inhibitors, a series of clinical experiments (clinical trials) eventually showed that lowering blood cholesterol reduced the progression of atherosclerotic vascular lesions and the complications of atherosclerosis (myocardial infarction, stroke, and death) (4).

Interestingly, the effects of the statins on halting the progression of atherosclerosis are far greater than with other means of lowering cholesterol. Although such observations do not invalidate the lipid hypothesis, they may well indicate that the mechanism of benefit is due to effects other than simple lowering of the blood cholesterol concentration. As in the fictional hypotheses H1 and H2, a well-designed experiment can prove that an *intervention* affects the manifestations of disease, and it can prove that the same intervention affects some function that is a logical mechanism for the intervention's effects, but proving that the change in *function* is what alters the manifestations of the disease is much more difficult. Rarely can that be accomplished within a single experiment.

The final experimental hypothesis to be tested in any particular study, then, is usually the result of much iteration. Although an observation (e.g., by an individual investigator, or as gleaned from the literature) may lead to an interesting initial question, the specific hypothesis often requires many adjustments before the "who," "what," "how much," "which," and "when" issues are resolved—each individually reflecting issues of feasibility, cost, and other factors. Although the big question (the overall or general hypothesis) may drive an investigator's interest in pursuing a particular research problem, it is the little (explicit) experimental hypotheses that actually move the research program forward.

Because so many decisions, and therefore choices, are necessary when a clinical study is planned and because the ethical conduct of research demands that such choices maximize the likelihood that the participation of human patients will provide useful information (see Chapter 14), these choices must be made wisely. The proposed experiment must build appropriately on information already available. This background information may come from literature sources (see Chapter 2) or from the investigator's own previously conducted research, or it may be necessary to perform a set of preliminary (pilot) studies to be able to finally specify the experimental hypothesis to be tested.

## GENERATING PRELIMINARY DATA

For many reasons, generating preliminary data may be useful, even necessary, before an investigator can formulate a precise experimental hypothesis. These studies often identify and quantify sources of measurement bias, variability, sensitivity, and specificity. Preliminary studies can also determine the likely size effect of any experimental intervention. This information is needed to estimate sample size in a power analysis (see Chapter 9). Although sample size estimates are necessary to appropriately *plan* a study after an experimental hypothesis has already been stipulated, they may also affect whether the study can be performed as originally planned, possibly leading to a refinement of the original experimental hypothesis—another example of the iteration that takes place as a study is conceived, planned, and finally implemented.

Similarly, preliminary studies may help the investigative team to work out or improve procedures or to train personnel in the use of specific techniques for measurement. Once again, this information may influence the final formulation of the hypothesis to be tested, and thus, ultimately, the design of the experiment.

Another compelling reason to generate preliminary data is to provide an acceptable justification for the proposed study. In clinical experimentation especially, investigators do not have the luxury of imposing an intervention on a human volunteer simply because it seems like an interesting idea.

Because all interventions carry risk (some trivial, others life threatening), the risk must be justified. Preliminary data are often the critical source of information used to defend the design of a specific human experiment.

Although preliminary data may include preclinical (e.g., animal) studies, some *clinical* data are almost always required before an experimental study can be appropriately proposed and properly designed. Sometimes the existing literature may provide a robust foundation for the proposed study. For instance, the first clinical studies of HMG-CoA reductase inhibitors to reduce blood cholesterol concentrations were preceded by numerous epidemiologic studies demonstrating a relationship between blood cholesterol levels and the risks of atherosclerotic cardiovascular disease, as well as by various experimental studies that tested (by other means) whether an active intervention (any intervention) that lowered blood cholesterol levels would reduce adverse outcomes from atherosclerosis (4). In many cases, however, the investigator must face the possibility of first generating his or her own preliminary data before an experimental study can be implemented.

The prospect of doing so can be daunting because the investigator must delay the study he or she actually wants to do. Accordingly, a premium is generally placed on efficiency (i.e., collecting the required data in the shortest time possible). In practice, to achieve this goal, such studies generally employ a retrospective cohort, case-control, or cross-sectional format (see Chapter 7).

A common variant of the cross-sectional study, one that is often used to justify subsequent clinical experiments, is one in which measurements are made in unrelated groups of subjects (e.g., those with the disease in question and others without it). Although this design may sound like a case-control design, from a classical epidemiologic viewpoint, it differs because case-control studies are generally accepted to be retrospective comparisons of two groups on the basis of measurements already obtained. Because the type of study being considered here includes measurements that are obtained prospectively at a single point in time, we will continue to refer to such studies as *cross-sectional*.

Cross-sectional studies of this type have several compelling features. For one, they are usually relatively easy to implement, which means that they can usually be completed in a relatively short period of time. Because their design is simple, they are often inexpensive in comparison with other study formats. They are also useful for describing the distribution (variation) of the outcome variable in one or more subject populations, which is often critical information for estimating the sample size required for a subsequent experimental study.

Consider once again, then, the hypothetical example of a study in which the investigator wants to eventually determine whether Disease D is causally related to Factor Q via its effects on cell Function F. The investigator plans to test this hypothesis using the newly developed Factor Q Inhibitor. The rationale for such a study would be strengthened if the investigator could first demonstrate that Factor Q levels are higher in patients with the disease than in healthy controls. Eventually, the investigator wants to demonstrate that Factor Q Inhibitor will normalize cell Function F, and so he or she also needs to demonstrate that measurements of that function can be made in patients with Disease D.

The investigator designs and performs a simple cross-sectional study. The results of this hypothetical study are shown in Figure 1–2. They clearly show that levels of Factor Q are higher in patients with Disease D than in patients without the disease, and that cell Function F is simultaneously reduced in patients with the disease. The details of designing and implementing such a study are considered in Chapter 7.

Commonly, results like those in Figure 1–2 would be reported as showing that Factor Q is "associated" with Disease D. However, *association* or *relational* studies are those in which two variables are related in one group. In this case two groups are being compared (and, as a consequence, comparison not correlation statistics would be used to analyze the data). Nevertheless, the language of association is often used when the results of these studies are described. The reason is simple enough: the alternative is to use the language of causation. Cross-sectional studies, however, cannot provide strong evidence for causation because it is unknown whether the putative risk factor preceded the development of disease, a necessary criterion of causation. In addition, cross-sectional studies provide little protection from multiple sources of confounding because the groups being compared are defined by the disease attribute, and not on the basis of a randomized intervention under the control of the investigator. Thus, the investigator cannot ensure that the two groups are similar in all respects *except* for the intervention.

What if the results shown in Figure 1–2 were different and showed instead that there was *no* difference in Factor Q levels between those with and without Disease D? This type of result is often interpreted to mean that a putative mechanism is unlikely to be involved in disease pathogenesis, but such an interpretation is potentially faulty because previously elevated levels of the mediator (Factor Q in this case) may have returned to normal before measurements were obtained, even as other events in the chain of causation continued to progress toward the eventual clinical manifestation of the disease.

An example of this phenomenon is the putative role of tumor necrosis factor-alpha (TNF-$\alpha$) in the pathogenesis of septic shock (8). Although the preclinical evidence that TNF-$\alpha$ is an important mediator of septic shock is extremely robust, clinical evidence has been much more difficult to establish. Numerous clinical trials of TNF-$\alpha$ inhibitors have failed to show any benefit in patients with septic shock. At first, these results raised the possibility that TNF-$\alpha$ was not an important mediator in human septic shock. Eventually, however, the increase in TNF-$\alpha$ was discovered to be relatively brief, despite persistent symptoms of shock. In other words, the proverbial "horse had already left the barn." The administration of TNF-$\alpha$ inhibitors after TNF-$\alpha$ levels had already fallen would of course be

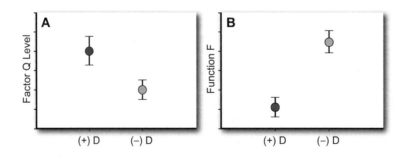

**FIGURE 1–2** ● Hypothetical results from a simple cross-sectional study comparing Factor Q levels (*A*) and a measure of cell Function F (*B*) in two groups of research participants, those with (+) and without (–) Disease D. The results are consistent with, and provide a rationale for a clinical experiment to test, the hypothesis that inhibition of Factor Q in patients with Disease D would restore Function F.

of little value. Of course, a cross-sectional study of TNF-α levels in septic shock patients at such a time would fail to show any differences compared with healthy participants.

Thus, rather than saying that a particular factor is *associated* (or not) with the development of disease, a more precise conclusion would be simply that the results of a study (like those shown in Figure 1–2) are *consistent* with the hypothesis that the factor is causally related to the disease in question—a hypothesis to be tested at a later time by an appropriate experimental intervention.

## WHEN IS A RESEARCH QUESTION *IMPORTANT*?

Young or new investigators are frequently advised not to work on a research problem unless it is important—but how are they to know which problems are important (9)? The frustrating answer is that they can not know for certain. The history of science is replete with stories of how what once seemed trivial turned out to be momentous and vice versa. Yet this history of error does not mean that anything and everything is worthwhile. After all, human participants in clinical experiments are not guinea pigs. If the experiment is not important, it should not be done. By whatever standard this conclusion is reached, and whether it is ultimately proven to be right or wrong, a decision that the research does not appear to be important is tantamount to saying that performing the research would be unethical (10).

Certainly, the research should be interesting to the investigator, and hopefully to others, especially the investigator's peers. Finding out that others who are respected in the field think that an answer to the investigator's question would be interesting is not a bad test of whether it would also be important. Conversely, if no one else seems to find the problem interesting, the investigator should consider why he or she thinks the problem is so important. This kind of feedback can be gained from presenting ideas to a mentor or at a research conference.

The answer to the proposed question should also advance understanding in the field. Although replication is at the heart of the scientific method, *novel* findings are generally valued more highly than those that merely replicate what is already known. An important study may or may not replicate previous findings, but it should *also* advance understanding.

Finally, any study that has or will have a clinically relevant impact is, almost by definition, important. This is not to say that *only* studies with immediate clinical significance are important, but

| **T A B L E   1 – 4** |
| :--- |
| **A "Getting Started" Checklist** |

| |
| :--- |
| State the overall objective(s) of the research |
| State the specific aim(s) of the proposed study |
| State the explicit or implicit mechanism |
| State the overall study hypothesis |
| State the specific experimental hypothesis |
| Determine that the hypothesis is testable, ethical, important |
| Translate the experimental hypothesis into a statistical one |

it is an acknowledgment that in the hierarchy of priorities, the purpose of biomedical research, is, after all, to improve *human* health.

## A "GETTING STARTED" CHECKLIST

Table 1–4 provides a checklist to help new investigators get started. The items do not need to be completed in order, but each item should be considered as a study question is initially conceived, adjusted, and finally formulated. As Claude Bernard said more than 150 years ago (1):

> *The true scientist . . . (1) . . . notes a fact; (2) a propos of this fact, an idea is born in his mind; (3) in the light of this idea, he reasons, devises an experiment, imagines and brings to pass its material conditions; (4) from this experiment, new phenomena result which must be observed, and so on and so forth (1).*

Defining—and refining—a research question is an iterative process. The answers to each question almost invariably raise new questions to be answered by carefully designed and conducted clinical studies.

## SUMMARY

- Questions suitable for study may be found from a variety of sources: an investigator's own observations, existing theories, and from the biomedical literature, among others. In addition, unresolved problems often require new technologies, which themselves must be appropriately studied and validated.
- Study questions are generally one of three types: descriptive, relational, or comparative. Each requires its own unique study design.
- Scientists basically make two types of observations. "Passive" observations are made without preconceived ideas. The fact that they weren't anticipated is part of what makes the observation

interesting and potentially important. They are often the seed idea for what later becomes a study question or hypothesis. By contrast, active observations are actually measurements that are made to confirm or refute a preconceived idea (i.e., a hypothesis).

- Questions that theoretically can be answered with a "yes" or "no" should be restated as a hypothesis, preferably one that includes the presumed underlying mechanism. Ideally, such questions should be answered with studies that incorporate an experimental design. When that is not feasible, additional preliminary data may be needed, or the question may need to be addressed in a study with a nonexperimental design.

- In designing a research study, the investigator should make an effort to move progressively from stating the overall objectives for the research to the specific aims, the general study hypothesis, and finally the explicit experimental hypotheses that will answer the "who," "what," "how much," "which," and "when" aspects of study design.

- Most clinical experiments require preliminary evidence to justify the need for the research (i.e., importance of proving or disproving the hypothesis) or to demonstrate the feasibility of performing the research. These data may come from existing literature, the investigator's prior studies, or newly designed studies. Cross-sectional study designs, in which measurements are obtained from the target human patient group and compared with those in one or more control groups (e.g., healthy individuals), are a commonly used format for such studies.

- An important study is generally one that is of interest to the investigator and the investigator's peers, and has the potential to favorably affect clinical care, either directly or by advancing understanding in the field.

## REFERENCES

1. Bernard C. An Introduction to the Study of Experimental Medicine. New York: MacMillan, 1927.
2. Kubinyi H. Chance favors the prepared mind—from serendipity to rational drug design. J Recep Sign Transduct Res 1999;19:15–39.
3. Morgan G, Harmon R. Research questions and hypotheses. J Amer Acad Child Adolescent Psych 2000; 39:261–263.
4. Thompson G. The proving of the lipid hypothesis. Curr Opin Lipid 1999;10:201–205.
5. Silverman W. Human Experimentation: A Guided Step into the Unknown. Oxford: Oxford University Press, 1985.
6. Smith G, Ebrahim S. Data dredging, bias, or confounding. BMJ 2002;325:1437–1438.
7. Inman K, Martin C, Sibbald W. Design and conduct of clinical trials in critical care. J Crit Care 1992;7: 118–128.
8. Riedemann N, Guo R, Ward P. The enigma of sepsis. J Clin Invest 2003;112:460–467.
9. Kahn C. Picking a research problem: the critical decision. N Engl J Med 1994;330:1530–1533.
10. Schulman K, Seils D, Timbie J et al. A national survey of provisions in clinical-trial agreements between medical schools and industry sponsors. N Engl J Med 2002;347:1335–1341.

# CHAPTER 2

# Searching the Literature

Christina Sullivan, Neville Prendergast

All research to some extent relies on the results of previous research endeavors and scientific inquiry. The record of these results in biomedical research is best found in the published health sciences literature. A search of this literature, therefore, should be an integral part of any research undertaking. It plays an essential role in creating the foundation on which the rest of the research process is built.

In Chapter 1, a systematic approach to generating a research question was described. A similar systematic approach should be applied to a search of the relevant scientific literature. The search topic(s) should flow naturally from the concepts and constructs that fashioned the initial research questions, and these may change and evolve depending on the literature findings.

In general, there are four major reasons to review the literature: (1) to determine the existing research on a topic, (2) to determine the relevant level of theory and knowledge development (including knowledge gaps), (3) to determine the relevancy of the existing knowledge base to a particular research inquiry, and (4) to provide a rationale for the selection of the research strategy (1). However, in clinical research, a fifth reason of paramount importance, to determine patient safety, transcends these more general reasons. The risks associated with a proposed experimental intervention must be carefully weighed against the value of the new information to be gained, making the accuracy of the literature search even more imperative.

## THE KEY TO GOOD LITERATURE SEARCHING: GET TO KNOW YOUR LIBRARIAN

The savvy investigator begins his or her search of the literature by contacting—in person (ideally), by phone, by e-mail, or on the Web—the nearest health sciences librarian (or information professional). An experienced medical reference librarian can direct the investigator to the most relevant available resources and services, many of which are free. An almost limitless number of possible information sources are available to researchers, but not all are created equal (and not all are best found on the search engine Google). Now, especially, in a climate where institutional review boards (IRBs) and human studies committees are requiring researchers to adhere to specific literature search guidelines and to provide detailed documentation of their findings, the quality of supporting evidence and the thoroughness of the search process are receiving closer scrutiny. Partnering with an information professional who is competent in managing information resources, managing information services, and applying information tools and technologies, streamlines the search process and provides direction to those information sources best suited to individual research needs (2).

The Medical Library Association has published a policy statement, "The Role of Expert Searching in Health Sciences Libraries," that defines expert searching and includes specific key skills and knowledge essential for the expert searcher. These qualities include knowledge of subject domain, database subject content and retrieval system interfaces, and the ability to effectively document the search process. The policy statement notes that this combined set of skills and knowledge is unique to the experienced librarian and not generally required of health care professionals and biomedical research personnel (3). The policy statement is available online at http://www.mlanet.org.

Academic medical centers invariably have library services within the institution. For individuals outside the academic community, membership in a local medical society frequently includes library privileges at nearby institutions. Also, the health sciences libraries that make up the National Network of Libraries of Medicine (http://nnlm. gov) offer services to physicians who do not have access to a local medical library.

Document delivery and photocopy services supply articles of interest generated by a literature search. Many journals are now available in electronic format so that pertinent articles the search identifies can be easily retrieved. Some electronic journals are freely available online; most charge a fee, but access is usually free to those electronic titles subscribed to by the library. Institutional subscriptions come with varied restrictions, including eligibility for accessing electronic resources. In sum, for the most efficient and effective search of the literature, form an alliance with an information professional as the first step.

The challenge of the 21st-century researcher is how to wade through excessive amounts of information to find those sources that are both valid and relevant to the proposed research question. No literature search, no matter how thorough and comprehensive, can guarantee that every relevant, or even important, detail on a topic will be unearthed. That something will be missing is almost guaranteed. However, a systematic approach to searching the literature, bolstered by collaboration with colleagues and consultation with information specialists, should minimize the number of inevitable oversights.

## INSTITUTIONAL REVIEW BOARDS AND HUMAN STUDIES COMMITTEES

Although investigators routinely undertake a thorough literature search in support of a proposed research topic, uniform research standards that ensure a comprehensive literature search have not yet been formally established. The absence of formalized guidelines for the literature search portion of a research proposal is cited among several factors that contributed to the unexpected death of a

healthy 24-year-old research participant at Johns Hopkins University in 2001 (4). In this now infamous incident, human volunteers inhaled hexamethonium. Its toxic effect on the lungs and the resultant pulmonary complications had been documented in both published journal articles and books—information a comprehensive literature search would have retrieved. Unfortunately, the researchers restricted their search to online databases in which, generally, the earliest cited literature is from the mid-1960s. At the time of the study, the MEDLINE database dated back to 1966, but the articles detailing the dangers of inhaled hexamethonium were published before that date and thus were not retrieved in the MEDLINE search.

In response to this event, Johns Hopkins created a committee made up of a diverse group of experts including scientists, pharmacists, and librarians to develop literature search guidelines for researchers and IRBs (5). The resultant "Guidelines for Determining an Adequate and Comprehensive Literature Search of Drug Safety for Use by Investigator and Institutional Review Boards" are available online from the Johns Hopkins University website at http://irb.jhmi.edu/Guidelines/LiteratureSearch .doc. The document provides guidelines only; currently, there are no published written standards for adequacy and comprehensiveness of literature searches of drug safety.

The guidelines describe a two-part process made up of a search for primary references followed by a critical evaluation of the retrieved information. A form for the required literature search log, summary, and bibliography is included, followed by an appendix outlining a model search process, examples of relevant databases, and a template for documenting the search path that the investigators followed. Also included are examples of reference or tertiary drug information sources, examples of secondary sources (e.g., abstracting and indexing services) for drug and chemical information, and a list of suggested search techniques. Additional guidelines have been made available by other universities, including Washington University (http://medicine.wustl.edu/~hsc/guidelines/) and Yale University (http://www.med.yale.edu/library/education/hic/).

## ONLINE DATABASES AND PRINT INDEXES

To find information that is both relevant and reputable, it is essential to understand the content, structure, and producer of the database in which the search is run. The traditional starting point for a literature search is the MEDLINE database, but there are several others (as described in following sections, see Tables 2–1 and 2–2) that are also important. In addition, comprehensive, retrospective literature searches may require a manual search of printed indexes. Additional information about the full range of online databases is available from Dialog (http://www.dialog.com) via the *Gale Directory of Online, Portable, and Internet Databases*. Dialog databases require a subscription, so access to the electronic version of the directory is restricted; however, many institutional libraries have subscriptions that are available to its academic community. The print counterpart to the database is the *Gale Directory of Databases, Volume 1: Online Databases*, another resource available in many libraries.

## MEDLINE

MEDLINE is produced by the National Library of Medicine (NLM), the world's largest medical library located on the campus of the National Institutes of Health in Bethesda, Maryland. Health sciences investigators have a unique advantage over researchers in other disciplines because MEDLINE, the main source of access to the published literature, is a government-produced resource that is free and publicly available. It is the primary bibliographic database for accessing the health sciences journal literature in the United States and features references to peer-reviewed journal articles in the life sciences with a concentration on biomedicine. MEDLINE also includes references to journal articles in nursing, dentistry, veterinary medicine, health care systems, and the basic sciences. MEDLINE, as stated earlier, is bibliographic: the database contains references and summaries of published articles, but not the actual article. Until recently, the years covered in MEDLINE ranged from 1966 to the present. However, the NLM has recently incorporated earlier references—1951 to 1965—from its former OLDMEDLINE database into PubMed (more about PubMed and other MEDLINE interfaces later). Retrospective indexing is an ongoing process, and earlier citations will continue to be added to MEDLINE for keyword and author searches.

Searching the health sciences literature before 1951 entails a manual search of *Index Medicus*, MEDLINE's print counterpart. The NLM has been publishing *Index Medicus*, a monthly author and subject guide to the health sciences journal literature, since 1879. MEDLINE, the expanded online version of *Index Medicus*, evolved from the introduction of computerization to the publishing industry.

Computers allowed the creation of an automated database that was used to create the printed *Index Medicus*. The NLM appreciated that vital health information could be more rapidly disseminated if the database could be searched directly before the printed *Index* reached the health sciences community. Thus, MEDLINE was at the forefront of the digital age. Its creation revolutionized the literature search process and forever changed the way medical professionals find information. It also served as a model for the creation of additional databases in the biomedical sciences, as well as other disciplines.

The sophisticated indexing process used by the creators of MEDLINE influenced the design of these other databases so that search techniques similar to those used in MEDLINE can be used in other databases. The MEDLINE data usually include an abstract of the article's content, in addition to such identifying information as title, authors' names, institutions, and journal name. In the indexing process, NLM contracts with subject experts who are trained indexers to read the journal articles in their area of expertise and index (i.e., describe the content, using specific descriptors known as Medical Subject Headings [MeSH]). This additional field of indexing terms is incorporated into the MEDLINE database where it can be searched along with author-supplied keywords and those from titles and abstracts. Also, not all of the references in MEDLINE have an abstract that summarizes the article (approximately 20% of the references do not have an accompanying abstract), so a reliance on title and abstract searching alone is likely to miss potentially important database content. Other databases in the health sciences use similar indexing processes whereby controlled vocabulary descriptors are assigned to references within the database and form a value-added searchable field. Also, the inclusion of MeSH headings in the index of searchable terms of databases other than MEDLINE provides consistency of vocabulary across databases.

The MEDLINE database is available from a multitude of different sources and information vendors; Medical Matrix, an online clinical medical resource service, lists 17 available versions of MEDLINE (6). What distinguishes one version from another is primarily the search interface. PubMed and Ovid are likely the two search systems most familiar to researchers because they are the most powerful and widely used. The PubMed database (http://www.pubmed.gov) comes directly from the NLM and is freely available over the Web. It includes MEDLINE along with some extras such as access to additional selected life sciences journals, links to the full-text of articles at

## TABLE 2–1

**Primary Databases for Clinical Research**

| Title | Producer | Description | Electronic Availability | Print Availability |
|---|---|---|---|---|
| MEDLINE | National Library of Medicine (NLM) | Primary bibliographic database to access health science journal literature in the United States. Features peer-reviewed articles in the life sciences with concentration on biomedicine. International in scope. Contains over 12 million citations; 10,000 new citations added weekly. | Free online via PubMed. Coverage from 1951 to present. Access at http://pubmed.gov. Fee-based resource via Ovid MEDLINE, etc. | Literature before 1951 in *Index Medicus*, published from 1879 (U.S. Surgeon General's Catalogue) to present. |
| EMBASE | Elsevier Science | European counterpart to to MEDLINE; 9.5 million biomedical citation references from 70 countries (more than half in Europe, a third is North American). Strong emphasis on pharmacy and pharmacology. Some overlap occurs between EMBASE and MEDLINE. | Fee-based resource at http://www.embase.com. Coverage: 1974 to present. Limited access to citations from 1963–1973. Subscription required. | *Excerpta Medica* 1948 to present. |
| Cochrane Library | Cochrane Collaboration, produced by Wiley InterScience, presented online by Update Software | Premier source of reliable evidence-based health care and research methodology. Consists of seven different databases. Features the Cochrane Database of Systematic Reviews. | Fee-based resource available at www.interscience.wiley.com/cgi-bin/mrwhome/106568753/HOME. Began 1996, with the reviews available since 1988. | Available as a serial publication, The Cochrane Library, 1996 to present, Oxford, UK; Update Software Ltd. |
| Web of Science (WoS) | Thomson ISI | Cited reference search capability points to other published papers that have cited a specific work or author. Three different databases combined; 1945 to present. | Extent of coverage varies by institutional subscription choice at http://isi10.isiknowledge.com/portal.cgi/wos. | Available in various editions and formats back to 1945. |

## TABLE 2–2

### Secondary Databases for Clinical Research

| Title | Producer | Description | Electronic Availability | Print Availability |
|---|---|---|---|---|
| BIOSIS Previews | BIOSIS—a nonprofit organization providing information services to the global life sciences community | International in scope. References to biotechnology, preclinical and experimental medicine, and pharmacology. Includes nonjournal reference sources (e.g., meetings, symposia, workshops, software, and patents). | Fee-based resource. Accessible at http:// www.biosis.org, from 1969 to present. | *Biological Abstracts*, since 1926, *Biological Abstracts/RRM* —a resource, since 1980– featuring references to research reports, reviews, and international meetings in biology and biomedicine. |
| TOXicology Data NET work (TOXNET) | NLM | A collection of databases that cover toxicology, hazardous chemicals, and environmental health. They are TOXLINE, DART/ETIC, HSDB, ChemIDplus, CCRIS, and GENE-TOX. Factual data are gathered from varying government research agencies (e.g., EPA, NCI). | Free of charge and accessed at http:// toxnet.nlm.nih.gov. | Via the NLM as numerous bibliographies and topical fact sheets on toxicology, hazardous substances, and environment issues. |
| Chemical Abstracts/ SciFinder Scholar | Chemical Abstracts Services (CAS)—a division of the American Chemical Society | SciFinder Scholar is a desktop research tool featuring software that accesses the CAS databases and the world of chemistry literature. The combined databases are CAplus, CAS Registry, CASREACT, CHEMCATS, and MEDLINE. | Fee-based and accessed at http:// www.cas.org. References for material date back to 1907, and some from before 1907. | CAS has published the printed index, *Chemical Abstracts*, since 1907, to monitor, abstract, and index the world's chemistry literature. |

## TABLE 2–2 (Continued)

### Secondary Databases for Clinical Research

| Title | Producer | Description | Electronic Availability | Print Availability |
|-------|----------|-------------|--------------------------|--------------------|
| CrossFire Beilstein | MDL Information Systems | Comprehensive database of organic chemistry—organic reactions and chemical facts. Comprises the most complete collection of structures, properties, and references to organic chemistry literature, including bioactivity records. | Fee-based and accessed at http://www.beilstein.com, it features over 8 million compounds and 9 million reactions from 1779 forward. | Crossfire's print counterpart is *Beilstein's Handbuch der Organischen Chemie* (Beilstein's handbook of organic chemistry). |
| Drugs in Clinical Trials Database | CenterWatch—a publishing and information services company specializing in the clinical trials industry | Detailed profiles of new investigational treatments in phases I through III clinical trials plus information on over 2,000 drugs to treat over 800 disease conditions. The website includes an extensive list of IRB- approved clinical trials being conducted internationally. Drug profiles include mechanisms of action, study phase status, and clinical trial results. | Fee-based and accessible at http://www.centerwatch.com. Personal subscription is possible or institutional subscription through a library. | No print counterpart. |

EPA, Environmental Protection Agency; IRB, Institutional Review Board; NCI, National Cancer Institute

participating publishers' websites, and links to the molecular biology databases maintained by the National Center for Biotechnology Information (NCBI) (7). Ovid MEDLINE (http://www.ovid.com) comes from Ovid Technologies, a subsidiary of the information services company Wolters Kluwer. Most medical center and medical school libraries subscribe to Ovid MEDLINE because librarians and information professionals, as well as their clientele, appreciate its sophisticated search interface. The Ovid system requires either an individual or institutional subscription, so access to Ovid MEDLINE is restricted; investigators should consult

their medical library to determine accessibility or contact Ovid directly.

Both PubMed and Ovid MEDLINE have basic and advanced search capabilities. The PubMed search interface is geared toward the broadest possible range of searchers. Every researcher should be able to enter a natural language phrase or question and generate some results. The more advanced search features need to be sought out and learned. In contrast, at most university libraries and medical centers, Ovid MEDLINE is generally entered through the advanced, rather than basic, search mode. Its search interface is geared toward the more sophisticated searcher (e.g., researchers and clinicians). Its interface offers the researcher more control over the search strategy and process; the PubMed interface does most of the work behind the scenes. Searching Ovid MEDLINE is like driving a car with a manual transmission; PubMed is like driving a car with an automatic transmission.

Unlike PubMed, Ovid MEDLINE does not respond to natural language queries or phrases. Rather, Ovid responds better to a conceptual approach. When a search query is formulated in Ovid, it is helpful to divide the topic into its different components, search the components separately, and then combine them. Nearly all databases (and Web browsers), including those that use natural language searching, allow the creation and combination of separate search sets with the Boolean operators AND and OR. Connecting terms with AND generates the overlap between or among sets of information and reduces retrieval. In contrast, connecting terms with OR generates the union of two or more sets of information and increases retrieval. Avoid using the NOT connector, as it can eliminate relevant citations.

Creating and combining search sets afford greater flexibility when searching because different sets can be combined in different ways and the results compared. Also, the same search logic applies across various databases and information systems despite differences in the specific content and search interface. The same strategy can be used across different systems. For instruction, PubMed features an overview, a help/FAQ (frequently asked questions) option, and a tutorial. Ovid MEDLINE has detailed, context-specific help screens, and the *Ovid Web Gateway Online Users Guide* and a Web-based tutorial are available at http://www.ovid.com/site/help/ovid_tutorials.jsp. A university-based tutorial is available from Washington University at http://becker.wustl.edu/computercourses/resources/tutorials.htm. (Additional tutorials can be found by searching the Web for "Ovid MEDLINE tutorials.")

## SEARCH STRATEGIES

While formal instruction and ongoing practice are the best means of developing and sharpening search skills, some general strategies and problem-solving suggestions can still be made. The MEDLINE database is used in the following examples, but the same general techniques and principles can be used in other databases. The identical search logic applies across all bibliographic databases.

Any search should include the steps shown in Table 2–3. To begin, research questions, as described in Chapter 1, should be both precise and answerable (e.g., Does either fish liver oil or vitamin E reduce the incidence of cardiovascular disease in high-risk middle-aged men?). This is a concrete question that will have an answer. Next, divide the question into key concepts that can then be searched separately. As mentioned previously, some search interfaces allow a natural language approach in which the question can be typed out verbatim, but many do not. However, all databases respond to conceptual searching (i.e., searching concepts separately and connecting them with the appropriate Boolean operator—AND for the overlap of concepts; OR for the union of concepts). The key concepts in our example include fish liver oil, vitamin E, cardiovascular disease, and middle-aged men. Depending on how much information is retrieved, it may also be useful to add the concept of high risk. Obviously, as qualifying terms are added and the concepts combined, the number of retrieved articles will decrease.

No matter which MEDLINE interface is searched, the underlying database structure remains the same. All bibliographic databases are made up of records that are made up of fields that are in turn composed of elements. Searches within a bibliographic database are done at the field level. A MEDLINE record is made up of multiple searchable fields and always include (but is not limited to) the following: journal source, Title, Language (if the article is not in English), Authors, Author Affiliation, Abstract (if present), Publication Types, and MeSH Terms. Subject searching is enhanced in MEDLINE and other databases that include a descriptor or indexing field like the MeSH Terms field. A keyword subject search can be expanded on or refined by including available or related MeSH terms. Most MEDLINE search interfaces include a thesaurus of MeSH terms (e.g., the MeSH Database in PubMed) and many

---

**TABLE 2–3**

**Key Elements in any Literature Search Strategy**

Specify the search topic

Prepare an initial search strategy

Select a database

Execute the search

Evaluate the references

Rework the strategy if warranted

also automatically map keywords to MeSH headings (e.g., the mapping feature in Ovid MEDLINE). PubMed automatically translates keywords to MeSH terms and adds them to the search strategy. Selecting the Details link from the PubMed search page reveals the keywords and translated terms. For example, the MeSH term for Heart Attack is Myocardial Infarction; a search of MEDLINE from 1996 to 2004 will retrieve 701 citations for the keyword phrase Heart Attack, compared with 24,862 citations for the MeSH descriptor Myocardial Infarction. (MeSH won't always retrieve more citations than text words; sometimes just the reverse. The most comprehensive subject search will combine keywords with MeSH terms, with the use of the Boolean OR connector.)

As described earlier, subject experts read articles from journals in their area of expertise and then assign MeSH terms that describe the article content, to the citation. The MeSH terms provide a kind of shorthand description of the entire article. Other features of the indexing process can enhance search retrieval. Indexers use the most specific MeSH descriptor available to describe a concept. This means that an article about Heart Arrhythmia

that does not discuss other kinds of cardiovascular disease or cardiovascular disease in general, will be assigned the MeSH descriptor arrhythmia rather than cardiovascular disease. When devising a search strategy, therefore, an investigator should choose the most specific terms possible so that the most relevant citations will be retrieved.

In addition, citation retrieval can be further refined and customized by exploiting the following software options in MEDLINE: Subheadings, Explode, Focus, and Limit.

## SUBHEADINGS

Subheadings are used by indexers to describe a certain aspect or aspects of a topic. For example, in our search question we want to know if there are published reports that Fish Oils help reduce heart disease in an at-risk population. Some relevant subheadings used in the indexing process and applied to the MeSH terms include Administration & Dosage (ae), Metabolism (me), Pharmacokinetics (pk), and Therapeutic Use (tu) (the two-letter abbreviations can be added directly during the search process) (Figures 2–1 and 2–2).

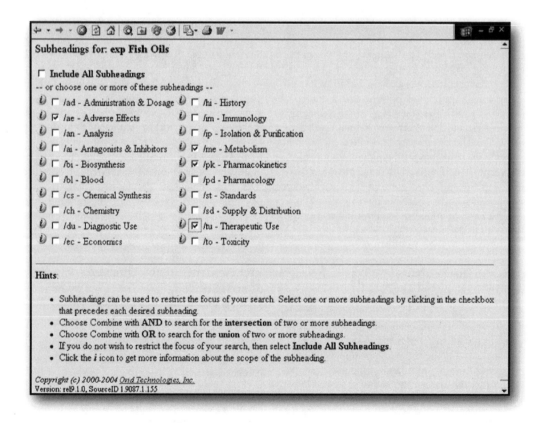

**FIGURE 2–1** ● Subheadings for Fish Oils. From Ovid Technologies, Inc., 2000–2004.

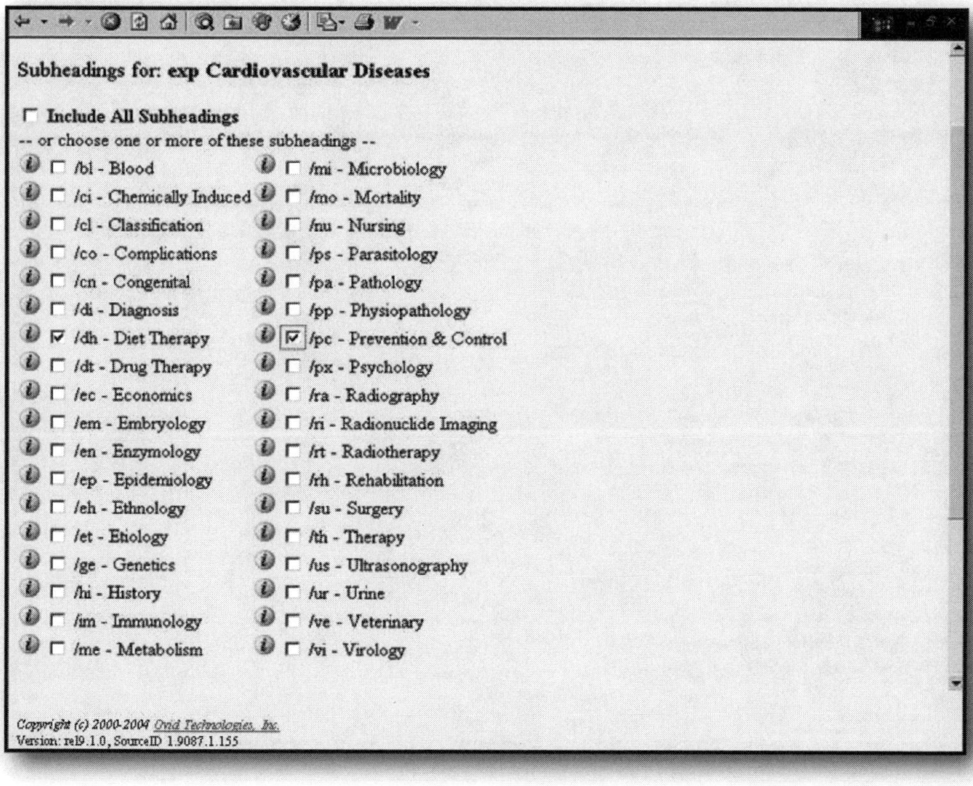

**FIGURE 2–2** ● Subheadings for Cardiovascular Diseases. From Ovid Technologies, Inc., 2000–2004.

Another aspect of our search concerns the prevention of cardiovascular disease in a target population. The MeSH descriptor cardiovascular diseases could therefore be further qualified by adding the subheadings Diet Therapy (DH), Drug Therapy (DT), or Prevention & Control (PC). The search interface used (e.g., the Ovid version of MEDLINE) includes a thesaurus of MeSH terms along with a list of available subheadings and instructions on how to incorporate them.

## EXPLODE

The Explode feature of MEDLINE allows an investigator to search for multiple related terms simultaneously; it always expands search retrieval. For instance, exploding the MeSH descriptor Fish Oils allows an investigator to simultaneously search for the more specific yet related terms Cod liver oil, Omega-3 Fatty Acids, Docosahexaenoic Acids, and Eicosapentaenoic Acid. Searching the unexploded heading Fish Oils generates 1,357 citations, while the exploded term generates 4,203 citations (Figure 2–3).

## FOCUS

The Focus feature limits retrieval to those citations where the concept (e.g., Fish Oils) is the major focus of the article. The MeSH terms assigned to an article are used to describe both those topics that are the major focus of the article and those that are significant but more peripheral. The Explode and Focus options can be performed simultaneously. For instance, if only articles with Fish Oils as the major focus of the article are retrieved, the number of citations drops from 1,357 to 780. If both the Explode and Focus options are used together, retrieval changes from 4,307 citations to 2,992 (Figure 2–4).

## LIMIT

Limiting search retrieval is always the last step before retrieving and evaluating references. Limits include language, publication year, publication type, age, gender, human, and full-text among others. In our search example, an investigator might limit the search to English Language, Human, Male, and

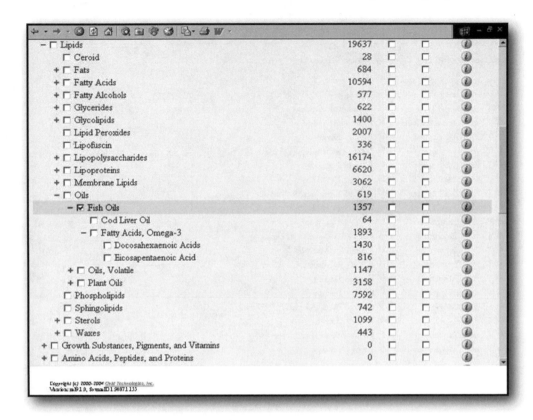

**FIGURE 2–3** ● Explode feature. From Ovid Technologies, Inc., 2000–2004.

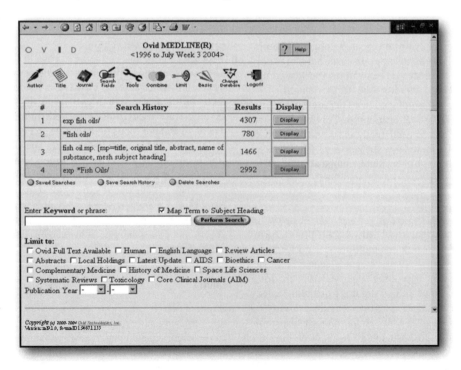

**FIGURE 2–4** ● Explode, focus, and keyword features. From Ovid Technologies, Inc., 2000–2004.

Middle Age. Figures 2–5 and 2–6 show limit options available in Ovid MEDLINE that could be applied to the search shown in Figure 2–4.

## BEYOND MEDLINE

Inevitably, some searches will retrieve too few citations, while others will yield too many. Some problem-solving hints to consider when encountering these situations are shown in Table 2–4.

Several additional databases are relevant to clinical researchers, including EMBASE, Web of Science, and the Cochrane Library. Summary information about these and other databases can be found in Tables 2–1 and 2–2. Note that several chemistry databases are included; these are especially useful for information about drugs, medical devices, and patents, and they contain much that is relevant to clinical research and medicine.

## EMBASE

MEDLINE has what is often referred to as its European counterpart, EMBASE, the online version of the printed *Excerpta Medica*. Both are produced by Elsevier, a publisher of scientific, technical, and health information products and services. There is overlap between MEDLINE and EMBASE, but remarkably (considering the size of each) only approximately 34% of the journals overlap. At present there are 1,881 titles unique to EMBASE and 1,937 titles unique to MEDLINE. EMBASE is especially strong in the areas of pharmacology and pharmacy. Studies that involve the administration of a drug should supplement the MEDLINE search with an additional search in EMBASE. EMBASE uses an indexing system similar to that of MEDLINE; thus, a field within the database composed of EMBASE-controlled vocabulary descriptors is available for searching. MeSH terms are searchable in EMBASE as well. EMBASE is proprietary with restrictions on access, depending on arrangements made at each library. EMBASE can also be contacted directly at its Web address (http://www.embase.com).

## WEB OF SCIENCE

Web of Science (WoS) (http://isi15.isiknowledge.com/portal.cgi) is produced by Thomson ISI, a

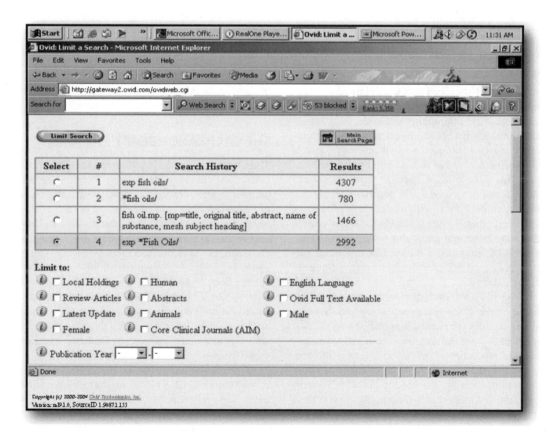

**FIGURE 2–5** ● Limit feature. From Ovid Technologies, Inc., 2000–2004.

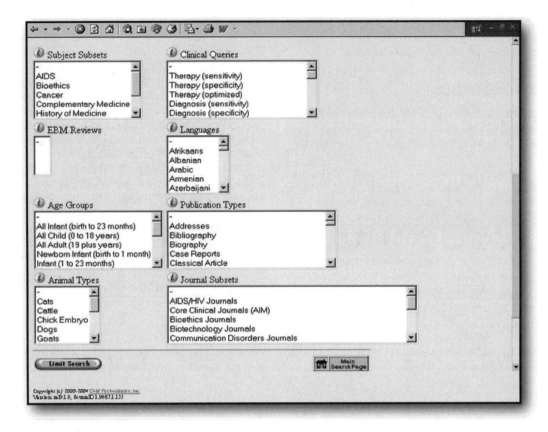

**FIGURE 2-6** ● Options available for limiting searches. From Ovid Technologies, Inc., 2000–2004.

subsidiary of the Thomson Corporation, a major information broker. WoS shares some features with other bibliographic databases like MED-LINE and EMBASE, but its cited reference capability makes it unique. A cited reference search allows the researcher to find other published papers that have cited a specific work or author. After a classic or especially pertinent article has been identified in a particular area, WoS allows an investigator to run a search for other papers that have cited that particular work. Journal articles, book chapters, published abstracts, or papers presented at scientific meetings, all appear in the database.

WoS is a vast, multidisciplinary resource containing three different databases of which Science Citation Index Expanded has the strongest biomedical content. Information about print counterparts is especially important in the case of WoS because institutions vary in the number of years covered by their online subscriptions. WoS covers over 150 disciplines, including medicine and biology, and contains cited references from 5,900 scholarly science and technical journals. It is broader in scope than MEDLINE or EMBASE and

includes references to published abstracts, which neither of the other two databases includes.

## THE COCHRANE LIBRARY

The Cochrane Library (http://www.update-software.com/clibng/cliblogon.htm) is self-described as the premier source of reliable evidence about the effects of health care. It is made up of seven different databases covering evidence-based health care and research methodology and features the Cochrane Database of Systematic Reviews—highly structured, systematic, evidence based, full-text reviews of the effects of health care. The reviews are generated by the Cochrane Collaboration, an international nonprofit organization founded in 1993. They are prepared by volunteer health care professionals who together make up over 40 Collaborative Review Groups.

Of particular interest to the clinical investigator is the Cochrane CENTRAL register of controlled trials. The register is free of date limitations and is therefore an important source of older studies and of new studies not indexed in MEDLINE. At present, Cochrane CENTRAL features over 300,000

**TABLE 2–4**

## Problem-Solving Suggestions

Too few citations
  Search for both keywords and MeSH terms
  Explode MeSH terms
  Eliminate specific subheadings (the default is usually to include all subheadings)
  Search additional years
  Consider synonyms
  Use the truncation device the search interface offers to retrieve alternate word endings
  Reduce the number of search concepts
Too many citations
  Search for either text words alone or MeSH terms
  Look for keywords in article titles
  Use the Focus feature
  Add specific subheadings
  Limit by publication year or publication type (e.g., controlled clinical trials or review articles)
  Bypass the Explode option
  Limit to a specific population or age group

reports of controlled trials including approximately 4,000 published between 1948 and 1966. "The Cochrane CENTRAL register has been described as probably the best single source of published trials for inclusion in systematic reviews, and thus should be seen as a vital resource for comprehensive literature searches" (8).

The Cochrane systematic review process entails finding, evaluating, and synthesizing evidence from as many relevant scientific studies as possible. This creates a useful compilation of all the available evidence on a particular topic. Unlike other review articles, systematic reviews are unique in that their explicit design ensures a more comprehensive review with minimal bias and greater reliability. All the available evidence on an intervention is gathered and summarized in one convenient place; thus, the systematic review is an invaluable part of the literature search.

## BOOKS

A health sciences literature search generally focuses heavily on journal articles because they afford the researcher access to the most up-to-date published information. As previously discussed, however, there are additional sources of supporting information such as the Cochrane systematic reviews. Books comprise another essential secondary source in the literature search, both for coverage of the topic under investigation and for references. The value of books as a resource in the literature search process is often downplayed because the information they contain is not as current as that in published in journals. They can, however, be an indispensable tool in accessing the earlier literature if a comprehensive, retrospective search is called for, as well as more current information. With the advent of electronic books, immediacy is diminishing as a drawback to their use because many books (available through vendors such as STAT!Ref, Books@Ovid, Health & Wellness Resource Center, MDConsult, and SKOLAR MD) can now be accessed online.

## THE GREY LITERATURE

If a specific topic is not adequately represented in the conventional resources just described, it may be useful to try the so-called "grey literature." Conn et al. define the grey literature as "studies with limited distribution (i.e., those not included in computerized bibliographic retrieval systems), unpublished reports, dissertations, articles in obscure journals, some online journals, conference abstracts, policy documents, reports to funding agencies, rejected or unsubmitted manuscripts, non-English language articles, and technical reports" (9, pp. 256–261). This same article cites publication bias in describing the differences between grey literature and the more broadly disseminated published literature. The outstanding difference is the likelihood that published research is more likely to report statistically significant findings. Furthermore, those studies demonstrating statistically significant findings are more likely to be published in English-language journals, in journals with high citation impact factors, in journals with wide distribution, and in those in online database indexes (9, p. 257). Getting to the grey literature is not as daunting as in the preelectronic era, thanks to the Internet and e-mail, but it is time consuming and effortful. Its usefulness will be determined by each investigator's unique research topic and the adequacy with which a particular topic is represented in the conventional published literature.

## EVALUATING REFERENCES

The literature search process is one of ongoing evaluation—of the research topic, the various sources accessed, and the resultant references. The literature search usually generates more information than is relevant to the topic at hand, resulting in some extraneous retrieval. As investigators scan the various lists of references generated by their search strategies, they next need to distinguish between those that warrant reading in their entirety and those that do not. An article's title is not necessarily an accurate description of the accompanying paper's content. Fortunately, most databases contain abstracts for most references, so if interest is piqued by a title, additional summary information is presented in the abstract. However, take heed against an overreliance on the information presented in a paper's abstract. "Because of the need to be concise, abstracts select only the highlights of a paper. They are also, quite understandably, an author's attempt to put one's best foot forward. Sometimes the summary of the article contains more wish than reality and presents a distorted view of the work that follows" (10).

At the same time a recent editorial in the *Annals of Internal Medicine* begins by stating "The abstract is, arguably, the most important part of an article in a medical journal because it is the only part of an article that many people read" (11). This quandary—abstract as essential but not necessarily dependable—is somewhat allayed by the inclusion of structured abstracts in most general medical journals. The structured abstract was introduced in 1987 in the *Annals of Internal Medicine* as a way to help clinicians discern articles that are scientifically sound and applicable to their practice from articles of less value. The authors of the proposal determined the key information that clinicians needed to select articles of high relevance and quality and recommended that this information be culled from the article and featured in the abstract. They proposed that abstracts feature the following parts, each clearly indicated and labeled: objective (a clear statement of the question addressed); design (a description of the basic plan of the study including duration of follow-up if applicable); setting (location and level of clinical care); patients (characteristics and number); intervention (the exact treatment); measurements and results (methods); and conclusions (clearly stated with clinical application) (12). In 1996 the *Annals of Internal Medicine* added a background section to the structured abstract. Beginning with the March 16, 2004, issue, authors were instructed to include a limitations section to briefly describe the principal limitations of their research. This section precedes the conclusions section in the structured abstract.

Most published papers follow a standard format of Introduction, Methods, Results, and Discussion (IMRAD format). This standardized format, like that of the structured abstract, further expedites the evaluation process. The Introduction provides background information and the reasons the study was undertaken. The Methods section describes the study design; the patient or subject characteristics; and how the data were gathered, analyzed, and evaluated. The Results section tells what happened, and the Conclusion/Discussion/Comments section sums up the results and offers the authors' interpretation of the results. It is especially important to review the Methods section before completely accepting the authors' conclusion. Information presented in the Conclusion section should be compared with the information presented in the Methods section to ensure that it is logical and accurate. Greenhalgh suggests asking three preliminary questions (13): Why was the study done and what hypothesis was the author testing? What type of study was done? Was this design appropriate to the broad field of research addressed? For more detailed information on critical appraisal please refer to the Journal of the American Medical Association's "Users' Guides to the Medical Literature" series, the "How to Read a Paper" series of articles by Trisha Greenhalgh published in the *British Medical Journal* (13), and to the relevant references at the end of this chapter.

## MANAGING AND ORGANIZING REFERENCES

Reference management software simplifies the creation of a personalized database of citations imported from various sources that can then be modified and formatted in a customized manner. The software creates a bibliography and automatically inserts references into manuscripts according to the journal's style or style manual. Some examples of the different reference management software packages include Biblioscape, EndNote, Papyrus, ProCite, and Reference Manager (there are many more). An excellent resource for comprehensive information about the commercially available reference management software packages, including reviews, is available from the University of Birmingham in the United Kingdom (http://www.ukolug.org.uk/content/public/links/refmanlinks.html#esprit). Most of these software producers offer free trial versions of their reference management software, which is very useful when comparing software features. In deciding which reference management software package to use, an investigator may find it helpful to determine whether the library or computer support group recommends or supports a specific package.

## PRESENT AND FUTURE TRENDS

Clinical research, literature searching, and the publishing process are constantly changing, buffeted by innumerable forces from what seems like every direction. The literature search process has evolved from a painstaking, time-consuming manual search of printed indexes and publications to an almost entirely online, electronic undertaking. Offsetting the convenience of automated searching is the tremendous increase in the amount of information available that investigators are obligated to sift through and evaluate. Along with a rise in the number of specialty journals published is an even steeper rise in the cost of purchasing scientific and health sciences journals across the board. Libraries faced with diminishing budgets and spiraling journal costs are in the midst of a serials crisis, whereby they can no longer afford to maintain their journal collections. To save money, they are cutting subscriptions, forgoing print copies for electronic-only format, and restricting access. To further stretch limited funds, libraries are canceling expensive MEDLINE subscriptions from commercial vendors (e.g., Ovid and Dialog) and making PubMed their sole MEDLINE interface. They are charging for services and resources that they offered for free in the past. A thorough literature search demands access to these resources, so investigators find they are obliged to pay for articles and databases formerly subsidized by their institutions.

The academic community is responding to the dramatically escalating costs of scholarly publishing by creating alternative means of scholarly communication. The Open Access movement encourages researchers to publish in journals whose funding model does not charge readers or their institutions for access or in journals that charge only the institution and not the individual author. *The Directory of Open Access Journals* (http:// www.doaj.org) currently lists over 1,000 open access titles including the *Journal of Translational Medicine* and the *Journal of Clinical Investigation*. The Public Library of Science (PloS) (http://www.plos.org) is a nonprofit organization of scientists and physicians committed to making the world's scientific and medical literature a freely available public resource. The organization currently publishes the journals PloS Biology and PloS Medicine. BioMed Central (http://www.biomedcentral.com/home) is an independent publisher committed to providing free access to peer-reviewed biomedical research. Authors retain copyright on their published material, and all of the BioMed Central journals are indexed in the PubMed database. Many institutions are creating repositories to permanently store the intellectual output of their researchers in local or regional digital archives. Researchers are being encouraged to retain copyright on their publications so that these publications, along with other research materials, can be deposited in these archives. The Association of Research Libraries has formed the Scholarly Publishing and Academic Resources Coalition (SPARC) (http://www.arl.org/sparc) to offer open-access publishing alternatives to the traditional commercial publishing model. Hopefully, the resourcefulness of the academic scientific community will help clinical investigators continue to pursue their research endeavors despite an ever more competitive and complex research and publishing environment.

## SUMMARY

- A systematic approach should be used in searching the medical literature. Consultation with an experienced research librarian should be part of the strategy.
- Five reasons to search the literature include (1) determining existing research on a topic, (2) determining the relevant level of theory and knowledge development (and knowledge gaps), (3) determining the relevancy of an existing knowledge to a particular research inquiry, (4) providing a rationale for selecting a research strategy, and (5) determining patient safety.
- MEDLINE is the most common database used to search the biomedical literature. Two commonly used online interfaces to access MEDLINE are PubMed and Ovid. Other databases of importance in clinical research include EMBASE, Web of Science, and the Cochrane Library. EMBASE is especially strong in the areas of pharmacology and pharmacy.

## REFERENCES

1. DePoy E, Gitlin LN. Introduction to Research: Understanding and Applying Multiple Strategies. 2nd Ed. St. Louis: Mosby, 1998:46–47.
2. Abels E, Jones R, Latham J et al. Competencies for information professionals of the 21st century. Information Outlook 2003;7:11–18.
3. Medical Library Association Expert Searching Task Force. Medical Library Association policy statement: role of expert searching in health sciences libraries. Available at: http://www.mlanet.org/resources/expert_search/policy_expert_search.html. Accessed March 3, 2005.
4. Ramsay S. Johns Hopkins takes responsibility for volunteer's death. Lancet 2001;358:213.
5. McLellan F. 1966 and all that—when is a literature search done? Lancet 2001;358:646.
6. Neely JG, Hartman JM, Wallace MS. Building the powerful 10-minute office visit, Part II: Beginning a critical literature review. Laryngoscope 2001;111:70–76.
7. National Library of Medicine Fact Sheet. PubMedr®: MEDLINE® Retrieval on the World Wide Web.

Bethesda, MD: National Library of Medicine, 2003. Available at: http://www.nlm.nih.gov/pubs/factsheets/pubmed.html. Accessed March 3, 2005.

8. Lefebvre C, Lusher A, Dickersin K et al. Literature searches. Lancet 2002;359:896.

9. Conn VS, Valentine JC, Cooper HM et al. Grey literature in meta-analyses. Nurs Res 2003;52:256–261.

10. Gehlbach SH. Interpreting the Medical Literature. 4th Ed. New York: McGraw-Hill, 2002:6.

11. The Editors. Addressing the limitations of structured abstracts. Ann Intern Med 2004;140:480-481.

12. Ad Hoc Working Group for Critical Appraisal of the Medical Literature. A proposal for more informative abstracts of clinical articles. Ann Intern Med 1987;106:598–604.

13. Greenhalgh T. How to Read a Paper: the Basics of Evidence-Based Medicine. 2nd Ed. London: BMJ/Publications, 2001.

# CHAPTER 3

# Variables and Measurements

Judith E. C. Lieu, Jay F. Piccirillo

Clinical measurement involves a two-step process: first, the construction of rating scales and other indices to convert observed phenomena into raw data, and second, the grouping of raw data for description and comparison (1). In this chapter, we introduce the types of variables that can be measured, some performance criteria by which measurements can be judged, criteria for choosing variables for measurement, approaches for describing how data are distributed, and criteria for departures of that distribution from an expected normal distribution. Some of these issues will be considered in greater detail in Chapter 23.

## TYPES OF VARIABLES

The types of variables used in a study and how they are defined influence both the descriptive and inferential statistics used during the study's analysis phase. Thus, careful thought should be given during the *planning* stages of a study about which variables to measure, their scale, and how well they can be expected to perform.

*Dichotomous* variables, also called binary or existential variables, are those limited to two responses, such as "yes/no," "present/absent," or "dead/alive." For instance, in a study of whether a novel neurotransmitter may be involved in the pathogenesis of epilepsy, one way of classifying patients is to document whether or not they experience seizures.

*Nominal* variables are those that are categorized without any inherent order or ranking. Examples include occupation (e.g., engineer, administrative assistant, nurse), race (e.g., Caucasian/white, African American/black, Hispanic/Latino), and tissue antigens (e.g., HLA types, blood types). Other examples of nominal variables include complications of

surgery (e.g., bleeding, wound dehiscence, infection), types of treatment (e.g., radiation, chemotherapy, surgery), and medical specialty (e.g., internal medicine, pediatrics, surgery, radiology).

*Ordinal* variables, also known as categorical variables, are those whose responses are ranked in ascending or descending magnitudes, but have unmeasured or arbitrary intervals or gradations between them. Examples of ordinal variables include pedal edema (1+ to 4+), TNM stage (I to IV), and highest education level (high school, college, graduate school).

*Dimensional* variables, also known as equi-interval variables, are data that possess inherent order, and the interval between successive values is equal. These variables are further subclassified into continuous and discrete types. *Continuous* variables are those with ascending or descending scales of measurement with equal intervals or gradations between two adjacent categories; data can take on any value in a continuum. Examples of continuous dimensional variables include age, weight, height, hematocrit, and serum sodium level. *Discrete* variables are data that can take on only integer values and are expressed as counts (e.g., number of seizures, number of pregnancies).

A particular variable may begin as one type of variable and be converted to another type, depending on how it is categorized. For instance, age is usually thought of as a dimensional variable. However, it is often divided into ordinal categories (e.g., <18, 18–34, 35–49, 50–64, 65–85, >85) or dichotomous categories (e.g., <55 vs 55 and older). (It may even be divided into nominal categories, such as odd or even ages, if one so chooses.)

Sometimes ordinal variables are treated as *pseudodimensional* variables; that is, although the variables have arbitrary intervals or gradations of measurement, they are treated as though their intervals or gradations are equal, usually in order to simplify the statistical analysis. For example, visual analogue scores (VAS) are often used to measure the severity of a symptom, such as pain. VAS can be constructed as a 10 cm long line, with 0 indicating no pain and 10 indicating the worst pain a patient ever experienced. When a patient circles a number on this line, pain can be analyzed as a pseudodimensional variable. In another example, satisfaction with care may be measured on an ordinal scale from 3 being extremely satisfied, 0 being neither satisfied nor dissatisfied, to –3 being extremely dissatisfied. When a patient chooses one of these scores, satisfaction with care can also be analyzed as a pseudodimensional variable.

## MEASUREMENT PERFORMANCE

The performance of measurements is assessed using four criteria: validity, reliability, responsiveness, and variation. The concepts of validity and reliability are illustrated in Figure 3–1.

### Validity

*Validity*, also known as accuracy, is defined as the degree to which the data measure what they were intended to measure, or that the results of a measurement correspond to the true state of the phenomenon being measured. For clinical observations that can be measured by physical means, it is relatively easy to establish validity because the observed measurement is compared with some accepted "gold standard." For example, serum sodium can be measured on an instrument recently calibrated against solutions made with known concentrations of sodium. Other measurements such as pain, nausea, and tinnitus cannot be verified physically, and thus the validity of measurement scales intended to measure these phenomena are more difficult to establish.

To establish the validity of difficult-to-measure phenomena such as pain, nausea, and tinnitus, three areas of validity must be addressed—content, construct, and criterion validity. *Content* validity refers to the extent to which a particular method of measurement includes all of the dimensions of the specific phenomena one intends to measure, and nothing more. For example, a scale for measuring pain should include questions about aching, throbbing, and burning, but not pressure, itching, or nausea. *Construct* validity is the extent to which the measurement is consistent with other measurements of the same phenomenon. For example, responses on a scale for pain should be related to other manifestations of the severity of pain, such as sweating, moaning, writhing, and asking for pain medication. *Criterion* validity is the extent to which the measurements predict a directly observable phenomenon. For example, responses on a scale for pain should bear a predictable relationship to pain of known severity: mild pain from minor abrasion, moderate pain from ordinary headache and peptic ulcer, and severe pain from renal colic.

### Measurements of Validity

#### Sensitivity and Specificity

These are statistical indices that refer to the ability of a measurement to detect the true condition or

**1.** Both accuracy and precision

**2.** Accuracy only

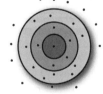

**3.** Precision only

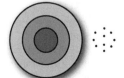

**4.** Neither accuracy nor precision

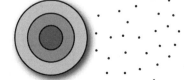

**FIGURE 3–1A** ● Two ways of illustrating the concepts of validity and reliability (accuracy and precision). Figure 3–1.A1 shows measurements that are both accurate and precise (closely clustered around the bull's-eye). Figure 3–1.A2 shows measurements that are accurate only (clustered around the bull's-eye, but widely scattered), whereas Figure 3–1.A3 shows measurements that are only precise (closely clustered together, but not near the bull's-eye). Figure 3–1.A4 shows neither accuracy nor precision (widely scattered measurements that are far from the bull's-eye). Similar concepts are illustrated in Figure 3–1.B, this time comparing the true value of some variable to the measured distributions of that variable, obtained during the course of a study.

**1.** Both accuracy and precision    **2.** Accuracy only

**3.** Precision only    **4.** Neither accuracy nor precision

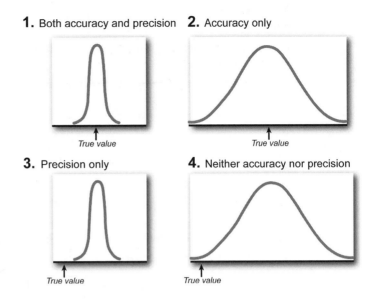

*FIGURE 3–1B* ● *(Continued)*

state being measured. For the assessment of diagnostic tests, sensitivity refers to the probability that a test will be positive when disease is present and specificity refers to the probability that a test will be negative when the disease is absent. When the true state of the clinical phenomenon is known, then sensitivity and specificity are the correct indices of validity for an independent observation. Because no test is perfect (i.e., no test always correctly identifies all patients with *and* without the disease), sensitivity and specificity provide a quantitative measure of test function. These indices can be simply derived from a 2 × 2 table, as shown in Table 3–1, in which the columns denote disease presence or absence, and the rows denote test positivity or negativity. *Sensitivity* is defined as the proportion of persons with the disease who are correctly identified as positive by the measurement or test, or the rate of testing positive given that the disease is present. *Specificity* is defined as the proportion of persons without the disease who are correctly identified as negative by the measurement or test, or the rate of testing negative given that the disease is not present. These values can be derived from making "vertical" calculations in a 2 × 2 table (see Table 3–1). More complicated calculations are necessary when the disease (e.g., Stage I, II, III) and measurement options (e.g., None, Mild, Moderate, or Severe) are more than two.

Tests with high sensitivity are helpful in the clinical scenario where there is an important penalty (e.g., significant morbidity or mortality) for missing a disease, such as with tuberculosis or syphilis. They are also useful during screening large populations of presumably asymptomatic people, where the probability of disease is low. In both situations, a negative result from a high sensitivity test helps a clinician to rule out disease. A helpful mnemonic to remember this is "SnNout"—with a high *Sen*sitivity test, a *N*egative result rules *out* the disease in question.

Tests with high specificity are especially helpful in the clinical scenario where a false positive result can result in harm to the patient physically, emotionally, or financially, such as with initiating cancer chemotherapy. In another example, a pulmonary angiogram may be indicated to rule in a pulmonary embolism in a patient who has just had major surgery, rather than using a ventilation-perfusion lung scan. In this situation, a positive result from a high specificity test helps a clinician to rule in disease. A corresponding mnemonic to remember this is "SpPin"—with a high *Sp*ecificity test, a *P*ositive result rules *in* the disease in question.

### Receiver Operating Characteristics (ROC) Curves

Optimally, an investigator would like a test with both high sensitivity and high specificity, but in many cases this is not possible. Whenever clinical data take on a continual range of values, a trade-off between sensitivity and specificity is required to decide what cutoff point is the dividing line between normal and abnormal. Consequently, for any given test result, one characteristic (e.g., sensitivity) can only be increased at the expense of another characteristic (e.g., specificity). This trade-off is reflected in the construction of a *receiver operating*

## TABLE 3–1

**2 × 2 Table Used to Assess Sensitivity and Specificity of a Diagnostic Test**

|  | Disease | No Disease | Total |
|---|---|---|---|
| **Test Positive** | a<br>True positive | b<br>False positive | a + b |
| **Test Negative** | c<br>False negative | d<br>True negative | c + d |
| **Total** | a + c | b + d | a + b + c + d |

$$\text{Sensitivity} = \frac{a}{a + c} \qquad \text{Specificity} = \frac{d}{b + d}$$

*characteristic* (ROC) curve, in which the sensitivity (true-positive rate) is graphed on the *y*-axis and 1-specificity (false-positive rate) is graphed on the *x*-axis (Figure 3–2). For example, setting a 2-hour postprandial blood glucose level at 80 mg/dL would have high sensitivity for diagnosing diabetes, but very low specificity. Conversely, a 2-hour postprandial blood glucose of 140 mg/dL would have very high specificity for diagnosing diabetes, but low sensitivity. The curve that is depicted corresponds to the pairs of true-positive and false-positive rates for each possible cutoff for a diagnostic test result. The upper left corner of this graph denotes a perfect diagnostic test (i.e., a true-positive rate of 1.0 and false-positive rate of 0.0). The point on the ROC curve that is closest to this upper left corner is the "best" cutoff in terms of making the fewest errors.

### Bland-Altman Plot

A graphical technique can be a useful way to identify where the differences between a new measurement technique and the gold standard differ

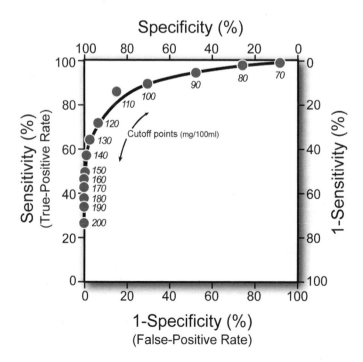

**FIGURE 3–2** ● Receiver operator characteristic (ROC) curve demonstrating the accuracy of 2-hour postprandial blood sugar as a diagnostic test for diabetes mellitus. This ROC curve shows the trade-off between sensitivity (true-positive rate, graphed on the *y*-axis) and 1-specificity (false-positive rate, graphed on the *x*-axis) that is required to decide what cutoff point is used as the dividing line between "normal" (no disease) and "abnormal" (disease present). (Data from Diabetes Program Guide, Public Health Service Publication No. 506, 1960.)

(Figure 3–3). The measurements by the two separate methods are plotted against the averages of the two techniques (2,3). The graph displays a scatterplot of the differences plotted against the averages of the two measurements. The plot is useful to examine a relationship between the differences and the averages, to look for bias, and to identify possible outliers. If the observed differences are within 1.96 standard deviations and are not clinically meaningful, the two methods of measurement can be used interchangeably. The Bland-Altman plot can also be used to assess reliability of measurements (see next section).

## Reliability

*Reliability*, also known as precision, is the extent to which repeated measurements of a stable phenomenon—by the same person or different people and instruments, at different times and places—obtain similar results. Random error, if large, results in lack of precision. The reliability of laboratory measurements is established by repeated measures, sometimes by different people and with different instruments. The reliability of clinical phenomena can be established by showing that different observers under different conditions similarly describe them. When the true state of the phenomenon is not known or a gold standard test does not exist, then the two observations are compared to each other with measures of reliability.

## Measurements of Reliability

### Intraobserver and Interobserver Variability

If the same investigator makes successive measurements of the same phenomenon, such as the blood pressure of the same person, the same radiograph, or the same histologic slide, there will usually be some differences in the measurements or their interpretation. These differences are referred to as *intraobserver variability*. If two or more investigators evaluate the same phenomenon, there will also usually be some differences in the measurements or their interpretation. These differences are referred to as *interobserver variability*. Although it is not unusual to find such differences, either by the same investigator or among different investigators in the interpretation of clinical data, an important challenge is to quantify the degree of agreement.

### Overall Percent Agreement

A relatively simple and common metric for agreement is to cite the overall percent agreement. If the test uses a dichotomous variable then the results can be placed in a $2 \times 2$ table as shown in Table 3–2. Cells $a$ and $d$ represent agreement and cells $b$ and $c$ represent disagreement. The overall proportion of agreement is measured as the sum of observations in the $a$ and $d$ cells divided by the total number of observations ($N$). One of the major weaknesses of reporting the overall percentage agreement is that

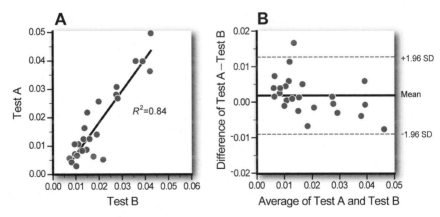

**FIGURE 3–3** ● **A**. Correlation of measurements of the same hypothetical biologic phenomenon by two different methods (Test A and Test B). **B**. Bland-Altman plot of the same data as in A. In this case, the mean difference is close to zero (no significant bias of one test compared to the other) and almost all the points lie within two standard deviations of the average difference between the tests. Thus, in this case, both the correlation and Bland-Altman plots indicate that the two methods are essentially equivalent. Note, however, that the Bland-Altman plot shows that at low values, Test A tends to be higher than Test B, and at high values, Test A tends to be lower than Test B. Such a trend may or may not be significant, depending on whether the range of values obtained represents the entire physiologic and pathophysiologic range of values likely to be encountered.

## TABLE 3–2

### Agreement Matrix for Radiologists Reading Mammography for Breast Cancer

| | Radiologist A | | |
|---|---|---|---|
| **Radiologist B** | **Yes** | **No** | **Total** |
| **Yes** | 21 | 43 | 64 |
| | *a* | *b* | |
| **No** | 3 | 83 | 86 |
| | *c* | *d* | |
| **Total** | 24 | 126 | 150 |

$$\frac{a + d}{a + b + c + d} = \text{Overall \% agreement}$$

$$\frac{21 + 83}{150} = .69$$

#### Proportion of Agreement

$$\text{Kappa} = \frac{P_0 - P_c}{1 - P_c}$$

$$= \frac{.69 - .55}{1 - .55}$$

$$= 0.31$$

considerable agreement could be expected by chance alone.

### Kappa Coefficient

The *kappa coefficient* is calculated to determine the extent to which the observed agreement between two physicians (or any two interpretations of data) improves on the agreement by chance alone (4). As shown in Table 3–2, the proportion of observed agreements ($P_o$) is $(a + d)/N$ or 0.69. The number of expected chance agreements for cells $a$ and $d$ is calculated by multiplying the corresponding row and column margin totals and dividing by the total number of agreements ($N$). For example, two radiologists may agree on the reading of a normal mammogram in a certain number of cases (cell $a$). In the example shown in Table 3–2, the row total is 64 and the column total is 24. For $N = 150$, the chance agreement would be expected to be $(64 \times 24)/150 = 10.24$ times. A similar calculation

is performed for the other agreement (abnormal mammograms, cell $d$) and the expected agreement due to chance would be 72.24 times. Thus, the sum of the expected chance agreements for cells $a$ and $d$ is 82.48. The proportion of agreement expected by chance alone ($P_c$) is $82.48/150 = 0.55$. The proportion of observations that can be attributed to reliable measurement (i.e., not due to chance) is defined by $P_O - P_C (0.69 - 0.55 = 0.14)$. The maximum possible nonchance agreement is $1 - P_C$ or 100% less the contribution of chance ($1.00 - 0.55 = 0.45$). Kappa is thus a ratio of the number of observed nonchance agreements to the number of possible nonchance agreements. In this case, the kappa is 0.31.

Kappa is a ratio that can go from –1 to +1. Landis and Koch (5) proposed criteria for the interpretation of strength of agreement denoted by kappa: Poor (–1 to 0), Slight (0 to 0.2), Fair (0.2 to 0.4), Moderate (0.4 to 0.6), Substantial (0.6 to 0.8), and Almost Perfect (0.8 to 1). If the data are ordinal (i.e., more than two values), a weighted kappa test is used.

### Correlation Coefficient

In situations of test–retest reliability or rater reliability, the Pearson product-moment correlation coefficient (for ordinal or continuous data) and Spearman rank correlation coefficient (for ordinal data) are often reported. Because there are several problems with this approach (pp. 508–509 reference [6]), an alternative index, the *intraclass correlation coefficient (ICC)* (7), is recommended. The *ICC* is a reliability coefficient that is calculated using variance estimates obtained through an analysis of variance. It should be noted that Bland and Altman argue that the concept of correlation is misleading when comparing measurements and their alternative approach, using graphic plots, is preferred.

### Responsiveness

*Responsiveness* refers to the extent that a measurement instrument's results change as conditions change. For example, the New York Heart Association scale—classes I to IV (no symptoms, symptoms with slight and moderate exertion, and symptoms at rest)—is not sensitive to subtle changes in congestive heart failure that patients would find to be symptomatically important, whereas measurements of ejection fraction can detect changes that are too subtle for patients to notice. Responsiveness can be assessed using measurements such as effect size (8) and standardized response mean (9).

### Effect Size

Effect size is defined as the difference in the mean score at baseline from the mean score at completion divided by the standard deviation of the baseline score. The effect-size statistic is a number that represents "how many standard deviations" the two groups differ by. The effect-size statistic is normally known simply as the effect size. Effect sizes greater than 0.8 are considered large and represent differences that are likely to be clinically meaningful. Medium effect sizes are defined as about one-half standard deviation and would represent differences that are likely to be noticeable. Small effect sizes are less than one-half the standard deviation and are not likely to be perceptible (10). The effect size is important when calculating the sample sizes needed for a study (see Chapter 9).

### Standardized Response Mean

The standardized response mean is defined as the difference in the mean score at baseline from the mean score at completion of the study divided by the standard deviation of the change score. It is often used to compare responsiveness to change between measurement instruments.

## Measurement Variation

Measurements of the same phenomenon can take on a range of values, depending on the circumstances in which they are made. To avoid erroneous conclusions from data, clinical researchers and clinicians should be aware of the reasons for variation in a given situation and know which are likely to play a large part, a small part, or no part at all in what has been observed. Overall variation is the sum of variation related to the act of measurement, biologic differences within individuals from time to time, and biologic differences from person to person. All observations are subject to variation because of the performance of the measurement instruments and observers involved in making the measurement. The conditions of measurement can lead to a biased result (lack of validity) or simply random error (lack of reliability). It is possible to reduce this source of variation by making measurements with great care and by following standard protocols.

There are several types of measurement error. *Bias* refers to systematic error, such as occurs with the miscalibration of instruments, design flaws, and systematic differences in interpretation. *Random* error occurs simply by chance. *Sampling error* refers to variations in measurement that occur because the sample misrepresents the whole. For example, a liver biopsy represents only about 1/100,000th of the liver. Because such a small part of the whole is examined, there is room for considerable variation from one sample to another. *Biologic variation* causes fluctuations in measurements because biologic changes occur within individuals over time. Most biologic phenomena change from moment to moment, so that a measurement at any one point in time is a sample of measurements during a period of time and may not represent the usual value of these measurements. For example, night-to-night variability in sleep studies occurs because intuitively we know that the quality of sleep can differ from night to night. Biologic variation also arises because of differences among people. For example, facial growth may differ among individuals of different racial backgrounds.

## CHOOSING VARIABLES

### Dependent, Independent, and Extraneous Variables

The main research question of a study governs which measurement should be used to determine the *outcome* of interest. These outcome measures become *dependent variables* in any statistical analysis. For instance, an evaluation of risk factors for mortality may use 5-year survival or age at death as its outcome measure; an evaluation of therapies to lower morbidity in cardiovascular disease may use time to recurrence of a cardiovascular event as the outcome measure; and an evaluation of quality of life may use the Medical Outcome Study SF-36 questionnaire or a disease-specific health status measure as its outcome measure.

Another set of variables, referred to as *independent variables*, are those variables that the investigator anticipates will impact or predict the value of the outcome measure. Independent variables may also be known as *exposures*; they may include therapies, interventions, habits, passive exposures, genetic status, and so on. In a clinical experiment, the investigator has control over the independent variable(s), such as when he or she assigns a given intervention in a randomized controlled study. In observational studies, the independent variables are those that are specifically expected to have an effect on the outcome. For example, patients with mutations in the BRCA1 and 2 genes have been found to have more aggressive breast cancer then women without those specific mutations (11). In this case, the status of the gene mutation is the independent variable predicting breast cancer outcome.

*Extraneous* variables are those variables (e.g., age, sex, tumor-node-metastasis [TNM] stage, comorbid conditions) whose presence or absence, or degree or severity may be used to describe the characteristics of the patients being studied; they may or may not impact on outcome.

The variables to be measured in a study other than the dependent and independent variables can be any factor that makes one patient or group of patients different from another, and that could potentially affect the outcome (sometimes referred to as covariates, confounders, or effect modifiers, depending on *how* they affect outcome). As long as these variables can be measured and recorded in a standard fashion, they can be evaluated as possible determinants of outcome.

An extraneous variable is referred to as a covariate if it is possibly predictive of the outcome under study. It is common in translational and experimental clinical research to measure many such variables at baseline, hopefully, to show that the experimental groups are similar. (If not, it may be possible to adjust for differences in covariates among the experimental groups by statistical means, using, for instance, an analysis of covariance).

These same (or possibly other) covariates may also be measured at various appropriate times throughout the study observation period (to show that changes, if any, are similar among the experimental groups). If differences among the experimental groups do exist, the covariate may be acting as a confounder or effect modifier (12).

A confounding variable is one that is systematically related to the independent variable (an "exposure") and to the outcome, yet does not lie on the hypothesized causal path from exposure to outcome (13). For instance, in investigating the association between maternal alcohol consumption and infant low birth weight, maternal cigarette smoking could be a confounder. Cigarette smoking is known to be an independent risk factor for infant low birth weight, and is associated with more alcohol consumption. However, cigarette smoking is not necessarily involved in the mechanism by which maternal alcohol use is purported to cause low birth weight.

In some cases, it may be possible to reduce or even eliminate the effect of a potential confounder by controlling the variable as part of the study's design. For instance, a glucose clamp is a procedure commonly used in metabolic research in which glucose levels are kept constant by infusing insulin intravenously and adjusting the dose as necessary (as dictated by repeated glucose measurements) to keep the plasma glucose concentrations steady throughout the observation period. This procedure, then, eliminates the potential confounding effect of varying glucose levels on some other metabolic outcome of interest.

Effect modifiers are variables that either affect the exposure or the outcome, but not both. For instance, smoking and increased age are known to increase the incidence of myocardial infarction (MI). However, because there is no difference in smoking rates based on age, then age is an effect modifier of the incidence of MI, but not a confounder.

## Hard versus Soft Data

Because of their selection and training, physician clinical investigators tend to prefer the kind of precise measurements the physical and biologic sciences provide, known as hard data (14). *Hard data* are data that have exact numerical values, such as age, hemoglobin level, weight, serum creatinine, survival rates, and so on. The importance of symptoms, functional status, quality of life, and other types of measurements, termed soft data, may be ignored or discounted. *Soft data* are often difficult to quantify, difficult to interpret, and may be partially or totally subjective (such as pain, patient satisfaction, or quality of life). Sometimes hard data may not be as objective as they appear. For instance, determining whether a pathologic specimen shows malignancy, or whether nodes on computed tomography scans are pathologic, is also subject to interpretation. Even so, such data are usually considered hard rather than soft, despite the problems with objectivity. On the other hand, it is often the relief of symptoms and promoting satisfaction and well-being that are among the most important outcomes of care. Ultimately, when the purpose of a research study is to guide clinical decisions, clinical research should include soft data to avoid distorting the picture of the whole patient. There should be no hesitancy to include soft data when it is appropriate for the research study in question.

## Primary versus Secondary Outcomes

*Primary outcomes* are the main outcomes or endpoints that drive a clinical study; they are the measurements that will be used to answer the main research question and to address the primary hypothesis. The primary outcome measurement drives the statistical calculation of sample size (see Chapter 9). *Secondary outcomes* are the other outcomes of interest that one hopes to measure and find significant, but are not the focus of the main hypothesis of the research study. They are the measurements used to answer secondary research questions and hypotheses.

## Surrogate Outcomes

*Surrogate* outcomes or measurements (also known as *proxy* measurements) are often used when the entity an investigator really wants to measure is inconvenient, difficult, or impossible to know, or considered soft data. For instance, an investigator may want to know when a patient is cured or responding to a new chemotherapeutic agent. The investigator cannot definitively know when a malignancy has been totally eliminated, or even when it is no longer enlarging, so surrogate measures, such as prostate specific antigen (PSA) levels, carcinoembryonic antigen (CEA) levels, and size of masses on CT scans, are used instead. Alternatively, an investigator may want to evaluate the efficacy of pain control, but have no objective measures, so surrogate measures—such as the number of doses of rescue narcotics used, the number of milligrams of morphine self-administered by a patient through a patient-controlled analgesia (PCA) pump, or how many feet a patient can walk after receiving analgesic medication—are used instead. Investigators often want to measure quality of life or return of function after using a new medication or undergoing a new procedure, but have no hard data to directly measure these entities. Instead, standard quality of life and functional measures, such as the Medical Outcomes Survey SF-36 (15) and Karnofsky Performance Scale (16), may be used to compare groups of patients.

Surrogate outcomes may also be used because they have the potential to save time and money. For instance, an investigator might want to know whether a particular intervention would ultimately result in fewer cancer deaths or longer survival. However, such studies can be difficult, time consuming, and expensive, especially if mortality is used as the primary endpoint. The investigator may instead use outcomes such as numbers of cancers detected, stage at which cancers are detected, rates of chemotherapy or surgical therapy used to treat patients, or rates of cancer recurrence.

The presence or absence of suitable, accurate, and easy-to-measure surrogate outcomes can sometimes determine the rate at which new therapies are developed, depending on whether consistent or accepted methods for measuring improvement or progress in a particular disease are available. In general, biomarkers of disease (e.g., serum levels, changes on imaging scans that are considered hard data) are more easily adopted as surrogate outcomes than clinical indices using symptoms and signs (soft data) because they seem less subject to bias, error, or interpretation. For instance, the rapid progress in finding therapies for HIV and AIDS has been made easier by the availability of reliable surrogate measures of disease activity (CD4 counts and viral loads) that are minimally invasive and easy to obtain (17). In contrast, the lack of progress in finding new therapies for

systemic lupus erythematosus has been at least partially attributed to the paucity of surrogate disease markers that are considered reliable and are well accepted (18). Thus, the search for suitable biomarkers as surrogate outcomes is a fertile and active area of translational clinical research.

Despite their usefulness, surrogate outcomes have limitations and hazards, especially when used as substitutes for definitive clinical outcomes in phase III clinical trials. For a surrogate outcome to be valid for phase III trials, the surrogate must not only be a correlate of the true clinical outcome, but it must also reliably predict the clinical benefit (or harm) of a therapy, and capture all the major effects of a new treatment (19). Therefore, surrogate outcomes, although commonly used in phase II trials that screen for potential benefit, are rarely used in phase III trials that are designed to evaluate benefit and adverse effects. Prentice developed statistical criteria for evaluating the validity of surrogate outcomes (20).

## DESCRIPTION OF DATA DISTRIBUTION

### Parameters of Frequency Distribution

Frequency distributions of data are described using *univariate* statistics (i.e., mean, median, mode, range, standard deviation). The distribution of data measured on dichotomous, nominal, and ordinal scales is represented as the number of participants in each group or value of the variable and the proportion of the total that this group comprises. Two types of measures define frequency distributions from continuous data: measures of central tendency and measures of dispersion.

### Measures of Central Tendency

Measures of central tendency (i.e., some type of "average" value) include the mode, median, and mean. The *mode* is the most commonly observed value (e.g., the value with the highest number of observations). A distribution may have more than one mode (e.g., bimodal distribution). The *mean* is the average value, calculated as the sum of all observed values divided by total number of observations. The advantage of using the mean is that it is simple to calculate and the sum of the deviations of observations from the mean should equal zero. The disadvantage is that it is sensitive to outliers. The *median* is the middle observation when data have been arranged in order from the lowest to highest value. For an even number of observations, the median is found halfway between the two middle observations. The advantage of using the median is that it is a better measure of central tendency for a non-normal distribution. However, the disadvantage is that it cannot be used to make statistical inferences about differences between experimental groups.

## MEASURES OF DISPERSION

Measures of dispersion describe the spread of data around any of the measures of central tendency. These measures include, but are not limited to, the mean deviation, standard deviation, percentile, and range. *Mean deviation* refers to the sum of the deviations from the mean divided by the number of observations. The problem with this measure is that it always equals 0. *Standard deviation* is a measure of the spread of data about their mean. It is based on the variance, which is the sum of the squared deviations from the mean divided by the number of observations minus 1. The standard deviation is then calculated as the square root of variance. As shown in Figure 3–4, for a normal distribution, 68.26% of a population will be within one standard deviation, 95.44% will fall within two standard deviations, and 99.72% within three standard deviations. *Percentile* refers to a number that indicates the percentage of a distribution that is equal to or below that number when all of the observations are ranked in descending order. It is not affected by a non-normal distribution of the data. Commonly used percentiles include the 50th percentile (which is equivalent to the median); the 75th percentile, the point below which 75% of the observations lie; the 25th percentile, the point

below which 25% of the observations lie; and the interquartile range (Q3–Q1), which is the distance between 75th and 25th percentile. The *range* refers to the difference between the largest observation and the smallest observation. For example, if in a cohort of patients at the time of diagnosis of head and neck cancer, the age of the youngest was 26 years and the oldest was 89 years, the range would be 63 years.

### Problems in Analyzing a Frequency Distribution

If a set of measurements for a population are normally distributed, then the mean = median = mode. In real life, measurements from clinical settings and biological systems are often not normally distributed. These aberrations from the normal distribution are described with the following terms: *skew, kurtosis*, and *extreme values*. *Skew* refers to the horizontal stretching of a normal distribution curve; *kurtosis* describes the vertical stretching of a normal distribution curve; and *extreme values* are those that are abnormally far above or below mean (often referred to as outliers), as shown in Figure 3–5. The impact of non-normally distributed distributions on the mean, median, mode is shown in Figure 3–6. As can be seen, as the distribution becomes more skewed the mean becomes less representative of the central tendency of the data. Data that depart greatly from a normal distribution may not be useful when applying some commonly used statistical tests (such as analysis of variance, see Chapter 24).

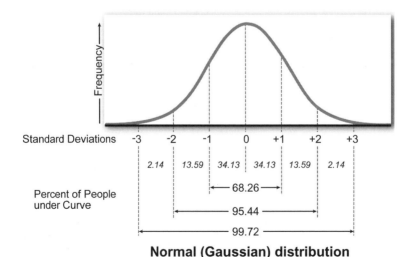

**Normal (Gaussian) distribution**

*FIGURE 3–4* ● Normal (Gaussian) distribution. For a normally distributed population, 68.26% of the population will be within one standard deviation, 95.44% will fall within two standard deviations, and 99.72% within three standard deviations.

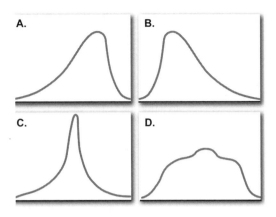

**FIGURE 3–5** ● Different examples of non-normally distributed data. Figures A and B represent a nonsymmetric skewed distribution (A—negative skew, B—positive skew); Figures C and D represent symmetric distributions; Figure C is a peaked kurtotic distribution and Figure D is a flattened kurtotic distribution.

## CRITERIA FOR ABNORMALITY

### Distribution-Based Versus Disease-Based Definition

It would be convenient if frequency distributions of lab values or other important findings from people with and without disease were so different that these distributions of values could be used to distinguish the distinct populations. However, most distributions of clinical variables from patients with and without disease overlap and thus it is not a simple task to define groups of patients into "normal" and "abnormal" categories based on lab values alone. In some cases, disease is acquired by degrees and so there is a smooth transition from low to high values with increasing degrees of dysfunction. For example, serum creatinine is often used to determine renal failure, but it is a dimensional variable with no clear demarcation between what is normal (no disease) and abnormal (disease). This distinction requires a clinical judgment that takes into account other patient factors such as age and overall health (21).

*Normal* often refers to the most frequently occurring or usual condition, so that whatever occurs often is considered normal or without disease, and whatever occurs infrequently is abnormal or with disease. This is a statistical definition, based on the frequency of a characteristic in a defined population, and is commonly used in medicine. However, there are problems with this strategy of defining disease status. For example, if all values beyond an arbitrary statistical limit, such as the 95th percentile, were considered diseased, then the prevalence of all diseases would be the same at 5%. This is inconsistent with the usual way of thinking about disease frequency. Many laboratory tests are related to risk of disease over their entire range of values, from low to high. For instance, there is an almost threefold increase in the risk of heart disease from the "low normal" to the "high normal"

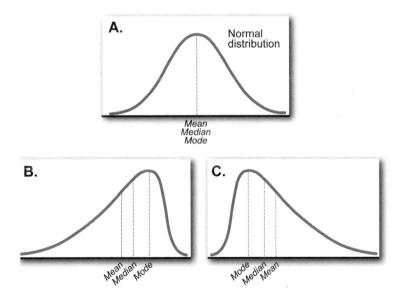

**FIGURE 3–6** ● Relationship between the mean, median, and mode in normal and non-normal distributions. Figure A shows the normal distribution where mean = median = mode. Figures B and C show negative and positive skew, respectively, in which mean ≠ median ≠ mode.

range of serum cholesterol. In other diseases, some extreme values are distinctly unusual but can be preferable to more usual ones. For example, who would not be pleased to have a serum creatinine of 0.4 mg/100 mL or a resting heart rate of 50 beats per minute? Sometimes patients have laboratory tests values in the usual range for healthy people, yet clearly have disease, such as with low pressure hydrocephalus, normal pressure glaucoma, and normocalcemic hyperparathyroidism.

Disease-based definitions of *abnormal* use the strategy of calling a condition a disease only when those observations that are regularly associated with disease, disability, or death are observed. Alternatively, a condition could be labeled a disease and a measurement abnormal only when treatment of such a condition leads to a better outcome.

### Regression to the Mean

When clinicians encounter an unexpectedly abnormal test result, they tend to repeat the test. Often the second test result is closer to normal. Analogously, if research participants in a study are selected because they exceed a certain threshold of measurement for inclusion (e.g., systolic blood pressure greater than 140), then on average, those patients tend to have a less extreme value when they are measured a second time, regardless of whether they received treatment or not. This statistical phenomenon is known as regression to the mean; it does not mean that the patients have necessarily improved. Regression to the mean is one example of why "time controls" may be necessary when the effects of an experimental intervention are compared to "baseline" values (see Chapter 8).

### Unit-Free Data

Data from normal frequency distributions can be described completely by the mean and standard deviation. However, even the same set of data provides a different value for the mean and standard deviation depending on the choice of *units of measurement*. For example, the same person's height may be expressed as 66 inches or 167.6 cm. To eliminate the distorting effect produced by the choice of units, data can be put into unit-free form, called Z *values* (or Z *scores*). Z *values* allow clinicians to easily make estimates of percentages of patients expected to have values higher or lower than a certain level, because they express the value of each observation as the number of standard deviations above or below the mean. A Z value is calculated as follows, where $x_i$ is the

value of the observation, $\bar{x}$ is the mean, and $s$ is the standard deviation:

$$Z_i = \frac{x_i - \bar{x}}{s}$$

A distribution of Z values always has a mean of 0 and a standard deviation of 1. For example, if a cohort of cancer patients has a mean age of 63 years and standard deviation of 11.3 years, then the Z values for 88-year old and 52-year-old patients are:

$$\frac{88 - 63}{11.3} = +2.21 \qquad \frac{52 - 63}{11.3} = -0.97$$

Without knowing anything about the *average* age of the cancer patients, an observer can immediately tell that the 88-year old patient with a Z score of +2.21 is significantly older than average, while the 52-year old, with a Z score of –0.97, is average.

## SUMMARY

- Types of variables—determine which descriptive and inferential statistics ought to be used in the study
  - Dichotomous—limited to two responses
  - Nominal—categorized without inherent order or ranking
  - Ordinal—categorical responses ranked in ascending or descending magnitudes without equi-intervals or gradations between them.
  - Dimensional—inherent order with equal successive interval values.

- Performance of measurements
  - Validity—the degree to which the data measure what they are intended to measure. *Sensitivity* and *specificity* are statistical indices that refer to the ability of a diagnostic test to detect disease. *Receiver operating characteristics (ROC) curves* and *Bland-Altman plots* are also quantitative measures of validity.
  - Reliability—the extent to which repeated measurements of a stable phenomenon obtain similar results. *Overall percent agreement, kappa coefficient,* and *correlation coefficient* are quantitative measures of reliability.
  - Responsiveness—the extent to which a measurement changes as the underlying condition being measured changes. *Effect size* and *standardized response mean* are quantitative measures of responsiveness.
  - Variation—the sum of variation related to the act of measurement and biologic differences within and between individuals. *Bias*

is systematic error while *random* error is due to chance.

- Choosing variables
  - *Dependent* variables—the outcome variable whose value is a function of other variable(s) (called independent variable(s)) in the relationship under study.
  - *Independent* variables—the variables representing an exposure, risk factor, or other characteristics that are thought to impact on the dependent variable.
  - *Covariates*—variables to be measured in a study other than the dependent and independent variables that can be any factor that makes one patient or group of patients different from another, and that could potentially affect the outcome.
  - *Extraneous Variables*—variables whose presence or absence, or degree or severity may be used to describe the characteristics of the patients being studied; they may or may not impact on outcome.
  - *Confounding* variable—a variable systematically related to the independent variable (an "exposure") and to the outcome, yet does not lie on the hypothesized causal path from exposure to outcome.
  - *Effect modifiers*—variables that affect either the exposure or the outcome, but not both.
  - Hard versus soft data—the choice of outcome measures in clinical research that reflect biological parameters that are measured in an (apparently) objective way (hard data) versus measures that represent clinical phenomena that are measured with patient-based questionnaires and other (apparently) nonobjective measures.
  - Primary versus secondary outcomes—primary outcomes are the main outcomes or endpoints that drive a clinical study; they are the measurements that will be used to answer the main research question and to address the primary hypothesis. Secondary outcomes are the other outcomes of interest that an investigator hopes to measure and find significant, but are not the focus of the main hypothesis of the research study. They are the measurements used to answer secondary research questions and hypotheses.
  - Surrogate outcomes—outcomes or measurements (also known as *proxy* measurements) that are used when the entity an investigator really wants to measure is inconvenient, difficult, or impossible to know, or considered soft data.

- Data distribution
  - Parameters of frequency distribution—*univariate statistics*
  - Central tendency—*mean, median,* and *mode*
  - Dispersion—*standard deviation, percentile,* and *range*
- Criteria for abnormality
  - Distribution-based versus disease-based definition
  - Regression to the mean—a repeated test often produces values closer to the mean than the original test result, especially when the original test result is unexpectedly abnormal.
  - Unit-free data—values of observations expressed as the number of standard deviations above or below the mean; useful when reporting or analyzing data with different units of measurement.

## REFERENCES

1. Feinstein AR. Principles of Medical Statistics. New York: Chapman & Hall, 2002.
2. Bland JM, Altman DG. Statistical methods for assessing agreement between two methods of clinical measurement. Lancet 1986;1:307–310.
3. Bland JM, Altman DG. Measuring agreement in method comparison studies. Statistical Methods in Medical Research. 1999;8:135–160.
4. Fleiss JL. Statistical Methods for Rates and Proportions, 2nd Ed. New York: John Wiley and Sons, 1981:212.
5. Landis JR, Koch GG. The measurement of observer agreement for categorical data. Biometrics 1977;33: 159–174.
6. Portney LG, Watkins MP. Foundations of Clinical Research: applications to Practice. East Norwalk, CT: Appleton & Lange, 1993.
7. Robinson WB. The statistical measurement of agreement. American Sociological Review 1957;22:17–25.
8. Kazis LE, Anderson JJ, Meenan RF. Effect sizes for interpreting changes in health status. Med Care 1989;27:S178–189.
9. Liang MH, Fossel AH, Larson MG. Comparisons of five health status instruments for orthopaedic evaluation. Med Care 1990;28:632–642.
10. Cohen J. Statistical Power Analysis for the Behavioural Sciences. 2nd Ed. Hillside: L. Erlbaum Assoc., 1988.
11. Nicoletto MO, Donach M, De Nicolo A et al. BRCA-1 and BRCA-2 mutations as prognostic factors in clinical practice and genetic counselling. Cancer Treat Rev 2001;27:295–304.
12. Last JM, ed. A Dictionary of Epidemiology, 4th Ed. New York: Oxford University Press, 2001.
13. Kramer MS. Clinical Epidemiology and Biostatistics. New York: Springer-Verlag, 1988.
14. Feinstein AR. Clinical biostatistics. XLI. Hard science, soft data, and the challenges of choosing clinical variables in research. Clin Pharmacol Ther 1977;22:485–498.
15. Ware JE, Snow KK, Kosinski M et al. SF-36 Health Survey Manual and Interpretation Guide. Boston: The Health Institute, 1999.

16. Karnofsky DA, Abelmann WH, Craver LF et al. The use of the nitrogen mustards in the palliative treatment of carcinoma. Cancer 1948;1:634–656.

17. Shaunak S, Davies DS. Surrogacy in antiviral drug development. Br J Clin Pharmacol 2002;54:75–80.

18. Mathews AW. Question hampers lupus drugs: what does better mean? FDA, industry seek markers of progress to break decades-long drought. harsh medicines, little hope. Wall Street Journal, April 15, 2004:1.

19. Fleming TR, DeMets DL. Surrogate endpoints in clinical trials: are we being misled? Ann Intern Med 1996;125:605–613.

20. Prentice RL. Surrogate endpoints in clinical trials: definition and operational criteria. Stat Med 1989;8:431–440.

21. Feinstein AR. Clinical Epidemiology: the Architecture of Clinical Research, Philadelphia: WB Saunders, 1985.

# CHAPTER 4

# Study Eligibility and Participant Selection

Roger D. Yusen, Benjamin Littenberg

In this chapter, we address the topics of sampling, developing study eligibility criteria, and collecting and reporting eligibility data.

## SAMPLING

A population has certain characteristics. Of the whole population, investigators may wish to apply their research to a target population, a group of people with common characteristics of interest that are eligible for study enrollment (Figure 4–1). From the target population, investigators try to enroll the accessible population. Investigators might only approach or choose to enroll a portion of the accessible people, and some accessible people might refuse to participate. The study sample consists of the individuals who consent to participate. For example, investigators may want to study a new anticoagulant for preventing recurrent blood clots in adults who have acute pulmonary embolism. The target population consists of the subgroup of adults in the whole population that has a diagnosis of pulmonary embolism. If the study has access only to patients admitted to the hospital, then eligible hospitalized adults with pulmonary embolism who consent to study participation comprise the study sample.

Researchers may or may not have access to an abundant accessible population. If the accessible population is small, the investigator may have inadequate statistical power to answer the research question, despite the enrollment of all individuals. If the accessible population is very large, the investigator may not want to study them all because of time and resource constraints. Even if it were practical, it is wasteful to enroll thousands of participants to answer a question that could be adequately addressed by a few dozen. In this case, the investigator should select a sample of eligible participants to enroll. Like all research design issues, the choice of a sampling strategy involves trade-offs between costs (in terms of time, money, and other resources) and validity (in terms of precision, statistical power, and potential bias). Methodologically appropriate sampling allows the investigator to draw valid conclusions about a population. Enrollment of a sample of participants that does not represent the target population limits study generalizability.

## SAMPLING DESIGNS

Just as random assignment to treatments minimizes bias in a controlled trial, random or probability sampling can protect against certain threats to validity. The threats to study validity that may occur with sampling come under the general heading of sampling bias. Sampling bias occurs when the probability of being entered into a study is associated with either the outcome or the predictors. For instance, if investigators enroll only those patients in the intensive care unit (ICU) who are able to respond to questions, the survival of the study cohort would likely be higher than that in a study that evaluates the survival of all patients admitted to the ICU. In the process of selecting individuals for study participation, investigators should aim to minimize such threats to validity.

More complex sampling methods may improve study generalizability, but they involve trade-offs in terms of costs, complexity, and acceptability. Various sampling techniques affect sample size requirements (Chapter 9) and require different statistical approaches during analysis. Researchers often classify sampling designs into nonprobability sampling designs and probability sampling designs.

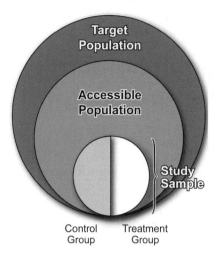

**FIGURE 4–1** ● Population and sample groups. A portion of the study participants from the accessible population make up the study sample. Ideally, the study sample represents the target population.

## NONPROBABILITY SAMPLING

With nonprobability sampling, individuals do not have an equal or known probability of being selected from the target population for study participation. Selective sampling may introduce systematic bias by enhancing recruitment and enrollment of participants with certain characteristics. The resulting sampling bias may produce a nonrepresentative sample of the population that hinders the generalizability of the study findings. For example, if the target population is all adults with lung cancer, but the sampling frame includes only veterans, it is likely that women will be underrepresented in the sample relative to the target population. The study question then changes its focus from adult patients with lung cancer to adult male veterans with lung cancer. Clinicians and other consumers of research who need to treat women and nonveterans may or may not find the results applicable.

Enrollment of an entire accessible population does not necessarily address sampling bias because the study enrollees might not fairly represent the target population. For example, enrollment of all patients with Wegener's granulomatosis seen in an outpatient clinic might not be generalizable to all patients in the world with the disease. This is especially true if the clinic is a national referral center for Wegener's granulomatosis that only evaluates patients with the most complex cases or the best-insured patients in the country.

Feasibility issues often lead to nonprobability sampling. Sometimes, researchers make practical decisions, and they choose to conduct a study that has a small sample size based on constraints of time, finances, and participant availability. This approach may be reasonable for preliminary data gathering, though it would not be recommended for more definitive studies. One of the most common nonprobability sampling methods for prospective studies is convenience sampling, especially in many translational or experimental clinical research studies. The reader is referred to other sources (1,2) for further details regarding nonprobability sampling schemes, such as those used in case-control and some epidemiologic study designs.

## CONVENIENCE SAMPLES

A convenience sample consists of easily accessible people who meet study eligibility criteria. For example, an investigating surgeon may enroll her patients who are easily accessible. Sampling bias could be significant if she excludes those patients who do not respond well to treatment, see her after hours, or have complex histories. Convenience samples have cost and logistical advantages: as the name implies, they are easy to enroll, and they tend not to disrupt busy clinical services. Convenience samples often lack generalizability to the target population, and the sample may not adequately reflect the intended target population due to selection bias.

Nonconsecutively enrolled convenience samples are usually not useful for anything more rigorous than a feasibility pilot study. Consecutive sampling, enrolling every eligible case for a period of time, decreases systematic bias associated with convenience sampling. During the enrollment period, every potential participant has a 100% chance of being sampled. Convenience sampling with a consecutive design is practical and acceptable for many clinical research studies (3). Phenomena of interest with seasonal or other time-dependent trends require caution when using convenience sampling, whether or not the sampling is consecutive. For instance, a study of respiratory complaints in which every patient seen in June was enrolled might have very different results than one conducted in December.

## PROBABILITY SAMPLING

Probability sampling involves a random process in which each potential participant has a known specified chance (probability) of being selected (3). The most straightforward approach is simple random sampling where all potential participants have the same or equal chance of being selected, although other weighting schemes are possible. Probability sampling designs avoid systematic bias because the chance of being selected is not associated with subject-related characteristics that may in turn be associated with the outcome.

Even with probability sampling designs, feasibility issues (e.g., time, money, access) greatly affect the sampling methods, and sampling bias may be introduced by quasi-probability sampling designs and quasi-consecutive convenience sampling. For example, potential study participants might only be available for recruitment at various times, or study staff might only be available during certain hours of the day or specific days of the week. "Off hours" eligible people, who are unavailable for enrollment, might have different characteristics compared with "on hours" eligible people, who are available for enrollment.

## SIMPLE RANDOM SAMPLING

The most common and gold standard approach to probability sampling for translational or experimental studies is the simple random sampling method. For the selection to be effectively random, each member of the study population should have the same chance of being included in the study sample (4), and nobody should be able to reliably predict who among the sampling frame will be enrolled. Methods used to randomly sample include computerized generation of random numbers or use of a random number table. For example, a researcher studying rheumatoid arthritis could theoretically obtain the list of all patients seen in the arthritis clinic with that diagnosis in the past year. Knowing the number of participants required for the study, the investigator could randomly sample from the accessible population by assigning each subject's name on the list to a number from a random number table or a computer-generated random number list. For instance, the first name will go to the first number, the second name to the second number, and so on. Next, the investigator could sort the list by ascending order of the random numbers. If the investigator needs to enroll a random sample of 35 people, then he or she would attempt to enroll the first 35 patients on the list. If all patients do not enroll, then the investigator would consecutively work down the list until he or she has enrolled enough patients to meet the sample size requirements.

Nonrandom sampling based on even or odd days or some function of the social security number, name, record number, birth date, or any other datum knowable by the investigators may introduce bias. For example, an investigator could choose to enroll people if the first letter of their last name ranges from A through K. If referring doctors know that patients whose last names begin with A through K will be enrolled in a study that they consider unattractive, they may refer such patients to another hospital to avoid enrollment. Though this extreme scenario is unlikely, the investigator could avoid the potential threat to validity with little cost or bother by using random sampling.

## STRATIFIED RANDOM SAMPLING

When a study population has distinct subgroups defined by important characteristics that potentially relate to treatment interventions and outcomes, stratified random sampling might be useful. With this approach, the study population is divided according to the stratifying factor. Within each stratum, a random sampling method is used to select patients for study participation (3,4). For example, investigators might think that gender has a significant impact on the issue that is being studied. Investigators could divide the study population into subgroups of males and females, and a random sample could be taken from each of these strata. Equal proportions of people are typically selected from the strata, though more complex methods might include using different sampling fractions or weighting schemas that allow disproportionate sampling from the subgroups. Stratified random sampling should not be confused with stratified random treatment assignment (Chapter 8).

## OTHER RANDOM SAMPLING METHODS

More complex methods of sampling exist, such as cluster random sampling and multistage sampling. These methods are not often applied to the types of studies being addressed in this book, and the interested reader is referred to other sources for further details (1,2).

## STUDY ELIGIBILITY CRITERIA

During the design phase of a study, investigators develop study eligibility criteria (Table 4–1). Investigators typically develop separate inclusion criteria and exclusion criteria, though this division of eligibility criteria often leads to confusion. Because using opposite wording for any given criterion makes the inclusion and exclusion criterion interchangeable, investigators may prefer to develop a single list of eligibility criteria (5). For example, in a study of airway epithelium in patients with asthma, the investigators might want to exclude patients with severe disease because of safety concerns related to bronchoscopic

## TABLE 4–1

### Issues to Consider When Creating Study Eligibility Criteria

**Methodology and Generalizability**
  Clarity of criteria
  Objectiveness of criteria (i.e., diagnosis of disease under study)
  Subgroups
    Disease stages
    Prognostic/risk factors
    Comorbidity/concomitant illnesses
  Rate of disease progression before enrollment
  Receipt of prestudy treatment
  Response to therapy before enrollment
  Nonrandomized treatment issues after enrollment
    Setting
    Geographic issues
    Temporal issues
    Ability to complete testing and follow-up
    Ability to complete treatment
  Need for demonstration of successful completion of prerandomization testing
  Need for demonstration of successful completion of prerandomization treatment
  Current enrollment in other clinical trials
  Previous enrollment in the same trial

**Safety**
  Risk of complications from study therapy
  Risk of complications from study evaluations

**Ethics**
  Study limitations on use of available alternative therapies
  Exclusion from enrollment in other future clinical trials

**Efficiency**
  Ease and speed of recruitment
  Costs to carry out the study
  Data quality
  Interpretability of results

sampling. Therefore, investigators would include only patients with nonsevere disease. To avoid having separate inclusion and exclusion criteria, the investigators could say that they will enroll only individuals with mild to moderate forms of asthma.

## CLEAR DEFINITIONS

Investigators should try to develop clearly defined objective eligibility criteria in order to enter appropriate participants into a clinical study and to have the same type of participant recruitment in different settings. Vague descriptions of eligibility criteria may lead to unwanted variability in the types of participants enrolled and difficulty in translating the criteria to the clinical setting. Clearly defining eligibility criteria differs from making an extensive list of eligibility criteria. Clearly defined criteria decrease ambiguity and confusion. Complicated lists create more work in the screening process, and long lists of eligibility criteria may significantly slow down the study enrollment (6). Similar to other aspects of study design, eligibility criteria should be expressed so explicitly and clearly that study staff can execute the protocol without specific guidance from the principal investigator (PI). If the PI is unavailable, the study can still go on, and the study staff members do not have to make judgment calls during the execution of the study that could introduce bias or imprecision. Clear and explicit criteria suggest that the protocol reviewed by the IRB, the funders, and others is a valid representation of what is likely to happen.

## GENERALIZABILITY AND EFFICIENCY

Generalizability, also called external validity, represents the extent to which the results of a study apply to individuals and circumstances beyond those studied. Though characteristics of enrolled participants help judge the generalizability of a study, other factors such as the trial setting, the treatment regimens, and the outcomes assessed also determine generalizability (7). For example, a study of joint fluid characteristics and functional status scores in men with rheumatoid arthritis undergoing treatment with a monoclonal antibody at a referral subspecialty clinic at a veterans administration (VA) hospital would not necessarily generalize to women undergoing care in a community hospital setting.

Efficiency refers to the ease of recruitment and data collection and the financial feasibility of conducting the study. During the study design phase, investigators need to create eligibility criteria that appropriately balance study validity and generalizability goals with efficiency concerns. Increased generalizability often produces a loss in efficiency and vice versa.

## RESEARCH PARTICIPANT HETEROGENEITY

Though broad eligibility criteria increase generalizability, enrollment of more heterogeneous participants might increase the number of participants needed to detect a difference in treatment effects because increased variation among participants decreases power (Chapter 9). A decision about whether to emphasize narrow eligibility with lesser generalizability or broader inclusion with more participant heterogeneity and greater generalizability depends on the research goals of the study. For instance, an explanatory study that seeks to answer questions about a mechanism of disease may not need to have great generalizability to convince the scientific community that the findings support or refute the hypothesis about the proposed mechanism. On the other hand, a pragmatic or outcomes trial of therapy for a common condition should probably include a very broad cross-section of the types of individuals that may be offered the treatment. Some clinical researchers have called for large, simple, relatively inexpensive, randomized trials to assess the effects of widely practical treatments for common conditions on important outcomes (e.g., mortality) (8). The intended research question (Chapter 1) should drive decisions about study design, and every decision about how to make the study go faster, cheaper, or easier must be balanced with the aims of the study.

The study design should dictate the characteristics of individuals appropriate for enrollment in a study. Enrollment of a very heterogeneous group of participants can sometimes dilute the value of the study's results, potentially resulting in a "negative" study. An example of this phenomenon can be seen in the National Emphysema Treatment Trial (NETT), in which the effects of lung volume reduction surgery were compared with medical therapy in participants with emphysema and severe chronic obstructive pulmonary disease (9). Although admittedly a multicenter efficacy trial (which is not the overall focus of this book), this study does illustrate the problem of potentially losing a "signal" when patient heterogeneity creates additional measurement "noise." The overall results of this study suggested that lung-volume reduction surgery does not confer a survival advantage over medical therapy (Figure 4–2 A–C), though surgery led to less dyspnea and increased exercise capacity compared to medical therapy. Investigators enrolled a broad sample of participants in whom the distributions of emphysema throughout the lung fields varied (10). Previous cohort studies (11), however, had suggested that narrower eligibility criteria (that would

only allow enrollment of individuals with an upper lobe predominance of emphysema) might produce a better surgical outcome. Indeed, a post hoc analysis of the NETT did show a survival benefit for surgical participants in the subgroup of participants with an upper lobe predominance of emphysema and a low preoperative postrehabilitation exercise capacity (Figure 4–2 D). Although the conclusions drawn from the post hoc analysis have been questioned (12), and the issue can't be resolved by NETT alone, the inclusion of the subgroups allowed for valuable hypothesis-generating analyses. Different study methodology, such as different eligibility criteria (e.g., enrollment limited to individuals with an upper lobe predominance of emphysema) or stratified randomization (Chapter 8) (e.g., separate randomized treatment assignment of those with and those without upper lobe predominant emphysema) could have provided stronger evidence of the effect of surgery within specific types of participants.

## DISEASE STAGES

Because broader inclusion criteria allow for better generalization of study results, a study of participants experiencing different disease stages (e.g., mild, moderate, and severe) has broader applicability than a study of participants who have developed a specific stage of disease (e.g., severe only). For example, if a study of pulmonary embolism treatment excludes patients with hypoxemia and hypotension, then the findings of the study may not apply to hypoxemic hypotensive patients.

## PROGNOSTIC FACTORS

To improve generalizability, investigators should consider including individuals with varied prognostic or risk factors for the outcome undergoing assessment. Investigators should not use eligibility criteria that exclude individuals based on factors unlikely to influence outcome, because such criteria interfere with recruitment and do not improve study precision. Each added criterion further restricts study recruitment and increases the number of individuals that must undergo screening to meet recruitment goals. This scenario leads to worsened generalizability and decreased efficiency. For example, patients with cancer who have venous thromboembolism have a higher risk of recurrent thrombosis than patients without cancer (13). In a pharmacogenetics study designed to evaluate the efficacy of anticoagulants in preventing recurrent venous thromboembolism as a function of genotype, recruitment of patients without cancer will likely decrease recurrent

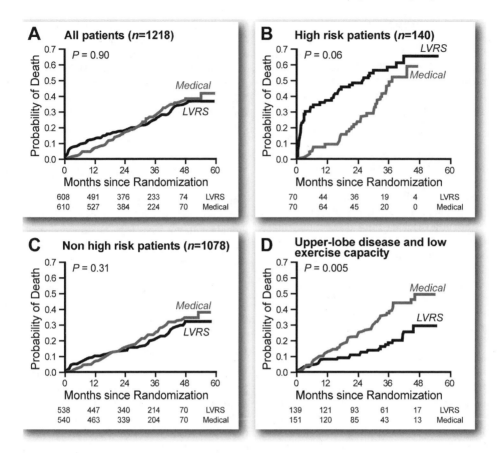

**FIGURE 4–2** ● National Emphysema Treatment Trial (NETT) Kaplan-Meier estimates of the probability of death as a function of number of months after randomization to lung-volume reduction surgery (LVRS) or medical therapy (Medical) in **(A)** all patients, **(B)** high-risk patients, **(C)** non–high-risk patients, and **(D)** a non–high-risk subgroup of patients with upper lobe predominant emphysema and low exercise capacity. High-risk patients were defined as those with a forced expiratory volume in 1 second that was 20% or less of the predicted normal value and either homogenous emphysema or carbon monoxide diffusing capacity that was 20% or less of the predicted normal value. A low baseline exercise capacity was defined as a maximal workload at or below the sex-specific 40th percentile (25 W for women and 40 W for men); a high exercise capacity was defined as a workload above this threshold. Using an intention-to-treat analysis, P values were derived by Fisher's exact test for the comparison between groups over a mean follow-up period of 29.2 months. Copyright 2003. Massachusetts Medical Society. All rights reserved. Adapted with permission from New Engl J Med 2003;348:2059–2073.

thromboembolism rates compared with recruitment of patients with cancer. The exclusion of patients with cancer from the study might increase the required sample size, the duration of the study, and the study costs.

## SUBGROUPS

If specific subgroups are expected to have different outcomes in a study, investigators should try to enroll an adequate number of participants to allow for planned subgroup analyses. For example, the Coronary Artery Surgery Study (CASS), a study of coronary artery bypass grafting compared with medical therapy in patients with coronary artery disease, found that patients with the combination of low left ventricular ejection fraction and triple vessel coronary artery disease had significantly better long-term outcomes after surgery compared with patients without these characteristics (14). If the CASS had not enrolled enough patients with these characteristics, then the investigators might not have detected the difference in outcome between the subgroups. Planned assessment of subgroups might significantly increase sample size requirements.

## GEOGRAPHIC AND TEMPORAL MATTERS

Practical geographic and temporal matters that affect eligibility criteria produce changes in study efficiency and generalizability. Some factors, such as study setting and study enrollment time frame, are sometimes implied but not explicitly stated in the eligibility criteria. For example, limiting study participation to hospitalized patients may improve efficiency, but the study results would not necessarily generalize to outpatients. Enrollment of and follow-up of participants during a limited time frame might affect efficiency and generalizability. For example, a study carried out in the summer season that assesses the impact of a vaccine on immune system markers in participants with and without influenza might be less efficient and less generalizable than a study carried out in the fall and winter seasons.

## DATA QUALITY, INTERPRETATION OF FINDINGS, AND STUDY FEASIBILITY

Investigators use eligibility criteria to exclude certain types of individuals in an effort to improve data quality, interpretation of findings, and study feasibility. Investigators want to enroll participants who will comply with testing, treatment, and follow-up. For example, many studies exclude individuals who are perceived as potentially noncompliant with medication use or follow-up. Also, studies that primarily assess nonmortality outcomes may have eligibility criteria that exclude individuals with an expected survival that is less than the duration of the study because of concerns about inadequate follow-up. To further address compliance concerns, investigators can design a study with a run-in period so patients can demonstrate good compliance in order to become eligible for the main study (Chapter 8). Once again, as eligibility criteria become more rigorous, the number of excluded individuals increases, and these exclusions may produce screening bias (see "Collecting and Reporting Eligibility Data," below), reduce generalizability, and slow enrollment.

## SAFETY

For the sake of participant safety, investigators should consider developing eligibility criteria that exclude people at high risk for complications from study interventions and testing. Investigators have an obligation to ensure that clinical trial participation will not expose individual research participants to undue risk (15). For example, investigators might develop criteria that exclude individuals with recent hemorrhagic stroke from anticoagulant studies, or investigators may develop criteria that exclude participants with allergies to intravenous contrast from studies that require radiologic assessment with intravenous contrast. Interestingly, large numbers of exclusionary safety criteria can paradoxically distract investigators from paying attention to other important

individual details (16). In addition, extensive numbers of criteria can hurt study generalizability, increase complexity and costs, and delay enrollment.

Though each investigator should believe that eligible people can proceed fairly with study entry on the basis of well-conceived eligibility criteria, sometimes an investigator concludes that it is not appropriate for an individual to enter the study despite meeting the eligibility criteria. Such exclusions will not affect the internal validity of the study if they occur before treatment assignment (randomization). The exclusion of eligible individuals based on subjective concerns may produce selection bias and affect generalizability (see "Collecting and Reporting Eligibility Data," below).

## ETHICAL CONSIDERATIONS

Ethical considerations also affect the development of eligibility criteria. Eligibility criteria should not unjustly deny individuals the potential benefits of research participation or place the burdens of participation on only a small group. Investigators might face significant criticism if the eligibility criteria exclude individuals based on factors such as age, gender, race, ethnicity, religion, and sexual orientation without explicit scientific rationale. In fact, the National Institutes of Health (NIH) requires investigators to address representative recruitment of individuals based on gender and race or minority status (17). Exceptions to this rule include diseases concentrated in certain types of individuals. For example, women are appropriately excluded from studies of prostate cancer. Otherwise, investigators often need to figure out how to improve recruitment of such subgroups. Recruitment practices also affect enrollment (Chapter 5). A lack of representative racial diversity may reflect referral practices, subject self-selection, access to medical care, poor community relationships, lack of trust, and a host of other issues.

Clinical studies should not unfairly burden vulnerable participants, such as children or individuals unable to provide uncoerced informed consent (Chapter 14). For example, pregnant women may be excluded from an anticoagulant study because of concerns about risk to the fetus. Some studies require women to provide proof of nonpregnancy (i.e., a negative beta human chorionic gonadotropin test) or an inability to become pregnant (i.e., history of bilateral oophorectomy or hysterectomy).

Eligibility criteria should exclude individuals who need a treatment that would be discouraged by the study protocol. For example, anticoagulant studies often appropriately exclude patients with acute pulmonary embolism if the individual is deemed in need of thrombolytic therapy.

As part of the informed consent process, investigators should inform potential participants about the consequences of enrollment in the trial. For example, enrollment in one trial may preclude their enrollment in another trial.

## DOUBLE ENROLLMENT

Eligibility criteria should not allow participants to enter the same study more than once if the planned statistical tests require independence of each observation from the others. Investigators may also need to exclude participants enrolled in other studies to avoid confounding. In addition, regulatory agencies might insist on such exclusions. Such criteria might threaten generalizability and delay enrollment. For example, a patient with advanced stage non–small cell lung cancer may wish to forgo enrollment in a Phase II venous thromboembolism treatment trial so that she may not lose the ability to enroll in a cancer chemotherapy trial that excludes individuals receiving other experimental therapies.

## CHANGING ELIGIBILITY CRITERIA

Investigators are sometimes tempted to change eligibility criteria after a study has started. They may choose to broaden eligibility criteria in studies with difficulty meeting recruitment goals. Safety concerns from an interim analysis could lead to a change in study eligibility criteria. For example, an interim analysis of the NETT revealed that a subset of high-risk participants with either very poor lung function or poor lung function associated with diffuse homogeneous emphysema had a significantly higher death rate after randomization to lung volume reduction surgery compared with participants randomized to medical therapy (Figure 4–2B) (18). Based on the recommendation from an independent data and safety monitoring board (Chapter 13), the study stopped enrolling these individuals.

Alteration of eligibility criteria might introduce bias and affect the internal validity of the treatment comparisons if the criteria undergoing change are related to study outcomes. A change in eligibility criteria might also affect the study's internal validity if it alters the proportion of participants allocated to the treatment group over the course of enrollment. Randomization procedures that balance the number of treatment assignments can usually address this latter issue. Changes to the eligibility criteria might also affect the generalizability of the study. Investigators should cautiously consider such changes to ensure that the final study is internally valid, precise, externally generalizable, and acceptable.

## COLLECTING AND REPORTING ELIGIBILITY DATA

Investigators should report the methods used for choosing research participants and the results of the recruitment process so that readers may assess the generalizability of the study. Though data collection is discussed in Chapter 12 and the reporting of data is discussed in Chapters 29 and 30, this section discusses a few key issues pertinent to choosing research participants.

The revised Consolidated Standards of Reporting Trials (CONSORT ) statement recommends that investigators in randomized controlled trials report the number of individuals assessed for eligibility, the number of individuals eligible for enrollment, and the number of individuals enrolled (19). Ideally, the investigators would also describe the number of ineligible individuals in each exclusionary category and the number of eligible nonenrolled individuals along with their reasons for nonparticipation (20). Researchers using other study designs should report similar eligibility data.

The types of patients enrolled in a study affect the ability to generalize the study results to other people and other settings. Selection bias, an error that arises in the process of identifying and enrolling the study sample, can harm study generalizability. Selection bias can also be introduced throughout the design and implementation phases of a study (21). Even after a study has been completed, investigators can introduce selection bias if they perform analyses that exclude enrolled participants. To address concerns about study generalizability, studies should be assessed for selection bias at various stages of the study. Before conducting a study, investigators should assess the potential of the study design for introducing selection bias. Investigators should redesign the study if significant concerns are present. To allow for post hoc assessment for the presence of screening bias, investigators should consider recording simple baseline information on all individuals screened. In the analytic and reporting phases of a study, investigators could then compare characteristics (e.g., age and gender) between enrolled (eligible) and all nonenrolled (eligible and noneligible) people. Investigators could also compare baseline characteristics of enrolled eligible and nonenrolled eligible people. Ideally, investigators would collect key demographic and prognostic baseline information. Investigators could potentially collect data that would allow them to compare outcomes of enrolled participants who received the control therapy with eligible individuals who were not enrolled in the trial (22). Significant differences in characteristics or outcomes between the groups would provide estimates about the presence and severity of screening bias. Reporting screening bias data allows the investigator to make judgments about the generalizability of the study. However, restrictions on collecting data without consent often limit access to such information.

The collection of data on nonenrolled individuals requires additional time and resources. To increase efficiency, rather than obtaining baseline data on all screened or eligible individuals, investigators could assess a sample of people. For example, investigators could collect baseline deidentified information on all individuals screened for the study in a log book. In a random sample of screened eligible nonenrolled individuals, investigators could collect more detailed baseline information after obtaining informed consent or permission from the IRB (Chapter 14). Again, appropriate sampling techniques would be necessary.

## SUMMARY

- Methodologically appropriate sampling allows the investigator to draw valid conclusions about a population.
- Enrollment of people who do not represent the target population limits study generalizability.
- The choice of a sampling strategy involves trade-offs between costs (e.g., time, money, and other resources) and validity (e.g., precision, statistical power, and potential bias).
- Clearly defined objective eligibility criteria ensure the enrollment of appropriate participants and enhance the application of study results to different settings.
- Broad eligibility criteria may improve generalizability at the expense of precision and feasibility.
- Narrow eligibility criteria may improve precision and feasibility at the expense of generalizability.
- Changes in eligibility criteria, like all other aspects of the study protocol, may effectively alter the research question, sometimes without the investigators realizing it.

## REFERENCES

1. Levy PS, Lemeshow S. Sampling for Health Professionals. Belmont, CA: Lifetime Learning Publications, 1980.
2. Peters TJ, Eachus JI. Achieving equal probability of selection under various random sampling strategies. Peadiatr Perinat Epidemiol 1995;9:219–224.
3. Kelsey JL, Whittemore AS, Evans AS et al. Methods in Observational Epidemiology. 2nd Ed. New York: Oxford University Press, 1996: 311–326.
4. Hulley SB, Newman TB, and Cummings SR. Choosing the study subjects: specification, sampling, and recruitment. In: Hulley SB, Cummings SR, Browner WS et al.,
   eds. Designing Clinical Research. 2nd Ed. Philadelphia: Lippincott Williams & Wilkins, 2001:30–31.
5. Fuks A, Weijer C, Freedman B et al. A study in contrasts: eligibility criteria in a twenty-year sample of NSABP and POG clinical trials. National Surgical Adjuvant Breast and Bowel Program. J Clin Epidemiol 1998;51:69–79.
6. Piantadosi S. The Study Cohort. Clinical Trials, A Methodologic Perspective. Indianapolis: John Wiley and Sons, 1997:187.
7. Jüni P, Altman DG, Egger M. Assessing the quality of randomised controlled trials. Pgs. 87–108 (pg. 93) Eds. Egger M, Smith GD, Altman DG. Systematic Reviews in Health Care: Meta-Analysis in Context. 2nd Ed. London: BMJ Books, 2001.
8. Yusuf S, Collins R, Peto R. Why do we need some large, simple randomized trials? Stat Med 1984;3:409–420.
9. NETT Investigators. A randomized trial comparing lung-volume—reduction surgery with medical therapy for severe emphysema. N Engl J Med 2003;348:2059–2073.
10. NETT Investigators. Rationale and design of the National Emphysema Treatment Trial: prospective randomized trial of lung volume reduction surgery. Chest 1999;116:1750–1761.
11. Slone RM, Pilgram TK, Gierada DS et al. Lung volume reduction surgery: comparison of preoperative radiologic features and clinical outcome. Radiology 1997; 204:685–693.
12. Ware JH. The National Emphysema Treatment Trial—how strong is the evidence? N Engl J Med 2003; 348:2055–2056.
13. The Columbus Investigators. Low-molecular-weight heparin in the treatment of patients with venous thromboembolism. N Engl J Med 1997;337:657–662.
14. Passamani E, Davis KB, Gillespie MJ et al. A randomized trial of coronary artery bypass surgery: survival of patients with a low ejection fraction. N Engl J Med 1985;312:1665–1671.
15. Weijer C, Fuks A. The duty to exclude: excluding people at undue risk from research. Clin Invest Med 1994; 17:115–122.
16. George SL. Reducing patient eligibility criteria in cancer clinical trials. J Clin Oncol 1996;14:1364–1370.
17. National Institutes of Health Office of Extramural Research. NIH policy and guidelines on the inclusion of women and minorities as subjects in clinical research—Amended, October, 2001. http://grants.nih.gov/grants/funding/women_min/guidelines_amended_10_2001.htm. Accessed March 3, 2005.
18. NETT Investigators. Patients at high risk of death after lung-volume—reduction surgery. N Engl J Med 2001; 345:1075–1083.
19. Altman DG, Schulz KF, Moher D et al for the CONSORT Group. The CONSORT statement: Revised recommendations for improving the quality of reports of parallel-group randomized trials. Ann Intern Med 2001; 134:663–694.
20. Meinert CL. Beyond CONSORT: need for improved reporting standards for clinical trials. JAMA 1998;279: 1487–1489.
21. Ellenberg JH. Selection bias in observational and experimental studies. Stat Med 1994; 13:557–567.
22. CASS Principal Investigators. Coronary artery surgery study (CASS): a randomized trial of coronary artery bypass surgery. Comparability of entry characteristics and survival in randomized patients and nonrandomized patients meeting randomization criteria. J Am Coll Cardiol 1984;3:114–128.

# CHAPTER 5

# Recruiting Research Participants

Janet B. McGill

S tudy recruitment has been called the rate-limiting step in clinical research. It is estimated that 25% of the delay in the clinical development of new therapies is due to difficulties with recruitment (1). In 1998, the average number of patients studied per new drug application (NDA) was 3,900, with projected increases of 7% per year. Industry-sponsored clinical trials required participation of about 140,000 persons in 1999; achieving that goal involved prescreening contact with 2.8 million individuals and on-site screening of nearly 600,000 (2). Volunteer participant numbers in clinical research sponsored by NIH or other agencies are not included in these figures. Estimates are that, as of 2005, 19.8 million volunteer participants will be needed for clinical research. Although healthy persons may participate in Phase 1 studies and in mechanistic translational research, the vast majority of volunteers in clinical research have an acute or chronic illness that is under study. Research volunteers who donate time and effort and who give permission for use of their protected health information (PHI), tissue, and genetic material are integral to the advancement of medical science. That they do so at a time of increased vulnerability, often under a cloud of negative publicity, demonstrates both the health concerns of average people and their willingness to contribute.

The earliest report of participation in a clinical investigation is recorded in the Old Testament. Daniel asked his Babylonian captors to observe him during a 10-day dietary intervention of vegetables rather than meats and wine. After successful completion of the study, the results were applied to others in the compound, with beneficial effects (3). More than two millennia later, during the 1900 yellow fever epidemic in Cuba, more than 30 men (including the four research physicians) volunteered to participate in a study of yellow fever exposure. Twenty-two developed yellow fever, which even today has a case-fatality rate of 20 to 50%, but there were no deaths (4). The study results implicated a mosquito vector and prompted health measures that ended the scourge in less than a year. The American volunteers were later listed in the Army Register's Roll of Honor for their participation (5). Today, Hoiyan Wan, Jesse Gelsinger, and Ellen Roche are remembered as enterprising young people who lost their lives while participating in translational clinical research (6). They, too, have changed history, prompting reform in many aspects of human research protection (7).

Medical research continues to rely on volunteer participation to populate the clinical laboratory. Examining the process of recruitment furthers the translation of breakthroughs in the basic science laboratory to treatments available to persons in need. Recruitment methods and results from large Phase 3 and 4 clinical trials are widely published and may be applicable to the needs of scientists who study human behavior and biology with cutting edge technology. This chapter focuses on the process and problems of recruitment for translational research.

## THE PLANNING STAGE

### Project Development

Accurate sample size estimates are critically important when planning any clinical research study (Chapter 9). Curiously, estimating the number of potential research participants that are needed to inform, contact, and screen to realize sample size goals is more difficult and less certain than doing the sample size estimate itself. Likewise, estimating the time, effort, and cost of recruitment is more difficult than budgeting for study personnel and procedures. Reports from large clinical trials are instructive, but they may or may not be relevant to smaller mechanistic and translational studies. Adding to the problem, the terminology used in published studies is inconsistent. In one study, screening participants might imply only a telephone call, whereas in another, screening refers to those who have signed a consent form and undergone on-site screening tests.

The following two examples illustrate some recruitment metrics. In a study of brain function, normal volunteers were needed as healthy controls. Of the 1,670 persons who responded to an advertisement, 23% were not interested, 51% did not meet the inclusion/exclusion criteria, 312 underwent on-site screening, and 157 ultimately participated in the study (8). In the second example, volunteers with Type 1 diabetes and microalbuminuria were needed for a clinical trial. A chart review of over 400 people with Type 1 diabetes uncovered fewer than 100 who were not taking excluded medications. Recruitment efforts produced 152 potential participants who underwent a prescreening 24-hour urine test, and 22 qualified for the study. Only 7 agreed to proceed to the next screening visit, and 5 were randomized (9).

In general, the number needed to contact (or charts needed to review) is 10 to 40 times the number needed to study (Figure 5–1). The number of interested people needed to screen by phone or on site is 2 to 5 times the number needed to study. Study planning (and grant writing) should include realistic estimates rather than statements of recruitment bravado: "We have access to a large population with elevated serum porcelain levels for the study of stiff Achilles tendons." Study budgets should be developed with recruitment challenges in mind.

### Sources for Research Volunteers

Investigators should carefully consider not only the numbers but also the potential sources of volunteers for a research study. Large projects may require a discussion of local and regional demographics, such as ethnic distribution by zip code and socioeconomic dispersion. Smaller translational projects often rely on convenience samples of research volunteers that may or may not be representative of the population in demographic and illness characteristics (Chapter 4). For NIH-sponsored research, the investigator

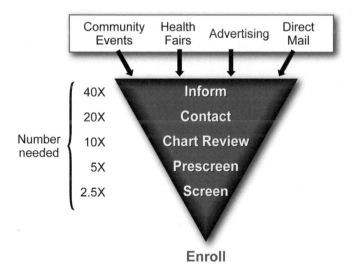

**FIGURE 5–1** ● The number of persons needed to be identified (or charts needed to be reviewed) may be as high as 40 times the number actually needed to be enrolled for any one study.

must outline the prevalence of the disease in question by ethnic group and describe whether the study population reflects that distribution of disease burden (10). If the sample of persons with a particular illness is to be drawn from a clinic population, grant reviewers expect to see a breakdown of the numbers of clinic or hospitalized patients who are affected by the illness in question and the percent who are expected to meet the study entry criteria. Letters of support from clinical colleagues who are invested in the project are useful. Translational studies that need healthy volunteers must rely on advertisements unless the investigator has an approved database of volunteers available. Recruitment plans that are well developed and adequate in scope will be noted during the grant review.

## REGULATORY REQUIREMENTS AND INCLUSION OF WOMEN AND MINORITIES

### Regulatory Requirements

Recruitment of people for purposes of experimentation is considered part of the research undertaking and therefore must meet the same regulatory requirements (Chapters 14 and 15) (10). The institutional review board (IRB) must approve the recruitment plan and each method of communication used in the recruitment process. Careful analysis of recruitment needs and advance planning are required to procure adequate funding, to draft the materials that will be used for recruitment, and to submit each piece of communication to the IRB for approval. The most important IRB mandates are that the tools used for recruitment purposes must inform the reader or listener that the purpose of the communication is research and that no promise of positive results or benefit is being made. The amount of detail required varies from one venue to another and from one IRB to another. Materials developed for multicentered trials for national distribution need local IRB approval. Even items that the study team views as educational should be submitted for IRB approval if they are to be used in the recruitment process.

The Health Insurance Portability and Accountability Act of 1996 (HIPAA) prompted the Department of Health and Human Services (HHS) to issue regulations regarding the use and disclosure of PHI (11). That set of regulations is known as the Privacy Rule. The Privacy Rule has provisions for the use of PHI for "preparatory research" in section 164.512(i)(1)(ii). These provisions allow covered entities such as hospitals or universities to permit researchers to review PHI to prepare research protocol or to aid in recruitment. Both activities require proper representation—meaning approval from the IRB (11). In order for a researcher to actually contact a patient, however, either the patient should have provided prior authorization, or the researcher can apply to the institutional IRB for a waiver of authorization. Physicians who have a treating relationship with a patient may introduce clinical research during a discussion of treatment alternatives.

The Privacy Rule also has a set of provisions for creating and using a database or repository for research (12). In general, a recruitment database should have IRB approval, and authorization from patients should be sought if PHI is to be used for research purposes. A database that contains PHI linked to personal identifiers should be electronically secure.

### Inclusion of Women and Minorities

In 1993, after decades of clinical research that involved predominantly white male populations, both the National Institutes of Health (NIH) and the Food and Drug Administration (FDA) issued guidelines for the inclusion of women and minorities in clinical studies. The NIH policy was amended in 2001 (13). The FDA provided guidance to ensure that new drugs are evaluated in women and removed the exclusion of women with childbearing potential from early phases of clinical trials (14). The NIH Revitalization Act instructed the NIH to monitor inclusion of women and minorities in clinical research. The stated intent of the guidelines is to remove barriers to participation by women and minorities, and they strongly recommend including women and minorities unless there is a compelling reason not to (13). Investigators and sponsors are expected to know whether the drug, device, or intervention is likely to show clinically important differences by gender, or race or ethnicity. If the answer is yes, the study should be powered to show or accommodate the differences in order to provide representation. If the answer is no, then inclusion of women and minorities is strongly encouraged so that differences will be detected if present. Recruitment plans should be designed to reach these groups regardless of the size of the proposed study. Often reaching these groups means increased recruitment effort and increased cost. For instance, in a study of bone loss and fracture risk, researchers found that minority recruitment required culturally sensitive strategies, and that the cost of recruiting a minority subject was five times the cost of recruiting a participant from the majority Caucasian population (15).

## Vulnerable Populations

Vulnerable populations include individuals or groups who lack autonomy by virtue of age (children), mental impairment, acute or severe physical or mental illness, pregnancy (the fetus is considered vulnerable), incarceration, or people who are economically or educationally disadvantaged. The Common Rule (45 CFR 46.111) (Chapter 14) contains regulatory language that mandates additional safeguards for research volunteers who are perceived to be "vulnerable to coercion or undue influence." (16) The investigator's relatives and immediate coworkers are now tacitly included in this definition and, in general, should not be recruited into the study. Although precise definitions and descriptions of process are lacking in the regulations, IRBs have become both more sophisticated and instructive in providing guidance for investigators. The NIH requires "that children (i.e., individuals under the age of 21) must be included in all human research, conducted or supported by the NIH, unless there are scientific and ethical reasons not to include them" (17). Both grant agencies and IRBs require a discussion of the appropriateness of including or excluding children in clinical research.

A pertinent question is: "How does an investigator recruit subjects who are considered vulnerable?" Often the first task is to determine decisional capability, which requires trained staff and may require additional observers for validation. Persons who are truly vulnerable generally have an advocate who is a parent, relative, or court-appointed guardian. Recruitment involves engaging both the potential volunteer and the advocate, and accommodating the needs of both. In the case of children, the parent must sign the informed consent, but the child will be asked to sign either the informed consent or an age-appropriate assent. Recruiting patients with acute physical or mental illness for research should involve the treating physician as well as the patient advocate.

Inpatient and outpatient medical settings are the prime sources for these individuals; however additional recruitment venues, designed specifically for some vulnerable populations, will be needed to meet the demand. Questions now being debated are asking whether it is ethical to contact children through schools or the Internet, for example.

## Stipends and Incentives

It is common practice to offer a stipend to volunteers for the time spent participating in a clinical study. This practice is particularly relevant to translational research where patients are likely to receive no other benefits and their time involved can be substantial. The ethics of offering payment have been debated, but in an empirical assessment Halpern et al. found that payment did not alter the perception of risk and did not have a differential influence on poorer patients (18). Clinical trials that offer testing, medication, and supplies do not always include monetary stipends. Regardless, the stipend should not be so large as to be viewed as an incentive to participation, and it must be prorated such that persons who withdraw from a study are not penalized. Stipend amounts should be approved by the IRB, specified in the consent, and included in the study budget.

## ATTITUDES: WHY DO PEOPLE PARTICIPATE IN CLINICAL RESEARCH?

### Attitudes About Participation

Attitudes toward clinical research are reported as generally, but not uniformly, positive by study participants and the public. Those interested in participating in clinical research cite both personal gain and altruism. Tolmie et al. found that among senior citizens, curiosity and self-interest are motivators to inquire about clinical trial participation, but the possibility of health screening and ongoing structured health monitoring may play a role in the decision to participate (19). A survey of over 1,000 study participants in Phase 2 or 3 clinical trials found that the most common reason for participation was finding an effective treatment (60%), followed by altruism (23%), monetary gain (11%), and hope of receiving better medical care (6%) (20). Such data emphasize the challenge of meeting recruitment goals in translational research studies where the possibilities finding a new effective treatment or better medical care are limited, if present at all. Nevertheless, a small study of pairs of psychiatrists and patients with schizophrenia in clinical trials showed that physicians were able to predict many of the patient concerns, such as ease of participation and privacy, but underestimated the patients' positive experience (21).

Surveys of persons who have actually participated in clinical trials represent a biased sample and may not reflect the attitudes of uninvolved persons in the community. For instance, a study of women who had received a mailed notice but declined to participate in the Women's Health Initiative Study of hormone replacement therapy reported that negative attitudes about clinical research in general and presumably non-caring clinical researchers were barriers to participation (22). Nonetheless, positive experiences as a participant in clinical research are commonly reported.

Among individuals with a positive perception of clinical research, not all elect to participate when information is presented. The gap between perception and action on the part of both individuals and practicing physicians who may decline to recommend study participation to their patients is often perplexing to clinical researchers. A physician-generated survey of women with breast cancer found that the main reason for failed enrollment among women who qualified for a variety of protocols was simply patient refusal (88%) (23). The underlying reasons for patient refusal and thus nonparticipation were not captured, and may or may not have been appreciated by the physician researcher. Understanding the barriers to study participation among informed persons is critical to the processes of recruitment and retention.

## The Personal Balance Account

An in-depth analysis of the determinants of patient participation using the Health Belief Model as a guideline found that patients employ a personal balance account in the decision-making process (24). Individuals project the physical and emotional value of study participation as compared to non-study treatment versus the risks and time of participation. The potential participant enters the clinical research arena with a unique frame of reference that includes a level of regard for medical experimentation in general, and beliefs and concerns about their illness, prior treatment, caregivers, and impact of the illness on the family. Verhaggen concluded that "Patient consent to trial participation can be explained by only a couple of variables, but the motivations for patient refusal are evidently quite diverse and patient-bound" (24). Reasons for nonparticipation in clinical studies include lack of awareness, uncertainty that the experimental treatment would be better than optimal treatment currently available, poor understanding of common clinical research methodology (such as randomization and use of placebos), concern about risk, and a variety of factors unique to the illness and the population in question. These factors, by necessity, are superimposed on life circumstances such as socioeconomic status, dependence on others, functional ability, time commitments, and family obligations.

The importance of patient factors was echoed in an interview-based study of patients' motivations to participate in Phase 1 cancer trials. Patients who are offered Phase 1 chemotherapy trials have generally exhausted other treatment possibilities and have progressive disease. Concerns about putative ethical dilemmas involving this population

were not supported by this study, which found that patients were well informed and generally positive about the experience. Moore stated, "Their current situation appeared to be the main factor in their decision-making, rather than any past values or attitudes towards experimental treatment" (25).

What motivates individuals to consider participation in clinical research? And how can investigators and sponsors effectively engage a person who might have an interest in becoming a study volunteer? Prochaska et al. developed a theoretical construct addressing health-related behavioral change (26). It contends that with regard to a particular health behavior, an individual may find himself or herself at one of five stages: precontemplation, contemplation, preparation, action, and maintenance. The personal accounting of the pros and cons of changing a behavior is termed decisional balance. According to this construct, certain things must happen for behavior to change, such as volunteering for clinical research. Moving forward from precontemplation requires that the pros of change increase. To move from contemplation, the cons of change must decrease. To engage in an action, the pros must exceed the cons (26).

Although not tested in clinical research, there are potential applications of this construct to the process of volunteer recruitment. Recruitment strategies may need to consider whether potential participants are likely to be ready for active participation in a clinical study. Key components in the process of moving someone from precontemplation to action might require communication of a sufficient information for decision making (increasing the pros), reassurance that the information is reliable and valid (decreasing the cons), and making a connection between the message about the clinical study in question to the disease state of the individual and the life issues that are ever present (helping to change the pro/con balance).

How well clinical investigators can communicate the need for participation and the procedures and risks of study participation while concurrently addressing concerns about an individual's personal balance account may determine the ultimate success of recruitment and retention in clinical research.

## BARRIERS TO RESEARCH PARTICIPATION

### Physical Barriers

Physical barriers to participation are not often considered in the literature but are well known to research staff and volunteers. For example, the vast majority of publicly funded translational research is done in universities, and most universities are located in congested areas of large cities. Within the university or hospital, the study location is often obscure, may lack signage, often has insufficient space, and sometimes compromises patient privacy. The distance from the parking lot or public transportation drop-off to the study site may be greater than the usual distance to a physician's office.

The location and appearance of clinical research facilities may have an impact on recruitment that is difficult to measure. It is appropriate for a potential volunteer to have questions, even suspicions, about the prospect of engaging in a research project. The location, appearance, and ease of use of the study site might be important factors to the volunteer with a personal balance sheet in mind. In one anecdote, a newly recruited research volunteer called from a portable phone to say that he was lost in the building and no longer interested in participating in the clinical study. In another instance, a motivated study participant, who was already randomized in a clinical trial, sent the study material back by courier to avoid returning to the study location, citing inconvenience and lack of privacy at the study site.

Investigators and institutions should collaborate to provide space that is accessible, pleasant, and private. Volunteers appreciate such amenities as coffee, a water cooler, reading material, and television for longer tests. Child care may be necessary for recruitment of a large cohort of women. Some sites provide videotapes and other educational materials about the illness under study so that family members can gain from the experience. Simple gestures, such as offering a coupon for a meal at the hospital cafeteria, may offset some of the irritation of fasting specifically and of participating generally. Volunteers appropriately expect that parking will be provided.

Research sites that are highly visible and accessible can be used for other activities like health screening and education. Focused health screening may increase the pool of individuals who are interested in participating in research and may be done in advance of the start-up of a study. Health screening can become an ongoing community outreach program that brings uninformed individuals into contact with a research environment and may help to reduce barriers to later participation. A key component for melding screening with recruitment is obtaining permission from the participant to call back for actual recruitment purposes, which implies using PHI for research. Although IRB approval is not generally necessary for general health screening, recruitment for current or future studies that asks for patient authorization for use of PHI should have IRB approval. In summary, if general information about research is handed to individuals

at a health fair, IRB approval is not needed. If the health-screening staff keeps identifiable PHI with the intent of contacting the person in the future, IRB approval and informed consent is required.

The most obvious physical barrier to research participation is distance from the study site. The vast majority of potential subjects live too far from university centers to consider participation in clinical research. Even within large cities, distances and travel time can be daunting for those who are ill or impaired. Creative solutions might entail enlisting local physicians as subinvestigators connected electronically to the research site, or the establishment of study centers in rural areas. Recruitment of ethnic minorities such as Native Americans requires accessible study locations. As research enters the realm of genomic testing, finding suitable candidates outside the usual referral area and making the study possible for the participant may require innovative solutions to distance problems.

## Attitudes Among Minorities and Women

African Americans' participation in clinical research has received considerable attention in the literature because of persistently low enrollment in clinical studies. For example, the Prostate, Lung, Colorectal and Ovarian Cancer Screening Trial enrolled only 5.1% African Americans despite the fact that they are disproportionately affected by some of these cancers and structured screening was provided at no cost (27). Barriers cited were lack of knowledge, mistrust, fear of exploitation, and the Tuskegee Syphilis Study. Based on a background of suspicion dating to medical misdeeds during slavery and the postbellum South, the Tuskegee study is viewed as validation of how uninformed minority individuals can be mistreated by the medical research establishment. Misconceptions about the process, the value of informed consent, and concern about the lack of individualization in research are troublesome to African Americans. Clinical research participation is generally perceived as another unwanted task for this minority population.

Changing the perception that research is "being done on you" to research as an important collaboration between physicians and participants is an ongoing challenge. Investigators who are able to communicate their interest in identifying individual illness conditions and responses to testing or treatment among persons from various backgrounds fare better than investigators who wish to fill categorical slots with minority participants. Increasing minority participation depends on establishing trust, developing closer ties to the community, and reexamining the benefits offered to participants. The addition of increased regulation and safety measures has not changed the pervasiveness of negative perceptions about clinical research among minority individuals. Culturally sensitive materials and research staff members are important to the process of engaging diverse minority populations.

Poor enrollment of women in clinical studies has a different set of concerns. Historically, women were not included in many large clinical trials and also were avoided in smaller translational projects. More recent cardiovascular trials have included women, but enrollment is typically less than 25% (28). Overall, it has been difficult to pinpoint the exact reasons for low participation rates of women. Some possibilities include a less frequent background in science among older women generally, less flexibility with work time, and more obligations at home (such as child care). Women may be somewhat less likely to encounter advertisements for clinical research in the newspaper and on the radio but more likely to open the mail. Women are more likely to need family support, whether emotional or physical, to participate.

### Attitudes of Treating Physicians

A component of recruitment that merits attention is the input of private treating physicians. A survey of African American physicians regarding their perceptions of clinical research revealed the following factors that influenced recruitment of African Americans: lack of awareness, concern about patient mistrust of the medical community, additional administrative tasks when a participant is enrolled in a study, and blinded treatment assignment (29). Investigators can understand the dilemma of a busy practitioner who is asked by a patient about a clinical research project that is unknown to the physician. The equipoise response is often reluctance to recommend participation when the risks of the study and the investigator are unknown to the treating physician. A vote of no confidence from a trusted caregiver has a powerful negative influence on an undecided individual, particularly in minority communities. In a study of attrition from the National Marrow Donor Program, the authors found that those who were discouraged from joining initially had more than double the attrition rate at 4 years and that those encouraged by professionals had half the expected attrition rate (30).

Communication between the research team and the treating physician should continue throughout the study, which will add to the overall safety of the patient. Although universities are happy to inform practicing physicians about the results of the latest research project, they have been less successful teaching physicians about the process and importance of participatory research. Treating physicians have a role in counseling patients about therapeutic misconceptions and acting as trusted advisors (31). Participation in clinical research should be viewed as an activity that will connect doctors and patients with researchers to promote the welfare of the larger community, including the next generation.

## STUDY DESIGN AND IMPLEMENTATION

### Inclusion, Exclusion, and Demographics

Study design plays an important role in whether recruitment will be successful. The high frequency of protocol changes in response to slow enrollment attests to problems in the initial design. The theoretical advantages of studying a homogeneous patient population (Chapter 4) relate to reduced measurement variation with a reduced sample size required to detect the effect of an experimental variation. However, by limiting enrollment to persons within a certain age range, with defined disease severity, and with a limited number of comorbid conditions and concomitant medications (or other restrictions), the difficulties in recruitment may actually make recruitment more difficult and prolong the enrollment phase of the study.

The most common exclusion criterion, and thus design barrier to recruitment, is age restriction. Underrepresentation of elderly patients has been well documented in cancer and cardiovascular studies (32). Many studies use an upper age cutoff of 70 years despite evidence that toxicity may not be increased in the elderly. This practice has changed recently, and it is now common for cancer studies in particular to report results by age categories. Poor accrual of older subjects across cancer types when age is not a specified exclusion speaks to other barriers for persons in older age groups. Socioeconomic variables have been posited but have not been clearly identified as barriers to elder participation in clinical studies. Additional study procedures might entail additional visits, tests, and drugs to combat side effects. Increased complexity, dependence on supportive relatives, and lack of remuneration are barriers to persons with functional limitations. Transportation is a pressing need, and expensive to provide for this population of patients. Investigators should consider the potential contribution of older patients before applying arbitrary age restrictions, even in mechanistic or early phase research.

There is an interaction between age restriction and the number of women enrolled in clinical studies of heart failure and acute coronary syndromes because women develop cardiovascular diseases at older ages (33). The typical heart failure study design requires a defined level of systolic dysfunction and may limit the level of renal impairment. African American patients are more likely to have hypertension-induced diastolic dysfunction and concomitant renal impairment. In retrospect, exclusion of persons with diabetes in both cardiovascular and kidney disease trials may have contributed to recruitment delays and may limit the application of results to the growing segment of the population affected by these disorders.

Although some proponents of inclusion favor the NIH requirements, others have called for additional studies to clarify treatment concerns in minority populations. The very successful African American Study of Kidney Disease and Hypertension (AASK) provided answers about the treatment of persons with hypertensive kidney disease (34). Low enrollment of African Americans in studies of heart failure and diabetic nephropathy has left similar questions unanswered, despite the excess disease burden in this group, leading to studies being planned that exclusively target the African American population (35).

Restrictive inclusion criteria can have unintended secondary effects. Weight loss trials commonly report results in percent loss of body weight and typically accept patients within a defined range of body mass index (BMI). Curiously, the most common reason for excluding a subject in weight loss trials is "too overweight." Diabetes trials are notorious for restrictive age and BMI criteria, which puts the studies off limits to segments of the population. For example, Asians are at risk for diabetes when their BMI exceeds 23 $kg/m^2$. Limiting the enrollment of persons with higher BMI may limit the recruitment of Asian Americans. Similarly, exclusions on the high end of the BMI spectrum may adversely affect enrollment in the Southeast and Midwest, and potentially impact participation among women and minorities. Many of these potential study participants are excluded during the initial phone interview; hence, they are not listed as screen failures at the study site and therefore are not identified as potential volunteers for future studies.

Careful examination of inclusion and exclusion criteria in light of changing population demographics, disease susceptibility, and study endpoints will allow more inclusive policies and should enhance recruitment and enrollment. When entry criteria are by necessity highly restrictive, methods to expand the pool of available participants should be planned and employed early.

## Disease State Criteria

Disease states that are narrowly defined can impede recruitment efforts. Finding volunteers with diabetes, hypertension, rheumatoid arthritis, glaucoma, HIV, and many other illnesses who are naïve to therapy or who have failed specific therapies can be difficult. Temporary withdrawal of proven therapy may be possible in some conditions (e.g., hypertension or acne) but presents an ethical dilemma for others, such as HIV or epilepsy. Prolonged withdrawal of therapy that requires a disease flare, as in arthritis or asthma, may be problematic. Smaller translational studies and early phase trials often require that participants have similar disease characteristics to limit variability. As "biologics" leave the laboratory and approach the clinic, it is common for both early and later stage testing to be done in persons with the disease in question, which is often narrowly defined with the intent of limiting the number needed to study.

Genomic testing of individuals for both disease characteristics and response to therapy is a field in its infancy. Currently, the use of this type of testing to define treatment is largely restricted to some cancers. It is possible to envision a time when therapies will be developed for resistant viruses or virus-host interactions, to modulate specific immune responses, to affect a receptor subtype, or to interact with a particular enzymatic pathway (and many more possibilities). Finding study participants with unique genotypic characteristics, infections, or tumors will require entirely new approaches for research recruitment (36). Projections for the numbers needed to inform, contact, and screen will need to be revised. Volunteer pools of the future may consist of deidentified DNA, which is screened in advance of screening the patient. Consent procedures will need to be reevaluated to accommodate these advances.

## Study Visits and Procedures

Deterrents to study participation in translational research are often found in the study protocol. In addition to typical medical procedures, such as physical examination, blood draws, imaging, and electrocardiogram, cutting edge studies often include invasive procedures such as infusions, endoscopy, colonoscopy, or biopsies of skin, nerve, muscle, kidney, liver, or fat tissue. Compensation for both time and procedures is limited by IRB mandates to avoid offering incentives. The time consumed and the rigid schedule of study visits can deter the most willing volunteer. Lack of scheduling flexibility may impede the recruitment of hourly workers and those with child care responsibilities. Clinical studies in diabetes, hypertension, lipids, and even arthritis stipulate fasting conditions for all visits, even though many interim visits are for safety rather than endpoint testing. Complex testing may require specialized facilities such as the NIH-sponsored General Clinical Research Centers, mass spectrometry, cyclotrons, PET scanners, or other specialized facilities. Scheduling study visits that are convenient is often not possible and thus limits the pool of participants to those who can meet the time demands of the study. Provision of overnight accommodations and meals will assist some volunteers who need to travel to the center.

## Screening Approaches

Staged or stepped screening over several visits has been used in some studies to minimize the time consumed by screening visits, to avoid unnecessary testing, and to allow time for the participant to develop a relationship with the study staff and familiarity with the study requirements. Some have touted staged screening as a method of reducing the dropout rate, while others have found the idea appropriate when large numbers of potential participants are needed and there is uncertainty about qualification. For example, the Diabetes Prevention Program used a four-step screening process (37). The first study visit used an abbreviated consent and tested only height, weight, and fasting blood glucose. The next step was an oral glucose tolerance test. The third step was a placebo run-in period to test compliance and compatibility. Sufficient time was allotted in the process for potential participants to formulate questions, discuss the study with their family and treating physician, and develop a relationship with the study staff before making a multiyear commitment. Industry-sponsored clinical trials often operate with an overriding sense of urgency, loading screening visits with expensive testing that will not be used if the patient is disqualified as the result of common, predictable laboratory abnormalities.

Phone screening is standard practice, and if done well reduces the time and expense of on-site screening. Documentation of every screening call is requested by grant agencies and industry sponsors in order to meet the requirements of the Consolidated Standard for Reporting of Trials (CONSORT). All persons evaluated for a clinical trial including screen failures, nonqualifiers, enrolled subjects, drops, and completers should be counted (38). Experienced study staff members are aware that phone screening is a good opportunity to establish a relationship with the potential volunteer, to answer questions about research in general and to identify whether the individual might be a candidate for a future study if he or she does not qualify for the current protocol. If the volunteer appears to qualify and has continued interest after the study procedures are explained, scheduling in the near future promotes the best adherence with the first visit.

Newer study designs select subjects for randomization based on response to therapy during the run-in phase in order to enrich the final cohort with subjects who are both compliant with and who respond to the therapy under study. Although the internal validity and applicability of this design has been debated, the impact on recruitment is clear (39). The recruitment to randomization ratio is increased along with the challenge of finding not just suitable, but ideal, study subjects. Both of these strategies increase the workload of recruitment and screening, which is less well reimbursed per hour spent than are follow-up visits of a randomized participant.

Emergency, intensive care and some cancer studies need rapid referrals and immediate decisions by the volunteer so that the treatment plan can be adjusted as part of the study. Any study with a narrow window of opportunity for recruitment and enrollment requires a well-organized and vigilant approach. Considerable time is spent educating colleagues and staff members to generate referrals. Study designs that permit longer lead times, allowing for a few doses of standard antibiotics, anticoagulation, pain medications, or the like before randomization, may be able to increase enrollment without compromising the validity of the study.

## Treatment Considerations

Randomized, placebo-controlled clinical studies have the most statistical rigor, but have been subject to some criticism. When no treatment exists or is approved for the condition in question, a placebo-controlled design is appropriate (40). However, informed persons may decline to participate in studies that are placebo-controlled, especially if the illness in question is serious or highly symptomatic. Several problems can be envisioned: the first is the ethical dilemma of depriving persons who are ill of effective therapy for more than short periods of time. IRBs are questioning the ethics of study designs that have been used for many years and are thus considered standard for the disease state. The recruitment problems of placebo-controlled studies are reflected in the interpretation of the study results. If only mildly affected participants are recruited for placebo-controlled studies, they may be more susceptible to both study and placebo effect. This effect has occurred in depression studies and may occur in other disease states (41).

As medicine moves from small molecules to biologic therapies, study participants will be asked to take investigational medications given by either intravenous or subcutaneous injections. The pharmacokinetics and risks of these therapies will differ from those of typical medications and monitoring the administration of some foreign proteins requires more attention from investigators. Recruiting participants for these studies, especially if they are told that the injections they receive might contain a placebo, will be challenging (42).

A second design issue that can impact recruitment is the use of either concomitant or rescue medications. Even in conditions as benign as allergic rhinitis, participants may be concerned about restrictions in the use of rescue medications. Trials of pain medications or interventions commonly include rescue medications, and the use of rescue therapy can be monitored as a secondary study endpoint. Any trial that is done in a disease state that is not life threatening but is highly symptomatic, whether from itching or shortness of breath, should consider planned rescue therapy that can be standardized and monitored. Investigators may find that in studies requiring concomitant medications, whether anti-emetics for chemotherapy or antirejection medications for experimental transplant procedures, the added expense is a deterrent to participation.

Realistic defined stopping points are appropriate for clinical studies of diseases in which current therapy is available, such as diabetes, hypertension, seizure disorders, HIV, and many others. Barriers to recruitment occur when the study-specified rescue medication or stopping point is far beyond current treatment guidelines. An example is the continued use of a fasting blood glucose level of 270 mg/dL (15 mmol/L) as the predefined stopping point in today's diabetes trials.

### Staff Time

A hidden cause of slow recruitment is the conflict for time experienced by many study coordinators. These critically important individuals to the research endeavor often have diverse duties, among the most time consuming is paperwork. The ever-increasing demands of IRBs, radiation safety boards, General Clinical Research Center applications, the contracts office, the sponsor, the NIH, and the FDA make starting any study a test of endurance. Once the study is under way and the few available participants have been enrolled, the coordinator or other staff member must tackle the unexpected duties of data entry. As standard office notes and noncarbon case report forms vanish from the scene, complex standard visit sheets and electronic data capture have taken their place (Chapters 10 and 11). Each system is a unique design, requires training, and results in extended monitoring visits from the sponsor's representative. Every error, question, or concern requires additional data entry from the staff. Some studies mandate double data entry, which is announced at the start-up meeting. Study sites that are successful tend to have a staff member dedicated to recruitment—in some cases, outsourcing the regulatory burden to centralized clinical research resources that are available at some institutions. (For information about one such site, see http://ccs.wustl.edu.)

## CURRENT RECRUITMENT PRACTICES

### The Investigator's Practice

The most common recruitment strategy for an investigational site is to call or contact potential participants with whom the investigators have a treating relationship. This strategy has advantages and disadvantages. The advantages are that the principal investigator (PI) has access to medical records that can confirm eligibility and may know whether the potential participant is sufficiently compliant with treatment and follow up to do well in a clinical trial. Many trials use the results from routine clinical testing and follow-up that is paid by third parties in conjunction with study medications and visits. Clinical trials in cancer; studies involving surgery, biopsies, endoscopy; and some HIV and cardiovascular studies may require this type of collaborative payment arrangement. (However, it is critically important that all research-related laboratory testing be strictly paid for by study funds and not by third-party insurance—see Chapter 15). People who have insurance carriers that are not accepted by the study physician or institution would simply not be eligible for the study. An unspoken concern is that uninsured people would not qualify due to lack of paid follow-up and testing. Although Medicare covers routine clinical care and testing that occur when a person is enrolled in a clinical trial, some insurance carriers do not and people may risk losing coverage if they agree to participate in research. State laws that govern the insurance industry are inconsistent. Uncertainty on the part of volunteers adds to recruitment difficulty.

If the PI is part of a group practice or university, the pool of eligible participants may be sufficiently large to provide adequate enrollment. Often, recruitment is slow because the cohort of potential participants is not as large as expected, and the accrual of new patients with the exact qualifications is uncertain. Investigators may not know in advance whether people will agree to participate in a clinical study and overestimation is common. Primary or specialty physicians from within or outside of the institution can be contacted using IRB-approved informational letters, brochures, and placards. Personal contact by the PI may be the most effective approach to elicit help from professional colleagues. It is important to remember that finder's fees generally are not acceptable to IRBs. These relationships can be built at low cost.

Experienced investigators recognize that people who have had a positive experience in one project will participate in subsequent clinical research. Persons with asthma, hypertension, diabetes, arthritis, GI problems, skin diseases, and many other disorders may become repeat volunteers. They value the relationship with the study physician and nursing staff as an "extra" to their usual health care. Inclusion and exclusion criteria typically specify the period of time that a person must be free of a prior investigational medication before starting another study. Individuals who donate blood or who participate in metabolic studies may require monitoring for anemia, while those who have received radioactive isotopes need counseling about radiation exposure before considering additional study participation.

Translational research may need volunteers with particular disease characteristics or genomic traits. The most direct way to access these people is to include a treating physician as part of the project. Experienced clinicians can be valuable partners to physician-scientists both for their expertise and access to patients.

## Institutional Resources

Investigators can often find assistance with recruitment of study participants within the institution. Some university clinical centers are able to generate lists of potential participants based on diagnosis codes, and to determine who has given authorization for use of PHI for research and permission to be called about a clinical study. Narrowing the search requires access to medical information on potential participants, a process that may require IRB approval. Alternatively, investigators can post placards in clinical areas, staff can hand cards to potential participants, and the treating physician can introduce the idea of study participation during a routine clinic visit. All of these materials need IRB approval. Nurses acting as recruitment coordinators may be needed for busy areas like emergency departments, cardiac catheterization labs, and cancer centers. Often the research fellow or PI must remind colleagues, nurses, and staff numerous times about an ongoing clinical study to maintain their interest. The major disadvantage to relying on others for recruitment or referral is that they may not know the details of the study, are certainly not as passionate about getting it done, or may neglect to mention it at all to potential participants.

Some institutions have recognized the need to assist investigators with recruitment efforts. Most hospitals and universities use public relations departments to publicize results of studies done by local investigators, but assistance with recruitment may be fragmented. One unique program, known as Volunteer for Health (VFH), began as a database for study subjects to support efforts of Diabetes Research and Training Center investigators (43). The program is now university-wide and maintains a database of over 20,000 potential volunteers who have provided contact information, health history information, health interests, and permission to be called for possible participation in appropriate studies. These persons have chosen to volunteer by contacting VFH in person, by phone, or via the website, http://vfh.wustl.edu. Investigators who register their studies with VFH get assistance with IRB approval for website information and designing posters, placards and other recruitment materials. The VFH phone number can be used for advertising campaigns, and the staff refers callers to the study coordinator or PI. VFH staff can also handle phone and mail prescreening.

A stated goal of VFH is to generate positive interactions between the university and the interested public. Serving volunteers as well as investigators is an unusual aspect of this university-supported program. The IRB reviews VFH annually, and all materials used for the program are approved before release.

## Media and Public Relations

Use of mass media to communicate clinical trial opportunities has become standard practice, both for publicly-funded and industry-sponsored clinical studies. The choice of communication varies depending on the penetration of potential subjects within a population, the cost, and the prior experience of the investigative site. Information about clinical studies is transmitted via print, radio, television, and the Internet. Occasionally billboards are used to advertise for clinical studies. Very large studies use direct mail for recruitment, which has the advantage of zip code selection. Advertising venues are selected contingent on factors such as prior experience of the study team, budget constraints, and the need to target a particular demographic subset of the population. For example, recruitment for an osteoporosis study might use a religious radio station and bulletins at senior centers or churches. Studies involving men only are often recruited with ads in the sports section of the local newspaper. Coordination of media efforts by an institution provides volume discounts and better placement of news spots. Communication with local physicians in addition to the public should not be overlooked.

Use of the Internet for subject recruitment has received considerable attention recently. Several sites list enrolling studies and provide contact information for the investigator. First on a list of nearly 100 sites is http://www.ClinicalTrials.gov, which is sponsored by the NIH. Interested persons can learn a lot about the listed trials and about the process of participation in clinical research. Some sites allow interested participants to register for studies by providing demographic and health information, which is forwarded to the investigator. Typically, if a person does not qualify for the selected study, the online interview ends abruptly. The overall utility of this venue in placing subjects in studies has not been reviewed, so the metrics are unclear. Most call centers and Web enrollment sites do not provide an opportunity to ask questions, which is an important part of building a relationship.

In the near future, all funded studies will be listed on websites. The International Standard Randomized Controlled Trial Number (ISRCTN) will be used to identify treatment trials globally, and may lead to greater accountability by the sponsors to make study results available at the conclusion of the trial. Clinical trials can be registered at http://www.controlled-trials.com. The value of public registries of clinical trials may be to verify information that is received through another source, whether advertisement or physician referral. The combined efforts of investigators, study teams, sponsors, granting agencies, and public intervention groups will be needed to meet the growing demand for research participation in the coming years.

## SUMMARY

- To be successful, planning for a clinical research study should include estimates of the numbers of potential research participants that are needed to inform, contact, and screen to achieve the desired sample size. Costs associated with these functions should be incorporated into budget planning.
- Not only the numbers, but the potential sources of volunteers for a research study should be considered.
- The IRB must approve the recruitment plan and each method of communication used in the recruitment process. These plans must take into account protection of private health information as regulated by HIPAA.
- Federally-sponsored research, and most national foundation research, must include women and minorities, or must give cogent reasons why such efforts cannot or should not be made.
- Reasons for nonparticipation in clinical studies include lack of awareness, uncertainty that the experimental intervention would be better than optimal treatment currently available, poor understanding of common clinical research methodology (such as randomization and use of placebos), concern about risk, and factors unique to the illness and the population in question.
- Other barriers to participation include physical barriers, attitudinal barriers by both volunteers and the treating physician, unnecessarily restrictive inclusion and exclusion criteria, disease states that are narrowly defined, and complex testing procedures.
- Some strategies for improving recruitment include staged or stepped screening, effective use of screening by phone, dedicated personnel, attention to protocol issues such as rescue therapies, collaboration with physicians with large practices in specific therapeutic areas, effective use of the media, and the use of institutional resources that support research recruitment.

## REFERENCES

1. Association of Clinical Research Professionals. Report on future trends. The Monitor 1998;12:13–26.
2. Kroll JA, ed. An Industry in Evolution. Boston: CenterWatch, 2001.
3. Old Testament. Daniel 1:8–18.
4. Pierce JR. "In the interest of humanity and the cause of science": the yellow fever volunteers. Mil Med 2003;168:857–863.
5. McCarthy M. A century of the U.S. Army yellow fever research. Lancet 2001;357:1772.
6. Steinbrook R. Protecting research subjects—the crisis at Johns Hopkins. N Engl J Med 2002;346:716–720.
7. Steinbrook R. Improving protection for research subjects. N Engl J Med 2002;346:1425–1430.
8. Shtasel DL, Gur RE, Mozley PD et al. Volunteers for biomedical research. Recruitment and screening of normal controls. Arch Gen Psychiatry 1991;48:1022–1025.
9. McGill, JB. Unpublished data.

10. NIH Grants Policy Statement. http://grants2.nih.gov/grants/policy/nihgps_2003/NIHGPS_Part5.htm#_Toc5 4600079. Accessed March 3, 2005.

11. Clinical Research and the HIPAA Privacy Rule. http://privacyruleandresearch.nih.gov/clin_research.asp. Accessed March 5, 2005.

12. Research Repositories, Databases, and the HIPAA Privacy Rule. http://privacyruleandresearch.nih.gov/research_repositories.asp. Accessed March 5, 2005.

13. NIH Policy and guidelines on the inclusion of women and minorities as subjects in clinical research— Amended, October, 2001. http://grants2nih.gov/grants/funding/women_min/guidelines_amended_10_2001.htm Accessed March 2, 2005.

14. Merkatz RB, Temple R, Sobel S et al. Women in clinical trials of new drugs. A change in Food and Drug Administration Policy. N Engl J Med 1993;329:292–296.

15. Marquez MA, Muhs JM, Tosomeen A et al. Costs and strategies in minority recruitment for osteoporosis research. J Bone Miner Res 2003;18:3–8.

16. Code of Federal Regulations. Title 45 Public Welfare DHHS NIH Office for Protection from Research Risks. Part 46 Protection Human Subjects. Effective December 13, 2001. http://www.intraining.com/ohsrsite/guidelines/45cfr46.html. Accessed March 3, 2005.

17. NIH Office of Extramural Research. Inclusion of Children Policy Implementation. http://grants1.nih.gov/grants/funding/children/children.htm. Accessed March 3, 2005.

18. Halpern SD, Karlawish JHT, Casarett D et al. Empirical assessment of whether moderate payments are undue or unjust inducements for participation in clinical trials. Arch Intern Med 2004;164:801–803.

19. Tolmie, EP, Mungall MMB, Louden G et al. Understanding why older people participate in clinical trial: the experience of the Scottish PROSPER participants. Age Ageing 2004;33:374–378.

20. Getz K. "Study volunteer behaviors and attitudes in industry-sponsored clinical trials" presented at the Institute of Medicine's Clinical Roundtable, Washington DC, September 25, 2000.

21. Warner TD, Roberts LW, Nguyen K. Do psychiatrists understand research-related experiences, attitudes, and motivations of schizophrenia study participants? Compr Psychiatry 2003;44(3):227–233.

22. Mouton CP, Harris S, Rovi S et al. Barriers to black women's participation in cancer clinical trials. J Natl Med Assoc 1997;89:721–727.

23. Simon MS, Du W, Flaherty L et al. Factors associated with breast cancer clinical trials participation and enrollment at a large academic medical center. J Clin Oncol 2004;22:2046–2052.

24. Verheggen FW, Nieman F, Jonkers R. Determinants of patient participation in clinical studies requiring informed consent: why patients enter a clinical trial. Patient Educ Couns 1998;35:111–125.

25. Moore S. A need to try everything: patient participation in phase 1 trials. J Adv Nurs 2001;33:738–747.

26. Prochaska JO, Redding CA, Evers KE. The transtheoretical model and stages of change.In Glanz K, Rimer BK, Lewis FM, eds. Health Behavior and Health Education:

Theory, Research, and Practice. 3rd Ed. San Francisco: Jossey-Bass, 2002: 99–120.

27. Andriole GL, Reding D, Hayes RB et al. PLCO Steering Committee. The prostate, lung, colon, and ovarian (PLCO) cancer screening trial: status and promise. Urol Oncol 2004;22:358–361.

28. Harris DJ, Douglas PS. Enrollment of women in cardiovascular clinical trials funded by the National Heart, Lung and Blood Institute. N Engl J Med 2000;343:475–480.

29. Lynch GF, Gorelick PB, Raman R et al. A pilot of African-American physician perceptions about clinical trials. J Natl Med Assoc 2001;93(12 Suppl):8S–13S.

30. Switzer GE, Dew MA, Stukas AA et al. Factors associated with attrition from a national bone marrow registry. Bone Marrow Transplant 1999;24:313–319.

31. Chen DT, Miller FG, Rosenstein DL. Clinical research and the physician-patient relationship. Ann Int Med 2003;138:669–672.

32. Lee PY, Alexander KP, Hammill, BG et al. Representation of elderly persons and women in published randomized trials of acute coronary syndromes. JAMA 2001; 286:708–713.

33. Heiat A, Gross CP, Krumholz HM. Representation of the elderly, women, and minorities in heart failure clinical trials. Arch Intern Med 2002;162:1682–1688.

34. Wright JT, Bakris G, Greene T et al. Effect of blood pressure lowering and antihypertensive drug class on progression of hypertensive kidney disease: results from the AASK trial for the African American study of kidney disease and hypertension study group. JAMA 2002;288:2421–2431.

35. African-American Heart Failure Trial. http://clinicaltrials.gov/ct/show/NCT00047775?order/1. Accessed March 3, 2005.

36. Lesko LJ, Rowland M, Peck CC et al. Optimizing the science of drug development: opportunities for better candidate selection and accelerated evaluation in humans. J Clin Pharm 2000;40:803–814.

37. The DPP Research Group. The Diabetes Prevention Program: recruitment methods and results. Control Clin Trials 2002;23:157–171.

38. Moher D, Schulz KF, Altman D, for the CONSORT Group. The CONSORT Statement: revised recommendations for improving the quality of reports of parallel-group randomized trials. JAMA 2001; 285:1987–1991.

39. Leber PD, Davis CS. Threats to the validity of clinical trials employing enrichment strategies for sample selection. Control Clin Trials 1998;19:178–187.

40. Emanuel EJ, Miller FG. The ethics of placebo-controlled trials—a middle ground. N Engl J Med 2001; 345:915–919.

41. Walsh BT, Seidman SN, Sysko R et al. Placebo response in studies of major depression: variable, substantial and growing. JAMA 2002;287:1840–1847.

42. Vincent-Gattis M, Webb C, Foote MA. Clinical research strategies in biotechnology. Biotechnol Ann Rev 2000; 5:259–267.

43. Schuster DP, McGill J. The right infrastructure can help you attract clinical trials to an AMC. Applied Clin Trials 2001;10:44–52.

# CHAPTER 6

# Reducing Bias

Bradley Evanoff

Of the many difficulties that can befall a clinical research study, bias is one of the most common and difficult to control. The term *bias* refers to *systematic* errors that can occur at any one of multiple points during the planning, conduct, analytic, or reporting stages of a research study. Bias occurs, for instance, when a procedure or measurement produces differences between groups that are consistently in the same direction. For example, if all participants in a study of weight loss were weighed on one scale, and all participants in the control group were weighed on another scale, a bias would be present if the two scales were calibrated differently. Nonsystematic errors, by contrast, are *random*. Importantly, random errors can be quantified and evaluated by statistical analysis and testing. Statistical analysis is of little value in managing bias.

Bias is also distinct from confounding and effect modification. As discussed in Chapter 3, confounding occurs if a variable, not thought to lie on the hypothesized mechanistic path between a cause and effect, is nevertheless systematically related to both the independent variable (e.g., the exposure or intervention in an experimental study) and the outcome. For example, a study showing an association between coffee drinking and myocardial infarction could be confounded by cigarette smoking, which is causally associated with the outcome (MI), and associated with the exposure (people who drink more coffee are more likely to smoke). The observed relationship between coffee drinking and MI might be spurious. Effect modifiers, on the other hand, are variables that can affect the relationship between the intervention (or the exposure to a risk factor) and the outcome. For example, a

medication may have different effects in smokers and nonsmokers, or a physiologic effect could change with the age of the subject. In other words, confounders and effect modifiers can lead to errors in interpretation of study results, but they are variables, not errors themselves.

Clinical experimental studies are subject to a wide range of such systematic errors. The clinical researcher must think through each step of a study, from initial conception to publication, to ensure that the results are not subject to one of the many types of bias that can plague it. The reason these types of errors are problematic is that they may appear to weaken what is otherwise a true association between an experimental condition and an outcome, or may produce a spurious association, or may distort the apparent direction of a relationship or association between variables. The inability to exclude a potential bias may limit the impact or generalizability of a study's findings, as reviewers and readers will be uncertain of the validity of the study's results.

As already noted, bias can occur at many different stages in a research study. Indeed, it can even occur before a study is conceived—for instance, if an investigator is not careful when performing the initial search of the relevant research literature (Chapter 2). Selectively reading literature that only supports the investigator's preconceived notions could obviously lead an investigator astray before a study is even planned.

Bias can also occur when specifying and selecting the study sample, for instance by selecting control participants who are systematically different from the study participants with the outcome of interest. Bias can occur in the execution of the experimental protocol in a variety of ways. In an unblinded study, an investigator may devote extra attention or otherwise treat the experimental group differently from a control group, thereby affecting the study's results. The measurement of experimental outcomes is another area in which a variety of biases may occur, if different procedures, measurement methods, or methods of interpreting data are used among different groups. Biases can occur in data analysis and data interpretation, particularly when investigators do not adhere to analytic plans that were described before the data collection, but perform post hoc analyses after the main study results are known. Such analyses are especially tempting if the results from the planned a priori study analysis are disappointing. Finally, bias may also occur when publishing the results, as investigators may be less likely to submit for publication, and journals less likely to accept for publication, "negative" studies. As Sackett points out (1), this type of publication bias brings us back to the first point, as bias in a study may begin with the review of existing literature.

These types of bias are common in translational and experimental clinical research, and they will be discussed in greater detail below, as well as steps that can be taken to reduce or eliminate them. However be aware that dozens of other types of bias are also important in observational or epidemiologic forms of clinical research (1).

## SAMPLING ERRORS

Translational and experimental clinical research depends on using a study sample to represent a larger population (Chapter 4). The generalizability of study findings (external validity) depends on being able to draw inferences from that sample population to the larger population of interest. Thus, any bias in the selection of the study sample (selection bias) can greatly affect a study's external validity.

The individuals chosen for a study can also have deleterious effects on the *internal* validity of the research. The choice of appropriate control participants can be particularly vexing, especially in nonexperimental observational studies in which the exposure to an intervention or risk factor is not under the control of the investigator. Both the procedures used to select study participants and the factors that influence a potential participant's decision to volunteer for a study can lead to selection bias. For instance, volunteers for a disease screening study may have symptoms or known predispositions for disease, leading to a bias toward a higher prevalence of disease. When different relationships between exposures and disease status exist between people who choose to participate or not participate in a study, or

people who are eligible or ineligible for a study, spurious associations can occur.

A commonly described form of selection bias is self-selection bias. Persons who volunteer for clinical studies, or who willingly participate in clinically recommended screening procedures, are likely to be systematically different from persons who do not volunteer or comply with recommended screening. The size of a clinical effect observed in a treated group of self-selected participants may be different from that seen when the treatment is later applied to the general population. Similarly, the prevalence of a given exposure or given disease outcome among self-selected participants may differ from that seen in the general population.

Another form of selection bias is termed *diagnostic bias* (1). Diagnostic bias can occur when physicians are more likely to consider certain diagnoses in patients who have another condition or another exposure. For instance, physicians may have a higher index of suspicion for some diseases in patients who take certain medications or have habits such as smoking. Particularly for conditions that may go undetected in many patients, there is the possibility of a spurious association occurring because one group may be subjected to more diagnostic procedures than another group. Likewise, diagnostic bias may occur among patients who are regularly seen or treated for one disorder. Because of greater contact with physicians, patients regularly treated for one disease may be more likely to be diagnosed with a second condition that otherwise would not have become apparent.

Both self-selection bias and diagnostic bias are primarily threats to external validity. In other words, these biases would yield sample populations that are not fully representative of the disease population that is the object of the study. Experiments performed with these volunteers may be *internally* valid, but lack generalizability to the larger patient population. Methods for choosing more representative populations for study were reviewed in Chapter 4.

## MEASUREMENT ERRORS

An important source of bias in translational and experimental clinical research are systematic errors that creep into measurements obtained during the course of a study. The greater the errors that occur, the less likely is it that the experimental study will show true associations that actually exist, and the more likely that the experiment will produce spurious results. Three main classes of measurement biases exist: observer bias, subject bias, and instrument bias.

*Observer bias* occurs when a measurement is consistently distorted by the person who is making the measurement. This distortion can be conscious or unconscious, and can occur in the perception of the measurement by the observer or in the reporting of the measurement. Observer bias is especially likely when the measurement requires a subjective judgment about the quality or severity of an outcome. Examples might include judgments about the degree of differentiation in a histologic sample, the degree of wound healing, or the level of functional recovery in a study participant. Even apparently quantitative measures are not immune to differential perception or reporting. For instance, observers might systematically round measurements up in one group and round down another group, especially if the distinguishing characteristic that differentiates the groups is known to the observer.

Observer bias can also occur when measurement instruments are systematically operated by different persons, for instance when one person makes the measurements in the experimental group and another makes the measurements in the control group. Observer bias can also result from more intensive measurements being performed in certain study participants. For instance, a more detailed medical history might be obtained from participants with a particular genotype compared to those without that genotype. Studies that rely on record review or history obtained by examiners should ensure that these data are obtained independent of knowledge of diagnosis or treatment status in order to avoid more persistent or specific questioning of participants with a specific outcome of interest.

To minimize observer bias, investigators should use automated measurement procedures requiring little subjective judgment whenever possible. The most effective way to eliminate the possibility of observer bias is "blinding" or "masking" (see the next section). Interestingly, successful blinding is difficult to achieve, and observers are often able to ascertain the treatment status of a research participant, even in studies that are double- or triple-blinded.

*Subject bias* occurs when there is a consistent systematic effect on study measurements, caused by the research participant rather than the observer. Perhaps the most well-known form of subject bias is differential recall of past events by persons who have had a certain disease outcome versus those who have not. This is known as recall bias, and has been particularly problematic in some epidemiologic studies. For instance, women who have had a child with a birth defect may be more likely to recall use of medications during pregnancy than are women who have had a normal pregnancy outcome. In translational research, a similar problem could occur in a pharmacogenetics study. This type of differential recall can lead to spurious associations between an exposure

and a disease outcome. To eliminate this type of measurement bias, information could be limited to that which was collected prior to the result of pregnancy being known. Such a study could be done by examining pharmacy records or physicians' office notes describing which medications were prescribed during pregnancy, or by using self-reported medical history information obtained before results of pregnancy were known.

Another example of a subject bias is the placebo effect, where study participants may report clinical improvements despite receiving no active treatment if they believe that they are being treated. This type of differential reporting is another reason for blinding in clinical research studies.

*Instrument bias* occurs when an instrument gives different readings over time, or different readings in different groups of study participants. Instruments such as cell counters or spectrophotometers may give different readings across time due to "drift" in calibration. Clinical laboratories change testing procedures over time; reagents or test strips may give different results with age. Great caution must be used when comparing tests performed at different points in time. This is why concurrent control groups are an important element of good experimental design, and why frequent instrument calibration and concurrent testing of blanks or known samples is an important procedure when performing some types of experimental measurements. Instrument bias can also apply to questionnaires or other data collection forms. For example, persons of different ethnic backgrounds or cultures may systematically give different answers on questionnaires or interviews even though they share the same disorder or severity of disorder.

## STRATEGIES FOR REDUCING BIAS

A number of approaches can be taken to reduce the possibility of bias in translational or experimental research. Perhaps the most powerful strategy is blinding (sometimes referred to as "masking"). Blinding typically involves two participants—the observer and the study participant—but can involve three, namely the person administering the intervention, the person obtaining the outcomes measurements (the "observer"), and the study participant. Blinding of study observers is used in both experimental and observational studies and seeks to disguise the assignment of exposure or treatment group from the person who is making the measurements of physiologic effects or other study outcome. As noted above, this blinding is particularly critical when there is any degree of subjectivity to assessments of study outcome. Some study outcomes, such as death, can be assumed to be free of observer bias. However, most other study outcomes should not be assumed to be free of this type of observer bias. Hence, blinding should be employed whenever feasible.

Blinding of study participants to treatment assignment is also an important design consideration. Sham injections or even sham surgery, which are meant to replicate the experience of the experimental group, can be considered a type of blinding analogous to the placebo group in a placebo-controlled clinical study. Blinding may at times involve ingenious or elaborate procedures. For example, in a recent study (2), arthroscopic surgery for osteoarthritis of the knee was compared to a control group that underwent sham surgery. The outcome of interest was a change in knee pain—obviously, a very subjective endpoint. Therefore, to preserve blinding in the event that participants in the placebo group did not have total amnesia after anesthesia, the standard surgical procedure was simulated. The knee was prepped and draped in the usual fashion and the usual number of incisions were made in the skin. The surgeon manipulated the knee as if performing arthroscopy. Saline was splashed to simulate the sounds of lavage.

Postoperative observation procedures were similar to participants actually undergoing arthroscopy, and nurses were unaware of the treatment-group assignment. Postoperative care also specified that all participants should receive the same walking aids, graduated exercise program, and analgesics. The use of analgesics after surgery was monitored; during the 2-year follow-up period, the amount used was similar in the study groups. In this carefully designed and executed study, with such elaborate procedures to preserve blinding, the treatment and placebo groups showed no differences in relief of pain—a very important result.

Another strategy to avoid bias, at least in some studies, is the use of unobtrusive study measurements. Intrusive observation procedures may make study participants act differently, perhaps in ways that are distinct between different treatment groups. For example, persons assigned to an educational intervention for smoking cessation may be less likely to report their true smoking status than persons not receiving this intervention; measurement of urinary cotinine (a nicotine metabolite) in both groups would eliminate the potential for differential reporting of smoking between groups. Measurements of blood hemoglobin $A_{1c}$ and urinary opioids would serve a similar purpose in studies that require a certain level of glucose control in diabetics, or the avoidance of narcotics in an addiction study.

After blinding, the other most important way to avoid bias is to insist that the research team adhere

meticulously to a predetermined study procedure protocol, including standardized, consistent, and repeatable procedures with the same instruments and same observers collecting data on people from all experimental groups. Careful attention to standardization of measurement methods, training and certifying observers, and automating and calibrating instruments can lessen the potential for bias that would otherwise result from differential measurements. In studies where multiple observers are used, common training of observers and tests of interobserver reliability should be performed. In studies using multiple labs performing similar techniques, tests of reproducibility of results between labs should be performed. Ideally, critical study measurements will be centralized as much as possible to avoid the possibility of variability of measurements between different observers in different centers. Large multicenter studies often employ a single center or set of observers for critical test elements such as interpretation of radiographic results or analysis of key samples. Highly automated and standardized measurements allow less scope for variable measurements between different groups.

In addition to making every possible effort to eliminate bias through sound experimental design, investigators can also attempt to estimate the extent to which bias may be present in their studies. Such quantitative assessments of bias can provide useful insights into the magnitude of various potential sources of error and allow better assessment of the uncertainty of study results. Such quantitative assessments are particularly useful when they demonstrate that certain sources of bias cannot plausibly explain their study result.

Some assessments of bias are simple and straightforward. For instance, investigators and research volunteers may become aware of treatment status, despite even the most detailed efforts to blind them. The degree to which unsuccessful blinding may have affected the study results can be estimated by assessing whether the study participants and the study investigators were truly blinded. This is done by asking participants and investigators to guess the treatment assignments. If a greater than expected proportion of participants or investigators correctly guess treatment assignment, investigators must take into account the possible effects of partial unblinding in interpreting and presenting study results. Although this statistical analysis of bias does not correct the problem, it is one instance in which the magnitude of the effect can at least be estimated.

Overall, however, addressing bias in the analytic phase of the study often requires additional data collection to validate study findings. Such data are often absent or limited. Methods for quantitative assessment of bias include sensitivity analysis and external adjustment. Basic methods for these procedures have been described by Rothman and Greenland (3).

## BIAS IN CASE-CONTROL STUDIES

Much has been written about potential sources of bias in case-control studies performed in epidemiologic research. In a classic case-control study, persons with a disease of interest are sampled and compared to an appropriately selected control population for the presence or absence of exposures of interest. The analysis of a case-control study typically results in the calculation of an odds ratio, which gives the odds of exposure among persons with the disease compared to persons without the disease of interest. Case-control studies offer an efficient and economical means for studying rare diseases, and to study multiple exposures that may be associated with a given disease. However, because the exposure status is ascertained after the disease status is known, there is always concern about the possibility of nondifferential misclassification of exposures in a case-control study. Also, the choice of an appropriate control population is not always straightforward, and inappropriate selection of controls can bias the results of a case-control study. For example, an investigator doing a case-control study of coffee consumption and heart disease might pick cases from a cardiology clinic. If controls were selected from among patients in a gastroenterology clinic, many of these patients may have stopped drinking coffee due to their digestive disorders. This would lead to a spurious association between coffee drinking and heart disease.

These issues are equally germane to some types of translational research, where persons with a disease or condition of interest are compared to a control population for differences in physiological measures, genotype, or other factors (referred to as a cross-sectional study design in Chapter 1). For instance, outcome measurements may be affected when the disease status of the research volunteer is known to the person making the measurement. Blinding the observer to disease status can readily be accomplished for procedures such as radiographs and analysis of laboratory specimens. For other procedures that involve an interaction with an observer, blinding may not be achievable.

Choice of case and control populations is a critical issue for case-control studies, and likewise for small clinical studies comparing diseased and nondiseased persons. The choice of representative cases is not always straightforward, particularly for diseases where persons with the disease do not always come to medical attention. Persons presenting to a hospital or clinic may thus be different from those persons with the condition who have not presented for treatment. For unbiased strategies to sample a patient population, see the discussion in Chapter 4.

For cases recruited from hospitals, particularly academic or tertiary referral hospitals, the choice of an appropriate control population is typically difficult. The controls should be persons who are representative of the population from whom the cases were drawn. The ideal controls can be thought of as those persons who would have come into the study as cases if they had the disease under investigation. However, it is often difficult to ascertain or to sample the representative population from which cases were drawn. This is particularly true for rare diseases seen in a referral hospital. An academic clinic studying a rare disorder may draw patients from a wide geographic area; it may be difficult to determine what the appropriate source population for sampling would be. Different strategies for recruiting controls are used, including the use of hospital- or clinic-based controls drawn from the same hospital or clinics from which cases were recruited; use of a population-based sample often recruited through random digit dialing; or use of more than one control group. Detailed discussions of these methods, as well as their advantages and drawbacks, can be found elsewhere (3,4).

The problem of choosing a control group can be illustrated as follows. Consider a study that attempts to determine whether a given genetic variant is more common in persons with a disease than without the disease. A sample of persons with the disease have their genotypes ascertained. What control group should be selected to compare the prevalence of given genotypes to those found in the case group? Certain genotypes vary widely by ethnic background and by geographic area; choice of an inappropriate control group could easily give spurious findings. Considerable literature exists on the choice of appropriate control groups for case-control studies. As yet, little such literature exists for translational research in small clinical studies, though the problems faced are very similar.

## OTHER ISSUES

Another source of bias that may affect translational research is bias resulting from the spectrum of disease severity. This spectrum bias occurs when the severity of disease in a study sample differs from that in a sample or group to whom the results are later applied. This phenomenon has been best described in the clinical epidemiology literature relating to clinical test performance. Usually, clinical tests are developed to distinguish between persons with a disease and persons without a disease, and are tested initially in persons who have an unambiguous or severe disease. The nondiseased persons used in early tests are typically different from people in whom the tests might be used in practice. (In fact, medical students or graduate students are often used as "normal" subjects in early stage tests, as many readers of this book can attest!) Early studies of a test may thus show that it can discriminate between persons with severe clinical manifestations of a disease and persons who are very healthy. However, the test may not be able to discriminate as well between persons who have less severe manifestations of a disease and persons who have symptoms consistent with the disease. This same potential bias holds true for physiologic measures that apparently differ between persons with a disease and persons without a disease, yet this study design is extraordinarily common in translational studies of new technologies (e.g., imaging studies).

A final potential source of bias, particularly in the analysis and interpretation of results, or in the failure to publish negative results, is financial conflicts of interest. An increasing concern in medical research is that financial ties between investigators and pharmaceutical or technology companies may provide financial incentives to investigators that may color their interpretation of studies (Chapters 14 and 15). This issue is of concern not only for investigators who may own stock or have other financial interests in pharmaceutical or technology companies, but for investigators who hold consulting arrangements or have other ties with commercial interests that might be affected by the results of research. Despite more stringent standards for reporting potential conflicts of interest, this potential source of bias is difficult to recognize or measure. Major medical journals have recently taken steps to reduce nonpublication of negative results by calling for all trials to be publicly registered, including the study protocols and results.

## SUMMARY

- Bias refers to systematic errors that occur during the design, conduct, or analytic phases of a study. Statistical analysis is useful for managing nonsystematic (random) errors, but not errors caused by bias.
- Self-selection bias and diagnostic bias are potentially important sources of bias in clinical research that especially threaten the external validity of the study. A related type is spectrum bias where the severity of disease in a study sample differs from the population to whom the results are meant to be applied. This may occur because of referral bias (e.g., only the sickest patients are referred to a medical center) or because of selection choices made by the investigator.
- Observer bias, subject bias, and instrument bias produce measurement errors caused by the person performing the measurement, by the research volunteer (e.g., the placebo effect), or by the instrument used to make the measurement (e.g., calibration drift).
- Masking and strict adherence to the protocol are the most powerful means of reducing bias.

## REFERENCES

1. Sackett, DL. Bias in analytic research. J Chron Dis 1979;32:51–63.
2. Moseley J, O'Malley K, Petersen N et al. A controlled trial of arthroscopic surgery for osteoarthritis of the knee. N Engl J Med 2002;347:81–88.
3. Rothman KJ and Greenland S. Modern Epidemiology. 2nd Ed. Philadelphia: Lippincott-Raven, 1998.
4. Hulley SB, Cummings SR, Browner WS, et al. Designing Clinical Research. Philadelphia: Lippincott Williams & Wilkins, 2001.

# CHAPTER 7

# Observational Study Designs

Brian F. Gage

In an experiment, the investigator controls the process by which some research participants are exposed to an intervention while others are not (Chapters 1,8). The intervention might be a drug, device, diet, or health-related habit. Randomization of the intervention can balance comorbid conditions and other risk factors that are present prior to group assignment while masking minimizes bias that occurs after allocation.

In observational studies, exposure is not under the investigator's control so randomization is impossible. However, by using appropriate study design and analysis the investigator can minimize the effect of confounding variables and other biases and maximize valid inference. Observational study designs include cross-sectional, cohort, and case-control studies. As summarized in this chapter, each of these study designs has strengths and weaknesses that depend on the study's goals, the prevalence and type of risk factor, and the disease frequency.

Observational studies have several virtues. First, they are versatile. The outcome can be the development or cure of disease or a surrogate outcome (e.g., blood pressure); the risk factor can be a genotype or gene expression pattern, an environmental agent, medical therapy, comorbid condition, medical image, or health-related habit. Second, observational studies can elucidate putative mechanisms of disease. For example, observational studies provided the first links between cigarette smoking and lung cancer and between elevated cholesterol and coronary artery disease. Third, they avoid ethical barriers inherent to human experiments involving environmental toxins or genes. Perhaps the greatest virtue of observational studies is that they can be completed more quickly and less expensively than experimental studies.

## CROSS-SECTIONAL STUDIES

In a cross-sectional study, the investigator studies a group of individuals at a given time (Figure 7–1). These individuals represent a sample of people taken from a population of interest. The time is usually just the date on which the key measurement or measurements have been made, but it can also be a time interval, such as the academic year 2005–2006. However, unlike cohort studies, cross-sectional studies do not evaluate the same participants over time.

Cross-sectional studies are especially useful for determining the *prevalence* of a risk factor or disease in a sample population, which is calculated as the number of affected individuals divided by the total number of individuals in the study sample. In translational research, the risk factor might be a particular genotype, data from a genomic or proteomic microarray study, or the results from a novel imaging study.

An example of a well-done cross-sectional study is a study by Finzi et al. (1). They tested the hypothesis that quiescent CD4+ T lymphocytes provide a reservoir for human immunodeficiency virus-type 1 (HIV-1) in patients taking antiretroviral therapy. They recovered replication-competent virus from resting CD4+ T lymphocytes in patients infected with HIV. The frequency (prevalence) of CD4+ T cells harboring latent HIV was not lower in participants who had been taking antiretroviral therapy for a longer duration. Most recovered viruses were sensitive to antiretroviral therapy.

Although cross-sectional studies accurately measure disease and risk factor prevalence, they

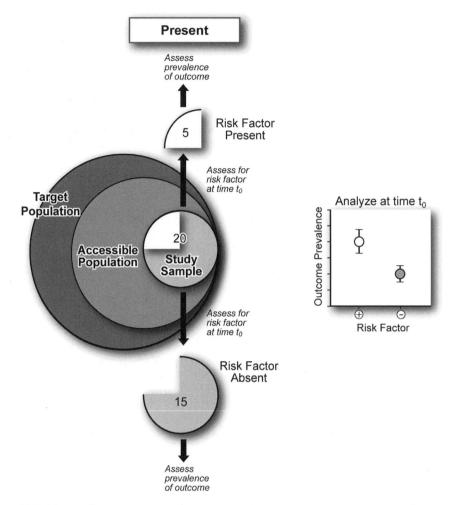

**FIGURE 7–1** ● Schematic representation of a cross-sectional study. After enrolling participants at study initiation (time $t_0$), the investigator simultaneously collects data on risk factors (e.g., a genotype or comorbid condition) and outcome (e.g., a disease).

cannot establish temporal relationships, which is a key criterion for establishing causation (Chapter 1). For example, in a recent cross-sectional study, Aviles et al. found an association between a laboratory marker of inflammation (C-reactive protein) and the presence of atrial fibrillation (2). From this cross-sectional study, they could not prove their hypothesis that inflammation predisposed to atrial fibrillation, because atrial fibrillation itself could have been the cause of an inflammatory response. To establish a temporal relationship between inflammation and the development of atrial fibrillation, they also did a prospective cohort study (see next section) of participants free of atrial fibrillation at enrollment. As hypothesized, participants with a greater C-reactive protein at baseline were more likely to develop the arrhythmia.

Although the inability to determine temporal relationships is the major weakness of cross-sectional studies, they also have several minor weaknesses. First, diseases (or disease stages) of short duration are underrepresented in cross-sectional studies. Second, cross-sectional studies that rely on input from the research participant (e.g., a patient survey) cannot be used to study fatal diseases. Third, *confounding variables* can cause apparent associations in cross-sectional studies (and in other observational studies). Confounding variables are associated with both the outcome and the risk factor but are not part of the causal pathway linking one to the other (Chapter 3). Finally, cross-sectional studies are inefficient when study outcomes or risk factors are rare. However, studying high-risk populations can improve efficiency.

## Execution and Analysis

In cross-sectional studies, investigators collect all key measures at one time. Thus, cross-sectional studies have no loss to follow-up and can be accomplished more quickly than prospective cohort studies. This simplicity in design is one of the most attractive aspects of the cross-sectional format and is one of the reasons this type of study is so common in translational clinical research. The key analytic measurement in a cross-sectional study is the calculation of risk factor prevalence.

The most difficult aspect of designing a cross-sectional study is often related to the choice of controls. Determining the prevalence of a risk factor in a diseased population is a first step, but the interesting question is whether this prevalence differs from an appropriate control group. Ideally, as outlined in Chapter 6, the controls should be a sample of persons who are representative of the population from whom the affected individuals were also drawn. The ideal controls can be thought of as those persons who would have come into the study as cases if they had the disease under investigation. More information about sampling strategies can be found in Chapter 4.

## PROSPECTIVE COHORT STUDIES

In a prospective cohort study, investigators follow participants with or without a risk factor forward in time and note the development (incidence) of outcomes. Because the study is conducted prospectively, the investigator can decide on the quality and quantity of data (and biological specimens, if applicable) that are collected at enrollment. The investigator then follows the participants longitudinally until the outcomes have occurred in some participants. Some prospective cohort studies have a single cohort and report only the natural history of disease. More commonly, the investigator follows multiple cohorts. For example, in a *dual-cohort study* (Figure 7–2), the investigator follows one cohort with and the other without the risk factor of interest, allowing any association between the outcome and risk factor to be identified and quantified.

As an example, Palareti and colleagues used a prospective cohort design in a study of 599 patients with a recent venous thromboembolism (3). After patients were treated with a standard course of anticoagulant therapy, the investigators determined the plasma D-dimer level. Because D-dimer is a fibrin degradation product resulting from activation of the coagulation and fibrinolysis process, they hypothesized that high levels would predict recurrence of venous thromboembolism. They followed participants with physical examinations every 3–6 months over the subsequent months. They found that one-sixth of participants who had an elevated D-dimer level (>500 ng/mL) had a recurrent venous thromboembolism while only 5.8% of participants with a normal D-dimer level had a recurrence over the same 1.5 years (mean) follow-up. Thus, they concluded the D-dimer was a valid predictor of recurrent venous thromboembolism.

Cohort studies must be planned and conducted *prospectively* when accurate information needs to be gathered that would not otherwise be available—for example plasma levels of a biomarker, surveys about health-related habits, environmental exposures, or details about medication use. At the time the study by Palareti et al was performed, for instance, D-dimer levels were not routinely obtained to manage venous thromboembolism. Thus, the study could only have been performed by prospectively planning to obtain the D-dimer levels on each research participant.

There are several advantages of using a prospective cohort study design. For one, this strategy is an efficient way to study outcomes associated with risk factors that are rare or infrequently documented. An advantage compared to case-control studies (see below) is that multiple outcomes can be evaluated during a single study. Finally, and by definition in a prospective cohort study, the risk factor is identified *prior* to the outcome, so that the temporal relationship is unambiguous, strengthening inferences about causality (Chapter 1).

Despite these advantages, prospective studies are often expensive because they are conducted over prolonged periods of time and can be impractical. In particular, if the incidence rate of the outcome of interest is low, then either the study has to be large or the length of follow-up has to be long to provide sufficient power to test the research hypothesis. Patients may also be lost to follow-up, potentially compounding the problem of insufficient outcome events. In addition, as in any observational study, observed associations may be due to baseline differences between the cohorts, silent preclinical disease, or unmeasured confounding variables.

## Execution and Analysis

Most new investigators should involve a biostatistician or epidemiologist when designing a prospective cohort study. The biostatistician or epidemiologist should help ensure that necessary information is collected to control for likely confounders and to allow for attrition of participants.

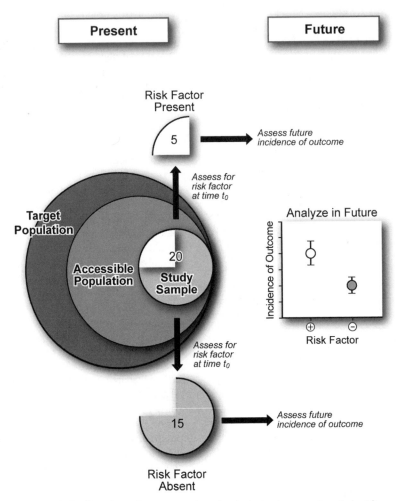

**FIGURE 7–2** ● Schematic representation of a dual-cohort prospective study. After enrolling participants, the investigator determines who has the risk factor and then follows participants into the future, noting incident disease (or other outcome). Incidence rates in participants with the risk factor (e.g., a genotype or comorbid condition) are compared to incidence in participants who lack the factor.

He or she can also help ensure that study information is collected in a manner that facilitates subsequent analysis.

In a dual-cohort study, the two groups should resemble each other as much as possible except for the presence or absence of the risk factor of interest. After potential volunteers consent to participate in the study, the investigator gathers baseline information, including important demographic information, data relevant to the risk factor of interest, participant contact information, and (often) biological specimens. Then, the investigator plans to have participants return for regular follow-up assessments during each year of the study. Ideally, outcomes should be assessed by someone who is unaware of the participant's risk factor status (masking). For example, laboratory assays should

be run or radiographic images should be reviewed while the evaluator is masked to the participant's risk factor status.

If a contemporaneous cohort is not available for comparison, the investigator can consider using historic controls or data from a registry or census, especially when the outcome is unambiguous, like all-cause mortality. Although historic controls provide useful comparisons, they can bias the study in favor of the newer cohort because of temporal improvements in health or other (unmeasured or immeasurable) variables between the contemporaneous and historic control groups.

Unlike cross-sectional studies, prospective cohort studies provide *incidence rates*, rather than prevalence data, because the frequency of developing the outcome accrues over a span of time. The number of *patient-years* in each cohort is the sum of each participant's length of follow-up ($\Sigma$pt-yrs), which may be uniform or variable across the different participants in the study. The average *incidence rate,* IR, is calculated by dividing the number of new outcomes by the number of patient-years, that is IR = Number outcomes/$\Sigma$pt-yrs. The *absolute risk reduction* is the difference between the IR in the two cohorts. The *relative rate* (also called the relative risk), RR, is the ratio of the exposed and unexposed cohorts (or its reciprocal). For example, in the Palareti et al. study, the incidence of developing venous thromboembolism recurrence was 2.6 times greater in participants with elevated D-dimer levels compared to others. Studies that compare rates using time-to-event analyses (e.g., Cox-proportional hazard regression) often report the *hazard ratio*, which is quantitatively and conceptually similar to the RR. When the exposure to the risk factor turns out to be protective, the data are often expressed as the *relative risk reduction*, 1 – RR.

To illustrate some of these metrics, consider a trial of 20 participants: 5 with the risk factor and 15 without it (Figure 7–2). If 4 participants with the risk factor develop the outcome after a total of 20 patient-years of follow-up, then their incidence rate is 4/20 = 0.2 event per patient year. If 3 participants without the risk factor develop the outcome after 60 patient-years, then their rate is 3/60 = 0.05 event per patient-year. The ratio between these two rates, the RR, is 4.0. Thus, patients with the risk factor were 4 times more likely to develop the outcome. The absolute risk increase was 0.15 event per patient-year.

## RETROSPECTIVE COHORT STUDIES

When existing data are available to answer the study question, retrospective cohort studies are faster and cheaper to conduct than prospective studies. At the start of a retrospective cohort study, investigators study existing medical records of nondiseased participants, some of whom were exposed to the risk factor of interest (Figure 7–3). As in a prospective study, the risk factor might be a genotype or gene expression pattern, environmental agent, therapy, comorbid condition, imaging data, or health-related habit. Investigators then continue to assess participants by examining later records, moving toward the present time. Obviously, the investigator lacks control over the information, or the quality of the information, that is available for review. Despite this disadvantage, retrospective studies are a commonly used design format because they avoid the delay inherent in prospective studies when an investigator has to wait for the event of interest to occur.

As an example, Lynch and colleagues recently used a retrospective cohort study design to quantify the association between activating mutations in the Epidermal Growth Factor Receptor (EGFR) and responsiveness of non–small cell lung cancer to the antitumor drug, gefitinib (4). They began with patients who had non-small cell lung cancer and had received gefitinib, a drug that inhibits the tyrosine kinase of EGFR. Then, they sequenced the exons of the EGFR coding sequence and correlated mutations with prior clinical response. They found mutations in the tyrosine kinase domain in 8 of 9 responders and in none of 7 nonresponders, suggesting that screening lung cancers for EGFR mutations would identify patients who would respond to gefitinib.

Retrospective cohort studies share several strengths with prospective cohort studies: they provide incidence rates, quantify how a risk factor correlates with the outcome, and are easy to interpret. The main advantage over a prospective study is that data are obtained starting from some point in the past, with additional relevant data obtained from that point toward the present. Obviously, in this way, results can be obtained without having to wait for outcomes to develop in the future.

On the other hand, with retrospective cohort studies, the investigator is at the mercy of the existing data about risk factors and outcome. When these data are incomplete or unreliable, potential participants may need to be excluded or missing values may need to be imputed (methods of imputation can be discussed in collaboration with a biostatistician).

If the investigator can find a prospective cohort that was assembled for another purpose, he or she may be able to answer additional questions retrospectively. For example, during the years 1948 to 1952, 5,209 residents of Framingham, Massachusetts, were recruited. These participants have been followed every other year for standardized assessment. The data and blood they provided have been used in hundreds of retrospective cohort studies that were not anticipated when the Framingham study was initiated.

### Execution and Analysis

Retrospective cohort studies are conducted in much the same way as prospective cohort studies, with the key exception that the required data must already be available. Like prospective cohort studies, retrospective cohort studies provide data to calculate patient-years and incidence rates. Likewise, when two or more cohorts are studied retrospectively, the investigator can calculate relative rates, absolute and relative risk reductions, or hazard ratios.

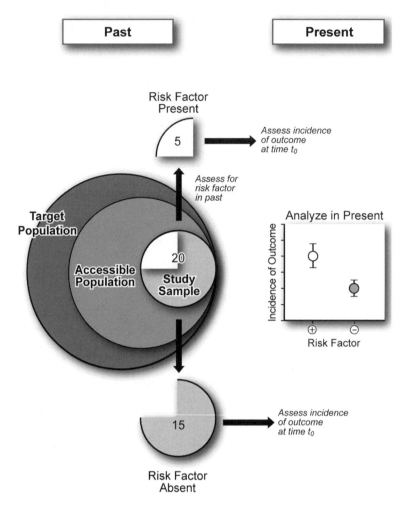

**FIGURE 7–3** ● Schematic representation of a retrospective cohort study. After enrolling participants, the investigator determines who had the risk factor in the past and then follows participants toward the present, noting incident disease (or other outcome). Analysis is identical to a prospective study.

## CASE-CONTROL STUDIES

Whereas cohort studies often begin with two groups, one with the risk factor and the other lacking it, case-control studies begin with patients who have already developed the outcome of interest ("cases") as well as a group of appropriate controls. Thus, by definition, cases have the disease or other outcome of interest and control patients do not. At the start of a case-control study, investigators identify cases and then typically match these cases to one or more controls from the same population sample (Figure 7–4). Then, the investigator determines the history of prior exposure to the risk factor in the case and control patients. As in a retrospective cohort study, investigators cannot control the quality of information available from the prior exposure. Despite this disadvantage, case-control studies are

also used commonly, especially for rare outcomes or diseases with long latency periods. Case-control studies are also ideal when the exposure of interest is a fairly common genotype and the disease of interest is not rapidly fatal (thereby allowing sufficient opportunity for cases to be identified and consented for genetic analysis).

An instructive example is a recent case-control study by Cipollone et al, who quantified the association between the -765G—>C variant of the cyclooxygenase-2 (COX-2) gene and the risk of myocardial infarction and ischemic stroke (5). They matched 864 patients with their first myocardial infarction or ischemic stroke with 864 hospitalized controls. The groups were matched for age, sex, body mass index, smoking, hypertension, hypercholesterolemia, and diabetes. The -765G—>C heterozygous genotype was 2.4 times more common among controls than cases and -765G—>C homozygosity

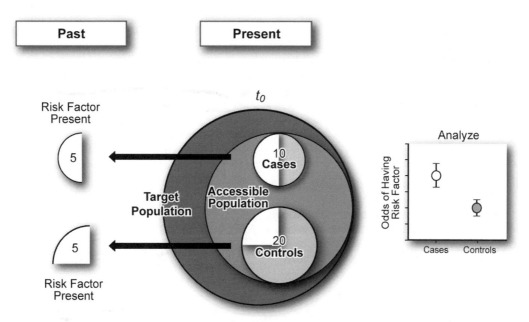

**FIGURE 7–4** ● Schematic representation of a case-control study design. After enrolling cases and unaffected controls (matched 2:1 in this example), the investigator determines which participants had the risk factor.

was 5.8 times higher in controls. They concluded that the -765G —>C polymorphism of the COX-2 gene is associated with a decreased risk of MI and stroke. By staining for metalloproteinase in a cross-sectional substudy, they showed that patients with the -765G—>C polymorphism had a lower activity level of metalloproteinase in atherosclerotic plaques. This substudy of metalloproteinase activity suggests that the COX-2 variant is causative, rather than merely being in linkage disequilibrium (Chapter 32) with some other causative gene.

Because case-control studies begin with cases, the investigator does not need to wait for the outcome events to accrue, as in a prospective cohort study. Likewise, case-control studies typically include more cases than could be captured by any other study design, thereby allowing for greater statistical power. They also allow matching on potential confounding variables to be employed in the selection of control participants (as in the study by Cipollone et al.), allowing these variables to be controlled for in the study-design phase (rather than in the analytic phase). Not only are case-control studies the most efficient study for rare diseases, but they are also ideal when the risk factor is difficult or expensive to ascertain. In cross-sectional (or cohort) studies, the risk factor has to be measured on all participants, even though few participants are likely to have (or to develop) the outcome. In contrast, case-control studies require risk factor assessments in only the cases and controls, typically a limited number of participants.

One caution about case-control studies is that once a variable is matched in the study-design phase, an investigator cannot later decide to quantify the association between the matched factor and outcome, because they will be equally represented in both cases and controls. A second caution is that when patients have an acute, fatal disease, they cannot be recruited as cases (because they don't live long enough to be identified as a "case"). Furthermore, because deceased patients often have severe disease, their omission from the study may dilute the apparent association that is observed between the risk factor of interest and the outcome in surviving evaluable patients (thereby biasing the results toward the null hypothesis). Occasionally, however, a family member or other surrogate can provide the needed information on the risk factor. Finally, except for a nested case-control study (see below), case-control studies do not provide incidence rates, although sometimes they can be estimated by applying epidemiologic methods to case-control data (6).

A major weakness of case-control studies is that information about risk factors is collected ex post facto. If the risk factor (e.g., a therapy or environmental toxin) has to be recollected by the patient (or a surrogate), then *recall bias* may inflate the apparent association between the outcome and risk factor. For example, mothers of diseased children are more likely to recall a risk factor during their pregnancy than are mothers of healthy children.

The second major weakness of case-control studies is the difficulty in selecting control patients. For example, the hospitalized controls selected by Cipollone et al might have been admitted to the hospital for some other disease that is associated with the COX-2 polymorphism (e.g., asthma, colon cancer, or non–small cell lung cancer), an example of *sampling bias*. For more on this topic, see Chapter 6.

### Execution and Analysis

To avoid recall bias, investigators often use case-control studies to study risk factors that are not susceptible to it, such as a genetic risk factor (e.g., the study by Cipollone et al). However, when studying a genetic risk factor, the investigator should match cases to controls at least on the basis of race and ethnicity, which decreases the risk of confounding by population stratification, whereby both allele frequency and risk of disease are correlated with race or ethnicity (see Chapter 32).

When studying nongenetic risk factors, masking the observer as to who is a case and who is a control when the key measurements are made can prevent bias. Often, however, the cases and controls are readily distinguishable—if not by themselves, then at least by the evaluator. Sometimes, everyone can be masked as to the risk factor of interest and sham questions (or similar controls) can be included to quantify the effect of *measurement bias* (where a risk factor is assessed differentially in controls vs cases, see Chapter 6). When masking is not possible, a useful technique is to obtain or corroborate the risk factor from a source that is not susceptible to recall bias. Thus, prior use of a drug therapy could be verified by review of pharmacy records; exposure of an environmental toxin could be corroborated by review of reports sent to the Environmental Protection Agency or by biochemical analysis of appropriate biological tissue donated by the cases and control.

The most important principle in selecting proper controls is that cases and controls should arise from the same population with an appropriate at-risk period (Chapter 6). The population might be a prospective cohort (e.g., participants in the Nurses Health Study), a geographic catchment area (e.g., residents of Olmsted County, Minnesota), or a roster (e.g., members of a certain health maintenance organization). When the risk factor is time dependent, then cases developing the outcome during a specific time interval should be matched to controls that did not have the outcome during the same or longer time interval.

The number of controls per case depends on the availability of cases and controls and the resources of the investigators. When cases are plentiful, it is more statistically efficient to match cases and controls one to one. However, because case-control studies are used to study rare diseases, the number of available cases is often limited. When this occurs, using more than one control per case increases statistical power.

Unlike cohort studies, incidence rates cannot be calculated directly from case-control studies. Thus, the relative risk (RR) and other types of risks cannot be calculated directly from case-control studies. However, a quantitatively similar measure, the *odds ratio (OR)*, can be calculated from a case-control study. In the analysis of a single risk factor, the OR is calculated from a standard $2 \times 2$ table; in the analysis of multiple risk factors, the OR is calculated from logistic regression (Chapter 25). Regardless of how the OR is estimated, it provides an estimate of the RR for rare outcomes. If the frequency of the outcome exceeds approximately 10%, then the OR exaggerates the relationship between the risk factor and outcome as compared to the RR (7). When calculating measures of effect, the analyst should use a statistical approach that takes into account the pair-wise nature of the data. For example, conditional logistic regression is appropriate for case-control data while ordinary logistic regression is not (8).

## NESTED CASE-CONTROL STUDIES

A nested case-control study is sometimes called a *prospective incident case-referent study* to differentiate it from a traditional case-control study. Participants in a nested case-control study have been followed in a prospective or (less commonly) in a retrospective cohort (Figure 7–5). At the study's completion, rather than analyzing all participants in the cohort, the investigator studies only cases (i.e., participants who have developed the outcome of interest) and a select number of controls. Nested case-control studies are ideal when the outcome is rare or when the predictor variable being evaluated would be too difficult or expensive to obtain on all participants.

A good example of a such a study was performed by Meigs and colleagues when they investigated the relationship between biomarkers of endothelial dysfunction and the risk of developing Type 2 diabetes mellitus (9). Their study was nested within the Nurses Health Study, which had archived blood samples from 32,826 women in 1989 to 1990. During prospective follow-up, 737 of these women developed new diabetes. Meigs et al. matched each of these women to at least one nondiabetic woman of

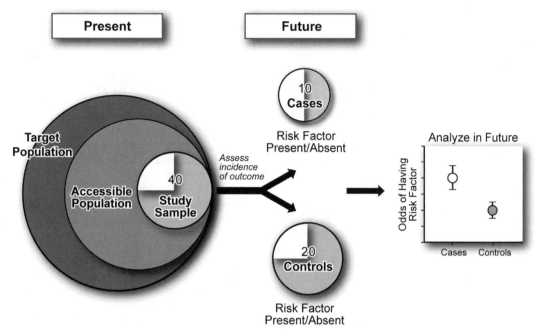

**FIGURE 7–5** ● Schematic representation of a nested case-control study design. After enrolling participants, the investigator follows participants into the future, noting incident disease (or other outcome). After completion of the prospective follow up, the investigator selects cases and unaffected controls (matched 2:1 in this example). Then, the investigator determines which participants had the risk factor.

similar age, date of blood draw, fasting status, and race. They found that biomarkers of endothelial dysfunction including E-selectin and intercellular adhesion molecule-1 (ICAM-1) predicted the subsequent development of diabetes.

Nested case-control studies combine the accuracy and versatility of prospective data collection with the analytic efficiency of a case-control study. In the example above, it would have been prohibitively expensive for Meigs et al to have measured biomarkers of endothelial dysfunction in all 32,826 nurses who donated blood. Even if the cost of the biomarkers had been inexpensive, it would have been wasteful to use plasma from all participants when only 737 of them developed diabetes.

As compared to traditional case-control studies, nested case-control studies offer two advantages: prospective data collection and ease in matching appropriate controls to the cases. The ease in matching arises because the cases and controls are drawn from the same population—participants in the cohort—and because information about the controls is collected at the same time and in the same manner as information collected from the controls. The prospective data collection in a nested case-control study eliminates the problem of information bias (e.g., recall bias) that can poison a traditional case-control study. Because of the potential advantages and efficiency of nested case-control studies, large

funding agencies (e.g., the NIH and the Veterans Affairs Cooperative Studies Program) encourage the storage of blood or other biologic specimens from trial participants for subsequent nested case-control studies.

Like a cohort study, a disadvantage of the nested case-control study is that it continues until enough outcome events are likely to have occurred. In addition, because case-control studies are usually done prospectively, they often cannot be used to study diseases that have a long latency period or a slow rate of occurrence. And again, as in any observational study, observed associations may be caused by baseline differences between the identified case and control cohorts, silent preclinical disease, or unmeasured confounding variables.

### Execution and Analysis

The execution of a nested case-control study initially resembles a cohort study: after consenting individuals within an appropriate cohort, the investigator collects baseline information, and sometimes biological specimens, and then follows the cohort prospectively (or gathers data retrospectively). Subsequently, only cases that develop the outcome of interest and controls are analyzed. Like a traditional case-control study, the statistical power is primarily a function of the number of participants who develop the outcome of interest (i.e., the number of cases). However, matching each case to more than one control can improve power.

Although used less commonly than a nested case-control study, a *nested case-cohort study* is executed similarly with one difference: control data are derived from a random sample of all participants in the study, instead of unaffectd patients. Data from cases are then compared to data taken from these participants selected at random. During the analytic phase, participants who were selected at random who turn out to have developed the outcome can be reclassified as cases. Case-cohort studies are useful when investigators wish to measure disease prevalence or desire a random sample of participants to serve as controls for multiple case-control studies.

Like traditional case-control studies, the key analytic measure in nested case-control studies is the odds ratio. However, because cohorts of patients are often followed over time, data from nested case-control studies can also provide incidence rates.

## CASE-CROSSOVER STUDIES

In case-crossover studies, the same participants are exposed to two or more conditions. Each participant then serves as his or her own control. The endpoint in these studies is often a biologic measure rather than an adverse event, and the study is more often experimental than observational in design. When case-crossover studies are observational in format (e.g. [10]), the investigator doesn't control the order of the exposure as he or she does in an experimental crossover study (Chapter 8).

Because participants served as their own control, case-crossover studies are an efficient method to determine how a transient risk factor (e.g., alcohol consumption, cigarette smoke, or vigorous exercise) acutely affects an outcome (11). Case-crossover studies also can be used to quantify the risk of transiently stopping an exposure, such as the risk of pregnancy or breakthrough bleeding when an oral-contraceptive tablet is inadvertently missed. In observational case-crossover studies, the main difficulty is in ascertaining each participant's usual (i.e., control) behavior (11).

### Execution and Analysis

The execution of a case-crossover study is similar to a retrospective cohort study, but the investigator must also quantify the duration of the exposure. Because participants are compared to themselves,

paired statistical techniques are often used to analyze case-crossover studies (Chapter 24).

## SUMMARY

- Observational studies are especially valuable when experimental interventions are ethically impermissible or logistically impractical (e.g., when the outcome is rare). They are also valuable as a relatively inexpensive and efficient means of collecting preliminary data to justify experimental studies.
- Common observational study designs include cross-sectional, cohort, and case-control designs.
- Cross-sectional studies are especially useful for determining the prevalence of a risk factor or disease in a sample. Their main disadvantage is that they provide weak evidence for causation because the temporal relationship between the risk factor and the outcome of interest cannot be determined with certainty.
- Cohort studies may be conducted either retrospectively or prospectively. These studies provide incidence rates. In dual-cohort studies, the investigator can calculate relative risks, relative risk reductions, and absolute risk reductions. As compared to prospective studies, retrospective studies are easier and less expensive, but the investigator cannot control the data quality in retrospective analyses. Thus, prospective studies are more rigorous but also more difficult and time consuming to complete than retrospective studies.
- Case-control studies are an efficient design for rare outcomes and common risk factors, but are especially susceptible to recall bias and sampling bias (unless the risk factor is a genotype). The frequency of risk factors in cases and controls are compared with the odds ratio.
- Nested case-control studies combine the accuracy and versatility of prospective-cohort studies with the analytic efficiency of a case-control study: patients are followed prospectively and those who develop the outcome ("cases") are compared to a subset of unaffected participants.

## REFERENCES

1. Finzi D, Hermankova M, Pierson T et al. Identification of a reservoir for HIV-1 in patients on highly active antiretroviral therapy. Science 1997;278(5341):1295–1300.
2. Aviles RJ, Martin DO, Apperson-Hansen C et al. Inflammation as a risk factor for atrial fibrillation. Circulation 2003;108(24):3006–3010.
3. Palareti G, Legnani C, Cosmi B et al. Predictive value of D-dimer test for recurrent venous thromboembolism after anticoagulation withdrawal in subjects with a previous

idiopathic event and in carriers of congenital thrombophilia. Circulation 2003;108(3):313–318.

4. Lynch TJ, Bell DW, Sordella R et al. Activating mutations in the epidermal growth factor receptor underlying responsiveness of non-small-cell lung cancer to gefitinib. N Engl J Med 2004;350(21):2129–2139.

5. Cipollone F, Toniato E, Martinotti S et al. A polymorphism in the cyclooxygenase-2 gene as an inherited protective factor against myocardial infarction and stroke. JAMA 2004;291(18):2221–2228.

6. Rothman KJ, Greenland S. Modern Epidemiology. 2nd Ed. Philadelphia: Lippincott-Raven, 1998.

7. Zhang J, Yu KF. What's the relative risk? A method of correcting the odds ratio in cohort studies of common outcomes. JAMA 1998;280(19):1690–1691.

8. Stokes ME, Davis CS, Koch GG. Chapter 10: Conditional Logistic Regression. Categorical Data Analysis Using the SAS System. 2nd Ed. Cary, NC: John Wiley and Sons, 2000:271–322.

9. Meigs JB, Hu FB, Rifai N et al. Biomarkers of endothelial dysfunction and risk of type 2 diabetes mellitus. JAMA 2004;291(16):1978–1986.

10. Redelmeier DA, Tibshirani RJ. Association between cellular-telephone calls and motor vehicle collisions. N Engl J Med. 1997;336(7):453–458.

11. Marshall RJ, Jackson RT. Analysis of case-crossover designs. Stat Med. 1993;12(24):2333–2341.

# CHAPTER 8

# Experimental Study Designs

Daniel P. Schuster

The great virtue of performing an experiment is that the investigator has control over the experimental intervention (e.g., a drug, a device, a change in the diet, or an exercise program).[1] This feature, more than any other, gives the investigator freedom to manipulate key aspects of study design, including the timing, dose, and duration of the imposed treatment. Ironically, control over the experimental intervention also allows the investigator to give up that control so that treatment allocation can be randomized and masked. Randomization minimizes bias by balancing factors that are present prior to the allocation of treatment that could bias outcome, while masking minimizes bias by balancing factors that occur after allocation that could bias the measurement of that outcome. These key elements (control over the intervention, randomization, and masking) are what distinguish experiments from observational studies (Chapter 7) and they are what provide the basis for any inference that the intervention itself is the cause of the measured outcome (Chapter 1).

The goal of every experiment, insofar as it is possible, is to create a situation in which the only source of variation among those participating in the research is whether or not they have been exposed to the experimental intervention, allowing the investigator to conclude that any measured differences after the exposure are because of that exposure. Randomization and masking are the experimentalist's two most powerful tools to minimize both known and unknown sources of bias that would prevent such an inference.

In the animal or bench laboratory, many options are available to the investigator to eliminate bias. Genetically identical animals may be used. All animals may be studied at essentially the same time. Known confounders (e.g., blood pressure, heart rate, blood sugar) may be controlled as part of experimental design. With this level of control, formal randomization and masking in laboratory research often seems unnecessary. In most cases, however, the clinical investigator just does not have this same level of control. And even if he or she did, individual responses to the same intervention vary. Presumably, this "biologic variation" is the result of unknown confounders that are left uncontrolled. For these reasons, randomization and masking assume greater importance in the conduct of clinical experiments.

Exercising such control does have its downside, however. The observed outcome may only occur if the very limited conditions of the experiment can be reproduced. Thus, although well-designed and conducted experiments have a high degree of internal validity, they may have little external validity, that is, the results may not extend to the target population that is really of interest. For an experiment to be externally valid, the study population, at the very least, must accurately represent the target population (as discussed in Chapter 4). In the animal laboratory, control over genetic strain, animal age and gender, environmental conditions, and similar factors render the need for random sampling from the animal population relatively unimportant (an experimental inference derived from a study sample of

---

[1]Note that here, as elsewhere in this book, the terms experimental intervention *and* treatment *are used interchangeably. The use of either term, however, is problematic. To some, an intervention implies an intrusion, or interference, and is a one-time event. On the other hand, a treatment clearly implies therapeutic intent, but many clinical experiments are performed only to elucidate a biological mechanism, with no reasonable prospect that the "treatment" (or "intervention") will benefit the research participant (who might not even be sick!). Here, we favor the use of the term* intervention *because the term* treatment *is so linked to the concept of drug efficacy trials—which are decidedly not the focus of this book. However, both terms are used, especially if overuse of one term or the other makes the writing cumbersome.*

Sprague-Dawley rats supplied by a commercial vendor will probably be true for all rats of this strain; it is not necessary that the rats represent a random sample of the Sprague-Dawley rat population). In clinical research, however, patients referred to an academic center for management of congestive heart failure may not be representative of the general population of such patients. Thus, inferences from studying such a sample have to be tempered.

Furthermore, when therapeutic interventions are tested, the treatment must be used in a way that can reasonably be used in a typical, not experimental, clinical setting for the study's conclusions to be externally valid. This constraint is less important in translational research, however, where the goal is to elucidate biologic mechanisms rather than to demonstrate therapeutic effectiveness.

Thus, it should be no surprise that it is usually not possible to accomplish everything in a single study. However, when the primary goal of the study is to demonstrate a cause-effect relationship between an intervention and outcome, the randomized, controlled, experiment remains the most powerful means of doing so. This chapter covers the basic features of this type of study design, some of its most common variants, and some cautions that should be understood when setting up to design and conduct a clinical experiment.

## BASIC EXPERIMENTAL DESIGN

To answer a research question, a study must be designed, measurements must be made, and the results must be analyzed. If data are simply collected but cannot be appropriately evaluated, the investigator has at the very least wasted his or her and everyone else's time and money—and at worst, has exposed a volunteer human being to an intervention that carries risks and side effects. So, part of proper design includes a plan for how the data should eventually be analyzed.

Standard statistical models used to compare groups (such as the *t* test or an analysis of variance) assume that the participants in each group represent randomly selected members of the target population, that the data extracted from the measurements follow a "normal" distribution, and that the data variances are equal across the groups (Chapter 24). Significant departures from these assumptions may invalidate the proper use of some statistical models used to compare groups, although others continue to perform adequately despite such violations (i.e., some models are more robust than others). As a result, some study designs, when analyzed with their appropriate statistical models, may be more powerful than others (i.e., more likely to detect statistically

significant differences between or among groups), while at the same time less robust than an alternative (i.e., more likely to produce a spurious result if the data violate the underlying assumptions of the statistical model). These and other tensions (such as feasibility or ethical concerns) must be taken into account before a final choice is made for one study design over another.

Despite a wide variety of available study formats, experimental study designs can actually be divided into two simple categories: between-subject and within-subject designs[2] (1). Studies with a between-subject format are sometimes called between-group or parallel group designs.

In the simplest between-subject study (Figure 8–1), a cohort of research participants is identified, recruited, and consented. Then, one-half of the participants will be exposed to the experimental intervention, while the other half will not. At a suitable time after the intervention, a measurement will be performed on each participant, and the data from the two groups will be compared.

In the simplest within-subject study (Figure 8–2), a cohort of research participants (perhaps a cohort identical to the one that would have been assembled for the between-subject study) is again identified, recruited, and consented. However, in this case, a baseline measurement is made before exposure to the intervention. All the participants then receive the experimental treatment, and again after a suitable time, the same measurement is obtained after the exposure. The investigator then compares data from before and after the intervention.

These most basic designs have many variations (some of which will be discussed later), but it's important to thoroughly understand the advantages and disadvantages of these two first.

To begin, note that in both types of design, only one trait distinguishes one experimental group from another. In a between-subject study, it's whether or not the research participant was exposed to the experimental intervention. In a within-subject study, it's whether the measurement was obtained before or after the intervention. In the between-subject case, it's the intervention itself; in the within-subject format, it's time. Attributes used to characterize and differentiate one group from another for purposes of analysis are often referred to as factors. A factor is

---

[2]In this book, we have assiduously avoided referring to research volunteers as "subjects" in an attempt to emphasize the voluntary nature of their participation. However, the terms between-subject and within-subject are firmly entrenched in the literature, and alternatives such as between-volunteers or between-participants seem unnecessarily cumbersome. Thus, this is one exception where we will use the term subject to refer to a human research volunteer.

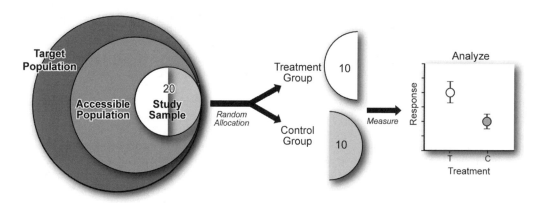

**FIGURE 8–1** ● Schematic representation of a between-subject study design. A study sample is enrolled, the experimental intervention ("treatment") is allocated to one-half of the participants by a formal process of randomization, a measurement is made of an appropriate response variable after a suitable time, and then finally, the data are analyzed statistically.

an example of a specific type of variable used to distinguish groups from one another, and both the between-subject and within-subject experiments are examples of single factor studies.

Factors can have levels (just like variables can have values). In the simplest between- and within-subject studies, there are only two levels: either the participant received the treatment or not, or the measurement was made before or after the treatment. But obviously, studies could be designed so that these same factors had more than two levels. For instance, different groups of research participants might receive the same drug,[3] but at different doses. Or, alternatively, the measurements in a within-subject study could be made at multiple times, before or after the intervention. A decision to

use more than two levels in either type of study has implications for both how the study should be designed and analyzed, as will be discussed later.

Just as factors can have more than two levels, studies can also have more than one factor. A study with a between-subject factorial design would be an investigation of multiple, independent factors (Figure 8–3). For instance, an investigator might design a study to determine whether an experimental intervention (say, a drug) had different effects in men than women. In this case, gender would be one factor and whether or not the participant received the active drug would be the other factor, resulting in four experimental groups. Alternatively, a study that investigated the use of two treatments would also be a between-subject factorial design. Thus, the multiple factors can include a combination of classification variables (not under the control of the investigator) and experimental interventions (by definition, under the control of the investigator), or can include only different types of experimental interventions.

---

[3]In this chapter, we will often use a drug as the experimental intervention, for convenience, even though other interventions would be equally germane. In translational research, drugs are often used as a probe of a particular biologic mechanism and not necessarily to demonstrate therapeutic efficacy.

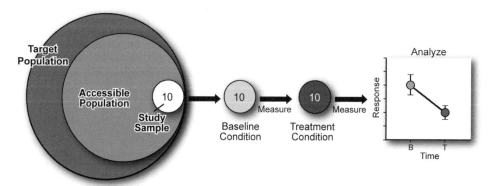

**FIGURE 8–2** ● Schematic representation of a within-subject study design. After enrollment, a baseline measurement of the primary response variable is made in all participants, then all participants are exposed to the experimental intervention ("treatment"), the measurement of the response variable is repeated, and finally the data are analyzed statistically.

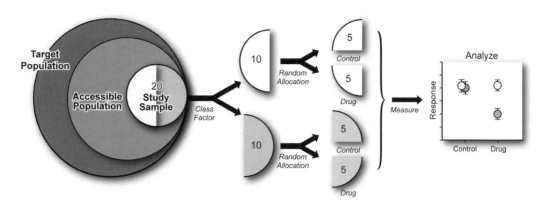

**FIGURE 8–3** ● Schematic representation of a between-subjects factorial design. In this example, research participants are first divided into two groups based on a classification variable (e.g., above or below a certain age). Then, the two subgroups are separately randomized as in a simple between-subject study (in this case, to receive either a control placebo or an active drug). Alternatively, the first separation into subgroups could have been based on a random allocation to one experimental intervention, with a second randomization within each subgroup to a second intervention.

Studies that combine elements of the between-subject and within-subject formats are called mixed factorial designs (Figure 8–4). Perhaps participants would be randomized to either receive a test drug or not (one factor), and measurements would be made before and after (another factor) the experimental intervention (active drug or placebo) in all participants. The result would again be four experimental groups. As will be shown, the mixed factorial design is one of the most common and important design formats in experimental medicine. Table 8–1 lists the most common experimental study designs.

## Between-Subject Designs

The defining characteristic of between-subject designs is a mechanism for deciding who should or should not be exposed to the experimental intervention. Ideally, this decision is made through the process of randomization, that is, a formal set of rules for allocating the intervention to different participants in an unbiased manner.

Randomized studies generally, but not automatically, have the same, or nearly the same, number of participants in each group. Such studies are referred to as balanced. When the number of participants is distinctly different in the experimental groups, the study is unbalanced.

Importantly, randomized, balanced, between-subject studies are very robust with respect to statistical analysis; that is, the models used to analyze such studies continue to perform well even if underlying assumptions about normality and variance equality are violated (Chapter 24). This feature is especially significant in translational clinical experiments because these studies tend to include

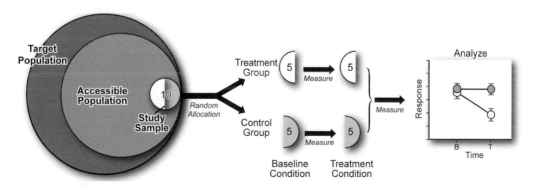

**FIGURE 8–4** ● Schematic representation of a mixed-factorial study design. As in the between-subject design, the experimental intervention is allocated to one-half of the participants by a formal process of randomization. However, a baseline measurement of the response variable is made in both active and control intervention groups, followed by exposure to the intervention ("treatment"), followed by a repeat measurement of the response variable. Finally, the data are analyzed statistically.

## TABLE 8–1

### Experimental Study Designs

| Basic | Variations |
| --- | --- |
| Between-subject | Between-subject factorial |
| | Run-in |
| Within-subject | Crossover |
| | Latin square |
| Mixed factorial | |

relatively small numbers of participants (<50, often much less) and it is difficult to ensure either normality or equal variance with such small numbers.

Unfortunately, between-subject studies are relatively inefficient and less powerful than alternative within-subject studies. The reason for this lack of efficiency is straightforward. Each measurement is made once on each research participant. Thus, as the levels of each between-subject factor increase (e.g., the dose of a drug), more volunteers must be recruited. As discussed in Chapter 5, perhaps as many as 40 people must be identified before a volunteer is successfully enrolled into a clinical experiment. Depending on the disease and the nature of the experimental intervention, among other issues, it may be impossible to identify the required number of volunteers for a multilevel, or multifactorial between-subject research study.

The relative lack of statistical power of the between-subject format further compounds the problem of identifying sufficient numbers of research volunteers for this type of study. If the only difference between two research groups is the allocation of the experimental intervention (as it is in a between-subject study), then any differences in the responses to the intervention among the individuals of the groups must be due to uncontrolled (and usually, unknown) confounding factors, loosely attributed to individual "biologic variation." In standard statistical models, these individual variances are summed to estimate a variance for the group as a whole (Chapter 24). If the sum of this individual variation within the groups is greater than the variation in response specifically due to the experimental intervention itself, then it can be difficult to detect a difference between groups with a high degree of confidence. It is because of this relative lack of power and efficiency that within-subject designs are often preferred in experimental medicine (see below).

Although the dropout of research participants before the study is completed is a problem for any research design, between-subject studies are especially susceptible to the selective dropout of research volunteers from one group more than the other groups. Although random allocation of the experimental intervention virtually ensures equal (or nearly equal) numbers of participants in each study group, it does not ensure that equal numbers of volunteers will finish the study. For instance, a drug may have side effects that some participants find intolerable. As a result, they simply fail to show up for follow-up evaluation as prescribed by the study protocol. (In the worst case, they die before follow-up observation is completed!) In nonrandomized studies, it might be tempting to simply add more volunteers who can successfully complete the protocol until there are equal numbers of participants in the control and treatment groups. However, this strategy would be a poor solution because those who can complete the protocol, despite receiving the drug in question, might be very different than the population of those who couldn't complete the protocol. In every clinical experiment, then, it is important to fully account for dropouts.

In general, the unit of experimentation in clinical research is the individual research participant. But in some circumstances, a distinction must be made between between-experimental units and observational units (2). For instance, in an asthma study, airway tissue biopsy samples might be obtained after some intervention designed to modulate airway inflammation. In such a case, the intervention is applied to the experimental unit (the person) and measurements are made on the observational units (the tissue samples). Treating each specimen as an independent observation would greatly increase the apparent "*n*" of the experiment, thereby increasing the likelihood of identifying a difference compared with data from tissue samples of research volunteers treated with a placebo. However, this difference would violate the assumption in such an analysis that the data points come from completely independent observations, because in fact multiple samples come from the same individual. Actually, this study is a good example of a mixed factorial study (as discussed later in this chapter) in which one variable is a between-subject factor (whether or not the active drug was administered to the person) and another variable is a within-subject factor (the number of biopsy specimens from each person).

A variant of this problem develops when more than one assay is to be performed on the tissue samples, but methodologic constraints mandate that each assay can only be performed once on each biopsy specimen. In this case, the best strategy is to formally randomize assignment of the different specimens to the different assay types in the same manner used to randomize individual research volunteers to an experimental intervention or placebo.

## Within-Subject Design

In contrast to the between-subject format, the defining characteristic of the within-subject format is not whether a research participant was exposed to the experimental intervention but when the measurement was made—either before or after the intervention. The implications of this difference are significant.

Because the major source of error in measuring the response to an experimental intervention (when bias has been minimized by randomization and masking of treatment assignment) is individual differences in those responses, making measurements from the same individual before and after the intervention, intuitively, should be free of that error variance. By effectively eliminating the influence of biologic variation, within-subject studies are more powerful than between-subject studies; that is, they are more likely to detect a difference that can be ascribed to the intervention. This increase in power means that within-subject designs are also more efficient, because fewer participants are needed to complete the research protocol. These advantages are particularly attractive for translational research studies because both the patient base and financial resources supporting the study may be very limited.

Importantly, in a within-subject study, there is no random assignment of treatment; every participant receives the experimental intervention. The control in this case is the data obtained prior to the intervention (baseline data). Unfortunately, there can be no guarantee that the group of volunteers is exactly the same in all respects after the intervention as it was before the intervention (except of course for the specific effects of the intervention itself, if any). Indeed, the longer the time interval between measurements, the more likely it is that the individuals will not be the same. For this reason, a simple within-subject study, while still an "experiment" in the sense that it includes an intervention under the control of an investigator, is sometimes called "quasi-experimental" (3) to signify the lack of randomization and the potential introduction of bias, in this case, caused by the effects of time.

There are no statistical methods for managing this problem per se. Rather, investigators attempt via experimental design to either control known confounders that may change over time (e.g., insulin clamping to control blood sugar), or they measure a variety of other variables (covariates) hoping to demonstrate that the individuals in the two states are similar (except for the variables that are hypothesized to be responsive to the intervention).

A good example of this problem is known as "regression to the mean." This phenomenon occurs when an abnormal value is used as an entry criterion to a study. Commonly, a second measurement will be closer to the population mean (i.e., less abnormal). The difference between the two measurements without any intervening treatment is simply another example of normal "biologic variation." Unfortunately, if an experimental intervention had been used prior to the second measurement, it would be tempting to attribute the change in the variable to the intervention itself. For instance, imagine a study in which the blood pressure had to be elevated to qualify for entry into the study. Second measurements of blood pressure at a later time are notorious for frequently being lower (an example of so-called white coat hypertension). Had a drug been given between the two measurements, it would be impossible to distinguish whether the effect was due to the drug or an example of regression to the mean. It is exactly because of experiences like this that other designs, like the mixed factorial design (see next section), are favored when possible.

Another problem with within-subject formats is that the statistical models commonly used to analyze data from these studies (e.g., a paired *t* test or a repeated measures analysis of variance—see Chapter 24) are less robust than the tests used to analyze between-subject formats. That is, these tests fail to perform adequately if assumptions such as the normality of the distribution and equal variance are violated. The result is an increased risk of Type I statistical error; that is, of making the inference that a difference exists between or among groups when one in fact does not exist. Thus, investigators should carefully inspect their data (and the computer output of programs that perform the related analyses) and if problems are identified, they should seek a biostatistical consultation.

Yet another problem develops with within-subject study designs when more than one level of a factor is tested on the same individual (e.g., dosages of a drug) or research participants are exposed to more than one experimental intervention (e.g., two different drugs). The risk here is that the effects of the earlier intervention will carry over to the second intervention. One method that addresses this problem is to wait until the effect of the first intervention has dissipated and measures of this effect have returned to control (baseline) levels (sometimes referred to as a washout period). However, there is still the possibility of unmeasured effects, which only become apparent after exposure to the second intervention. An additional strategy is to counterbalance the order of the interventions in a randomized way, such that the order of the interventions is not the same for all participants. There are many counterbalancing schemes, but two of the most common are the crossover and Latin square designs, which are discussed in greater detail in the following section. However, note that counterbalancing doesn't eliminate the carryover effect if it exists; it simply allows the investigator to isolate, analyze, and quantify the impact of any carryover effect (by comparing subgroups based on the order of the interventions received).

A variation of this general carryover phenomenon is the differential carryover effect (sometimes called a "treatment by period interaction" by statisticians), which occurs when the order of the interventions determines whether a carryover effect will be present (e.g., the effects of drug B are different if they are given before or after drug A, but the effects of drug A are the same). Unfortunately, counterbalancing won't be useful in this circumstance.

These issues of general and differential carryover effects are sufficiently troublesome that within-subject factorial studies are often controversial, limiting their use overall.

## ADVANCED EXPERIMENTAL DESIGNS

A number of more complex variants of the basic between-subject and within-subject study formats have been developed, primarily to improve efficiency; that is, the ability to answer the experimental question with the fewest number of research volunteers. Given the rarity of some diseases and the costs of some sophisticated assays (e.g., imaging), this motivation is understandable. However, many problems in execution, cost, and interpretation accompany these more complex designs, including possible interactions among interventions (when multiple interventions are studied as part of one experiment), failure to complete the study because of problems (e.g., side effects) associated with one intervention (making it impossible to study the other intervention even though it itself is not a problem), and failure to adequately adhere to the protocol (because of the increased complexity).

### Nesting

A factor is said to be *nested* within another factor when it is restricted to one level of that factor (1,2). For example, in a simple between-subject format, the individual participants are nested within the group to which they are randomized, because they are in that group and that group only (each group

representing one level of the factor group). Examples of non-nested studies, then, include cases where each participant is exposed to all levels of a factor, such as the simple within-subject design (each volunteer participates in all levels of the "time" factor). Crossover studies and some factorial studies (like the Latin square design) (see below) are other examples of non-nested studies.

### Mixed Factorial Designs

Despite the previous cautionary remarks about complex study designs, the so-called "mixed factorial design" is one of the most commonly employed formats in translational research because it maintains the efficiency and power of the within-subject study design while allowing time-related effects (which is the major problem of the within-subject design) to be evaluated. The simplest form of the mixed factorial study is limited to two factors (one between-subject and one within-subject factor). The between-subject factor would be the experimental intervention, and the within-subject factor would be time. In this way, it is possible to assess the impact of time by simultaneously studying two groups, one that is exposed to the active form of the intervention and a control group that is identical in every respect except that none of the participants are exposed the intervention (Figure 8–4). For instance, after a volunteer is enrolled into a study, he or she would first be randomized to a group that would either receive a drug (or other active intervention) or get the placebo. The allocation could (and should) be masked so that neither the volunteer nor the investigator knew the assignment. Then, baseline measurements would be made, followed by administration of the active drug or placebo (again masked to conceal its actual identity). Afterward, an additional measurement (or measurements) would be made at an appropriate time (or times) to assess the response to the intervention. The measurements would be made at the same predetermined times in all participants. The statistical model that would be used to analyze these data (Chapter 24) would take into effect these two main effects: group assignment and time (the latter accounting for the "repeated measures"). It would also take into account any possible interaction between these two main effects; that is, that one group would behave differently than the other only at some, not all, of the measurement times.

Obviously, as additional between- or within-subject factors are added, the number of potential interactions among the factors can quickly become overwhelming. For instance, consider a mixed factorial study in which the key response variable is cardiac output and assume that the hypothesis to be tested is that a drug will increase cardiac output. Say that the plan is to make a baseline measurement of cardiac output, followed by administration of either the new drug or a placebo, followed by hourly measurements of cardiac output over 5 hours (six total measurements in each participant). Now, also assume that the measurement of cardiac output by the method to be employed is known to be variable, and that to account for such variability, the measurement is to be repeated three times at each hourly time point. The main factors in such a study include group, time, and measurement number. To analyze this study, a three-way statistical model would have to account for one between-subject comparison, two within-subject comparisons, three two-way interactions, and one three-way interaction. Additional factors would obviously add yet more complexity. In the example just given, one common method of reducing the complexity would be to average the cardiac output measurements before using them in the statistical analysis. This "solution" may not always be possible or appropriate.

The potential disadvantages of the mixed factorial format are similar to those of any within-subject study, namely carryover effects and greater restrictions on the statistical models used for data analysis. There is also some loss of efficiency, as well as increased cost, because an additional control group must be recruited and studied at multiple times, just as the interventional group is studied. Thus, estimates of sample size that take into account the expected effect size of the intervention should be balanced against this loss of efficiency (Chapter 9) before making a final decision about whether or not to employ this format (or any other, for that matter).

### Between-Subject Factorial Designs

In two general situations it makes sense to consider studying more than one factor as part of the same experiment. In one instance, the two factors are both of interest in terms of their potential effect on a particular outcome or response, and both are known (or assumed) ahead of time to not interact with one another to affect that outcome or response. In this case, it is possible to design a study with a between-subject factorial design that would evaluate the two factors more efficiently than would two separate studies. However, if the two factors are indeed found to interact with one another, it is likely that the study will be underpowered to evaluate main effects of each factor because these represent subgroups of the whole.

In the other situation, the two factors are known (or suspected) to interact such that their effects together on the outcome or response is different than their separate effects. Ironically, in this setting, the same between-subject factorial design is actually well suited to study such interactions.

As an example, consider a circumstance in which preclinical studies suggest that the effect of a drug may be different in patients who possess a specific single nucleotide polymorphism (SNP) in a gene, the gene product of which is thought to be important in the downstream effects of the drug. This problem could be addressed as a type of pharmacogenetics study (see Chapter 21). To determine whether a similar effect is true in humans, a randomized between-subject study could be designed in patients identified with the SNP, and then separately in those without the SNP. However, if the studies are done separately and at different times, any differences between the two groups in the effect of the drug could be due to differences that developed during the time interval between the two studies (e.g., changes in study personnel or changes in assay techniques). A between-subject factorial design would efficiently address this problem by designing the study so that both factors (the drug and the SNP) were evaluated at the same time.

Alternatively, consider the example of a study in which it's suspected that the effect of drug B depends on whether or not the patient is also receiving drug A. Separate between-subject studies of drug A versus placebo, and of drug B versus placebo, would not reveal such an interaction. In a between-subject factorial study, however, one-quarter of the patients would receive two placebos, one-quarter would receive drug A and placebo, one-quarter would receive drug B and placebo, and one-quarter would receive both drug A and drug B. The analysis of the results from these four cells would not only reveal the relative effects of each drug but also of their effects when combined, if any.

An important principle of factorial design is that when more than one intervention is to be tested, each intervention must be evaluated by a distinct outcome or response. For instance, if an investigator were testing the effects of two drugs, one of which was being evaluated as an antihypertensive, the other drug should not also affect blood pressure, or it would obscure the extent to which each was responsible for the change in blood pressure.

In some circumstances, it may be appropriate to exclude certain cells when interactions are known to be unimportant, yielding so-called partial or fractional factorial designs. In other situations, the interactions may not be feasible for ethical or toxicity reasons, yielding so-called incomplete factorial designs (4). Investigators are advised to obtain expert biostatistical advice before deciding to employ one of these designs.

## Crossover Designs

A between-subject factorial study is one strategy for improving the efficiency of studying more than one factor at a time. The factors involved may be classification factors (gender or genotype) or experimental interventions under the control of the investigator (drug dosage or different drugs).

As an alternative, the crossover study (Figure 8–5) is a variation of the within-subject study design with the same intent, namely to study the effects of more than one factor, in this case all experimental interventions under the control of the investigator, while retaining the advantages of the within-subject format (primarily, improved efficiency and greater statistical power, resulting in fewer participants to achieve the goals of the study). In a crossover study, unlike a two-factor between-subject study, participants are exposed to more than one factor in sequence (although the sequence varies among the participants). However, none of the participants are exposed to both (or more) factors at the same time (which distinguishes this study design from the between-subject factorial design). Thus, the two-factor between-subject design can be used when it is hypothesized that no interaction will occur (and analyzed statistically to prove that that is the case) or can be used when specifically an investigator wishes to determine the nature and magnitude of an interaction. By contrast, the crossover design should only be used when it is known or hypothesized that no interaction will occur as a result of carryover effects.

As mentioned earlier, the principle motivation for undertaking a crossover design (as opposed to a simple within-subject design) is when an investigator is concerned about carryover effects. By randomizing the order in which participants are exposed to the interventions, any bias that might develop because of one intervention affecting the other can be identified and analyzed. However, this end result depends on the power of the statistical methods to detect such interactions, and this ability has been questioned by some (5), resulting in recommendations that, in general, the crossover design be avoided.

Crossover designs become less desirable when the treatment period or the washout periods are lengthy. Not only does this lengthen the study duration overall, but the longer these periods are, the more likely it is that something may have changed in the participant during the time between treatment periods. Research participants are also less likely to adhere to protocols, or even to complete protocols, which are lengthy in duration. And, of course, lengthy trials are usually costly.

As with factorial designs, more complex crossover designs are also possible. For example, the Latin square is a design in which the initial intervention is randomized, but the sequence of interventions is not (1). Because of their complexity (including duration of time required to complete all interventions and washout periods) and associated costs, these designs are rarely used in most translational experimental research. The interested reader can find more detailed discussions of these designs in the references (1-4,6-8).

## Run-in Periods

Adherence to a research protocol, of course, is critical to whether or not a study is likely to be successful.

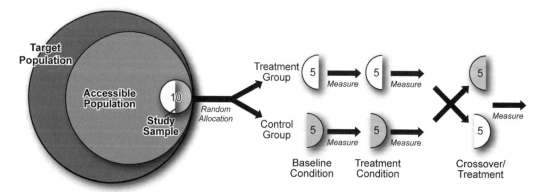

Treatment Group

Control Group

Baseline Condition    Treatment Condition    Crossover/ Treatment

**FIGURE 8–5** ● Schematic representation of crossover study design. In this variant of the within-subject design, research participants are first randomized to receive either the active or control intervention. A baseline measurement is made, followed by exposure to the intervention, followed by a second measurement of the response variable. After a suitable washout period, another baseline measurement is made, followed by exposure to the alternate intervention, followed finally by another measurement of the response variable.

This criterion applies to both the investigative team and the research participant. A significant number of volunteers may fail to complete some protocols, by their nature, more than others, wasting resources and making interpretation of final results difficult. To reduce this occurrence, studies can be designed with a run-in period in which it is determined whether a particular volunteer is likely to adhere to the protocol (Figure 8–6). Studies that depend on diets or exercise routines, for instance, may employ a run-in period to screen out those patients who are unlikely to comply with the protocol.

Both placebo and active interventions can be used during the run-in period, but for different reasons. Placebos are typically used when the goal of the run-in period is to determine whether or not the volunteer will adhere to the protocol itself. Of course, there is no guarantee that protocol compliance will remain high if the participant is subsequently randomized to the active intervention and experiences unpleasant side effects. However, chances of successfully completing the protocol are presumably increased if the participant successfully completes the run-in period of observation.

Alternatively, the active intervention itself can be used during the run-in period, especially if the overall desired response to the intervention is expected to be low. For instance, perhaps an investigator would like to test the effect of prolonged cholesterol reduction below a certain threshold on atherosclerosis, using imaging techniques to measure the lumenal diameter of the carotid artery as a surrogate measure of atherosclerosis. A run-in period would help select those individuals who could achieve this magnitude of cholesterol reduction before taking the additional time to determine whether prolonged reduction would have an effect on atherogenesis.

Clearly, then, when a run-in period is used, strict criteria must be applied to determine which patients will be allowed to continue in the study.

## RANDOMIZATION

### Types of Randomization

As has been emphasized repeatedly, random assignment of the intervention is the best protection against bias in experimental studies. Although the method of randomization can be as simple as flipping a coin, such methods do not guarantee that at the end of the study, equal numbers of participants will have received the various interventions—they only guarantee an equal chance of receiving each intervention. It is true that as the number of volunteers increases (say, >100), it is increasingly likely that, by chance alone, equal numbers of participants will receive either the active intervention or the control. However, the converse is also true: in small studies (<30), there is a significant chance that with simple randomization, the groups would be imbalanced. Intuitively, the chances of ending up with 7 tails and 3 heads with 10 coin tosses is much more likely than 70 tails and 30 heads with 100 tosses—a consequence of the "law of large numbers" (9).

A related problem is the likelihood that, even if the same number of participants were exposed to the intervention, they would be imbalanced with respect to some important known confounder (sometimes also called a covariate). For example, if age is known to be a factor that can influence the outcome of a particular intervention, simple randomization is less likely to produce groups with equal numbers of old and young participants in studies of small

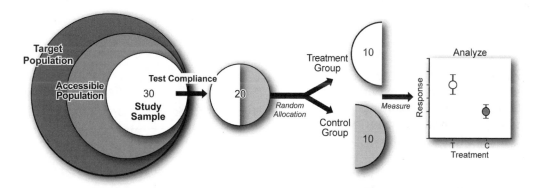

**FIGURE 8–6** ● Schematic representation of a study with a run-in design. In this variant of the between-subject design, all research participants first receive the placebo to test their compliance with the protocol. After review, the subset of compliant participants is selected and the study proceeds as in a simple between-subject study. Alternatively, all research participants could receive the active intervention first to identify those who will respond to a necessary threshold level before proceeding.

size than in studies of large size. Although it is possible to use statistical methods (e.g., analysis of covariance, see Chapter 24) to adjust for imbalances in baseline characteristics, reducing the likelihood that they will occur through study design is much preferred.

An alternative to simple randomization, especially for studies of small size, is the strategy of performing randomization on so-called permuted blocks. The primary purpose of blocked randomization is to ensure equal numbers of participants in each of the planned study groups. Generally, the blocks are twice the size of the number of groups (but they can be any multiple of the number of groups). So, if an experimental intervention is being compared to a control, the block size would be four research participants. Within each block, the number of participants who receive the intervention and control are equal (in this case, two each). Then, the assignments are permuted in a random manner, for example, as shown in Table 8–2. The research participants are assigned to their group as they are listed in the table (the exact sequence of which, as well as the block length, are kept masked from the investigators and research team). In this case, the first volunteer would receive the experimental intervention E, the next one would get the control, the third one would get the control, the fourth one would get the intervention E, the fifth one would get the control, and so on.

Another alternative to simple randomization is to employ stratification. The primary purpose of stratification is to ensure that important covariates that may affect the outcome or response variable (confounders) are equally distributed among the planned study groups. Usually only one or two covariates at most are used for stratification. Thus, a factor, like age, is first identified as an important covariate; then, separate randomization schedules are used within the groups identified by that factor. Even so, stratification only guarantees that at the end of the study, the treatment groups will be balanced with respect to that factor; it does not guarantee that equal numbers will end up being exposed to the experimental intervention versus control, especially in small studies. Thus, stratification is usually employed at the same time with blocked randomization.

Yet another strategy is randomization on matched pairs. This approach differs from stratification, even though it is also based on first identifying a factor, like age, that is known to influence the outcome of interest. Pairs of volunteers similar with respect to that factor are then assembled. Finally, the treatment assignment is randomized within each pair so that in all cases one participant will be exposed to the experimental intervention and one serves as the control. Obviously, for such a system to work, it is necessary to assemble such pairs prospectively, which may be inconvenient, because volunteers may have to wait until a match can be found before they begin their participation in the study. In some cases, natural matches are available, say when a study can use either eye or either limb for the active intervention and the contralateral eye or limb for the control.

Many other randomization schemes are available, including so-called adaptive procedures which adjust the odds of receiving the intervention based on interim looks at the data. Although these are generally unusual in most translational studies, they may be appropriate for trials of very small size, as discussed in Chapter 18. Table 8–3 lists the most common types of randomization.

## Mechanics of Randomization

Although randomization means unpredictable, it does not mean chaotic. The randomization scheme should be reproducible, and it should be well documented so that violations can be detected if the study is audited.

| TABLE 8–2 |
|---|

**Example of Permuted Block Assignments in a Study with 20 Volunteers, 10 Receiving the Experimental Intervention (E) and 10 Receiving the Control Placebo (P)**

| Block 1 | Block 2 | Block 3 | Block 4 | Block 5 |
|---|---|---|---|---|
| EPPE | PEEP | PEEP | PPEE | EPEP |

| TABLE 8–3 |
|---|

**Types of Randomization**

Simple
Permuted blocks
Stratified
Stratified with permuted blocks
Group

For most small experimental studies, a computer can generate a set of random numbers for allocation of research volunteers to the study groups. Typically, the assignments are placed individually into sealed, opaque envelopes at the beginning of the study by someone who will not be opening them at the time of enrollment to determine treatment allocation. The envelopes should be numbered, again facilitating an audit trail to be generated at the end of the study. The number of the envelope should be recorded onto the study case report form.

## MASKING

Although randomization minimizes bias due to confounders that may be present prior to and including treatment assignment, it does not prevent bias that can occur once the participant has been exposed to the intervention. To minimize postrandomization bias, it is important to employ masking (blinding). Ideally, the treatment assignments will remain unknown to the research participant, the person administering the intervention, and the person evaluating responses or outcomes (triple blind).

Even though the value of masking is just as important as randomization, its implementation is much more difficult to achieve, especially in investigator-initiated experimental research. In some cases, such as when testing a diet or an exercise program, it is not possible to conceal the nature of the intervention. Even when placebos can be manufactured, it can be virtually impossible for the academic investigator to obtain them without the resources and cooperation of a pharmaceutical company.

In these cases, a special effort should be made to at least mask the treatment assignment from the person performing the outcome evaluation, especially for the primary outcome if possible. Investigators should not assume that objective outcomes (perhaps, with the exception of death—although this is an unusual outcome for most investigator-initiated, single center, nontherapeutic clinical studies) are less prone to measurement bias than soft outcomes, such as pain assessments. Observer judgment is almost always required, even when scoring a chest radiograph or cardiac ejection fraction. When the treatment assignment is known to the person evaluating outcome, it can be very tempting to re-evaluate the outlier, to see why the data don't fit as well as data from other participants. Such bias is virtually impossible to detect. Its execution can occur for all the best of intentions, without a need to resort to accusations of fraudulent intent. It is still a bias, nevertheless.

## CHOOSING A TRIAL DESIGN

If serial measurements are possible and desirable, especially of an outcome that can be measured on a continuous scale, then a mixed factorial design is the most efficient and powerful scheme for most translational studies. However, it requires more resources (financial and otherwise) than either of the two basic research designs. When only a single endpoint will be measured (e.g., an assay on a tissue biopsy obtained after exposure to a drug), then the simple between-subject format is usually preferred. As noted throughout this chapter, the other, more complex designs are preferred especially when resources (including patient numbers) are limited.

## SUMMARY

- Most experimental designs employed in translational experimental medicine are either of a between-subject or within-subject format. The mixed factorial format is a combination of these two.
- In a simple between-subject study, a cohort of research participants is identified, recruited, and consented. Then, one-half of the participants are exposed to the experimental intervention while the other half is not. The allocation of the intervention can be decided by a process of formal randomization (true experiment) or in a nonrandomized manner (quasi-experiment).
- In a simple within-subject study, after volunteers are enrolled, preintervention (baseline) measurements are obtained, then all participants are exposed to the intervention, followed by repeat measurements.
- More complex (factorial) study designs incorporate exposures to different levels of an intervention, to different interventions, or classify patients into separate categories prior to exposure to the intervention.
- In general, between-subject studies are relatively robust with respect to the underlying assumptions of statistical models used to analyze these studies. Within-subject designs, although more restrictive with respect to the use of appropriate statistical models, are more efficient and statistically powerful than between-subject formats.
- Between-subject factorial studies are an efficient way of studying more than one intervention at the same time, and are the only way to study interactions among factors directly.
- Carryover effects, where the effects of the intervention during one measurement time period carryover to the next measurement time period,

are a major concern of within-subject studies. Mixed factorial and crossover study designs can help identify and quantify, but not eliminate, these effects.

● Randomization and masking are important strategies for eliminating bias, that, whenever possible, should be incorporated into the design of experimental studies.

## REFERENCES

1. Zolman J. Experimental design. In: Zolman J, ed. Biostatistics: Experimental Design and Statistical Inference. New York: Oxford University Press, 1993:38–76.
2. Piantadosi S. Clinical trials as experimental designs. In: Piantadosi S, ed. Clinical Trials: A Methodologic Perspective. New York: John Wiley and Sons, 1997:61–105.
3. Morgan G, Gliner J, Harmon R. Quasi-experimental designs. J Am Acad Child Adolesc Psychiatry 2000;39: 794–796.
4. Piantadosi S. Factorial designs. In: Piantadosi S, ed. Clinical Trials: A Methodologic Perspective. New York: John Wiley and Sons, 1997:388–403.
5. Friedman L, Furberg C, DeMets D. Basic study design. In: Friedman L, Furberg C, DeMets D, eds. Fundamentals of Clinical Trials. 3rd Ed. New York: Springer, 1998.
6. Morgan G, Gliner J, Harmon R. Randomized experimental designs. J Am Acad Child Adolesc Psychiatry 2000;39:1062–1063.
7. Hulley S, Cummings S, Browner W et al. Designing an experiment: clinical trials I. In: Hulley S, Cummings S, Browner W et al., eds. Designing Clinical Research: An Epidemiologic Approach. 2nd Ed. Philadelphia: Lippincott Williams & Wilkins, 2001.
8. Gliner J, Morgan G. Research Methods in Applied Settings: An Integrated Approach to Design and Analysis. Mahwah, NJ: Lawrence Erlbaum, 2000.
9. Lavori P, Louis T, Bailar III J et al. Designs for experiments—parallel comparisons of treatment. N Engl J Med 1983;309:1291–1298.

# CHAPTER 9

# Estimating Sample Size

Steven Goodman, Amanda Blackford

## THE PURPOSE OF THE SAMPLE SIZE CALCULATION

The need to calculate a sample size—for a grant proposal, study protocol, or some other study-planning purpose—is one of the most common reasons an investigator will use statistical software or will contact a statistician. It is also a widely misunderstood exercise. Some investigators question the need to perform such a calculation, because they can only afford (in terms of time or money) to study a fixed number of research volunteers; the purpose of calculations that merely follow a circuitous logic to "justify" that number is unclear. It is also not unusual for an investigator to claim complete ignorance about the basic inputs required for a sample size calculation; simply studying an accessible or affordable sample seems more reasonable than studying a higher number based on speculative estimates. The misconception that statistical formulas generate a sample size "requirement" or "justification" for a particular experimental design is also prevalent.

Each of these perspectives reflects different misunderstandings about both the role of statistics and statisticians in the planning of studies. In this overview of technical methods to calculate sample size, the chapter also addresses these deeper issues, because understanding these issues is more important than the formulas themselves.

### Implications versus Justification

Quite frequently, the language surrounding sample size suggests that the associated procedures are designed to justify a particular sample size choice. The objections noted above are directed at the fact that many practical reasons that govern the choice of sample size—particularly in the translational setting where there are many unknowns—preclude justifying a choice in statistical terms. If the study budget restricts an experiment to 10 subjects, how does the investigator justify that statistically? But every choice of sample size, regardless of its motivation, has implications. Even if a sample size is chosen for completely nonstatistical reasons, the consequences of that choice can be quantified. It may well be that an investigator, faced with the implications of a too-small experiment, will decide that his or her study needs to be redesigned or other avenues of study need to be pursued. So, it is often more constructive to speak of sample size implications, rather than justifications or requirements.

## CLARIFYING THE QUESTION

The first thing that a sample size calculation requires is a clear and operationally explicit hypothesis (Chapter 1). Once this hypothesis has been established, it is often a trivial matter to calculate a sample size. In reality, a sample size consultation is typically the discussion of various ways to clarify and operationalize the study hypothesis. Sample size implications can critically shape the choices made, and these choices affect the sample size.

To demonstrate, first consider a general hypothesis that might be posed as the basis for a study: "Methotrexate improves the course of rheumatoid arthritis (RA) by inhibiting the autoimmune-mediated destruction of the joint."

Although clear in some respects, this hypothesis is not nearly precise enough for the purposes of calculating a sample size. To start, it suggests three possible endpoints for the study. The first endpoint would be a clinical one that could be used to define the "course of RA." This definition might be measured by visual analog pain scores, an index of of activities of daily living, or some functional measure (see Chapter 3). A second possible class of endpoints is related to the autoimmune mechanism, which could involve measurements of cytokines, antibodies, or other markers of autoimmune activity. Finally, the investigator might want to look at the degree of joint destruction, as measured radiographically.

The choice of endpoint is just a beginning. The investigator must next consider how to convert the measurement of that endpoint into a number (Chapter 3). Typically, the choice is whether to make it a continuous measure (e.g., cytokine levels), an ordinal one (degrees of radiographic severity), or binary ($>50\%$ reduction in pain score). Each of these measures will have different variability within and between participants and a different degree of effect that might be expected from the intervention (methotrexate administration). *It is the ratio of the plausible effect size to the between-subject variability that drives the sample size calculation.* The smaller the signal (the effect) relative to the noise (the variability), the higher the number of participants required to distinguish between the two. In the section that follows, these basic concepts are discussed in more detail.

It should be clear from the example above that a given experiment or hypothesis does not have a single mathematically dictated sample size. Each choice of outcome measure, effect size, and analytic method has sample size implications, and each sample size in turn affects how an investigator might choose, measure, and analyze an outcome. To add to this mix, investigators have choices about purely statistical parameters that determine "how sure" they want to be about being able to distinguish between signal and noise of a certain magnitude. As is apparent below, investigators can manipulate these many dimensions to justify almost any sample size. But if the choices made are not realistic, a price is paid at the end of the study. In the discussion of sample size, this chapter will show how to make this projection so that price is apparent from the beginning.

## BASIC PRINCIPLES

Many books, chapters, articles, and software programs have been written for the purpose of showing investigators how to calculate sample size. Formulas for different purposes can be quite complex, but their essence is quite simple and always similar. This chapter will not recapitulate what has been reported in detail in these many places, nor try to present the full array of sample size formulas for all situations. Rather, it provides formulas that

demonstrate general principles and leaves it to statistical software to execute the details. Investigators should always use standardized software to calculate sample size, so the details of the formulas are helpful only insofar as they enhance understanding.

Many of the statistical principles discussed here will be repeated in part in the section on Analyzing and Reporting Results (Section 3). However, the perspective is different. The focus here is on understanding these principles in the context of estimating the appropriate sample size needed to test an explicit hypothesis during the design phase of a research project.

## Standard Deviation and Standard Error

The purpose of studying groups of people instead of one or two is to increase the ability to see a signal amid noise. The *signal* is some typical characteristic or measure of a group of people, and the *noise* is the natural variability among people that produces deviations from that typical value. Increasing the signal over the noise means the investigator can be confident that the measure accurately reflects an underlying biologic phenomenon, and it is not simply the result of individual or chance variation.

Statistical principles allow investigators to quantify exactly how the variability among individuals relates to the variability in the average of several individuals; that is, how much taking an average of several measurements reduces noise. The variability among *individuals* is measured with the standard deviation (the square root of the average squared difference between individuals in a group and the true underlying group mean), as follows:

**Equation 1**

$$\text{Standard Deviation} = \sqrt{\frac{\text{Sum[(Individual values} - \text{True mean})^2]}{N}}$$

$$N = \text{Number of individuals in group}$$

Because the true mean is typically unknown, it is estimated with the group average and a small price is paid by dividing by $N - 1$ instead of N:

**Equation 2**

$$\begin{array}{l}\text{Estimated}\\\text{Standard}\\\text{Deviation}\end{array} = \sqrt{\frac{\text{Sum[(Individual values} - \text{Group average})^2]}{N - 1}}$$

The SD of a collection of values can be estimated regardless of how they are distributed—its calculation does not presuppose a normal or bell-shaped distribution. The critical relationship for the purpose of sample size determination is the relationship between the standard *deviation* (SD) and the standard *error of the mean* (SEM) (often shortened to "standard error"), two terms that are often confused. The SEM is a measure of the variability or imprecision of a group's *average*. That is, where the SD tells how much an *individual* measurement might deviate from its underlying true mean value, the SEM reveals how much an *average of N individuals* deviates from the underlying true mean. There is a very convenient relationship between these two quantities:

**Equation 3**

$$SEM = \frac{SD}{\sqrt{N}}$$

This equation shows how much the variability of an estimate is reduced by increasing the size of the group that is averaged. This relationship plays a central role in setting sample size.

A second statistical fact that is used to help set sample size is based on the *central limit theorem* (Chapters 3 and 23). This theorem posits that no matter what the distribution of individual values in a sample looks like, the distribution of their average will look approximately like a bell-shaped curve (i.e., a normal distribution). Thus, regardless of the distribution of the data, if summarized by averaging, it uses the well-defined properties of the normal curve to help set the sample size, or to

describe uncertainty in the estimated mean. For example, if a group of measurements is distributed normally, the precision with which the true mean can be estimated, using the conventional 95% confidence level, is approximately:

**True mean = Sample average ± 2 SEM**

(The actual multiplier is 1.96, but statisticians typically round this off to 2 for clarity and simplicity.)

Equation 3 shows that the larger the sample size (N), the smaller the standard error in the estimated mean; as a result, the larger the sample size, the more precisely can the true mean can be estimated. The relationship between SD and SEM shows that the precision (1/SEM) varies as the square root of the sample size, so that to double the precision, the sample size must increase by 4. Figure 9–1 illustrates this relationship. The dotted vertical lines represent the 95% confidence intervals for the mean. When the sample size is quadrupled from 25 to 100 subjects, the precision is doubled, corresponding to a halving of the width of the confidence interval.

## Features of the Normal Distribution

The central limit theorem allows investigators to exploit the properties of the normal distribution to help design studies even when the underlying data are quite non-normal. The normal distribution is a bell-shaped curve that is centered at its mean, $\mu$. The spread of the curve is determined by the standard

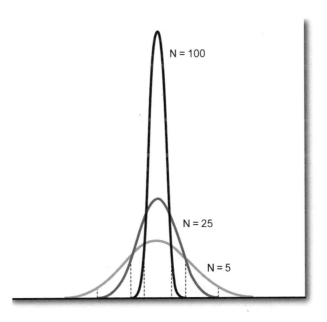

*FIGURE 9–1* ● Distributions around the average of samples of increasing size. As sample size increases, the precision of estimating the true mean improves. In this case, increasing the sample size by a factor of 4 improves the precision by a factor of 2.

N = 100

N = 25

N = 5

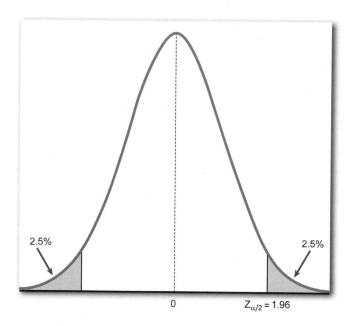

2.5%                                                    2.5%

0          $Z_{\alpha/2} = 1.96$

**FIGURE 9–2** ● Normal distribution curve with 2.5% tail areas.

## TABLE 9–1

### Tail Areas and Z scores

| Tail Area (one-sided) | Z score |
| --- | --- |
| 2.5% | 1.96 |
| 5% | 1.64 |
| 10% | 1.28 |
| 20% | 0.84 |

error. One standard error around each side of the mean includes 68% of the area under the curve; that is, it cuts off 32% from both tails combined or 16% from each separately. The number of standard errors from the mean is usually represented statistically by the Z score, with a subscript indicating the proportion of the area in the tail. The Z score for a two-sided tail area of 5% is sometimes written as $Z_{0.05/2}$, because it means $0.05/2 = 0.025$ of the total curve area will be in each tail. The Z score corresponding to a two-sided 5% area is 1.96, which is often rounded up to 2 for simplicity. Figure 9–2 illustrates this, as 2.5% of the null distribution is shaded in each tail. Other key Z scores are in shown Table 9–1.

## SAMPLE SIZE BASED ON PRECISION (CONTINUOUS MEASURES)

The previous simple relationships shown in equations 1–3 can be used to calculate sample sizes that will produce a certain degree of precision with an outcome measured on a continuous scale. For example, suppose an investigator wants to measure an average cotinine level (a measure of tobacco exposure) within 5 ng/mL. Assume further that in previous populations, the SD for cotinine was measured at 20 ng/mL. For a 95% confidence interval to be ±5 ng/mL, which is equal to ±2 SE, the SE must be 2.5 ng/mL. Rearranging equation 3 gives:

$$N = (SD/SEM)^2 = (20/2.5)^2 = 64 \text{ subjects}$$

### What to Do When You Don't Know the Standard Deviation

A difficulty can occur when there are no data on which to base a preliminary guess about the standard deviation. The investigator may know the desired precision, but not know the underlying variability. There are several ways to approach this common problem in translational clinical research. First, a literature search (Chapter 2) may uncover estimates of the standard deviation in other populations or experimental settings that may plausibly inform the researcher about this one.

Second, the investigator may know more than he or she realizes. Say he can make a guess about the highest and lowest values likely to be observed in a population. Then, because ±2 SD should encompass 95% of the values in that population, a rough estimate of the SD could be taken as (highest value − lowest value)/4. Third, if the investigator really has no clue as to the variability or the range of the data, then either a small pilot study needs to be done to estimate the variability, or the experiment can proceed until a given degree of precision is reached, without prior knowledge of what N will achieve that. Depending on safety concerns, it might be appropriate to incorporate a sequential one-at-a-time study design, as discussed in Chapter 18. Finally, for reasons that are outlined below, if the measurement can be converted from estimating a mean to estimating a proportion, the variability estimate will take care of itself.

## How to Choose a Desired Precision

Although the mathematics of the cotinine example were simple, the more difficult question is how, in general, to choose the desired degree of precision. This question can only be answered by posing it as a practical question; for example, if the true cotinine level is 30, what are the consequences of overestimating it as 35? Or underestimating it as 20? The desired precision is ultimately governed by the purpose of the estimation in the first place; the minimum degree of under- or overestimate that has material adverse consequences should be the basis for deciding what the desired precision should be.

## SAMPLE SIZE BASED ON PRECISION (DICHOTOMOUS MEASURES)

The formula for estimating proportions is very attractive for many sample size purposes because the standard error is derived from the proportion being estimated. It is of value to note that a proportion itself is an average; if the value "1" is assigned to an event and "0" to a nonevent, the proportion can be viewed as the average of N outcomes. This shows how powerful the central limit theorem is; even though the underlying data of only 1s and 0s is distinctly non–bell-shaped, the observed proportion is quite normally distributed for N > 20 (and proportions between 0.10 and 0.90).

In discussing proportions, the SEM notation is shortened to simply "SE," because a mean is not being estimated. The formula for estimating the SE of an observed proportion, *p*, is:

**Equation 4**

$$SE = \sqrt{\frac{p(1 - p)}{N}}$$

There are several important consequences and implications of this formula:

- It should only be used for sample sizes over 20 (better, over 30), when the normal approximation becomes accurate.
- It is symmetric about $p = 0.5$; that is, the SE of a proportion of 0.8 is the same as one of 0.2.

- Its maximum value occurs at $p = 0.5$ (i.e., SE $= 0.5/\sqrt{N}$).
- Except for large N, its use for setting sample size becomes less accurate for *p*'s near 0 or 1.
- For very small *p*, formulas based on the *arcsin* transformation yield better normal approximations, and these are often found in standard statistical software.

This formula can be used to very easily find a sample size that will estimate a proportion with a given precision. Rearranging the SE equation:

**Equation 5**

$$N = \frac{p(1 - p)}{SE^2}$$

Suppose the investigator wants to estimate a population proportion within ±10%. This requires the standard error to be half of 10%, or 5%. Further suppose that the investigator believes the proportion to be around 30%. The required N would be:

**Equation 6**

$$N = \frac{0.3(1 - 0.3)}{.05^2} = \frac{.21}{.0025} = 84$$

Because the maximum SE (and therefore maximum sample size) is produced when p = 0.5, a conservative rule of thumb to find a proportion within ±D%, is:

**Equation 7**

$$N \leq \frac{0.5(1 - 0.5)}{(D/2)^2} = \frac{1}{D^2}$$

So, to estimate a proportion within 10%, the investigator would need a maximum of 100 subjects. Within 5%, at most 400 are needed, and within 20%, at most 25.

## HYPOTHESIS TESTING FRAMEWORK

The approaches just discussed assume that the primary goal of a study is to estimate a specific quantity with some specific degree of precision. But if a formal hypothesis test is to be applied to the data to address a study question, the required precision is driven by the desiderata of that test. The statistical test requirements themselves may appear to have little to do with precision issues. This section, however, shows that the requirements of the hypothesis test are intimately linked to precision considerations. Retaining the precision perspective can help introduce clarity into the procedure for estimating sample size.

An hypothesis test introduces a notion of decision into an analysis. The purpose of the testing exercise is to decide between two hypotheses, usually a null hypothesis of no effect, and an alternative hypothesis that the effect differs from the null value to at least a specified extent. Obviously, when the null hypothesis is true, an investigator wants to decide in its favor fairly frequently, and conversely, when the alternative hypothesis is true, an investigator wants the statistical verdict to favor *it* most of the time. The hypothesis test framework assigns specific numbers and names to the two possible errors associated with the decision making. A conclusion to reject the null when the null is true is called a Type I error (or sometimes alpha, $\alpha$, error). Its value (alpha) is typically set at 5%. A one-sided criterion says that the null will be rejected if the difference is either positive or negative, but not both. A two-sided Type I criterion is one in which the null hypothesis would be rejected by a significant difference in either direction.

A decision to accept the null when a sizable difference actually exists is called a Type II or beta error. Its value (represented by beta $\beta$), is typically set at 5% to 20%. Its complement, $1 - \beta$, is called power: the probability of correctly rejecting the null hypothesis when a specified alternative is true. If the value for $\beta$ is between 5% and 20%, the power is between 80% and 95%. It is important to note that the power is always stated with respect to a specified difference, for example, "80% power to detect a 20% difference." To say that an experiment has "80% power" is literally meaningless, because all experiments have 80% power to detect *something*—the relevant issue is *what*. (Additional discussion about hypothesis testing is given in the section on Analyzing and Reporting Results.)

## How to Choose $\alpha$ and $\beta$

The values of $\alpha$ and $\beta$ are theoretically at the investigator's discretion, but an $\alpha$ of 5% is used almost universally, and $\beta$ is usually set between 5% and 20%. Any beta higher than 20% (i.e., power less than 80%) will be questioned (and the study characterized pejoratively as underpowered). Of course, an investigator can always raise the apparent power by increasing the difference of interest. Although this alternative strategy is rarely questioned, to do so merely to achieve a given power per se is inappropriate. In some cases, it might be advantageous to have low (<80%) power; in others, power should be high (>95%) For example, if a researcher is testing a new treatment against standard therapy—and the standard method is preferable in terms of cost, convenience, and efficacy—it might be acceptable to increase $\beta$ (raise the evidential bar). Increasing $\beta$ decreases power. This means that it will be harder to

detect a significant difference between the standard therapy and the new treatment. In other words, the new treatment will have to be much better than standard therapy. On the other hand, if the new treatment is something that is safe and low cost, or the investigator is designing a hypothesis-generating experiment, then it might be acceptable to lower $\beta$, or increase power, lowering the bar. In this case, the investigator might be more willing to take the chance of concluding that the new treatment works when it actually doesn't (1).

## What Are We Doing in a Sample Size Calculation?

Figure 9–3 shows what is going on in a sample size calculation under the hypothesis-testing paradigm and how it is linked with precision. The curve on the left represents the null distribution, the distribution of all possible observations (e.g., treatment differences) when the null hypothesis is true. The curve on the right is an alternative hypothesis distribution—all possible observations when some alternative hypothesis represents the real truth. As sample size increases, the observed average becomes more likely to be near the true mean, which is shown in Figure 9–3 as both distributions become narrower with increasing sample size. What is also happening is that the thresholds that cut off $\alpha$% of the null distribution and $\beta$% of the alternative distribution are moving closer together. In each plot, $\beta$ and $\alpha$ are the same—20% and 5%, but the observed effects that correspond to these cutoffs are different. As N gets larger, decreasing the standard errors and the narrowing of the curves, each cutoff moves toward the center of its respective distribution, bringing them closer to each other. The desired sample size is reached (N = 100 in this case) when the two thresholds coincide, forcing the null distribution to have 5% of its potential observations to the right of the same threshold where the alternative distribution has 20% of its potential observations to the left. So, one way to look at the procedure of setting a sample size is as an effort to increase the precision until the specified tails of the two distributions are defined from the same point. This perspective allows investigators to mathematically link the power and precision perspectives.

Figure 9–4 shows the curves in more detail when N = 100. For simplicity, it is assumed that the standard errors under the null and alternative hypotheses are the same. The standardized distance between the centers of each distribution is $Z_{\alpha/2} + Z_{\beta}$, or $1.96 + 0.84 = 2.8$ standard errors. Standard errors of 1.96 correspond to the 5% two-sided alpha error, and 0.84 corresponds to a

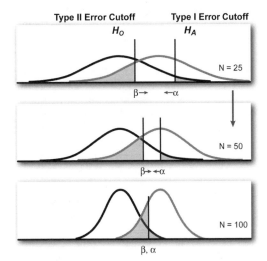

**FIGURE 9–3** ● A graphical representation of what a sample size calculation under a hypothesis testing model aims for; the overlapping of the thresholds for a given Type I ($\alpha$) and Type II ($\beta$) error.

one-sided 20% beta error. These numbers mean that the required sample size forces the difference of interest (i.e., the alternative hypothesis) to be 2.8 standard errors from the null whenever the power is 80%. (The corresponding number for 90% power is $1.28 + 1.96 = 3.24$ standard errors.) This allows investigators to predict approximately what the width of this experiment's confidence interval will be. Because 1.96 standard errors corresponds to 70% of the 2.8 standard errors (and 60% of 3.24 standard errors), the predicted 95% confidence interval is:

Observed Difference ± 0.70 ×
Difference detectable with 80% power

or

Observed Difference ± 0.60 ×
Difference detectable with 90% power

Both of these expressions yield the same answer. For example, suppose that an investigator designs a study to detect a 20% absolute difference between two interventions. The precision of outcome will be ±0.70*20% = ±14%. Also an observed difference of 14% will be just significant at p = 0.05. An observed difference of 0% would be reported as having a 95% confidence interval (CI) of −14% to +14%, an observed difference of 10% would be reported as 10%, 95% CI −4% to 24%, and an observed 14% difference would be reported

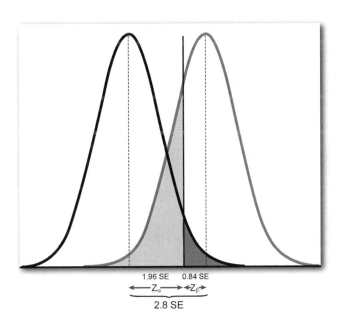

**FIGURE 9–4** ● Relationship between $\alpha$, $\beta$, and precision.

as 14%, CI 0 to 28%. This way of framing sample size implications can be very useful in understanding or communicating the implications of various inputs into the sample size equation. Researchers can see the consequences of using a difference of interest that is too large, or a study with too-small power. Predicted intervals can be a very important adjunct to traditional sample size calculations (2).

*It is a common misconception that a study designed to "detect" a certain difference means that any observed difference smaller than the "detectable" difference will not be statistically significant.* The above example shows that this is not true. When an experiment is designed to "detect" a 20% effect with 80% power, any effect larger than 14% will be statistically significant. It is the difference between the 20% and 14% that gives high power; if the *true* effect was really 20%, investigators would be very confident (80%, in this case) that they would *observe* an effect larger than 14%, leading them to declare that the null hypothesis was not tenable.

## Sample Size with Two-Group Comparisons, Continuous Outcomes

In the two-sample case, the goal of the sample size calculation is to estimate how many individuals are needed in each group to test the null hypothesis with Type I error probability $\alpha$ and Type II error probability $\beta$. Some examples of scientific questions that would motivate using the two-sample situation are:

- Can an investigator detect a 15 lb. difference in body weights of cancer patients treated with fish oil and those treated with placebo?
- How many individuals are needed to detect a 20 ng/mL difference in mean cotinine levels between heavy smokers and light smokers?
- What is the sample size to detect the effect on pain scores in arthritis patients treated with methotrexate versus placebo?

Once the motivating question is identified, all of the requirements for the sample size calculation can be put into place. For the two-sample case, the ingredients are shown in Table 9–2.

Sample size for the two-sample situation is calculated as:

**Equation 8**

$$n_1 = n_2 = \frac{2(Z_\alpha + Z_\beta)^2}{\left(\dfrac{\text{Treatment difference}}{\text{Standard deviation}}\right)^2}$$

The denominator, expressed in this way, is also referred to as the *standardized effect size,* or $\Delta$, the number of standard deviations difference that the experiment is designed to detect. This expression assumes equal variances and equal sample sizes in both groups. If these assumptions are not valid, the expression becomes more complicated (see below).

Substituting the conventional values $Z_\alpha = 1.96$ (two-sided 5% error) and $Z_\beta = 0.84$ (80% power) and $Z_\beta = 1.28$ (90% power) into the above expression gives:

**Equations 9a–b**

$$n = \frac{16}{\Delta^2} \text{ for 80\% power} \tag{a}$$

$$n = \frac{21}{\Delta^2} \text{ for 90\% power} \tag{b}$$

where $\Delta$ is the standardized effect size.

Notice that N is inversely proportional to the square of the effect size, $\Delta$. So, as this difference to be detected gets smaller, a larger sample size is required. The sample size needed to detect one standard deviation difference with 80% power is 16 in each group, 32 total. The sample size required to detect a standardized effect of 0.5 is $16/(0.5)^2 = 64$ per group, or 128 total.

**Example:** An investigator wants to test the effect of treating patients with drug A compared to drug B on serum cholesterol. She believes that a difference in mean cholesterol levels of 10 mg/dl would be plausible and clinically important. The between-subject standard deviation of cholesterol levels is reported in previous studies as 15 mg/dl.

With $2\alpha = 0.05$, $\beta = 0.20$, SD = 15, the total sample size required is $\frac{16}{(10/15)^2} = 35$ per group, 70 total. Investigators decide to recruit around 80 patients to account for noncompliance or dropouts. The predicted 95% confidence interval for this two-sample case is $\pm 0.7*10 = \pm 7$ ng/mL.

Using the cancer patient body weight question and assuming that the standard deviation of the body weights is 25 lbs., to detect a 15 lb. difference with 80% power, an investigator would need a sample size of :

$$\frac{16}{\left(\dfrac{15 \text{ lbs}}{25 \text{ SD}}\right)^2} = \frac{16}{0.6^2} \approx 44 \text{ patients/group}$$

Using this treatment and sample size, the predicted 95% confidence interval for possible observed differences of 5, 10, and 15 lbs. would be

5 lb. difference $\pm 0.7*15 = (-5.5$ to $15.5)$
10 lb. difference $\pm 0.7*15 = (-0.5$ to $11.0)$
15 lb. difference $\pm 0.7*15 = (4.5$ to $25.5)$

This same calculation shows that any observed difference less than 10.5 lbs. (i.e., 0.7*15 lbs.) will not be statistically significant.

So far it has been assumed that the number of individuals required in each group is equal. However, in some situations unequal sample sizes are required, such as when research participants of one type are much more common or accessible than another, or when a treatment is thought to be efficacious enough to justify giving it to more research volunteers. Table 9–3 gives sample sizes for control and treatment groups needed to detect a difference in LDL cholesterol of 0.7 with standard deviation 0.6 and $\alpha = 5\%$ and $\beta = 20\%$. In this table, the ratio of number of controls to number treated changes (the calculations for situations where sample size of the two groups will be different can be performed using many currently available statistical software programs).

In the example in Table 9–3, the total sample size does not increase substantially up to 2 to 1 controls treated (24 total vs 26 total), but beyond that, the total sample size can increase substantially. Note also that the number of subjects decreases in the smaller group as the allocation ratio rises, given a constant power. Depending on the relative costs of intervention or recruitment, the overall cost can be lower with unequal allocation even as the total number of subjects is higher.

## Sample Size Calculation for One-Sample Comparison, Continuous Outcome

In the one-sample case, the sample size needed for a single group whose average endpoint will be compared to some reference or historical control is calculated. Examples of situations when a sample size calculation for a one-sample case would be needed are:

## TABLE 9–2

### Requirements for Calculating Sample Size in a Two-Sample Study with Continuous Outcomes

- Clear statement of endpoint and measure of effect
- Treatment difference to be "detected"—usually the minimum important difference
- $\alpha$ (one- or two-sided) and ß
- Standard deviation of the measurement
- Allocation ratio $n_1 \, n_2$ (usually 1 to 1)

- In a crossover experiment, the same subject takes each of two treatments. Is the difference in effect between the two treatments different from 0?
- Is growth rate of a group of children treated with growth hormone different from established norms?

In the one-sample case, the ingredients are slightly different than in the two-sample case (Table 9–4).

The formula for the sample size is:

**Equations 10 a–c**

$$N = \frac{(Z_\alpha + Z_\beta)^2}{\left(\dfrac{\text{Treatment difference}}{\text{Standard deviation}}\right)^2} \quad \text{(a)}$$

This simplifies to:

$$N = \frac{8}{\Delta^2} \text{ for 80\% power} \quad \text{(b)}$$

$$N = \frac{10.5}{\Delta^2} \text{ for 90\% power} \quad \text{(c)}$$

## TABLE 9–3

### Sample Sizes Required for Varying Ratios of Number of Controls to Number of Treated with 5% and 20% Type I and II Error Rates

| Allocation Ratio (C/T) | Controls | Treatment | Total | Ratio of Total Sample Sizes |
|:---:|:---:|:---:|:---:|:---:|
| 1 to 1 | 12 | 12 | 24 | 1 |
| 2 to 1 | 17 | 9 | 26 | 1.1 |
| 3 to 1 | 23 | 8 | 31 | 1.3 |
| 5 to 1 | 35 | 7 | 42 | 1.75 |
| 10 to 1 | 64 | 6 | 70 | 2.9 |

| TABLE 9–4 |
|---|
| **Requirements for Calculating Sample Size in a One-Sample Study with a Continuous Outcome** |
| • Clear statement of endpoint and measure of effect<br>• Treatment of difference to be "detected"–usually the minimally important difference<br>• $\alpha$ (one- or two-sided) and $\beta$<br>• Standard deviation of the measurement |

| TABLE 9–5 |
|---|
| **Requirements for Calculating Sample Size in a Two-Sample Study with a Binary Outcome** |
| • Clear statement of endpoint and measure of effect<br>• Expected or minimal important success probability, $p_1$, in the treatment group<br>• Expected success probability, $p_0$, in the control group<br>• $\alpha$ (one- or two-sided) and $\beta$<br>• Allocation ratio, $n_1/n_2$ (also usually 1 to 1) |

This calculation is the same as that for the two-sample case, except that the total sample size is one-quarter as much. This reduction results from assuming perfect knowledge in the comparison group, thus eliminating half the uncertainty, and not having to include a separate comparison group, eliminating half the sample.

## Sample Size for Binary Outcomes, Two Samples

When the endpoint is binary (i.e., "yes" or "no"), its distribution can be modeled with a binomial distribution with success probability $p$. Some examples of endpoints that follow this distribution are:

- Vital status (alive/dead)
- Achieved complete remission after treatment for leukemia versus did not achieve complete remission
- Tumor reduction <50% versus ≥50%

In the two-sample case, the goal is to calculate a sample size that is large enough to detect a difference between the null hypothesis outcome probability, $p_0$, and the alternative hypothesis outcome probability, $p_1$. Some examples of when this method is used are:

- How many patients are needed to detect a difference of 30% versus 50% in survival rates of patients who had surgery versus those who did not?
- What is the sample size required to detect a 15% versus 25% difference in number of patients who improved in exercise capacity after undergoing physical therapy for 2 versus 4 days per week?

The requirements needed to calculate the sample size are shown in Table 9–5.

When the group sizes are equal, the required sample size is:

**Equation 11**

$$n_1 = n_2 = \frac{16\overline{p}(1 - \overline{p})}{(p_0 - p_1)^2}$$

where $\overline{p}$ is the average of $p_0$ and $p_1$. Sample size is maximized when $\overline{p} = 0.50$. Because the values of $p(1 - p)$ do not vary much for values of between 0.30 and 0.70, we can derive a rule of thumb for the two-sample case. Plugging in 0.5 for the average response rate gives:

**Equation 12**

$$n_1 = n_2 = \frac{4}{(p_0 - p_1)^2}$$

## One-Sample Case, Binary Outcomes

The one-sample case for binary outcomes is very similar to the one-sample case for continuous outcomes. The observed outcome is again compared to a historical or standard control. Some examples of scientific situations that would motivate the one-sample case are:

- Investigators are interested if taking calcium and vitamin D supplements together for 12 weeks increases muscle strength by 10% compared to the expected increase of 5% with calcium alone.
- A researcher wants to know if a new drug to treat breast cancer produces a remission rate of 35% compared to the expected remission rate of 20%.
- Investigators are developing a crossover design where each patient is his or her own control.

<table>
<tr><td>

**TABLE 9–6**

## Requirements for Calculating Sample Size in a One-Sample Study with a Binary Outcome

- Expected or minimal important success probability, p, in the experimental group, $p_1$
- Historical or external control outcome probability, $p_0$
- $\alpha$ (one- or two-sided) and $\beta$

</td></tr>
</table>

The requirements for the one-sample size calculation are shown in Table 9–6.

The sample size required for this one-sample experiment is:

**Equation 13**

$$N = \frac{\left(Z_\alpha \sqrt{p_0(1 - p_0)} + Z_\beta \sqrt{p_1(1 - p_1)}\right)^2}{(p_0 - p_1)^2}$$

Again, this formula can be simplified by calculating the maximum number it will produce, substituting 0.5 for all $p$'s. This produces a formula quite similar to that for the continuous case:

**Equation 14**

$$\text{Maximum N} = \frac{\left(Z_\alpha + Z_\beta\right)^2}{4 (p_0 - p_1)^2}$$

For $\alpha = 5\%$ and power = 80%, this simplifies to $2/(p_0 - p_1)^2$.

**Example:** If a researcher wants to test if a response rate of 40% after an intervention is significantly better than the expected response rate of 25% after the intervention, with 80% power and 5% Type I error rate, the required sample size required is:

**Equation 15**

$$N = \frac{\left(1.96\sqrt{.4(1 - .4)} + 0.84\sqrt{.25(1 - .25)}\right)^2}{(0.4 - 0.25)^2} = 76$$

The simple formula for the maximum sample size produces:

**Equation 16**

$$\frac{2}{(0.4 - 0.25)^2} = 89$$

## Survival Outcomes

With survival data, investigators are not only interested in a binary outcome (i.e., an *event*), but also the time to event, or survival time. The discussion thus far has relied on the assumption of normally distributed data, so the next example will assume a distribution for survival time. The most common assumption is that the distribution is exponential; that is, that participants experience an event at a steady relative rate, h, also known as the hazard rate. At any time *t* we can express the proportion of survivors remaining as $e^{-ht}$. The hazard rate is like a bank's interest rate, which compounds daily, so doubling the hazard rate will produce many more than double the number of events over time. Note that "survival" is a somewhat technical statistical term, and that these methods apply to any event where the time to achieving it is important to assess. This could be time to recovery of an immune parameter to normal levels or the time to reappearance of a tumor. Investigators use "survival" methods when not all of the outcomes are observed; that is, there are some patients who don't have tumor reappearance within a specified period, or the immune parameter stays abnormal in some patients during the experiment. These incompletely observed patients are called "censored" observations.

For the sample size calculation, assume that the hazard ratio is the same at all points in time. If $p_1$ is the proportion of treated experimental units who are event-free at time *t* and $p_0$ be the proportion of controls who are event-free at time *t*, then the hazard ratio, $h = \log(p_1)/\log(p_0)$. This ratio also equals the inverse of the ratio of median event times. So if the median survival time is doubled, it corresponds to halving the hazard rate.

The sample size formula for this simplified case is:

**Equation 17**

$$\text{Events per group} = \frac{2(Z_\alpha + Z_\beta)^2(h + 1)^2}{2(h - 1)^2}$$

The reason that the basic sample size formula is in terms of events and not units is because in survival studies researchers can get a lot of events by observing a lot of units for a short time or few units for a long time. Exactly how many units should be enrolled and how long they should be followed requires a series of judgments that are beyond the scope of this discussion, and should be made in conjunction with a statistician. The important message of equation 17, however, is it is not the starting population but the actual number of events generated in the course of the study that is critical to the statistical power.

Equation 17 leads to the following rules of thumb:

$$\text{Events per group} = \frac{4(h+1)^2}{(h-1)^2} \text{ for 80\% power}$$

$$\text{Events per group} = \frac{5.2(h+1)^2}{(h-1)^2} \text{ for 90\% power}$$

For 90% power, the number to detect a survival doubling (or halving) is about a total of 90 events in the two groups together. If the average mortality rate is about 10%, this translates into a sample size near 900.

## SAMPLE SIZE FOR EQUIVALENCE OR NONINFERIORITY STUDIES

Often, the goal in a study is not to demonstrate a difference between two groups, but to show that they are equivalent, or that one group is not worse (i.e., noninferior) than another. In quantitative terms, this means demonstrating that most or all of the confidence interval will fall in an "equivalence" or "noninferiority" region if the null hypothesis is true. For such a calculation, an investigator needs to specify exactly how wide that region is.

It is not sufficient to make the predicted CI equal in width to the equivalence region, because the CI will end up lying entirely within the equivalence region only if the observed effect is exactly zero. The sample size needs to produce a predicted precision that is narrower than the equivalence or non-inferiority boundaries. There are a number of approaches to setting sample sizes for these situations, and one of the more widely used is quite similar to the methods already presented, except for the following important differences:

1. The null and alternative hypotheses are switched, and defined as:
   i. Null hypothesis: The intervention group differs by more than $d$ from the control group.
   ii. Alternative hypothesis: The intervention group differs by less than $d$ from the control group.
2. The meaning of alpha, Type I error, is the probability of concluding equivalence when groups are different. Beta, or Type II error, is the chance of concluding nonequivalence when the groups are equivalent.
3. Beta is usually set much lower, e.g., at 0.05 or 0.10, instead of 0.1 to 0.2.

A widely used formula for binary outcomes is:

**Equation 18**

$$N = \frac{2(Z_\alpha + Z_\beta)^2\, p(1-p)}{d^2}$$

Where:

$p = $ expected response in both equivalent groups
$d = $ difference in response that would be deemed important
$\alpha = $ (probability of declaring equivalence when different by more than d) (one-sided)
$\beta = $ (probability of declaring difference when equivalent) (usually two-sided)

A very typical equivalence region on the probability scale is an absolute difference of 5% or 10%. For instance, assume a 10% equivalence region, a one-sided alpha of 5% and a two-sided beta of 10%, and a predicted response rate in both groups of 50%. This yields a sample size of:

$$N = \frac{2(1.64+1.64)^2\, 0.5(1-0.5)}{0.1^2} = 538 \text{ per group}$$

This total sample size of 1,076 (538*2) is moderately larger than that in Table 9–7 (816) for a superiority assessment of two groups with anticipated responses of 0.5 and 0.6. This is to be expected. If the bounds for equivalence are set tighter than those for declaring a difference, as they often are, equivalency assessments can often require sample sizes far greater than tests of superiority (3).

## PRINCIPLES FOR CHOOSING ENDPOINTS

We will now return to the questions posed at the beginning of this chapter about how the choice of endpoints affects sample size and show how it might work for the hypothesis presented; that is, for the effects of methotrexate on the course of rheumatoid arthritis. The basic message is that the more assumptions one makes about the data that are true, the easier it is to design an experiment that extracts maximum information from each subject's data and the smaller the required sample size. However, it is often the case that investigators are quite unsure about these assumptions (which might concern normality, variability, or effect size) and might need to buy some "insurance," in the form of sample size formulas that require fewer assumptions. The insurance comes in the form of a larger sample size, a cost that can be quantified via the sample size calculation process.

Using that example, assume that the primary clinical endpoint will be pain, as measured on a visual

## TABLE 9–7

**Total Sample Sizes (2n) for Comparison of Probabilities under the Null ($P_0$) and Alternative Hypotheses ($P_1$) with Two-Sided 5% Type I and 20% Type II Error Rates**

| | | .1 | .2 | .3 | .4 | $P_0$<br>.5 | .6 | .7 | .8 | .9 |
|---|---|---|---|---|---|---|---|---|---|---|
| | .1 | – | 438 | 144 | 76 | 50 | 34 | 26 | 20 | 16 |
| | .2 | 438 | – | 626 | 182 | 90 | 56 | 38 | 26 | 20 |
| | .3 | 144 | 626 | – | 752 | 206 | 98 | 58 | 38 | 26 |
| | .4 | 76 | 182 | 752 | – | 816 | 214 | 98 | 56 | 34 |
| $P_1$ | .5 | 50 | 90 | 206 | 816 | – | 816 | 206 | 90 | 50 |
| | .6 | 34 | 56 | 98 | 214 | 816 | – | 752 | 182 | 76 |
| | .7 | 26 | 38 | 58 | 98 | 206 | 752 | – | 626 | 144 |
| | .8 | 20 | 26 | 38 | 56 | 90 | 182 | 626 | – | 438 |
| | .9 | 16 | 20 | 26 | 34 | 50 | 76 | 144 | 438 | – |

analog scale from 0 to 10. The study will use a between-subjects group randomized study design (although a crossover study design would bring in yet different issues). This example will show how various assumptions affect the sample size.

Let's start with the study design itself. The statistic of interest at the end of this study could be a change in the magnitude of joint destruction for each research participant, measured as a radiographic score on a scale from 1 to 10. Perhaps these measurements will then be correlated against concomitant changes in the cytokine profile measured in fluid aspirated from the joint. The first question would be what difference would be considered biologically significant enough to merit treatment with methotrexate, a drug with significant adverse effects. Assume that the difference settled on is a difference of 2 (out of 10).

The next question is what is the degree of variability of the change in this measure between persons? If there is literature on this measure, the answer is easy. Operating as though there is no external information, assume that there is sufficient imprecision in the radiographic interpretations that a conservative assumption would be that the SD for the change score would be 2. Considering the width of the scale, this is a fairly safe assumption, because it assumes that 95% of individual scores would change within ±4 points without exposure to the drug. The width of this interval is 8 points, which encompasses nearly the whole scale. Plugging this into equation 8, the minimum sample size to provide 80% power for the 2 point difference would be 16 subjects per group, or 32 overall.

Now consider that instead of an average change in radiographic score, the goal was to determine whether exposure to the drug would reduce below a certain threshold the proportion of patients with a certain radiographic score. This strategy would mean converting the continuous radiographic score to a binary indicator: 0 if the score is less than the threshold, 1 if the score is equal to or greater than the threshold level (i.e., the sample size calculation would be based on proportions instead of a continuous measure).

Figure 9–5 shows the effect of setting this threshold at various cutoffs, with the difference between the two populations being 1 SD, the same difference assumed in the previous sample size calculation. Table 9–8 shows the sample size implications of these and other cutoffs. As the cutoff increases, the proportion in both populations that exceeds that cutoff decreases, and the sample size changes. The minimum sample size is 64—double the previous number, and it almost doubles yet again if attempts are made to distinguish the effects at the extremes, which may be an area of high clinical importance (i.e., the people in most pain.)

Even more variability is thrown into the mix when we consider that the power is not fixed, nor is the difference of interest. But even if these variables are held constant, this example shows an almost fourfold variation in the estimated sample size. So a natural question is which sample size is the "right" one? The answer is that this depends on what the experimenter thinks is biologically and clinically most important. If every change in change score is equally important, as it might be if the investigator

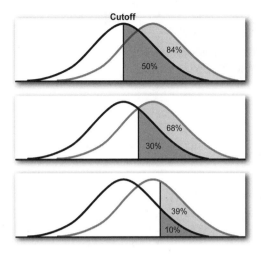

**FIGURE 9–5** ● Changes in the proportions due to exposure to methotrexate (left curve) and control (right) as the cutoff threshold for the radiographic score on the continuous scale increases.

were asking a primarily biological question, then the small sample size corresponding to the continuous change score analysis would be appropriate. However, if it is mainly a degree of joint destruction (measured radiographically) beyond a certain threshold that is associated with a material difference in a clinically relevant outcome (e.g., pain or ability to perform certain tasks), then the smaller sample size might not be sufficient to demonstrate that outcome. So, as stated in the introduction, the question of the "right" sample size is in some ways similar to the question physicians confront when asking themselves what is the "right" therapy for a particular patient; in different circumstances, with different kinds of patients, the investigator might tailor therapy differently, targeting different benefits and minimizing different side effects. The sample size formulas provide some constraints, but where in the wide range allowed by these formulas the sample size should be chosen is a question that can only be answered with a combination of biological, clinical, and statistical (and financial!) expertise.

## REPORTING THE SAMPLE SIZE CALCULATION

Any report of the sample size calculation should contain all of the following:

- The basic type of study design (e.g., single arm, randomized control trial, crossover)
- The operational definition of the primary endpoint, or any secondary endpoints that might be used to determine the sample size (if that sample size is larger than the primary endpoint)
- The statistical measure of effect that will be used (e.g., relative risk, risk difference)
- The nature of the hypothesis being tested (e.g., precision, superiority, equivalence, noninferiority)

## TABLE 9–8

### Sample Size Implications of Setting a Radiographic Score Threshold at Different Cutoffs

| Total Sample Size | Treatment Proportion Exceeding Cutoff | Control Proportion Exceeding Cutoff |
|---|---|---|
| 70 | 0.50 | 0.84 |
| 64 | 0.40 | 0.77 |
| 64 | 0.30 | 0.68 |
| 66 | 0.20 | 0.56 |
| 80 | 0.10 | 0.39 |
| 110 | 0.05 | 0.26 |

- The difference of interest, for which the power will be calculated
- If relevant, the source (e.g., other studies, informed guesses) of the estimates of effect size and variability

Here is a sample size section that has these components:

The hypothesis being examined is that treatment with an ACE inhibitor improves cardiac function, defined as echocardiographically measured ejection fraction, in patients with congestive heart failure. The design of the study is a parallel two-group between-subjects comparison with congestive heart failure treated with ACE inhibitors or placebo. Ejection fraction is measured as a continuous variable. Based on prior experience in this population[a,b], the ejection fraction in these patients averaged 35%, with a standard deviation of about 5%. An absolute difference of 2.5% (i.e., ejection fraction of 37.5%) in the ACE treated group was deemed the minimally important biologic effect. The two-sided Type I error was set at 5%, and the power at 90%, with a 10% increase in sample size to accommodate for loss to follow-up or attrition for other reasons. The Stata[c] "sampsi" routine was used for calculation. The sample size that fulfilled these criteria was 85 in each group, with a 10% increase yielding 93. This will also produce a predicted precision (i.e., 95% CI) in estimation of the ejection fraction difference of ±1.7%.

## SOFTWARE

There are many computational resources for easy calculation of sample size, from freeware on the Web to fairly expensive proprietary packages. The capacities range from simple "calculators" to programs that generate quite sophisticated text reports that can be placed directly into protocols or proposals. Most standard statistical packages, such as STATA, SAS, S-Plus, and others, have functions for basic sample size calculations. In general, only dedicated packages have the full range of options and flexibility. None of these tools, however, is a substitute for a consultation with an expert in study design. As indicated in the first sections, the actual calculation of sample size is only a small part of the sample size setting process; appropriate endpoints and analytic statistical approaches must be selected to calculate sample size implications, and no sample size software can offer that kind of assistance. Following is a noncomprehensive list of resources, in addition to the routines in commercial statistical software, that are currently available:

**Web-Based Freeware (Very Small Sampling)**
Vanderbilt university:
www.mc.vanderbilt.edu/prevmed/ps/
University of Calgary: www.health.ucalgary.ca/~rollin/stats/ssize/
UCLA Department of Statistics:
calculators.stat.ucla.edu/powercalc/
Southwest Oncology Group: www.swogstat.org/statoolsout.html

**Proprietary Software**
Power Analysis and Sample Size (PASS)
Power and Precision II
nQuery Advisor
StudySize

## SUMMARY

- All sample size choices have statistical implications that must be explored, even if the sample size was chosen for nonstatistical reasons.
- Sample size calculations must be motivated by clearly expressed and operationally explicit hypotheses.
- Each choice of outcome measure, effect size, and analytic method has implications for the sample size and sample size in turn affects how an investigator might choose, measure, and analyze an outcome.
- The two main components of a sample size calculation are the plausible effect size and between-subject variability. Smaller effects and larger variability both increase the sample size.
- The components of the sample size calculation can be manipulated to justify any N, but if the choices are unrealistic, a price may be paid at the end in the form of imprecise results leading to inconclusive findings. It can be very helpful before the study to portray the implications of sample size choice in the form of predicted confidence intervals.
- Choosing a sample size involves balancing many factors that are not found in the equations, and it can be very helpful to consult with an expert in study design.

## REFERENCES

1. Piantadosi S, ed. Clinical Trials: A Methodologic Perspective. New York: John Wiley and Sons, 1997.
2. Goodman S, Berlin J. The use of predicted confidence intervals when planning experiments and the misuse of power when interpreting results. Ann Intern Med 1994;121:200–206.
3. Blackwelder WC. "Proving the null hypothesis" in clinical trials. Control Clin Trials. 1982;3:345–353.

# SUGGESTED READINGS

Donner A. Sample size requirements for stratified cluster randomization designs. Stat Med 1992;11:743–750.

Freedman LS. Tables of the number of patients required in clinical trials using the logrank test. Stat Med 1982;1:121–129.

Lachin J. Introduction to sample size determination and power analysis for clinical trials. Control Clin Trials. 1981;2:93–113.

Lachin J, Foulkes M. Evaluation of sample size and power for analyses of survival with allowance for nonuniform patient entry, losses to follow-up, noncompliance, and stratification. Biometrics 1986;42:507–519.

Lee ET, Wang JW. Statistical Methods for Survival Data Analysis, 3rd Ed. Hoboken, NJ: Wiley-Interscience, 2003.

Machin D, Campbell MJ. Statistical tables for the design of clinical trials. Oxford: Blackwell, 1987.

Rees DG. Foundations of Statistics. Boca Raton, Fla.: Chapman & Hall, 1987.

Rosner B. Fundamentals of Biostatistics. New York, NY: Duxbury Press, 1999.

Shuster JJ. Handbook of Sample Size Guidelines for Clinical Trials. Boca Raton, Fla.: CRC press 1990.

van Belle G. Statistical Rules of Thumb. Hoboken, NJ: Wiley-Interscience, 2002.

# CHAPTER 10

# Database Development

David A. Mulvihill, David W. Gibson, Thomas G. Cole

Recording and maintaining the data collected during a research study is critically important to its success. The purpose of developing a formal database is to store data in such a way that ease and speed of retrieval is maximized while neither security nor integrity is diminished. By designing database tables (entities) and related fields (attributes) appropriately, the database is expandable, modifiable, and easily maintained. Of course, the amount of time, personnel, and finances required for the design of a database is directly proportional to the size and complexity of the data. A well-developed database leads to minimally redundant and more accurate data. Redundant data in a database is generally undesirable, because it increases the likelihood of data inconsistencies and the complexity of updating data stored in multiple locations.

Whole courses are given on database theory, development, and maintenance. This chapter, then, is meant as a brief introduction to the topic, to orient the beginning investigator to the benefits—and challenges—of developing useful databases for clinical research.

## TYPES OF DATABASES

A database model is a mathematical algorithm that describes a container to house data and a methodology for reading and writing to the container. There are four main types of database models: flat file, hierarchical, network, and relational. The strengths and weaknesses of these models, of course, should determine which format will best meet the needs of the investigator and the research itself (1).

### Flat File

An address book, data in a checkbook, or research participant information in a spreadsheet is representative of a flat file type database. Basic features, such as searches, calculations, and sorting are available, but become tedious as the size of the database grows. More importantly, data redundancy can easily develop when such files become large. For example, tracking participant data for multiple visits throughout a clinical study would require that a participant name such as "John Doe" be repeated for every visit instance in the file. Why would it matter if the data were duplicated on multiple rows in a spreadsheet? It is certainly not because of lack of physical space, which might have been a concern in the past, because electronic storage is large and inexpensive now. The main concern would be that the participant information was entered as "John Doe" for one visit and "Jon Doe" for another. Which participant name is correct? Are they the same participant? What happens when a name change is required? The name would have to be changed for every instance that it exists in the database, which could possibly lead to additional errors. Typically, a flat file works well for a small database that does not require special reporting or queries and where data redundancy is not a concern.

### Hierarchical

A good visualization of the hierarchical database model is an upside-down tree (sometimes called a balanced tree or b-tree) with the root of the tree being the single table from which other tables branch. This design supports what can be called a parent-child relationship. Each table farther down on the branch can be thought of as a child table of the parent. An example of this model is a file manager such as the Microsoft Windows Explorer. Parent folders can have multiple children but a child folder can have only one parent. This works well for a file manager, but turns out to be a poor model for data that needs multiple relations, such as the case of study participants with multiple visits. The model works well with data that requires a one-to-many relationship but not with a many-to-many relationship (many participants in a clinical study, each of which can have many visits). In terms of the Windows Explorer for example, a folder called NAME1 can have many children called VISIT1, VISIT2, and so on, but how could VISIT1 be related to another parent folder called NAME2? This type of relationship across parents is not possible, but an investigator could copy the child folder VISIT1 into the parent folder NAME2, creating redundant data that is desirable to avoid. Changing a visit name in this case would require changing the name for every participant folder in which the visit name exists.

## Network

The network model was designed to solve the problems of the hierarchical model. Although this model is better at describing many-to-many relationships than the hierarchical model, it has generally proved too cumbersome to use for the end user and has been mainly implemented by computer programmers for special purposes.

## Relational

In 1970, E. F. Codd at IBM first introduced the concept of a relational database model. One of the most important breakthroughs of the relational database model was the introduction of tables, consisting of fields (vertical columns) and records (horizontal rows). Every row and column position contains exactly one datum value. The difference between relational and other databases is that the tables in the relational database can be *related* to one another by a defined key value. These relationships are defined during logical modeling of the database prior to the physical database creation. Figure 10–1 shows a relationship between the Name and Adverse Events tables. Even though the tables are independent and contain different types of data, it is easy to see the relationship between the two; that is, the name in one table is related to the name in the other (2). A relational database can contain a huge number of tables, which have a finite number of columns. IBM, Informix, Microsoft, Oracle, and Sybase are some of the vendors that offer relational database management systems (RDBMS). The advantages or disadvantages of one product over another are all relative to the scope of the project because of factors such as reliability, availability, cost, customer service, and personal preference. Several considerations guide the choice of a specific product: Will the database contain only participant demographic information or will it contain laboratory results as well as support decision making and archive graphical data? What percentage uptime is required? How many users will be accessing the database simultaneously? What type of security and user access schema is needed? Answers to these types of questions determine which RDBMS is a more appropriate match to the task.

RDBMSs benefit from a relational database programming language called Structured Query Language (SQL—pronounced "sequel"). Even though the American National Standards Institute (ANSI) and the International Standards Organization (ISO) have standardized SQL, each vendor tends to extend the language with its own proprietary additions. The main benefit, however, is that any SQL92-compliant

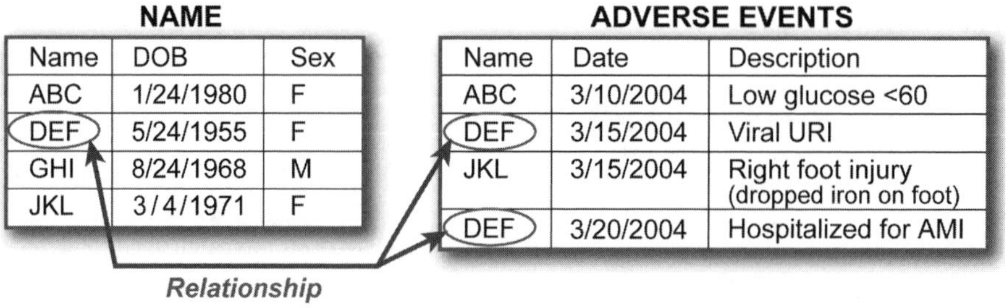

| NAME | | | | ADVERSE EVENTS | | |
|------|-----|-----|---|------|------|-------------|
| Name | DOB | Sex | | Name | Date | Description |
| ABC | 1/24/1980 | F | | ABC | 3/10/2004 | Low glucose <60 |
| DEF | 5/24/1955 | F | | DEF | 3/15/2004 | Viral URI |
| GHI | 8/24/1968 | M | | JKL | 3/15/2004 | Right foot injury (dropped iron on foot) |
| JKL | 3/4/1971 | F | | DEF | 3/20/2004 | Hospitalized for AMI |

*Relationship*

**FIGURE 10–1** ● Relational databases consist of tables with columns and rows. A one-to-many relationship is shown between the Name and Adverse Events tables based on the name field.

code can be used to access data from any SQL92-compliant vendor's RDBMS, which offers flexibility and code reuse. A SQL statement such as *SELECT * FROM Name* would produce the same output regardless whether the table was created with an Access, SQL Server 2000, or Oracle9i database.

## GOOD DATABASE DESIGN

Following an established database design process can decrease development time and lead to a well-designed database that provides efficient access to stored data (3). The most important and usually the most difficult phase of the process is conceptualizing the logical database model. A logical design is an abstract view of how data will be stored in a database, which allows for manipulation of the design *on paper* prior to the creation of the database. If the design is created ad hoc and without a set plan, the resulting database will most likely not meet the user requirements for performance and data integrity (4). Although the flat file database is often implemented in the clinical research setting because it is easy to use and does not require a computer programmer to make column or formula changes, the relational database offers the flexibility, security, and scalability of an enterprise-wide system and can be implemented in a clinical site setting with minimal planning. Due to the aforementioned limitations, design of a network or hierarchical database model is outside the scope of this chapter.

Selection of the appropriate type of database starts with an understanding of the type of data that is to be stored in it. A typical decision to make is whether the database needs to store participant demographic information such as date of birth, address, and phone number or just a participant name. Certain data, such as calculated data, should

not be stored, because every time a component of the calculation changes, cascading updates of all the related calculated fields would have to be performed. For example, it would be preferable to perform an age calculation for a report at the time it is printed using the participant's date of birth and the date the sample was collected.

The second step in the design processes can be thought of as data grouping. This crucial step can help determine whether a flat file database, such as a spreadsheet, is adequate or whether a relational database would be a better fit. The easiest way to describe the effects of grouping is to show an example of data that is not grouped. Table 10–1 shows an example of data inconsistency that can occur because of lack of grouping. For this example, assume that a data entry error occurred where name "ABC-0001" (record 5) should be "ABC-001" (record 2). Sorting the data by "Name" would treat these entries as being from different participants. Imagine the time that would be spent correcting problems such as this with participants and multiple visits in a spreadsheet, and the errors that would occur if they were not corrected. In contrast, Figure 10–2 shows similar data that is grouped and, as a consequence of the grouping, participant name information is stored only once in the Name table and related to the Visit table by the common PatID identifier. Thus, if a participant name is updated, it needs to be changed in only one place, the name table.

A value that uniquely identifies a record in a table is called a *primary key (PK)*. A *foreign key (FK)* is a value stored in a table that refers to the primary key of a different table. By adding the PatID foreign key to the Visit table, the Name table and the Visit table can be related via the PatID link. Adding the primary key of one table into another is a common strategy

## TABLE 10–1

**Example of a Common Data Entry Error Due to a Lack of Grouping**

| | A | B | C | D | E |
|---|---|---|---|---|---|
| 1 | Name | Visit | Systolic | Diastolic | Pulse |
| 2 | ABC-001 | Screen | 140 | 80 | 65 |
| 3 | DEF-010 | Screen | 130 | 80 | 70 |
| 4 | GHI-100 | Screen | 160 | 90 | 55 |
| 5 | ABC-0001 | Visit 1 | 130 | 70 | 60 |

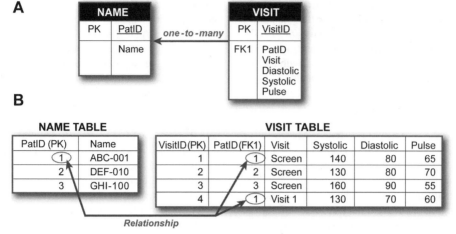

**FIGURE 10–2** ● **(A)** Shows the logical model of a two-table relational database with data grouped into "like" categories, one for participant demographics (Name) and one for visit information (Visit). A one-to-many relationship exists between the primary key (PK) value in the Name table (PatID) and the foreign key (FK1) value in the Visit table (PatID). **(B)** Values that are representative of data that might be stored in the database. This type of relationship (one-to-many) allows the Name to be stored once in the Name table and related to multiple Visits in the Visit table.

with relational databases. In a spreadsheet, data can be grouped by creating additional worksheets; however, setting relations is not possible. Two records in the Visit table (VisitID 1 and 4 in Figure 10–2B) relate to participant ABC-001 because these records both have a PatID of 1. This is described as a one-to-many relationship because one unique record in the Name table can have many matching records in the Visit table. A record in a table that matches only one record in another table is a one-to-one relationship. If a one-to-one relationship is identified in the logical design process, consideration should be made to combine tables because by definition data would not be duplicated. A many-to-many relationship is comprised of two one-to-many relationships that are linked by a third table called a *junction table* (Figure 10–3). Many-to-many relationships are useful for cases such as many participants with many visits. In this case, participant information would be stored in one table, visit information would be stored in another, and foreign keys from both tables would be stored in a third table. Although at first viewing, such a relationship seems complex, use of such relationships makes complex queries of data possible. This is where SQL plays a critical role. Consider the Name and Visit tables in Table 10–2A. A typical SQL statement used to query the two tables for all instances where the PatID equals 1 would be *SELECT * FROM Name INNER JOIN Visit ON Name.PatID=Visit.PatID*

*WHERE Name.PatID=1.* The resulting dataset would look like Table 10–2B. The *INNER JOIN* condition of the SQL statement retrieves rows from the Name and Visit tables where the PatID values are equivalent and the *WHERE* clause filters the results so that only records with PatID equal to 1 are returned. Notice that because an asterisk was used between *SELECT* and *FROM,* all the fields from both tables appear in the resulting dataset. Specifying desired fields in the SQL statement acts as a filter for the fields in the dataset. For example, the SQL statement *SELECT Name, Visit, Pulse FROM Name INNER JOIN Visit ON Name. PatID=Visit.PatID WHERE Name.PatID=1* would only have the name, visit, and pulse fields in the resulting dataset (Table 10–2C).

Data normalization, a fundamental concept of relational database design, deals with separating data into multiple related tables. A typical normalized relational database has multiple related narrow tables (few columns) with similar data that is grouped and not duplicated (5). When appropriate indexes are available, data normalization often increases the speed of queries; however, the complexities of the SQL join statements increase. Consideration should be given to balance the level of normalization with the types of queries required.

The last step in designing a working database would be to select and implement an appropriate database, relational or flat file, which best fits the logical model. Keep in mind, however, that identifying a

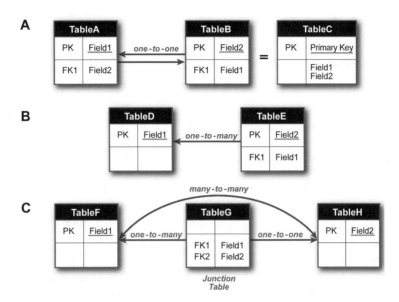

FIGURE 10–3 ● **(A)** TableA and TableB show a generalized, logical, one-to-one relationship between the primary key (PK) values and the foreign key (FK1) values in each table. One-to-one relationships provide no relational advantage because fields can be combined into one table with no duplication of data (TableC). **(B)** TableD and TableE show a generalized, logical, one-to-many relationship between the primary key (PK) value in TableD and the foreign key (FK1) value in the TableE. **(C)** A generalized, logical, many-to-many relationship exists between TableF and TableH. TableG is a *junction table* that links two one-to-many relationships between TableF–TableG and TableG–TableH.

## TABLE 10–2

### Output Tables Resulting from Queries of the Many-to-Many Relationship Example Shown in Figure 10.3

**A**

| NAME TABLE | | | VISIT TABLE | | | | |
|---|---|---|---|---|---|---|---|
| PatID (PK) | Name | VisitID (PK) | PatID (FK1) | Visit | Systolic | Diastolic | Pulse |
| 1 | ABC-001 | 1 | 1 | Screen | 140 | 80 | 65 |
| 2 | DEF-010 | 2 | 2 | Screen | 130 | 80 | 70 |
| 3 | GHI-100 | 3 | 3 | Screen | 160 | 90 | 55 |
| | | 4 | 1 | Visit 1 | 130 | 70 | 60 |

**B**

| | | | DATASET | | | | |
|---|---|---|---|---|---|---|---|
| PatID (PK) | Name | VisitID (PK) | PatID (FK1) | Visit | Systolic | Diastolic | Pulse |
| 1 | ABC-001 | 1 | 1 | Screen | 140 | 80 | 65 |
| 1 | ABC-001 | 4 | 1 | Visit 1 | 130 | 70 | 60 |

**C**

| | DATASET | |
|---|---|---|
| Name | Visit | Pulse |
| ABC-001 | Screen | 65 |
| ABC-001 | Visit 1 | 60 |

relationship does not necessarily mean that a relational database is desirable, particularly if the total quantity of data stored is small and not indicative of a multitable, normalized, relational database.

## THE USER INTERFACE

Regardless of the application manufacturer, a spreadsheet has an intuitive user-friendly interface and many users will be familiar with spreadsheets from use on other projects. Data in the rows and columns is easy to manipulate. Rows and columns are easily added and subtracted or moved and cells can be specifically formatted for data types. The rigid format of a spreadsheet does offer basic data entry features; however, it would be difficult to offer advanced functions such as viewing records from multiple worksheets in one consolidated area, data lookup, or record validation without significant user intervention.

In contrast, relational database management systems (the back end) are designed to manage data and not as an interface for the end user. A user interface application (the front end) that displays, adds, modifies, and deletes data from the database is required for the end user to interact with the data. Separating the database from the application allows for advanced programming techniques, such as separate business logic and multiple user interfaces. These techniques can extend the functionality of a relational database and are not available for a flat file database.

## SAMPLE PROTOCOL SETUP

To illustrate these principles of database design, consider two sample study protocols and how a database

### TABLE 10–3

**Example of a Simple Clinical Research Protocol**

|  | Visit 1 |
|---|---|
| Basic lipid panel (Chol, Trig, LDL-C, HDL-C) | ✔ |
| Vitals, weight, and height | ✔ |
| Pregnancy test | ✔ |

design might be developed from each protocol. For simplicity's sake, assume that there are 50 participants in each sample study. Table 10–3 shows a very simple sample clinical research protocol that contains only one visit per participant with laboratory results, vitals, weight, and height collected. Table 10–4 is an example of a flat file database (spreadsheet) that would be adequate for this type and size of data. Because no one-to-many relationships are indicated, all data can be grouped together without the risk of duplication. Spreadsheets such as this offer an intuitive user-friendly interface that typically works well with small datasets.

Table 10–5, on the other hand, shows a very complex protocol example with different types of data occurring at different visits. For this example, a relational database would be the best solution. Figure 10–4 is an example of a logical model using a relational database that could be implemented to meet the needs of this protocol. Note that individual tables for Adverse Events, Medications, and Medical History have been logically modeled, because each of these tables have information that could have many rows for each participant stored in the Name Demographics table. Likewise, each of these tables has information that is not related

### TABLE 10–4

**Example of a Spreadsheet with Participant Demographic and Results Information That Would Be Obtained When Following the Simple Protocol in Table 10–3**

|  | A | B | C | D | E | F | G | H | I | J | K | L | M | N |
|---|---|---|---|---|---|---|---|---|---|---|---|---|---|---|
| 1 | Name | Sex | DOB | Coll Date | Chol | Trig | LDL-C | HDL-C | Weight (lbs) | Height (in) | Systolic | Diastolic | Pulse | HCG |
| 2 | ABC-1 | F | 4/4/70 | 2/10/04 | 190 | 230 | 140 | 45 | 140 | 67.5 | 140 | 80 | 65 | Neg |
| 3 | DEF-2 | M | 8/1/80 | 2/10/04 | 170 | 190 | 145 | 38 | 190 | 73.2 | 130 | 70 | 60 | NA |
| 4 | GHI-3 | F | 10/22/72 | 2/15/04 | 160 | 245 | 138 | 55 | 132 | 62 | 130 | 80 | 70 | Neg |
| 5 | ... | | | | | | | | | | | | | |

## TABLE 10-5

### Example of a Complex Clinical Research Protocol

| | Screen | Q1 | Q2 | Q3 | W0 | W4 | W8 | W12 | W20 | W32 | W44 | W56 | W68 | W80 or ET |
|---|---|---|---|---|---|---|---|---|---|---|---|---|---|---|
| Informed consent signed | ✔ | | | | | | | | | | | | | |
| Medications washout | ✔ | | | | | | | | | | | | | |
| Current medication query | ✔ | | | | | | | | | | | | | |
| Treadmill familiarization/compatibility test | ✔ | | | | | | | | | | | | | |
| Medical history | ✔ | | | | | | | | | | | | | |
| Medical history update | | | | | ✔ | | | | | | | | | |
| Social History | ✔ | | | | | | ✔ | | ✔ | ✔ | ✔ | ✔ | ✔ | ✔ |
| Vital signs, weight, height | ✔ | ✔ | ✔ | | ✔ | ✔ | ✔ | ✔ | ✔ | ✔ | ✔ | ✔ | ✔ | ✔ |
| Diet instructions & logs dispensed | ✔ | ✔ | | | ✔ | ✔ | ✔ | ✔ | ✔ | ✔ | ✔ | ✔ | ✔ | |
| Diet logs collected & reviewed | | ✔ | | | ✔ | ✔ | ✔ | ✔ | ✔ | ✔ | ✔ | ✔ | ✔ | ✔ |
| Physical examination | | | | | ✔ | | | | | ✔ | | | | ✔ |
| Noncontinuous 12-lead ECG | ✔ | | | | | | | | | | | | | |
| Graded treadmill test/continuous ECG | ✔ | ✔ | ✔ | ✔ | | | | | ✔ | ✔ | | ✔ | | ✔ |
| Ankle-brachial pressure index | ✔ | ✔ | | | | | | | ✔ | ✔ | | ✔ | | ✔ |
| QoL measurements | | | | | ✔ | | | | ✔ | ✔ | | ✔ | | ✔ |
| Serum chemistries | | ✔ | | | | ✔ | ✔ | ✔ | ✔ | ✔ | ✔ | ✔ | ✔ | ✔ |
| Lipid panel | ✔ | ✔ | ✔ | ✔ | | ✔ | ✔ | ✔ | ✔ | ✔ | ✔ | ✔ | ✔ | ✔ |
| Hematology | | ✔ | | | | ✔ | ✔ | ✔ | ✔ | ✔ | ✔ | ✔ | ✔ | ✔ |
| Special chemistries | | ✔ | | | | | | | ✔ | ✔ | ✔ | ✔ | ✔ | ✔ |
| Pregnancy test | ✔ | | | | ✔ | | | ✔ | | ✔ | | | | |
| Serum and plasma reference samples | | | | | ✔ | ✔ | ✔ | ✔ | ✔ | ✔ | ✔ | ✔ | ✔ | ✔ |
| Dispense study medication | | | | | ✔ | ✔ | ✔ | ✔ | ✔ | ✔ | ✔ | ✔ | ✔ | |
| Collect study medication | | | | | | ✔ | ✔ | ✔ | ✔ | ✔ | ✔ | ✔ | ✔ | ✔ |
| Study medication compliance check | | | | | | ✔ | ✔ | ✔ | ✔ | ✔ | ✔ | ✔ | ✔ | ✔ |
| Adverse events query | | | | | | ✔ | ✔ | ✔ | ✔ | ✔ | ✔ | ✔ | ✔ | ✔ |
| Concomitant medication query | | | | | | ✔ | ✔ | ✔ | ✔ | ✔ | ✔ | ✔ | ✔ | ✔ |
| Schedule next visit | ✔ | ✔ | ✔ | ✔ | ✔ | ✔ | ✔ | ✔ | ✔ | ✔ | ✔ | ✔ | ✔ | |

directly to each other and is best placed in separate tables. In the same way, multiple visit orders can exist for each participant in Name Demographics, so the visit orders are placed in a separate table. For each scheduled visit of the protocol, multiple instances of the visit will occur, at least one for each participant. Thus, the relationship of the Visit Name table to the Name Demographics table is a many-to-many relationship, because it combines two one-to-many relationships, the Name Demographics to Visit Orders and the Visit Name to the Visit Orders.

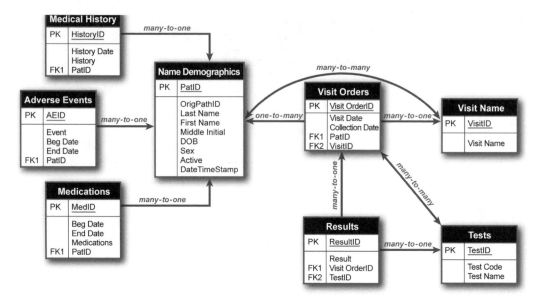

**FIGURE 10–4** ● One possible logical relational database design based on the protocol listed in Table 10–2. This model shows the Name Demographic table separate but related to the Medical History, Adverse Events, Medications, and Visit Orders tables. This arrangement allows one participant to have many entries in any of the connecting tables. The many-to-many relationship shown between the Name Demographics and Visit Name tables is desired because many participants can have many visits. The same logic is used for the many-to-many relationship between the Visit Orders and Tests tables. Many orders (linked back to the Name Demographics table via the PatID foreign key) can have many tests associated with them. In other words, a participant can have many visits, and each visit can have many tests.

## IMPLEMENTATION

Erroneous data can be introduced into a database from many sources. Taking preventative measures to avoid inclusion of erroneous data is key to having a valid database (6). Duplicate manual data entry and record level validations are some techniques that can be used to trap bad data or flag data to be double-checked. It is critical that the end user follow the *rules* of the database design. For example, if the data model indicates that a field for participant weight contains only numeric values, the end user should not enter a numeric value with units. Training the end user on appropriate field values, defining a cell format in a spreadsheet, or setting an input mask for a data entry field can prevent these types of problems. Checks for accuracy and correctness of data should be performed to validate the data being stored and serve as a second check for data types in tables. Mixed data in a field would result in added cleanup of data prior to performing calculations or reporting. It might also be necessary for researchers to retrieve, select, and combine results from separate but related clinical studies for the purpose of statistical analysis, a technique called meta-analysis. Data that is missing, incomplete, or implausible is very time consuming and expensive to correct as opposed to data that is valid

and accurate, which is arguably more scientifically valuable to researchers and their partners (7).

## DATA SECURITY

Medically sensitive data, protected health information, and working environment are some factors that can influence the level and type of security required. The Health Insurance Portability and Accountability Act (HIPAA) Privacy rule might influence the level of security required for information systems; for more information on this topic visit http://privacyruleandresearch.nih.gov/. Other regulatory bodies, such as the FDA, may also impose additional security requirements. Computer users in general should be aware of current practices that minimize the chance of exposing data to unauthorized parties. An innocent act such as opening an email attachment that contains malicious code could give an unauthorized user administrative access to the operating system and files. For computers that are part of a network or have a direct connection to the Internet, firewalls, and virus scanning software should be implemented and updated frequently. Operating systems should be updated frequently to obtain the latest security patches. Access to spreadsheet files can be password protected; RDBMSs however, offer a wide array of security schemes and access rights. Control of personnel, access to storage media, system access, internal audit trails, and off-site data backups should be considered (8).

## SUMMARY

- The database is a critical component of any clinical study and appropriate attention must be given to the format and design of the database, or entry and retrieval of data will be compromised.
- There are four main types of database models: flat files, hierarchical, network, or relational. In most clinical research applications, the choice is primarily between the flat file model (simple but restricted) and relational databases (potentially complex but flexible).
- A spreadsheet design that is suitable for a simple study becomes unruly and difficult to manage for more complex research projects.
- Key steps in database design are to determine the type of data that are to be stored, whether to group the data, and whether normalization is required (i.e., separated into multiple related tables). Answers to these questions help determine whether a flat file or relational database

will best meet the research needs of the study.
- Other issues to consider include the user interface and data security to protect private health information regulated by HIPPA.

## REFERENCES

1. Good P. Data Management. In: The Design and Conduct of Clinical Trials. Hoboken, NJ: John Wiley & Sons, Inc., 2002:125–153.
2. Loney K, Koch, G. Sharing Knowledge and success. In: Oracle 8i: The Complete Reference. Berkeley, CA: Osborne/McCraw-Hill, 2000:4–16.
3. Microsoft. Microsoft Visual FoxPro 6.0 Programmers Guide. Redmond, WA: Microsoft Corporation, 1998: 91–109,111–124.
4. Petkovic D. Database systems and SQL server. In: SQL Server 7: A Beginner's Guide. Berkeley, CA: Osborne/McGraw-Hill, 1999:3–19.
5. Microsoft. Microsoft SQL Sever Database Design and Implementation. Redmond, WA: Microsoft Corporation, 2001:1–42,45–96.
6. Day S, Fayers P, Harvey D. Double data entry: what value, what price? Control Clin Trials 1998;19:15–24.
7. Schmid CH, Landa M, Jafar TH et al. Constructing a database of individual clinical trials for longitudinal analysis. Control Clin Trials 2003;24:324–340.
8. Hasson AM, Fagerstrom RM, Kahane DC et al. Design and evolution of the data management systems in the prostate, lung, colorectal and ovarian (PLCO) cancer screening trial. Control Clin Trials 2000; 21:329S–348S.

# CHAPTER 11

# Case Report Form Development

## Janet Voorhees, Mary Ellen Scheipeter

I know that you believe you understand what you think I said, but I'm not sure you realize that what you heard is not what I meant.

—Robert McCloskey, 1960s

The Food and Drug Administration (FDA) defines a case report form (CRF) as "a printed, optical, or electronic document designed to record all of the protocol-required information to be reported to the sponsor/investigator on each trial subject" (1). Although CRFs are standard data collection tools for therapeutic clinical trials, they are unusual for investigator-initiated translational and experimental clinical research. Nevertheless, investigators would be well served by adopting many of the standards accepted by the pharmaceutical industry with respect to clinical research documentation. This chapter will describe the types of data that should be collected in case report forms (CRFs), why they should be collected, and how CRFs should be designed.

Forms serve various purposes, and several functions may be combined in a single form. CRFs may include questionnaires, dietary assessments, patient diaries, laboratory results, or any other set of clinical information. Because CRFs are used to record the research data generated by the study, they in effect end up controlling the scope of data analysis. The computer age adage of "garbage in, garbage out" applies here as well; that is, the results of any analysis can only be as good as the quality of the data used in the analysis. The goal of a well-designed CRF should be that the data collected will be complete and consistent. Clearly, investigators must give considerable thought to the development and pilot testing of the CRF during the planning phase of the research protocol (Table 11–1) (2).

Well-designed case report forms unambiguously capture the research data in a manner that clearly describes what happened with each research participant, where it happened, when, and what was the involvement of members of the research team. Well-designed CRFs come with unambiguous instructions, and are clear and easy to read. They are appropriate for the data being analyzed without capturing excessive data that will not contribute to answering any of the research questions or will never be analyzed. Well-designed CRFs can be completed quickly and efficiently and are not redundant in the data collected.

The basic items that need to be captured in CRFs include those required to answer the scientific questions specified in the research protocol and those required by government and local regulation of research. CRFs must capture data related to:

1. Study endpoints
2. Adverse events
3. Potential confounding variable that might affect an endpoint or safety
4. Protocol compliance, including, but not limited to, compliance with inclusion and exclusion criteria, subject follow-up, concurrent medications, modifications to the experimental intervention (e.g., study drug dose, dose interruptions), and management of participants who experience adverse events (3)

Ideally, case report form design should involve both those who use the forms to record data in the clinical research setting and those who will eventually be analyzing the data.

Case report forms may be paper forms, used for later data entry, or may be electronic forms entered directly into an electronic database (see Chapter 10).

## TABLE 11–1

### Principles of Form Design

**Parsimony**
Gather only the relevant data.
Ensure that each piece of data collected has a specific purpose.

**Logic**
Questions should be presented in a logical sequence.
Response codes need to be consistent.

**Space**
Allow appropriate format and space to facilitate data collection.

**Instruction**
Instructions should be provided on the forms where appropriate.
Units of measure and decimals should be printed on the forms.

**Pretest**
Field test and revise the form before the launch of the trial.

**Security**
Make duplicate copies and electronically back up the data forms.
To protect the confidentiality of research participants and data integrity, access rights to the data forms should incorporate a secure location with access limited to authorized persons. For electronic data, a secure network and password protection is necessary.

Although paper forms are still regarded as the standard for CRFs, increasing use of computerized systems to reduce the storage of paper documents is to be expected (4–6).

Data collection is typically one of the most time-consuming parts of the research process (7). The quality of CRF design can affect the amount of clinician time required to complete the study as well as the clarity or ambiguity of the data collected. Poor CRF design can result in poor participant management, coordinator burnout, and ambiguity in determining the study results.

## DESIGNING FORMS TO ANSWER THE RESEARCH HYPOTHESIS AND EXPEDITE DATA ANALYSIS

The ability to analyze the collected data easily and efficiently should be the primary goal guiding creation of the CRFs. Ideally, based on the data in the CRFs alone, it should be possible to reconstruct the who, what, when, where, and how the research was implemented and the research participant managed.

In pharmaceutical trials, CRFs serve as the principal data collection instruments, yet all data collected on them must also be verifiable through original source documentation. For instance, a blood glucose may be a piece of data entered into a field on CRF, but the *source document* for that laboratory result is the specific part of the medical record that documents the blood glucose value. Once again, a similar standard is not mandatory for non–FDA-regulated research, but adopting this standard voluntarily is a wise procedure.

To do so, in every case, the investigator must be able to trace the data in the CRF back to its original source documentation. Other examples of source documents include the signed and dated informed consent document, hospital records, clinic records, notes, correspondence, lab reports, radiographs, or electronic data. Clinic records may be specifically designed as source documents for a clinical study. In this case, the clinical records will in many ways reflect the design of the case report forms. However, CRFs, being research documents, should never take the place of clinical records, which include protected health information (covered by HIPAA regulations, see Chapters 14 and 15) such as participant's name, date of birth, and contact information. When electronic CRFs (e-CRFs) are used to collect data directly at the time of the subject visit, the electronic data become the "source" document for those data (8).

It is important to be frugal when choosing study variables that will be collected. Each measure that is collected adds to the complexity and cost of implementing the study and analyzing the data. However, it is equally important to make every attempt to collect the data that will be needed prospectively, rather than trying retrospectively to recapture needed data via a chart review. With the exception of data required by regulatory agencies (if any), all data collected should be justified in the protocol. Collection of additional data not directly related to the protocol objectives should be limited. Many studies have collected superfluous data that is ultimately never analyzed. For example, in one of the first large NIH trials of treatment for HIV positive patients, only 2% of the data base was utilized for scientific papers. It was estimated that the study collected more than 30 times more data on CRFs than was needed for study analysis (9).

It can be helpful to organize the forms for data collection by the study objectives to be achieved. Each item of data to be analyzed should be categorized into its role in answering the research questions. The data to be collected should fit into the following categories: predictor variables, outcome variables, or potential confounders of the outcomes (Table 11–2) (10). The data collection should not

only include information that will be used to answer the study question(s), but also pertain to demographic information required by regulatory agencies to demonstrate fair and equitable study enrollment, medical history and disease severity data to confirm eligibility of the volunteer for participation in the study, and safety characteristics (such as liver function in participants who will be given an intervention that may affect liver function).

After identifying the variables that need to be measured, CRF design should be broken down temporally to capture the data required for capture at each of the participant's study visits (e.g., Screening, Baseline, Follow-up, Study termination). *Baseline case report forms* capture information prior to study intervention. *Follow-up CRFs* should be labeled by the study time point at which they will be collected (i.e., Study week 4, Study week 8, Study termination, or visit 1, visit 2). The follow-up forms should be designed to collect pertinent safety information, adherence to the study protocol, the status of the primary and secondary outcome variables, and any other variables that could confound interpretation of the outcome.

## TABLE 11–2

### Example of Variables for a CRF in a Study of HIV-Related Peripheral Neuropathy

| Predictor Variables | Outcome Variables | Potential Confounders |
|---|---|---|
| Age | Symptoms of pain in feet | Exposure to drugs known to cause |
| Sex | Symptoms of numbness in feet | peripheral neuropathy (e.g., alcohol, |
| Date of HIV infection | Symptoms of tingling in feet | metronidazole) |
| CD4 lymphocyte count | Clinical signs of neuropathy: Bilateral | Exposure to toxic chemicals known to |
| HIV plasma viral load | distal decrease in sharp sensation | cause peripheral neuropathy (e.g., |
| D-drug exposure | Clinical signs of neuropathy: Bilateral | industrial solvents, heavy metals) |
| Investigation drug (study | distal decrease in vibratory sensation | Vitamin B12 deficiency |
| intervention) | Clinical signs of neuropathy: Bilateral | History of nerve injury |
| | distal decrease in ankle jerk reflex as | Systemic disease known to be associated |
| | compared to knee. | with peripheral neuropathies (e.g., |
| | Nerve conduction studies/Quantitative | diabetes, lupus) |
| | sensory testing | |
| | Adverse experiences | |

## DATA CODING GUIDELINES FOR THE RESEARCH VARIABLES

In response to the call for an advisory board, the Clinical Data Interchange Standards Consortium (CDISC), an open multidisciplinary nonprofit organization, has been created and has developed "industry standards to support the electronic acquisition, exchange, submission, and archiving of clinical trials data and metadata for medical and biopharmaceutical product development" (11,12). Although NIH-sponsored research are not held to these standards, they nevertheless serve as a useful template that can be applied to any translational or experimental research study.

Forms should be consistent with regard to questions. The questions should be asked in the same way and the same order across forms. Codes within forms should be standardized. An example would be dichotomous variables that capture answers to "yes" or "no" questions. If "no" = 0 and "yes" = 1, this same format should be continued throughout all the forms. If, on an ordinal Likert-type scale, "0" means "strongly disagree" and 5 means "strongly agree," then for all questions related to agreement and disagreement, "0" should always mean "strongly disagree" and 5 should always mean "strongly agree." This applies to all categorization of variables, such as "all of the time" at one extreme of a scale with "none of the time" at the other end of the scale.

The described scales above are ordinal measures. An example of collecting similar information using a continuous variable is the use of a *visual analogue scale (VAS)*. As noted in Chapter 3, continuous variables are preferred whenever possible over categorical variables. Continuous variables contain more information and result in a study allowing a smaller sample size (10). Visual analogue scales are usually designed with a continuous range from 1 to 100. For example, in a study of HIV-related neuropathic pain, a pain scale may depict 0 as "no pain" at one end of a line (usually 10 cm in length for simplicity and standardization with the measuring) and 100 at the other end of the line, depicting completely intolerable pain. The participant is asked to mark an "X" on the line at the spot that best represents the answer. The data is captured by measuring the distance of the "X" from the end of the line. A "faces scale" (Figure 11–1), on the other hand, would be an example of a visually presented ordinal scale designed to capture the subject's response whether it would be an adult or a child.

Questions to be answered in a CRF may be either open-ended or closed-ended. Open-ended questions allow the respondents to convey their thoughts. (A respondent is the person completing the questionnaire, and may be either the research volunteer or the research coordinator.) An example of an open-ended question is the following:

***What triggers do you believe increase a person's chance of having an asthma attack?***

*Open-ended questions* leave the respondent free to answer with fewer limits imposed by the researcher. This type of question prompts the respondent's understanding in a conceptual format. The chief disadvantage of open-ended questions is that they usually require qualitative methods to code and analyze the responses, which take more time and subjective judgment than coding closed-ended questions.

Closed-ended questions are more common in translational and experimental clinical research studies and form the basis for most standardized

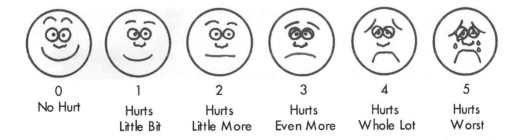

**FIGURE 11–1** ● Example of a visually presented ordinal scale designed to semiquantify the amount of pain being experienced by a research participant. From Wang DL, Hockenberry-Eaton M, Wilson D, Winkelstein ML, Schwartz P. Wong's Essentials of Pediatric Nursing, ed. 8 St. Louis, 2001, Mosby. P 1301, Copyright Mosby. Reprinted by permission.

measures. These questions ask the respondent to choose from one or more preselected answers, such as the following:

> Which asthma trigger do you think is the most likely to increase a person's chance of having an asthma attack? (Check one.)
>
> Smoking ☐
> Animal dander ☐
> Weather changes ☐

Closed-ended questions provide a list of possible alternatives from which the respondent may choose. These questions are quicker and easier to answer and the answers are easier to tabulate, enter into formal databases, and to analyze.

Closed-ended questions are not without their disadvantages. Respondents' answers to closed-ended questions are subject to a kind of observer bias. The responses provided on the form (essentially by the "observer," that is, a member of the research team) may not be the best answer for the respondent. Whenever there is a chance that the set of answers is not exhaustive, which means they may not include all possible options, it is important to include an option such as "Other (please specify)" or "None of the above" (10). "Other" responses may be hard to code for later analysis. For example, in 1992, the ACTG reported that almost 5,000 different "other" responses had been submitted on their "Signs and Symptoms" forms (13). When a single response is desired, the set of possible responses should also be mutually exclusive, which means that the categories should not overlap, to ensure clarity and parsimony.

When multiple responses are offered in a question, it is important to instruct the respondent to mark each possible response as either "yes" or "no." Instructing the respondent to mark "all that apply" is not ideal, because it does not force the respondent to pause at each individual option. Consider the following example:

> *Which of the following increases the chance of having an asthma attack?*
>
> |               | Yes | No  | Don't Know |
> |---------------|-----|-----|------------|
> | Smoking       | ☐   | ☐   | ☐          |
> | Animal dander | ☐   | ☐   | ☐          |
> | Weather changes | ☐ | ☐   | ☐          |

## REGULATORY COMPLIANCE ISSUES THAT SHOULD BE INCORPORATED INTO CRF DESIGN

One function of case report forms is documentation of compliance with federal and state laws, institutional, and IRB requirements. Federal regulations apply to all research that has received federal government funding and all research submitting new drug or device applications to the Food and Drug Administration. Many universities and IRBs also require that all research on human subjects at the institution follow federal regulations.

Although federal regulations focus on IRB approval and informed consent for the protection of human subjects, several aspects of the regulations are important to consider in case report form design.

## REQUIREMENTS FOR STUDIES FUNDED BY THE NIH

According to 45CFR Part 46, which addresses the protection of human research participants, the IRB approval of research must meet specific criteria. The following criteria impact case report form development:

- The risks to the participants are minimized.
- The risks to participants are reasonable in relation to the anticipated benefits.
- The selection of research participants for participation in the study is equitable.
- The research plan makes adequate provisions for monitoring the data collected to ensure the safety of participants.
- There are adequate provisions to protect the privacy of participants and to maintain the confidentiality of data.
- Additional safeguards are included to protect the welfare of protected vulnerable individuals (pregnant women, fetuses, prisoners, children, those who are cognitively impaired).
- "No human subjects may be involved in any project supported by these awards until the project has been reviewed and approved by the IRB" (14).

An approvable research protocol already addresses these regulations. Following is a description of how these regulations should be addressed in the case report form design. Once again, these are not mandatory, and they may not apply to all investigator-initiated translational research studies. They should be considered and employed as appropriate.

### Dates

Each CRF should contain the date of data being recorded. This information should capture dates of study visits and tests, as well as medication start and stop dates, and onset and resolution dates of illnesses and adverse experiences. Dates also confirm that participant enrollment into the study is after the date of IRB approval.

## Research Participant ID Number

Each case report form should be coded with an ID number unique to that individual participant. No participant name, address, birth date, or other direct participant identifiers should be entered into CRFs. Use of a participant ID number protects the privacy of study participants and helps to maintain the confidentiality of the data.

## Inclusion/Exclusion Criteria and Verification of Eligibility

Including a CRF checklist for study eligibility demonstrates that each volunteer who was enrolled met the criteria for participation. The checklist helps confirm enrollment only of those for whom participation would be safe, and those from whom appropriate data will be obtained.

## Demographic Information

Demographic information helps to identify differences in study outcomes that may be related to age, race, gender, or location. The NIH also requires this information be collected in order to document that study recruitment was equitable and that no groups were excluded from participation that would otherwise be eligible for study enrollment (15). For NIH-sponsored studies, the NIH criteria for ethnic/minority classifications should be used.

## "Baseline" and "On Study" Status Information

Data from before and after a study intervention is information that will be used to analyze the study hypothesis. In addition, the before and after intervention information should contain measures that document the state of health of the participant before and after the intervention in order to determine the study risk to participants. The baseline status may include results of participant screening evaluations and tests as well as baseline health characteristics that are not necessarily considered requirements for study eligibility. Participant status information usually includes the *medical history*, and includes *concurrent medications, concurrent illnesses, physical exams including height and weight (weight is usually required by regulatory agencies for reporting adverse experiences), laboratory data,* and *other tests or evaluations.* These forms document changes in the participant's health status during the course of the study, which helps to determine

the risk versus benefit of study participation to the subjects.

## Protection of Vulnerable Groups

Protection of pregnant women and fetuses are specifically addressed in the federal laws. In order to document that women of childbearing potential are eligible for participation in a clinical study that may have risk for the pregnancy or for the fetus, it is important to document pregnancy testing and compliance with birth control for those who are of childbearing potential. In studies that involve potentially cognitively impaired participants, having participants complete a questionnaire that demonstrates their understanding of the study, can help to demonstrate that they were competent to sign the informed consent. If the questionnaire demonstrates that participants are unable to provide evidence of their understanding of the study, a legal representative should be sought for consent, or the participants may be ineligible for study participation.

## Adverse Experiences and Serious Adverse Experiences

An adverse experience occurs whenever a research participant's status worsens during study participation, whether or not it is directly related to study participation. When assessing the participant's risk versus benefit of study participation, it is important to track this information in a timely manner. Case report forms should collect information on both serious and nonserious adverse experiences. *All* adverse experiences should be *documented* although the NIH and IRB may only require *reporting* of serious adverse experiences and unexpected events. The adverse experiences should be documented in the case report form by providing the following details:

> *Participant ID, description of the event, the severity of the event (serious, severe, moderate, or mild), the likely cause of the adverse experience, whether the experience was related to study participation or interventions, what interventions were used to treat the adverse event, and dates of onset and resolution. If the adverse experience did not resolve, the form should capture information about what happened, and if there were sequelae.*

## Study Medication/Treatment Dispensing

Forms that document the dispensing of study drugs and treatments confirm compliance with the study protocol. In addition to tracking dispensing of the intervention, case report forms that record the participant's return of unused study medication can be helpful not only in understanding the failure of a drug to have its intended effect but can also help to identify any risk from a participant's noncompliance with the study intervention. All treatments dispensed should be tracked and documented, even when done in error or not in compliance with the protocol design.

### Missed Visits, Exams, Tests

Case report forms must reflect not only the results of protocol-directed evaluations, but whether the evaluation occurred.

### Participant Study Termination and Dropout Information

Information about why research volunteers discontinued their study participation should be recorded. Such information may provide insight into safety issues, or possibly problems with the protocol design or implementation.

### Essential Documents

As explained in Chapters 14 and 15, good clinical practice (GCP) are a set of standards that govern the conduct of FDA-regulated clinical trials. Increasingly, GCP is being adopted by NIH as well as its standard for clinical trials. Although GCP may not be a regulatory standard for investigator-initiated translational and experimental clinical research (even if sponsored by NIH, as long as the study doesn't qualify as a "clinical trial" by NIH definitions), investigators would still be wise to use the GCP standards in the conduct of their own research. Section 8 of the International Conference on Harmonisation: Good Clinical Practice addresses "Essential Documents for the Conduct of a Clinical Trial" and states that "Any or all of the documents addressed in this guideline may be subject to, and should be available for, audit by the sponsor's auditor and inspection by regulatory authorities." Case Report forms are specifically discussed in the ICH/GCP, Section 8.3 (16). Those documents that are related to CRF design include the following:

- *Source documents* are required to document that each individual has volunteered to participate in the research and to substantiate the integrity of the trial data collected.
- *Case report forms* indicate investigator or designee confirmation of the observations recorded. Case report forms are required to be signed, dated, and completed.

- All *change, additions, and corrections to CRFs* must be documented.
- Documentation of *notification* to regulatory agencies and sponsors *of all serious adverse experiences, unexpected drug reactions,* or *other safety information*.
- *Screening logs* must be maintained to identify individuals who entered pretrial screening and should indicate the reason for screening failure for those who do not enroll in the study.
- The *identification code* protects the confidentiality of participants. The code is used to identify individual participants on case report forms, allowing the data to be collected and analyzed while keeping identity private.
- *Enrollment log* should document the chronological enrollment of volunteers into a clinical trial.
- *Investigation product(s) accountability* at the site.
- A *signature sheet* of all persons authorized to make entries or corrections on the CRFs.
- Record of *retained body fluids/tissue samples,* if any.

Investigators can create standardized forms that capture the data required by the regulatory agencies and can be used for any study. The basic regulatory requirements are consistent for all clinical trials. Examples of CRFs that can be standardized include Medical History, Diagnosis, Signs and Symptoms, Concomitant Medications, Adverse Experiences, Serious Adverse Experiences. With standardized forms, there is less need to train coordinators how to use forms from study to study, and the data entry does not have to be redesigned for each study.

### THE ROLE OF CRFs IN STUDY MONITORING OVERSIGHT

Formal study monitoring by third parties (from the investigator's institution or from a sponsor like NIH) has not been routinely performed for investigator-initiated translational or experimental clinical research, even though oversight is mandated by 45 CFR Part 46.111 (Chapter 14). It is likely that such monitoring will become more routine in the future. Once again, standards set by the clinical trial industry are likely to be used as a benchmark in this setting. The International Conference on Harmonisation: Good Clinical Practice section 5.18 has guidelines for monitoring. After reviewing completed CRFs, study monitors should be able to verify that:

- The rights and well-being of the participants were protected.
- Reported data on CRFs are accurate, complete, and verifiable from source documents.

- The trial was conducted in compliance with the currently approved protocol, GCP, and applicable regulatory requirements.

One of the responsibilities of monitoring is checking the accuracy and completeness of the CRF entries. Monitors are required to confirm that:

- The required data are reported accurately on the CRFs and are consistent with the source data.
- Any therapy modifications are well documented for each volunteer.
- Adverse events, concomitant medications, and intercurrent illness are reported on the CRFs.
- Missed study visits, tests, and exams must be clearly reported on the CRFs.
- All study withdrawals and dropouts of enrolled volunteers must be documented and explained on the CRFs (14).

## REQUIREMENTS AND METHODS FOR ARCHIVING CRFs

IRBs, institutions, sponsors, and other applicable regulatory requirements detail how long CRFs should be kept available for review (often 2 years or longer after completion of the research study). The records that should be retained include the case report forms (including records of all changes and corrections within the CRFs) and all supporting source documents including, signed and dated informed consents, medical records, progress notes, and lab reports (16).

## ANATOMY OF A CASE REPORT FORM

### Basic Requirements

The object of a case report form is to record observations about research participants. Many CRFs can be created as flow sheets. An example of the use of flow sheets is for the collection of concurrent medications. When flow sheets are used, at each study visit, the coordinator reviews all concurrent medications. All new medications are added to the flow sheet with the dosing and start date. If a medication is ongoing, this information is reflected by lack of a stop date. If that medication is stopped at a later visit, the stop date is added to the flow sheet. When flow sheets are used, it is important to have fields for data entry to sign off across from each data field. This signature is to confirm when the data has been entered, because the data should be entered at each study visit, or whenever there is a change in the data captured by a flow sheet.

The completed CRFs for a study, when combined, should provide concise data for analysis of the research hypothesis. When developing a form, it is important that the information captured should be reliable and reproducible for the study analysis. Following are the key components of a case report form.

### Headers

The header of a case report form should include the name of the study, and the name of the form (Figure 11–2). If the investigator is using standardized CRFs, the forms may be coded to differentiate them from study specific forms (i.e., "GMEDHX" may be a code for a standardized generic medical history form, whereas "PMEDHX" may indicate a protocol required medical history form that targets the respiratory system). The key fields of the form should include the clinic or site ID, the participant ID, the date of the report or visit, the sequential visit ID, the identification of the person completing the form, and when more than one of the same type of form will be required to capture data at a single visit, the form sequence number.

The instruction box should include the purpose of the form, when to use the form, and instruct the person on how to complete the form. When an instruction box is used, it should include information about the form that is concise and easy to follow. If this information is too lengthy to incorporate into the form, separate instruction pages should be created and incorporated in a study procedure manual (see Chapter 12).

### The Body of the Forms

The body of the form, of course, is where the actual study data are collected. The form may be designed to collect data about the participants' medical history, their medication history, symptoms, the severity of the illness that is being studied, specimens that have been collected, or administrative information (Figure 11–3). The body of the form should include instructions specifying what data needs to be entered. Checklists, pull-down menus, and skip boxes can help guide the clinician in the specific data collection required for each visit. In general, skips are indicated by an arrow and give instructions to either stop or skip to another data entry item.

The body of the form may include general instructions for how to enter the data. These instructions may be in italics and appear either above or below each question. There may be "yes" or "no" checkboxes, which must be checked for each item. If there is a checklist, it is very important that the form provides clear directions for answering the

## Study Eligibility Checklist

### Neutrophil glucose utilization during acute lung injury using radiolabeled fluorodeoxyglucose and PET imaging

Participant ID ☐☐☐☐☐☐☐    Date of Visit ☐☐☐/☐☐/☐☐
                                          m  m  m   d  d   y  y

Protocol ID ☐☐☐☐☐    Staff ID ☐☐☐

Study Day ☐☐☐    Form sequence # (if more than 1) ☐    Data Entry Code ☐☐☐

---

**Inclusion Criteria** (*if any inclusion criteria is marked "NO", the patient is not eligible for enrollment*)

Yes  No
☐  ☐    1. Participant is a healthy volunteer, male or female, any race or ethnicity.
☐  ☐    2. Participant is > 18 years old, but < 45 years old.
☐  ☐    3. Screening FEV1 and FVC must be > 80% of predicted.
☐  ☐    4. Participant must be capable of lying still and supine within the PET scanner for approximately 2 ½ hours.
☐  ☐    5. Participant must be capable of fasting for 6 hours.
☐  ☐    6. Participant has signed informed consent

**Exclusion Criteria** (*if any exclusion criteria is marked "Yes", the patient is not eligible for enrollment*)

Yes  No
☐  ☐    1. Participant is pregnant (positive qualitative urine hCG pregnancy test) or lactating.
☐  ☐    2. Participant has history of cardiopulmonary disease or asthma.
☐  ☐    3. Participant has history of tobacco use or smoked other illicit drugs (marijuana, cocaine) in the past year.
☐  ☐    4. Participant is currently taking any prescription medications.
☐  ☐    5. If Day 1 screening evaluations reveal health problems:

| Normal | Abnormal | | Normal | Abnormal | |
|---|---|---|---|---|---|
| ☐ | ☐ | H&P | ☐ | ☐ | CBC |
| ☐ | ☐ | Spirometry | ☐ | ☐ | BMP |
| ☐ | ☐ | ECG | ☐ | ☐ | PT, PTT |
| ☐ | ☐ | Chest x-ray | ☐ Neg | ☐ Pos | urine pregnancy test ☐ NA |
| ☐ | ☐ | H&P | | | |

☐  ☐    7. Participant is at increased risk for radiation exposure such as air flight personnel, radiation worker, or is enrolled in another study involving the use of radioisotopes.
☐  ☐    8. Participant is enrolled in another research study of an investigational drug.
☐  ☐    9. Participant is allergic to a TMP/SMX  and amoxicillin.
☐  ☐    10. Participant is allergic to Atropine, meperidine (Demerol), hydroxyzine (Vistaril), Lidocaine, Midazolam (Versed) or Fentanyl (Duragesic).
☐  ☐    11. Diagnosis of diabetes or fasting glucose at time of PET study is > 150 mg/dl.

**Is participant eligible for participation in this study?**
☐  Yes
☐  No

**Study Dates:**    GCRC dates ___/___/___ till ___/___/___

♦  **Baseline Spirometry:**    ___/___/___ at _____
♦  **Bronchial instillation of endotoxin:**    ___/___/___ at _____
♦  **Day 3 Spirometry:**    ___/___/___ at _____
♦  **PET scan:**    ___/___/___ at _____
♦  **Bronchoalveolar Lavage:**    ___/___/___ at _____

Version 3.2 (9-15-04)    page 1 of 1

**FIGURE 11–2** ● Example of the inclusion/exclusion criteria page from a case report form.

### Medical History and Physical Exam

**Neutrophil glucose utilization during acute lung injury using radiolabeled fluorodeoxyglucose and PET imaging**

Subject ID ☐☐☐☐☐☐☐    Date of Visit ☐☐☐/☐☐/☐☐
                                          m  m  m   d  d   y  y

Protocol ID ☐☐☐☐☐    Staff ID ☐☐☐

Study Day ☐☐☐    Form sequence # (if more than 1) ☐    Data Entry Code ☐☐☐

## Medical History

**Allergies**: _____

**List clinically significant diagnosis or surgeries below:**

1. _____    5. _____

2. _____    6. _____

3. _____    7. _____

4. _____    8. _____

## Physical Exam — baseline

Height: _____ in _____ cm     Weight: _____ lb _____ kg

Temperature: _____ F ____ C     Respirations: _____ RR/min

Heart rate: _____ /min     BP: _____ / _____ mm Hg

Oxygen saturation: _____ %     Oxygenation: **Room Air**

*Indicate Normal or Abnormal*

**Cardiovascular**
[  ] normal*          *(Underline: General: well developed, alert,
                        Heart: RRR, no murmur.
                        Extremities: warm, brisk capillary refill, no edema
                        Pulses: strong and equal bilaterally).

[  ] abnormal  (specify)_____

**Pulmonary**
[  ] normal*          *(Full, equal excursion, breath sounds clear, no adventitious
                        sounds, no retractions)

[  ] abnormal  (specify)_____

**Comments:** _____
_____
_____

Physical exam completed by:_____

Version 1.0 (9-15-04)                                           page 1 of 1

**FIGURE 11–3** ● Example of a medical history page from a case report form.

specific questions. Users of the form may need to check only the answer that applies, or they may need to check "all that apply." It is very important to try to imagine all possible clinical scenarios when designing the CRFs. If the data are not collected, it will not be analyzed. If information is collected in the source document but there is no corresponding data field on the CRFs in which to place it, the information will not be included in analysis. Often it is helpful to create a "free text" field at the end of the form to collect the qualitative information that would otherwise not be captured. The free text field may be designed as a section labeled "comments," with space allowed for written comments. Free text fields may create problems in coding data for future analysis (see above).

When designing the form, proper formatting is essential. To improve the flow of the form, questions concerning major subject areas should be grouped together and introduced by headings or short descriptive statements (Figures 11–2 and 11–4). If the instructions include different time frames, it is sometimes useful to repeat the time frame at the top of the new set of questions. For example:

1. How many times have you had asthma symptoms in the past year?
2. How many times have you seen your primary doctor in the past year?
3. In the past year, how many times have you needed emergency care?

Can be shortened as follows:

1. During the past year, how many times have you:

   • Had asthma symptoms?
   • Seen your primary doctor?
   • Needed emergency care?

The visual design of the form should make it as easy as possible for respondents to complete all questions in the correct sequence. If the format is too long, respondents may unintentionally skip questions or provide wrong answers. However, if a long form is squeezed onto too few pages, small font size and crowding, or cluttered space will lead to difficulty reading the forms and less accuracy in their completion. Response scales should be spaced widely enough so that the respondent can easily circle or check the correct response without accidentally marking the answer above or below. When asking open-ended questions, plenty of space should be included. Possible answers to closed-ended questions should be lined up vertically and preceded by boxes or brackets to check, rather than open blanks (Figures 11–2 and 11–4).

In the design of the form, it is important to remember that every word in a question can influence the validity and reproducibility of the responses. Standardized instruments that have already been tested for validity, specificity, and sensitivity should be used whenever possible. Making the forms readable and aesthetic encourages careful attention among those who will use them. The objective should be to construct questions that are simple, and encourage accurate and honest responses. Questions must be as clear and specific as possible. Concrete words are preferred over abstract words. Questions should use simple, common words that convey the idea and avoid technical terms and jargon (10). Forms created for the collection of data that is new or difficult to collect should be tested and evaluated before the start of the study. Pretesting ensures clarity of meaning and ease of use. Pretesting the completion of the CRFs can help identify confusion in the design or instructions, and allow time for troubleshooting the form prior to subject enrollment. Labeling every page with the date, study name, and ID number of the participant safeguards the integrity of the data should the pages become separated.

## Footers

The footer is where the form identification should be inserted. Form identification may use an abbreviation or number. The footer should also include the form version number, the date the form version was activated, and the page number of the form. Form version identification is important to data collection because forms may undergo many revisions during the course of the study. If a form changes during the course of the study, it is critical to insert the new version number and date. If this update does not occur, the incorrect form version may be used causing complications with data entry.

One general rule for identifying form version is to use a number, a decimal point, followed by another number. The number to the left of the decimal point should be changed if the revision affects data entry. The number to the right of the decimal point should be changed if the revision only affects text that has been edited, such as correcting a typo, or adding new directions to the form. When the data entry has not been affected, only the number to the right of the decimal should be changed.

## ADVANTAGES OF ELECTRONIC CASE REPORT FORMS

An electronic case report form is an auditable electronic record designed to record data that has been collected on each trial participant (17). There are a number of advantages to using computer-assisted data entry over paper case report forms:

<u>**Instructions for GCRC admission, Day 1 and evaluations**</u>

**Neutrophil glucose utilization during acute lung injury using radiolabeled fluorodeoxyglucose and PET imaging**

Participant ID ☐☐☐☐☐☐☐  Date of Visit ☐☐☐ / ☐☐ / ☐☐
                                            m  m  m    d  d    y  y

Protocol ID ☐☐☐☐☐  Staff ID ☐☐☐

Study Day ☐☐☐  Form sequence # (if more than 1) ☐  Data Entry Code ☐☐☐

**Pre-admission**
☐ Confirm that participant has transportation home.
☐ Instruct participant to arrive at 2:00 PM on day 1.
☐ Completed, signed orders.
☐ A copy of the signed informed consent.
☐ Admit data sheet.
☐ Procedure Evaluation sheet.
☐ Copy for participant's record.

**Day 1**
Complete Baseline evaluations:

☐ MD discuss consent with participant.
☐ Medical & Social History.
☐ Targeted Physical Exam (Ht, Wt, VS, Cardiovascular, and Pulmonary exam).
☐ Labs (CBC, BMP, PT, PTT).
☐ Urine hCG (Females of child bearing potential only)   Date: _____ / _____ / _____
    ☐ Positive
    ☐ Negative
    ☐ N/A
☐ Spirometry
    ☐ Escort participant to 8th floor CAM bldg.
    ☐ Get copy of report
☐ Chest x-ray
☐ ECG
☐ 1st dose of oral antibiotic. **ALLERGY:**_____

    ☐ SMZ/TMP (80/400)
      or
    ☐ Amoxicillin (500)

    Time given: _____

☐ NPO after midnight

Version 1.2 (9-15-04)                                          page 1 of 1

**FIGURE 11–4** ● Example of data to be collected from a patient admitted to a general clinical research center (GCRC) from a case report form.

1. **Error reduction.** The necessity to recode and reenter case report forms is all but eliminated. Errors are reduced as a result. Errors that do exist are more easily detected and corrected.
2. **Open-ended reporting.** If during the course of the study, the "other" category on a pull-down menu reveals that "shortness of breath" is being written frequently, then "shortness of breath" can later be added to the options on the pull-down menu.
3. **Quality control.** Even the best-designed forms can contain confusing information that can have unexpected consequences. Problems can be detected as the data are entered, and corrected by the system at that time.
4. **Ease of access.** The data entry software needs to be user friendly allowing both the research team and reviewers access to clinical trial data. Using a database can be less cumbersome than searching through the bulk of clinical files involved in paper case report forms.
5. **Data retention.** Data are not lost due to human error.
6. **Data verification.** When the data field is entered, there can be checks that do not allow out of range values or missing data. An example would be entering the pulmonary function testing results for "Peak Flow Rate." Peak flow normally ranges from 50 to 800. Database logic checks can help identify entries that do not appear logical for the data field. For example, if the number entered for "Peak Flow Rate" is lower than 50 or higher than 800 the data system will not accept the value and the data entry person will have to reevaluate the data.

## CASE REPORT FORM COMPLETION

The general rule for completion of paper case report forms is to use black or blue ink only. This makes photocopying of the data easier. *Never* use pencil or white-out, because a clear trail of all corrections is required. Abbreviations should be used sparingly. Similar abbreviations may have different meanings in various fields of health care. For example, BA could mean barium, blood alcohol, bone age, bronchial artery, or bronchial asthma. Whether the form is completed by a research volunteer or study coordinator, after completion of the form, it should be reviewed by the study coordinator for accuracy and clarity for later data entry.

All data collected on case report forms must be substantiated by a source document, where the original information is found.

Whoever completes the CRF should fill in their identifying information (initials or code number) in the header of the CRF. The correct way to change entries on CRFs is to draw a line through the incorrect response, then write the correct response next to or above the original entry. The correction is then initialed and dated by the person who made the correction. The person who made the correction may write a brief explanation in the margin of the form as to why the entry was changed. This same procedure should be used to track changes as a result of data queries.

If at later review it becomes evident that there are missing data in some of the CRF fields, review of the source documents may provide the information needed to complete the form. If the data were not collected, the entry should be completed with a code that indicates missing or unavailable data (i.e., "not done" can be coded as "ND"). It may be helpful during later analysis if the coordinator writes an explanation in the margin of the form as to why the information was missing, for example: "Participant does not know the answer," "participant refused to answer," or "not applicable to this participant." It is important when CRFs are being designed that many possible scenarios are taken into consideration in order to reduce the possibility of missing data (18).

## RESEARCHERS COMMENT ON CASE REPORT FORM DESIGN

In 1992, when the forms committee of the AIDs Clinical Trials Group (NIH), asked coordinators for comments regarding case report form design, hundreds of responses were received from across the country. Many of the responses were emotional, indicating a great degree of frustration on the part of the research coordinators.

The feedback from study coordinators included several common requests:

- If there is a list of choices for a question, the choices need to be mutually exclusive.
- Use the same term to describe the same data item from form to form.
- A list of forms for the study should be available.
- A forms manual that has been tested and piloted with the forms would be helpful.
- Use "generic" (i.e., standardized) forms where possible.
- Flow sheets for ongoing data, such as signs and symptoms, diagnoses, and concurrent medications would decrease the need to repeat the data entry at each study visit.

- Time is valuable. Only ask for the collection of information that will be analyzed.

## SUMMARY

- Design forms to answer the research hypothesis and expedite data analysis. Be frugal when choosing the data to collect in CRFs. Excessive data collection stretches resources and decreases the overall quality of the data collected. Identifying the study variables to be analyzed (predictor, outcome, and confounding) should help determine what CRFs will be needed. CRFs are designed to capture baseline and follow-up data. Coding needs to be consistent to reduce errors during completion of the forms.
- Regulatory compliance issues should be incorporated into CRF design. CRFs should contain date and participant identification number. Forms should be designed to capture eligibility, demographic information, baseline and follow-up status, adverse experiences, and compliance with the study intervention and protocol requirements.
- A large part of research monitoring oversight focuses on the data collected in CRFs to assure compliance with the protocol, the safety of the research participants, and proper adverse experience reporting. All data entered on CRFs must be supported by source documents. CRFs must be stored securely to preserve study data for later inspection. Sponsor regulations determine the time frame for required data storage.
- It is important understand the anatomy of a case report form. Forms are the foundation for the data collected in the study. The basic requirements for case report forms are the headers (which contain critical identifying information), the body of the form (where the actual study data is collected), and the footer (that directs the coordinator to the form version number, page number, and the date the form was activated). Electronic case report forms have the advantage of identifying the mistakes entered in the data field at the time of data entry, as well as open-ended reporting, quality control, and ease of access.
- A list of all CRFs to be used in the study is necessary for the research team. Whether paper or electronic forms are used, there must be a clear trail of documentation identifying who completes or changes the data. Any change to the data captured on a CRF should not obscure the original information.

- Training personnel in the completion of case report forms and written instructions are critical to the quality of data collection. Quality checks are necessary to reduce the risk of error.

## REFERENCES

1. U.S. Food and Drug Administration, Center for Drug Evaluation and Research, Drug Information Branch. Rockville, MD ICH Good Clinical Practice: Consolidated Guideline (E6), Federal Register, May 9, 1997. http://www.fda.gov/cder/guidance/959fnl.pdf.
2. Monsen ER. Research: Successful Approaches, 2nd Ed. Chicago: American Dietetic Association, 2003:92–94.
3. ACTG Forms Committee. Standard Operating Procedure: ACTG Forms Development (DRAFT). NIH, NIAID, AACTG, June 6, 1991.
4. CDISC. Core Principles. Austin Texas: Clinical Data Interchange Standards Consortium, Inc., 2003. http://www.cdisc.org/about/index.html
5. CDISC. Glossary: Clinical Trials terminology. Austin Texas: Clinical Data Interchange Standards Consortium, Inc., 2001. http://www.cdisc.org/glossary/ CDISCGlossary TerminologyV2.pdf
6. U.S. Food and Drug Administration, Office of Regulatory Affairs Guidance for Industry: Computerized Systems Used in Clinical Trials, April 1999.
7. Portney L, Watkins M. Foundations of Clinical Research: Applications to Practice, 2nd Ed. Upper Saddle River, NJ: Prentice Hall, 2000.
8. U.S. Food and Drug Administration, Office of Regulatory Affairs. Guidance for Industry: Part 11, Electronic Records: Electronic Signatures—Scope and Application, February 2003.
9. Voorhees J. Notes from first meeting of the ACTG Forms Committee, NIH, NIAID, AACTG, November 1991.
10. Hulley SB, Cummings SR, Browner WS et al. Designing Clinical Research: An Epidemiologic Approach, 2nd Ed. Philadelphia: Lippincott Williams & Wilkins, 2001.
11. CDISC: Mission Statement Clinical Data Interchange Standards Consortium, Inc., Austin Texas, 2003. http://www.cdisc.org/about/index.html
12. Christiansen D, Kubick W. CDISC Submission Metadata Model, Version 2.0 – 26, November 2001, © CDISC 2001.
13. Memo to ACTG Forms Committee, NIH, NIAID, AACTG. August 1992.
14. 45 CFR Part 46.
15. National Institutes of Health. Amendment: NIH policy and guidelines on the inclusion of women and minorities as subjects in clinical research—October 2001. http://grants.nih.gov/grants/guide/notice-files/NOT-OD-02-001.html. Accessed March 13, 2005.
16. The International Conference on Harmonisation: Good Clinical Practice Section 4.9.
17. Good P. A Manager's Guide to the Design and Conduct of Clinical Trials. Hoboken, NJ: John Wiley and Sons, 2002.
18. Batavia M. Clinical Research for Health Professionals: A User Friendly Guide. Boston: Butterworth-Heinemann, 2001.

# CHAPTER 12

# Data Collection and Quality Control

Janet T. Holbrook, David M. Shade, Robert A. Wise

Collecting accurate and reliable data, free of bias is crucial for the internal validity of a research study. Quality assurance considerations are crucial in every phase of a study (design, conduct, analysis) to ensure internal validity. Investigators need to be pragmatic about the volume and complexity of the research effort: study documentation needs to be detailed and clear; data collectors and analysts, trained and conscientious; information systems, reliable and accessible; and time and resources have to be set aside for quality assurance activities. This chapter focuses on design considerations, data collection procedures, personnel training, and analysis procedures that promote collection of accurate and reliable data. In general, the most important data to collect to ensure quality control for a clinical study is information related to eligibility, assignment of the experimental intervention (when present), protocol adherence, and outcome.

In large measure, quality assurance principles and procedures have been developed in the context of multicenter randomized clinical trials because of the need to control variability among centers (1). Many of the principles and procedures used to assure quality of data collection developed for multicenter trials can be adapted for a single-center translational and experimental research. Indeed, as the scrutiny of clinical research continues to increase, all studies, regardless of size, should include design features and monitoring procedures to ensure that research objectives are being met.

## DOCUMENTATION

### Protocol

For many investigator-initiated translational research studies, formal study protocols are not required by the IRBs or potential sponsors like the NIH. Rather, these regulatory bodies require that information be provided in response to specific questions. Yet, ensuring that relevant, reliable data are collected starts with a complete and carefully written protocol. The protocol should be specific and detailed about the essential components of a study; at a minimum, this protocol should include eligibility requirements, assignment of the experimental intervention, details about how the intervention is to be administered, and outcome assessments (2). Vague language in the protocol can lead to variable implementation and, at its worst, to significant errors in implementation. The CONSORT guidelines, designed for reporting the results of therapeutic clinical trials, are nevertheless a useful tool for the design of any human research project (3).

Eligibility criteria should precisely define the population of patients to be included in the study (Chapter 4). Criteria should be as unambiguous and as detailed as possible. Procedures should be ordered in such a way as to minimize the number of evaluations a patient must undergo before eligibility can be determined.

In studies that involve evaluation of an experimental intervention, the protocol should include a plan for unbiased assignment of that intervention (e.g., randomization) (4–7). A clear plan for treatment implementation should be specified with contingencies for likely events that may require changes to the study treatment, for example, drug toxicity or disease flare.

Objectives should be precisely articulated in hypothesis statements with defined metrics for evaluation; that is, outcome measures that can be evaluated in all patients. Ideally, outcome measures should have been shown to be valid and reliable before the study. The validity of outcomes that rely on evaluation of questionnaire data, new measurement techniques, or indices that are composites of multiple measurements should have been established by independent studies performed, ideally, in a population similar to the one under study. Even seemingly unambiguous clinical outcomes, for example, myocardial infarction, require specific criteria to be used as a study outcome (5).

If the primary outcome for the study relies on grading of tissue slides, radiographs, fundus photographs, echocardiograms, or other type of specimens or tests, there should be ongoing evaluation of the performance of those procedures and the grading results to monitor for agreement among graders and measurement drift over time. These evaluations may involve independent readers evaluating the same outcome on a standard set or from materials collected during the study. Kappa statistics or correlation coefficients may used to evaluate agreement (6).

For some outcomes that are known to have high variability, for example, blood pressure or lung function, it may be advisable to perform replicate measurements (6). The protocol and the manual of operations and procedures (MOP) should specify how replicate measures will be obtained and handled. For example, studies that use blood pressure as an outcome frequently specify the outcome as the average of multiple measurements and protocols for measurement of pulmonary function often require that measurements be replicated and reproducible (7).

The protocol should be planned in such a manner that the majority of enrolled patients can complete the study without major deviations from the protocol. Study evaluations should be performed according to a common follow-up schedule for all study groups to protect against ascertainment bias. Avoid turning events that result in unanticipated encounters with research staff into additional "interim study visits." Obviously, data need to be collected at these times about adverse events or key study outcomes, but such events should not be viewed as an opportunity to collect unrelated study data because it will be unlikely that the comparison group will have data collected at similar times. In addition, this type of practice may lead to ascertainment bias if the frequency of interim visits is different for each study group ("the more you look, the more you see").

A related issue is the follow-up observation of research participants, especially if a study involves a randomized experimental intervention. The number and type of follow-up visits should be the same for all study groups (8,9). The interpretation of some outcome results can be difficult if this principle is violated. For instance, if follow-up ends once the administration of an experimental intervention is terminated, an "intention-to-treat" analysis of data becomes problematic if the duration of follow-up differs for those for whom the intervention was prematurely stopped (10). The follow-up plan should be that all research participants be observed to the same planned outcome or time span.

Plans for study closeout, final data collection, and communications with participants should be outlined in the protocol.

## Manual of Operations and Procedures

The protocol is the key document describing the overall design and objectives, the case report forms (CRFs) and the manual of operations and procedures (MOP) are the key documents for procedural implementation of the study. Detailed information about how to design and use CRFs is given in Chapter 11.

Any study that involves more than a few individuals or that is going to be conducted over more than a few weeks should have an MOP. The MOP may range from a handout describing eligibility criteria, data collection schedule, and procedures for the study to a document that is of publishable quality. A well-developed MOP serves as the coordinator's guide to the protocol, a training tool, and also a historical record for the study. The MOP has the advantage of being easier to change than the protocol. An error or clarification can usually be added to an MOP without having to submit it to IRB for review and approval prior to implementation. Because the persons preparing the MOP necessarily focus on operational issues for the protocol, they often identify vagueness and inconsistencies in the protocol in the process of developing the MOP.

Among the items to be included in an MOP (Table 12–1) are a design summary with a data collection schedule and visit schedule overview; visit descriptions summarizing the timing, procedures, and forms completed at each visit (or visit type); instructions for administration of the experimental intervention including interruption and stopping criteria; instructions for completing evaluations (e.g., visual acuity assessment, expired breath condensate collection); instruction on study procedures (e.g., registrations, consent, randomization, data entry and editing, ordering supplies); and coding schemes.

MOPs should be concise; bulleted or numbered lists, flowcharts, and tables can make information more accessible (Tables 12–2 to 12–4). Bulleted lists and charts enable readers to scan the pages for quick reference and to easily incorporate checklists for step-by-step instructions. A standard set of

## TABLE 12–1

### Essential Items in Any Manual of Operations and Procedures (MOP)

- Participant eligibility criteria
- Data collection schedule
- Visit schedule
- Visit descriptions
- Experimental intervention
  - Instructions for administration
  - Instructions for interruption
  - Instructions for stopping
- Instructions for completing evaluations
- Instructions for each study procedure
- Coding schemes

formats should be used to develop MOP sections so that each section is organized in a similar manner. Navigation aids are important, so a detailed table of contents is desirable (Table 12–2). An index is ideal (although many software programs don't offer this feature easily or sometimes at all). A glossary is useful for applying standard definitions to the inevitable list of acronyms and jargon that are used as shorthand for communication. Creating an MOP as a series of individual documents that are merged together at the end allows multiple people to participate in developing it and makes it easier to update individual sections if the need arises.

### Document Revisions

In almost every study, investigators can anticipate that after the start of the study changes will occur to the protocol, the consent document, the CRFs, or to various procedures. Keeping all key study documents updated and making sure the most current versions are accessible is a challenge. Beware of "backing down" during the revisions process. Backing down happens when newer revisions are incorporated into an older version of the document. It is an easy and relatively common mistake to make. Document-naming and storage schemes, including back-up procedures, are essential and will help prevent backing down or other document disasters. Many schemes will work, but success usually depends on identifying someone to take responsibility for coordinating revision of documents, having procedures that are discussed and known by all personnel, and easy identification of the document version on electronic and paper copies.

Both electronic and paper archives of study documentation should be maintained. The archive should include all official versions of study documentation as opposed to every draft ever circulated. Electronic archives need to be updated regularly and backed up. Paper copies should be organized according to a filing system. The paper copies may be more robust in the long run because it is difficult to guarantee that new software will always be able to read older files.

A system should be in place at the start of a study to record implementation of document changes. One effective method has been to establish numbered memoranda that serve to communicate the information and to provide an indexed study record of the information. Numbered memos should have distribution lists that include all study personnel directly or indirectly affected by the change and be readily accessible to study personnel; accessibility can be achieved by keeping these in notebooks, as appendices to the MOP, or on a study website. A list of the title and date of numbered memoranda is a useful tool for training new personnel and can also be used as a historical record for the study (Table 12–5).

### TRAINING AND CERTIFICATION

Training for study personnel is an opportunity to educate study personnel on the overall goals and significance of the protocol as well providing training on specific study procedures. Data collectors may need two or three types of training: for specific evaluation procedures (e.g., visual acuity assessments or spirometry), for recording data on study forms, and for data processing. As mentioned earlier, a detailed MOP with tables and lists outlining data collection schedules and step-by-step instructions for specific procedures can serve as a training document. Such documentation can be supplemented with training examples and standard cases, including if necessary, didactic presentations and hands-on experience.

After training and demonstration of functional proficiency, personnel should be certified to perform specific functions. Ideally, functional proficiency can be demonstrated by evaluation of standard test cases in the actual study setting. Other ways to evaluate functional proficiency are to observe evaluations (e.g., visual acuity assessments), or to require submitting several evaluations from test case(s) that meet guidelines for acceptable results. For key positions, back-up personnel should also be trained and certified. Back-up personnel are important for filling in when primary staff are absent and for facilitating an orderly transition if primary staff leave. The certification process also serves as a way to document training and track data collectors. Personnel that stop

## TABLE 12–2

### Example of Table of Contents from a Manual of Operations and Procedures (MOP) for an Asthma Study

**Contents**

*(Continued)*

## TABLE 12–2 (Continued)

### Example of Table of Contents from a Manual of Operations and Procedures (MOP) for an Asthma Study

*(Continued)*

## TABLE 12–2 (Continued)

**Example of Table of Contents from a Manual of Operations and Procedures (MOP) for an Asthma Study**

## TABLE 12–3

**Example of Visit Time Windows and Data Collection Schedule for a Manual of Operations and Procedures (MOP) in an Asthma Study**

| Clinic Visit Schedule | V1* | V2* | V3* | V4* | V5* | V6* | V7* | V8* |
|---|---|---|---|---|---|---|---|---|
| Time Window (weeks)[5] | –6 to –4 | –3 to –1 | 0 | 1 – 3 | 3 – 6 | 6 – 10 | 10 – 14 | 14 – 24 |
| Target (weeks) | –4 | –2 | 0 | 2 | 4 | 8 | 12 | 16 |
| **Procedures/Data form abbreviation** | | | | | | | | |
| Baseline Asthma and Medical History (BA) | BA | . | . | . | . | . | . | . |
| Clinic Visit (CV) | . | . | $CV^6$ | CV | $CV^6$ | CV | CV | $CV^6$ |
| Diary Cards (DC) | | | | | | | | |
|  Distribution | DC | . | $DC^1$ | $DC^1$ | $DC^1$ | $DC^1$ | $DC^1$ | |
|  Collection | . | . | DC | DC | DC | DC | DC | DC |
| Drug Dispensing and Counting (DD) | DD | . | DD | $DD^1$ | DD | DD | DD | DD |
| Enrollment (EN) | EN | | | | | | | |
| Exit Interview (EI) | . | . | . | . | . | . | . | EI |
| Missed Data[1] (MD) | | | | | | | | |
| Methacholine Challenge (MC) | $MC^2$ | . | $MC^3$ | . | $MC^3$ | . | . | $MC^3$ |
| Participant Information (PI) | PI | . | . | . | . | . | . | . |
| Phone Contact (PC) | . | PC | . | . | . | . | . | . |
| Physical Exam (PE) | PE | . | . | . | . | . | . | . |
| Pulmonary Function Testing (PF) | PF7 | . | PF | PF | PF | PF | PF | PF |
| Randomization (RZ) | . | . | RZ | . | . | . | . | . |
| Serious Adverse Event Report (SR) | | | | | | | | |
| Treatment Failure Worksheet (TFW)[1] | | | | | | | | |
| Treatment Termination (TT)[1] | | | | | | | | |
| Unmasking (UM)[4] | . | . | . | . | . | . | . | UM |
| Unusual Event1 (UE)[1] | | | | | | | | |

*(Continued)*

## TABLE 12–3 (Continued)

**Example of Visit Time Windows and Data Collection Schedule for a Manual of Operations and Procedures (MOP) in an Asthma Study**

| | | | | | | | | |
|---|---|---|---|---|---|---|---|---|
| **Questionnaires** | | | | | | | | |
| Asthma Control Questionnaire (AC) | AC | . | AC | AC | AC | AC | AC | AC |
| Asthma Symptoms Utility Index (AS) | . | . | AS | AS | AS | AS | AS | AS |
| Asthma Therapy Assessment Questionnaire (AT) | . | . | AT | AT | AT | AT | AT | AT |
| Mini Asthma Quality of Life Questionnaire (QL) | . | . | QL | . | QL | . | . | QL |
| Pediatric Asthma Quality of Life Questionnaire (QP) | . | . | QP | . | QP | . | . | QP |
| **Specimens** | | | | | | | | |
| Exhaled Breath Condensate (BA, CV) | BA$^{10}$ | . | CV | . | CV | . | . | CV |
| Serum for ECP (CV) | . | . | CV | . | CV | . | . | CV |
| Whole blood for eosinophil count (CV) | . | . | CV | . | CV | . | . | CV |
| Whole blood for PCG (CV)$^9$ | . | . | CV$^9$ | . | . | . | . | . |
| **Logs/Administrative Forms** | | | | | | | | |
| Drug Accountability Log (DA) | DA | . | DA | DA$^1$ | DA | DA | DA | DA |
| Drug/Peak Flow Meter Order Form (DO)$^1$ | | | | | | | | |
| Methacholine Order Form (MO)$^1$ | | | | | | | | |
| Specimen Transmittal Sheet (ST)$^1$ | | | | | | | | |

* V1= enrollment, V2 = telephone, V3 = randomization, V4–8 = follow-up visits
[1] as needed
[2] Methacholine challenge is conducted on participants who cannot demonstrate 12% $\beta$-agonist reversibility
[3] Substudy participants only. V3 challenge test performed 1–3 days prior to Visit 3.
[4] At end of trial, unless required due to adverse event
[5] NOTE: Visits must be spaced at least one week apart
[6] Expired breath condensate and blood specimens procedures at V3, V5, and V8 only
[7] Post-bronchodilator test needed if $\beta$-agonist reversibility test conducted
[8] Optional. To be completed prior to Visit 1
[9] Procedure is pending at this time. If blood for PCG is not collected at V3, then collect at V5 or V8
[10] Pending IRB approval

working on a particular study should be decertified, so that they are no longer able to collect or access study data.

Periodic retraining and, possibly, recertification should be considered for key study procedures (11). Training and certification of staff is likely to be an ongoing need because of staff turnover; procedures should be in place to meet the ongoing need.

Investing in standard equipment reduces data variability (Chapter 3). If nonstandard equipment is to be used, procedure standardization can usually help control measurement variability. However, even that can be difficult when personnel not associated with the study (e.g., laboratory personnel affiliated with a hospital) perform procedures.

Laboratory tests should rely on standard specimens to establish calibration. Investigators should recognize these limitations when defining key variable for the study.

## PROCEDURES

### Visit Preparation

Study visits should be organized to flow as smoothly and efficiently for study participants as possible. To ensure a high rate of compliance with follow-up, clinic schedules should not be overbooked. CRFs and other materials required to complete the visit should be organized beforehand.

## TABLE 12 – 4

**Example of Task List for a Specific Study Visit from a Manual of Operations and Procedures (MOP) for an Asthma Study**

**Visit 4 (V4—follow-up)**
**Time Frame**

1. Target—2 weeks after Visit 3 (randomization)
2. Window—1 to 3 weeks after Visit 3

**Tasks**

1. Review returned Diary Cards. Distribute additional Diary Cards and return envelopes as needed
    a. Complete an interim medical history report
    b. Conduct spirometry procedure (pre-bronchodilator only)
    c. Participant completes questionnaires AC, AS, and AT
    d. Dispense one study kit, ONLY if needed
2. Confirm time for next scheduled visit
3. Key forms into data system within 5 working days, as applicable

**Forms (abbreviation)**

1. Clinic Visit Form (CV)
2. Diary Card (DC)
3. Drug Dispensing and Counting (DD), ONLY if additional drug needed to be dispensed†
4. Pulmonary Function Testing (PF)

**Questionnaires (abbreviation)**

1. Adult Asthma Therapy Assessment Questionnaire (AT)
2. Asthma Control Questionnaire (AC)
3. Asthma Symptom Utility Index (AS)

**Log (abbreviation)**

1. Drug Accountability Log (DA),* if applicable

**Clinic Worksheet**

1. Treatment Failure Worksheet (TFW)*

* Not entered into database
† Study drug should not need to be distributed at this visit. Drug distributed at V3 should last until V5

### TABLE 12–5

**Example of a Listing of Numbered Memoranda Relating to Study Developments**

| Memorandum # | Subject | Date |
|:---:|:---|:---:|
| 1 | Establishment of PPMs | 24-Apr-2004 |
| 2 | Protocol version 1.0 | 14-Nov-2002 |
| 3 | Questionnaires and scripts | 02-Apr-2003 |
| 4 | Consent forms: required elements | 30-Jul-2003 |
| 5 | Release statement concerning asthma care provider | 09-Oct-2003 |
| 6 | Revisions to consent form | 15-Dec-2003 |
| 7 | Certification requirements | 26-Feb-2004 |
| 8 | Pregnancy test procedures | 12-Mar-2004 |
| 9 | Changes to drug distribution procedures | 24-Apr-2004 |
| 10 | Adherence substudy | 24-Apr-2004 |
| 11 | Form revisions: RZ, SR, UE, KA, CC | 24-Apr-2004 |
| 12 | Additional of new questionnaires (KR, KO, EE) | 15-Jun-2004 |
| 13 | Revised protocol, version 2.0 | 15-Jun-2004 |

## Randomization

Randomization is a key feature to ensure the quality of a clinical experiment using multiple intervention groups (or a control group) and should be used whenever possible for all such experiments, regardless of their size. Uncontrolled studies often yield inadequate evidence to support the experimental hypothesis (12). Historical controls are rarely adequate as comparison groups and nonrandom assignment schemes of an experimental intervention are vulnerable to bias (13).

Random assignment protects against selection bias and ensures, but does not guarantee, that there is balance across the study groups with regard to known and unknown confounders (2,8). The hallmarks of a good randomization scheme are an unpredictable list of assignments for the experimental intervention; concealment of assignment until issued; strict adherence to the schedule; documentation of the method for generating and administering assignments; and a clear audit trail for issued assignments.

Procedures for generating treatment assignment should be secure, documented, and reproducible. Small studies can generate treatment assignment schedules that meet these criteria with random number tables. Statistical software makes generation of randomization tables relatively easy for standard designs (parallel, crossover, or factorial designs) and some even generate documentation. More complex designs may require customized programming. In any study that will require enrollment over several months or longer, permuted blocks or minimization techniques should be used to ensure that there is balance in treatment assignments over time. Blocking must be used to effectively implement a stratified treatment assignment schedule (8). Choice of block sizes is a trade-off between maintaining balance across time in treatment assignments and preserving the unpredictability of future assignments. Use of variable block sizes is helpful in maintaining integrity of randomization process by making the assignment schedule less predictable. Electronic back-up and paper documentation of the method used to generate randomization tables are essential. Optimally, the person(s) responsible for generating and maintaining assignment schedules should be entirely independent of those responsible for evaluating eligibility and requesting treatment assignments—but this goal may not be practical in investigator-initiated translational studies of small size.

The randomization process itself can be conducted in a number of ways including sealed envelope systems, numbered or coded drug packaging, systems administered by third parties such as a pharmacist, or online randomization systems. Regardless, it is essential that the order of the assignments be concealed to avoid selection bias (4,14).

Assigning treatment by randomization is antithetical to many clinicians, so safeguards to ensure that the pending assignments are unpredictable are essential (13,15). Envelope systems have the advantage of simplicity but are the easiest to circumvent. At a minimum, the envelopes should be sequentially numbered, opaque, and sealed.

All baseline and eligibility data should be collected prior to randomization and the penultimate step in any randomization procedure should be to check that all these data are collected and that all eligibility criteria are met. Laboratory analyses that are not required to determine eligibility do not have to be performed before randomization, but all specimens should be collected. Checking data completeness and conformance to the protocol can be done by inspection or, preferably, by keying essential data and relying on programmed checks of the data.

Deviations from eligibility criteria should almost never be allowed. Eligibility criteria are agreed on by investigators and reviewed and approved by other groups such as safety monitoring boards. There is almost no reason to disregard them, especially because disregarding them can put the study's practitioners in a precarious position should an "ineligible" participant have a significant problem. If necessary, protocols can be changed and eligibility criteria modified to enhance recruitment—once the amendments have been reviewed and approved by the appropriate regulatory committees.

The assignment process itself should be documented with information on who made the assignment, participant identifiers, date the assignment was made, stratum information (if applicable), and sequence number of assignment. Ideally this information will be stored in an electronic database and a hard copy of the information will be printed out for the file at the time the assignment is made.

## Masking

Ideally research participants, research coordinators, evaluators, and data recorders are masked (synonymous with blinding) to study group assignment. Masking the actual identity of the assignment is distinct from ensuring that assignments are concealed prior to randomization, both types of masking are important. Masking of assignment once issued protects against biases related to treatment adherence or outcome ascertainment. Masking is more important for outcomes that involve evaluations and judgment than for objective outcomes such as mortality (4).

Sometimes, masking research volunteers and coordinators is too expensive, logistically impossible, or unethical. Some interventions are difficult to mask because of distinctive side effects (e.g., color of a diluent) and creating a matched control (e.g., a placebo) can be expensive, impractical, or impossible (16). Regardless of whether research volunteers or coordinators are masked, the evaluators should be masked to study group assignment. This may be accomplished by using central reading centers or laboratories, or having personnel independent of those administering the intervention evaluate outcomes.

The integrity of masking, at whatever level, should be evaluated. For example, were there obvious differences between the appearance of active and control interventions? Does the occurrence of adverse events lead to unmasking? Some technique for masking should be considered and used when possible for any study having multiple intervention groups.

## DATA SYSTEMS

Once the data have been recorded, typically on paper CRFs, they will generally be collected and organized in some form of a *data system*. Data systems can range from the very simple (a folder in a desk drawer) to the very complex (dispersed computers employing large-scale databases and sophisticated networking). The design of a particular data system will be based on the complexity of the study, weighing factors such as duration, geography, funding, frequency of interim analyses, and size. More information about creating such data systems can be found in Chapter 10. Here, we simply address several issues related to quality control.

It is possible to consider a data system that is nearly completely paper based. For example, a small observational study conducted at a single site with little numeric data might collect data on paper data forms and do nothing more. However, it is far more likely that even the simplest study will ultimately need to have data accessible in some electronic format.

No matter what approach is taken, a data system should be designed from the very beginning to accomplish its primary objectives. First among these objectives is, of course, to capture the relevant data, completely and accurately, in a form suitable for analysis. Toward this end, it is useful for design of the data system to be well coordinated with the design of the CRFs. Another goal of a well-designed data system is to improve the quality of the study data, both by detecting and preventing mistakes during the data entry process and by identifying problems with the data previously recorded on the forms. In fact, the earlier in the process that problems are detected, the more likely it is that they will be able to be corrected. Among the strategies that can help reduce data entry errors are double data entry, selected data redundancy, and form validation. In double data entry systems, each data form is keyed twice, sometimes by different operators or at different sittings. Discrepancies between the two sessions are flagged and the data are not accepted until the problems are resolved. Although this strategy may appear to be onerous, good data entry personnel learn to rely on the double data entry system to help detect simple keyboarding mistakes. Data systems can also employ data redundancy, where selected (usually important) data items are collected more than once (often on different forms), to detect inconsistencies. This requires advance planning during the CRF design process. Form validation can reduce both data entry errors and data recording problems.

Perhaps the most important quality control step in any study is to design good data forms, as discussed earlier. For example, providing spaces only for the expected number of digits can help prevent reporting of values in the wrong units (e.g., height measured in centimeters cannot be recorded on a form expecting inches and having only two digits). The data system can help enforce and supplement this strategy by validating data at three levels. First, field-level validation looks at each field entry and looks for errors, using accepted ranges for numeric data or data format for other types of data (e.g., dates following a study convention format). Some systems employ multiple levels of minimum/maximum, with inner thresholds for "warnings" and outer thresholds for more important "errors." Second, intraform validation inspects related data elements on a single form and identifies possible discrepancies. For example, a form recording both height and weight might trigger an error on a height of 72 inches and a weight of 50 pounds. Finally, interform validation inspects data elements across data forms, either different forms at the same visit or forms from multiple visits. For example, a participant's height that was entered as 6 inches different on visits 3 months apart could trigger an error, as could a heart rate reading on a physical exam form that conflicted with an electrocardiogram data form recorded at the same time. It is helpful to include a method to override some or all of the validation checks for those inevitable situations where what was originally thought to be invalid or impossible turns out to be correct (this often comes to light at very inopportune times, making it worthwhile to consider this possibility in advance).

Many of the errors that a good data system can help detect are items that can and should prevent the data from being accepted, or marked as pending,

until the problem is resolved. However, there will undoubtedly be a need to allow for the editing of data already entered, because of a problem detected during some later data cleaning stage, because of a discrepancy noted during an audit, or because someone becomes aware of an error during the recording or data entry steps. The data system should make it easy for data to be edited so as to encourage corrections whenever needed. The best approach for data edits is to store the edited data in addition to, and not in place of, the original data, providing an absolute audit trail for all changes to the data. One technique is to store each entered data form with a date/time stamp, using the most recently entered data for final analysis but retaining all the older versions of the data records should a question later arise. It is also recommended that each version of a data record have a field that identifies the person entering the data.

Audits, in which source documents (usually medical records or data forms) are compared with the electronic data records, are another important component of data quality control (see section later in this chapter). There are no hard and fast rules for how much auditing should be done; the answer depends on the nature of the study. In any event, audits should take place as early as possible during a study to identify and correct problems with the data system before too much data have been collected. A system of continuous auditing, perhaps at a lower intensity, may be more likely to identify systematic problems earlier than would more intense periodic audits.

Finally, the data system should be clearly documented. Changes to the data entry and data collection software should be tracked, and copies of all versions of the software used should be archived. Access to the data system should be limited with passwords (or some other form of security), and passwords should only be issued or activated for personnel needing access to the system. The databases themselves should be archived frequently. This requires careful planning for distributed data systems without network data transfer capabilities. Early in a study the databases should be subjected to a "dummy" analysis to confirm that the data formats are correct and that the planned analyses will in fact be possible on the collected data.

Many of the foregoing approaches may seem cumbersome or overkill for small studies, such as those conducted by a single investigator or a small team at a single institution. However, thought should be given to each of these suggestions even for the smallest of studies at the earliest possible stage. Investigators in small studies often design data collection forms on an ad hoc basis, making changes along the way as the study proceeds, with the expectation of getting them all entered into some electronic format when the study is completed (often using a spreadsheet or small database program, such as Excel or Access). It is only then that they realize that the various versions of the data forms will make it very difficult to combine into a single analysis dataset. The most important quality control principles apply uniformly to studies of any size and only the means by which they will be achieved differ between large scale multisite clinical trials and small bedside translational studies with a single-digit N. Moreover, even the smallest study involving human subjects is worthy of extra attention to quality control to ensure both the safety of the study participants and the protection of the information that their efforts have helped produce.

The electronic tools used to capture and manipulate data are varied and their choice depends greatly on personal preference and experience. Spreadsheet programs are a popular choice because they are widely available and easy to use. They also allow for at least some simple statistical analysis of entered data. However, implementation of good quality control practices can sometimes be more difficult using spreadsheets. Designing specialized data entry screens with field-level and intraform checks is not a common task using a spreadsheet and can take more skill than may be available. Maintaining audit trails and implementing double data entry can be even more difficult. Desktop database programs are more amenable to the design of data entry screens and the implementation of data checks, although perhaps fewer investigators have experience using them and thus additional expertise may need to be obtained. Large studies often employ professional statistics packages (such as SAS), enterprise database products (such as Oracle), or dedicated research data collection systems, usually in combination with custom in-house programming.

One common mistake made in smaller studies that should be avoided whenever possible is the temptation to simplify the electronic data either by failing to capture all of it or by segmenting it by patient. If information is worth capturing on the hard copy CRF, it is almost certainly worth the small additional effort to have it entered for electronic analysis. Likewise, even though it might be natural to think of collecting all the information for each patient in a separate file (or a separate sheet in a spreadsheet), this is almost always a bad idea. Calculating even the simplest group statistics will require a great deal of tedious and error-prone combining or copying of data. Instead, similar data for all subjects should be collected and stored together, allowing for much easier application of good quality control principles.

No matter which approach is taken, a good data system will employ a variety of field-level, form-level, and system-level checks to help identify data discrepancies. Furthermore, it will, when possible, have a complete audit trail of edits made to the data and provide documentation as to who entered or edited data and when it was done. A secondary function of more complex data system is to provide management tools that help clinical personnel track data collection and participant follow-up and provide study leaders with data on the overall quality and completeness of study data.

## REPORTS

Regular reports on study performance (e.g., recruitment, completed visits, missing data, data entry, protocol deviations) are important tools for identifying problems and tracking their resolution. Although many data systems are capable of producing performance statistics in real time, there are advantages to compiling periodic reports that focus attention on performance issues and trends. Most investigators and other stakeholders are interested in recruitment, which can be slower and more difficult than anticipated (see Chapter 5). However, timely collection, keying, and editing of data are also essential for a successful study. Reports summarizing study performance help focus attention on these issues. Report content and frequency are important considerations.

Detailed periodic (e.g., monthly) reports should summarize completed visits, missed visits and outstanding data for each participant enrolled in a study. Tables 12–6 to 12–8 provide examples of data status reports. The tables summarize participant-visit data (Table 12–8), status of forms keyed for specific visits including which items were marked as missed or pending (Table 12–7), and a list of missing specimens for individual patients (Table 12–6). These tables can be scanned by personnel to identify missing and pending data items. For small studies, these reports may be generated from a spreadsheet that tracks the data collection on each patient or even actual data listings for each patient. For studies of long duration with many patients, it may be more effective to limit the detailed listings of completed and missing data to the most recent interval because a cumulative listing becomes voluminous and hence more difficult to use as a tool for identifying missing data that are still retrievable.

Other reports that have proven to be effective tools for managing clinical research studies include listings of participant visits that should occur in the next month, lists of protocol deviations, reports of

## TABLE 12-6

### Example of a Data Status Report of Missing or Expected but Not Received Blood Collection Specimens

| ID | Visit | Visit Date | Specimen not received at bank |
|----|-------|------------|-------------------------------|
| xxxx | F03 F04 | 07FEB03 18MAY03 | plasma cells |
| xxxx xxxx | F05 F06 | 18AUG03 17NOV03 | plasma, cells |
| xxxx | F02 | 11MAY03 | cells |
| xxxx | F04 | 09NOV03 | cells |
| xxxx xxxx | F02 | 15NOV03 08MAR04 * | plasma cells |
| N = 8 | | | |

ID = patient identifier
*Form set not received; date is target date, not actual visit date
"F" refers to visit number

data queries, drug distribution and inventory, specimen repository transactions, or IRB status. Automated generation of these reports involves considerable, ongoing investments of programming time and may not be feasible for smaller, shorter term studies.

Global performance reports are typically generated less frequently (if at all), perhaps quarterly or semiannually, and can include summary statistics on recruitment, completed visits, missed visits, missing key data, time to keying forms and other measures. For studies that continue over an extended period, it is advisable to look at overall performance as well as performance in the last period, for example, 3 to 6 months, to evaluate whether systems are improving, remaining constant, or deteriorating. In multicenter studies, performance should be examined by center.

## DATA AUDITS

Although data audits are a regular feature of industry-sponsored clinical trials, they are also becoming increasingly common for investigator-initiated research sponsored by the NIH or national foundations. Investigators should be prepared to have their clinical research records audited.

## TABLE 12-7

### Example of a Data Status Report Showing Incomplete Forms

| ID | Visit | Visit date | Pending Forms | Form set status | Missed forms/procedures* |
|----|-------|------------|---------------|-----------------|--------------------------|
| xxxx | V7 | 18APR04 | incomplete | CV PF AC AS AT QL | |
| xxxx | V8 | 22OCT04 | missed visit | | QL |
| xxxx | V8 | 25OCT04 | incomplete | | PF |
| xxxx | V4 | 06JUN04 | missed visit | QL | |
| xxxx | V3 | 15FEB04 | incomplete | MC | |
| xxxx | V5 | 13JUN04 | incomplete | MC PF | |
| xxxx | V6 | 26JUL04 | incomplete | | AL |
| xxxx | V7 | 08AUG04 | incomplete | AS QL | |

ID = patient identifier
"F" indicates a visit number; each two letter designation in the pending forms column indicates a different form (see Table 12–3)

## TABLE 12-8

### Example of a Data Status Report of Visit Status

| ID | Enr date | BL | F01 | F02 | F03 | F04 | F05 | F06 | F07 | F08 | F09 |
|----|----------|----|-----|-----|-----|-----|-----|-----|-----|-----|-----|
| xxxx | 10/26/01 | | * | * | * | * | * | * | * | * | F09 |
| xxxx | 01/07/02 | | * | * | * | * | * | * | * | * | F09 |
| xxxx | 01/25/02 | | * | * | * | * | * | * | * | * | F09 |
| xxxx | 02/01/02 | | * | * | * | * | * | * | * | * | F09 |
| xxxx | 03/05/02 | | * | * | * | * | * | * | * | F08 | F09 |
| xxxx | 04/02/02 | | * | * | * | * | * | * | * | F08 | |
| xxxx | 04/09/02 | | * | * | * | * | * | * | * | F08 | |
| xxxx | 05/07/02 | | * | * | * | * | * | * | F06 | F07 | |
| xxxx | 07/18/02 | | * | * | * | * | * | * | F06 | | |
| xxxx | 09/24/02 | | * | * | * | F03 | * | F05 | | | |
| xxxx | 10/07/02 | | * | * | * | * | F04 | F05 | | | |
| xxxx | 10/07/02 | | * | * | | | | | | | |
| xxxx | 10/31/02 | | * | * | * | * | * | F05 | * | | |
| xxxx | 03/31/03 | | * | * | * | F03 | | | | | |
| xxxx | 03/31/03 | | * | * | * | F03 | | | | | |
| xxxx | 02/09/04 | BL | | | | | | | | | |
| xxxx | 03/08/04 | BL | | | | | | | | | |
| xxxx | 03/29/04 | BL | | | | | | | | | |
| xxxx | 04/09/04 | BL | | | | | | | | | |
| xxxx | 05/04/04 | | | | | | | | | | |
| N = 21 | | | | | | | | | | | |

*Indicates that data have been entered
ID = patient identifier
"BL" and "F" indicate a visit for which data are expected but not yet received
"BL" is "baseline form"
Enr = enrollment date

Documents that may be inspected include IRB records, pharmacy records, and medical records. IRB files should be up to date and include copies of all correspondence regarding initial review and approval, revisions, safety reports, and other required communications. Pharmacy records should be complete, match current inventory, and should be consistent with patient-level data on drug distribution. Study data records on individual patients can be compared to patients' medical records, that is, data audit.

Data audits are useful tools for verifying the integrity of the data collection process, but such audits are rarely a complete check of data accuracy because many data items collected for study purposes are not routinely documented in a patient's medical record and it is expensive and labor intensive to do a complete audit on all patients. The purpose of the audit is to check for systematic problems in data collection, although specific errors may be found in the process that can be corrected. The completeness of the audits will depend on the number of research participants enrolled and the quantity of data collected. The audit should focus on data related to eligibility, assignment and administration of the experimental intervention, and outcome assessment. Some errors and inconsistencies should be expected; however, patterns of mistakes and sloppiness should be followed up with efforts to detect the source of the problem and implement corrective procedures. Ideally, audits should include a complete review of participant consent statements to ensure that all participants have appropriately signed and dated forms. Data edits should be inspected to check that queries are being resolved both in the study documentation and study database. Copies of all documentation should be filed as part of the study record.

## ANALYSIS

### Creating an Analytic Database

In any study with an experimental intervention that may cause harm, it will usually be necessary to look at least at some portion of the data collected during the study, for treatment effects monitoring (see Chapter 13), for performance monitoring, or other special purposes. Each analysis that is included in a study report (e.g., data monitoring report, progress report to sponsor) should be associated with an archived database. Archived databases enable verification of results at a later date and the ability to respond to questions or provide additional analyses based on the same data as the original analysis. These databases should include the complete set of available interim data from the study and the analytic datasets created from those interim data.

The first step in the construction of the analytic datasets is to copy primary datasets in which data are keyed to another storage device so they can be manipulated. Depending on how the data system is organized and the software used, there may be several conversion and merging steps to create a common database. A critical step is mapping any revisions of a particular data form to a common database for that data form. For large studies, one programmer should be responsible for creating the common databases with independent review of the procedures by another programmer. The common database should then be stored and archived. Analysts should make copies of the common database to use to construct analytic datasets. Programs used to create the analytic datasets and those datasets should also be archived. Key analysis results for reports or publications should be independently replicated by two analysts using the same common database but completely independent of each other, that is, individual analytic databases and programs.

### Role of Interim Analyses

Data monitoring serves many functions (see Chapter 13). A function not commonly mentioned, but which is essential, is that it gives investigators practice analyzing and interpreting their data. One of the most useful and important quality control practices, no matter what the size or scope of the experiment, is to perform one or more dummy or interim analyses of the most important questions addressed by the study, as early in the study as practicable, to ensure that the data are correct, valid, and in a form suitable for the primary analysis. An early run through the data can help detect unforeseen problems in data collection or analyses and may lead to new edit checks, alteration in training procedures, or forms revision. Such analyses do not need to be by study group assignment to be useful (thus, they do not have to violate masking or rules regarding the number of allowable looks at the data). However, a complete analysis by treatment assignment is the best way to ensure that there are no mistakes in the data coding, analysis, or interpretation of the data.

## SUMMARY

- Quality assurance should be a part of every phase of a clinical study, including study design and the development of study documents, monitoring of the protocol adherence and data collection efforts, checks of key data analyses, and the interpretation of results.
- Design features and procedures developed for quality assurance in multicenter trials may seem burdensome in the single center setting but design features such as precise definitions of outcomes, randomization, or masking are directly applicable to single center studies.
- The following checklist identifies key components that should be part of every quality assurance effort:
  - Clearly specify primary components of the study
    - Hypothesis to be tested
    - Eligibility criteria
    - Treatment protocol
    - Evaluation protocol
  - Adhere to clinical study design principles
    - Unbiased treatment assignment, typically randomized
    - Concealment of treatment assignment
    - Masking for evaluators for outcome assessment
    - Unbiased follow-up schedule
  - User friendly documentation
    - Train personnel on specifics of protocol and data collection procedures
    - Coordination of data system with CRF
    - Use data system to validate data at entry
    - Start data audits early
    - Archive and document analyses
- Monitoring of procedures and data can be accomplished by having staff members not directly involved in the conduct of the study act as monitors for key functions or by assigning staff specific responsibilities for performing certain

tasks and monitoring other tasks. Even small, single-center clinical studies require enormous efforts on the part of the investigator to plan, obtain funding, get approvals for, and conduct. Hence, implementing strategies to ensure that the data collected are unbiased and accurate is well worth the additional effort.

## REFERENCES

1. Blumenstein BA, James KE, Lind BK et al. Functions and organization of coordinating centers for multicenter studies. Control Clin Trials 1995;16:4S–29S.
2. Meinert CL, Tonascia S. Clinical Trials: Design, Conduct and Analysis. New York: Oxford University Press, 1986 (chap. 11).
3. Altman DG, Schulz KF, Moher D et al. for the CONSORT Group. The revised CONSORT statement for reporting randomized trials: explanation and elaboration. Ann Intern Med 2001;134:663–694.
4. Juni P, Altman DG, Egger M. Systematic reviews in health care: assessing the quality of controlled clinical trials. BMJ 2001;323:42–46.
5. Col NF, Pauker SG. The discrepancy between observational studies and randomized trials of menopausal hormone therapy: did expectations shape experience? Ann Intern Med 2003;139:923–929.
6. Kelsey JL, Whittemore AS, Evans AS et al. Methods in Observational Epidemiology, 2nd Ed. New York: Oxford University Press, 1996:345–347.
7. American Thoracic Society. Standardization of spirometry, 1994 update. Am J Respir Crit Care Med 1995; 152:1107–1136.
8. Piantadosi S. Clinical Trials: A Methodologic Perspective. New York: John Wiley and Sons, 1997.
9. Lewis SC, Warlow CP. How to spot bias and other potential problems in randomized controlled trials. J Neurol Neurosurg Psychiatry 2004;75:181–187.
10. Hollis S, Campbell F. What is meant by intention to treat analysis? Survey of published randomized controlled trials. BMJ 1999;319:670–674.
11. Anderson MM Jr, Boly LD, Beck RW for the Optic Neuritis Study Group. Remote clinic/patient monitoring for multicenter trials. Control Clin Trials 1996;17: 407–414.
12. Chalmers TC. Randomize the first patients. N Engl J Med 1977;296:107 (letter).
13. Chalmers TC. The need for early randomization in the development of new drugs for AIDS. J Acquir Immune Defic Syndr. 1990; 3(suppl 2):S10–S15.
14. Altman DG, Schulz KF. Statistics notes: concealing treatment allocation in randomised trials. BMJ 2001; 323:446–447.
15. Schulz KF, Grimes DA. Allocation concealment in randomised trials: defending against deciphering. Lancet 2002;359:614–618.
16. Holbrook JT, Wise RA, Gerald LB for the American Lung Association Asthma Clinical Research Centers. Drug distribution for a large crossover trial of the safety of inactivated influenza vaccine in asthmatics. Control Clin Trials 2002;23:87–92.

# CHAPTER 13

# Monitoring Experimental Interventions

## Robert A. Wise, Janet T. Holbrook, Curtis L. Meinert

Treatment effects monitoring is the process of reviewing accumulated outcome data by study group to determine if the research study should continue unaltered. The body that conducts this procedure goes by various names (Table 13–1). We prefer the title treatment effects monitoring committee (TEMC) in that it more accurately describes the role of the committee. The most commonly used terms are data monitoring committee (DMC) or data and safety monitoring board (DSMB). In translational medicine, treatments are often administered for the purpose of elucidating a mechanism of disease or pathophysiology as well as the treatment of a disorder. Accordingly, we use the term *experimental treatment* to incorporate all aspects of participation by a human volunteer in an experiment.

The general process of treatment effects monitoring requires periodic harvesting and summary of accumulating data. This process serves not only to provide periodic review of the research data for the evaluation of safety and efficacy, but also requires the regular review and cleaning of the dataset permitting early detection of data anomalies and quality defects. These interim analyses serve, in effect, as "practice" for the final analysis that may take into account unanticipated anomalies in the data collection.

The primary purpose of treatment effects monitoring is prevention of harm to current or future participants in the research project. Such harm may involve treatments or other procedures involved in the research study. Protection from harm is provided by cessation of the research or alteration of the research procedures. Harm from treatment may involve active harm from the adverse effects of one of the research treatments or passive harm when it is clear that one of the treatments is inferior. In practice, prevention of such harm may involve cessation of the entire study, or one of the treatments, or termination of treatment in a subgroup of patients. Research procedures, that is, those that are not provided as a component of the standard of care, may cause injury beyond what is anticipated or justified by the benefits of participation in the research study. Protection from harm may, in such cases, require modification of the research protocol or cessation of the research altogether. A second purpose of treatment effects monitoring is to ensure that the research objectives are being met. Poor execution of a well-conceived study may alter the risk–benefit balance for individual participants and diminish the value of the research effort. Hence, review of performance data, for example, participant recruitment and retention, are typically incorporated into the monitoring process.

The policies and procedures for treatment effects monitoring is an evolving field that is not codified. Most of the experience with treatment effects monitoring has been developed in the execution of multiple site clinical trials, rather than single-center clinical trials or translational research. However, the ever-increasing scrutiny over research involving humans has led to increased use of monitoring committees for all types of human research including both single-site and nonrandomized interventional studies.

The history and development of these practices has been strongly influenced by the need to protect human research volunteers during therapeutic clinical trials. However, experimental interventions, including the use of both FDA-approved and nonapproved drugs, are frequently employed

| TABLE 13-1 |
| --- |
| **Names Used for Data Monitoring Committees** |
| Treatment effects monitoring committee (TEMC) |
| Data monitoring committee (DMC) |
| Data and safety monitoring committee/board (DSMC / DSMB) |
| Independent data monitoring committee (IDMC) |
| Safety monitoring committee (SMC) |
| Policy and data board |
| Policy board |

in translational clinical research. In such studies, the intervention is often used to take advantage of its putative mechanism of action, and not to demonstrate therapeutic efficacy or effectiveness per se. Nevertheless, such interventions may expose research volunteers to the same risks and hazards. As a result, TEMCs are frequently required during all types of translational clinical research, and the treatment language employed when describing the structure and function of TEMCs should be understood in the wider context of any experimental intervention that may pose a safety risk to research volunteers.

## HISTORY AND CURRENT STATUS OF TREATMENT EFFECT MONITORING

Oversight committees have been involved in the review of human research since the first modern-day clinical trials were conducted after World War II. For the most part, however, this responsibility was vested in the steering committee that was composed of investigators who were participating in the trial and had a self-interest in the outcome. The notion of an independent monitoring board to oversee the propriety and conduct of clinical research was first proposed in the so-called Greenberg report which was commissioned by the National Institutes of Health, National Heart Institute (1). The 1967 Greenberg committee was constituted to recommend appropriate structures for the conduct of large-scale cooperative clinical trials. This report recommended the development of an external expert policy or advisory board. Originally, the role of such independent policy boards was proposed to review the scientific merit of the proposed protocol and to make recommendations to the sponsor regarding the conduct of the study. Over time, this

policy board took on monitoring the interim study data to protect the integrity of the research and the safety of the participants.

The NIH Clinical Trials Committee issued three recommendations on data monitoring in 1979. The recommendations were that (1) all clinical trials should have a plan for data and safety monitoring that might include oversight by the principal investigator for small studies; (2) the plan should be approved by the IRB; and (3) multicenter clinical trials with masked investigators should have a multidisciplinary safety monitoring group not including investigators administering study treatments (2).

In 1998, the NIH issued a policy that all phase III multicenter clinical trials should have an independent external data and safety monitoring committee to protect the safety of the participants and ensure the validity and integrity of the data collection (3). Subsequently, in 2000, this policy was extended to phase I and II trials such that "a DSMB may be appropriate if the studies have multiple clinical sites, are blinded (masked), or employ particularly high-risk interventions or vulnerable populations" (4). Since 2000, all NIH applications for research involving human volunteers must be accompanied by a plan for treatment effects monitoring. Although the guidances issued by the NIH (5) (below) about data monitoring focus on therapeutic clinical trials, similar scenarios are encountered, and are applicable, in any type of investigator-initiated clinical translational research.

The following provides examples of appropriate types of monitoring and oversight for different types of studies. These are illustrative only. The ICs [Institute or Center, sic] must develop and implement monitoring activities and oversight of those activities appropriate to the study, population, research environment, and the degree of risk involved.

*Phase I:* A typical phase I trial of a new drug or agent frequently involves relatively high risk to a small number of participants. The investigator and occasionally others may have the only relevant knowledge regarding the treatment because these are the first human uses. An IC may require the study investigator to perform continuous monitoring of participant safety with frequent reporting to IC staff with oversight responsibility.

*Phase II:* A typical phase II trial follows phase I studies and there is more information regarding risks, benefits and monitoring procedures. However, more participants are involved and the toxicity and outcomes are confounded by disease process. An IC may require monitoring similar to that of a phase I trial or supplement that level of monitoring with individuals with expertise relevant to the study who might assist in interpreting the data to ensure patient safety.

**Phase III:** A phase III trial frequently compares a new treatment to a standard treatment or to no treatment, and treatment allocation may be randomly assigned and the data masked. These studies usually involve a large number of participants followed for longer periods of treatment exposure. While short-term risk is usually slight, one must consider the long-term effects of a study agent or achievement of significant safety or efficacy differences between the control and study groups for a masked study. An IC may require a DSMB to perform monitoring functions. This DSMB would be composed of experts relevant to the study and would regularly assess the trial and offer recommendations to the IC concerning its continuation.

## WHEN IS A TEMC REQUIRED?

Monitoring in some form is required whenever there is some avoidable risk to research participants, either from participation in study procedures, from adverse experiences from an experimental treatment, or from withholding an effective treatment. In accordance with U.S. federal law, IRBs are charged with safety monitoring of clinical research. However, the level of oversight is typically limited to individual reports of severe adverse events and annual reports of patient enrollment, adverse events, and interim information that alters the balance of risk and benefit. It is generally recognized that IRBs are ill prepared to monitor complex clinical research. In masked treatment studies, investigators typically present the IRB with aggregate data not sorted by treatment group. Furthermore, because of the diversity of what they review, IRBs do not typically have expertise in all of the fields comprising their oversight. In many cases, the workload of IRBs does not permit the type of detailed data review that a dedicated TEMC can perform.

Ultimately, it is incumbent on the study investigators to ensure that a research study involving human volunteers is adequately monitored for safety and data validity. In many circumstances this responsibility does not require establishing a formal TEMC. For short-term or unmasked studies, investigators may assume this responsibility. In larger or more complex studies, it may be sufficient to have data reviewed by a panel of investigators or an independent person designated as a safety review officer. At present, there is little formal guidance for monitoring beyond IRBs for human experiments that do not involve testing of therapeutic agents; however, it is likely that this requirement will become mandated in the future because of highly publicized adverse outcomes from human experimentation.

The most straightforward approach is to accept that independent monitoring is necessary in all situations in which experimentation on humans involves more than minimal risk. In such cases, monitoring should be done unless it can be convincingly argued that the absence of such monitoring does not carry increased risk of harm.

## WHAT ARE THE FUNCTIONS OF A TEMC?

The tasks of the TEMC are straightforward. It must review accumulating data from a research study at specified intervals to determine whether the research should continue as planned, should be modified, or should be terminated. The first responsibility of the TEMC is to protect the safety of participants in clinical research. The second responsibility of the TEMC is to ensure the scientific validity of the research endeavor. The acquired data should be useful enough to the medical establishment to justify potential risks to patients. Although these two responsibilities are not mutually exclusive, it is often the case that the TEMC must rely on expert opinion and value judgments to weigh the risk to research volunteers against the value of the knowledge acquired from the study.

Reasons for terminating a study early may include:

- Convincing evidence of superiority of one treatment over another
- Evidence indicating that the experimental intervention may be harmful to participants
- Low probability that the research study can be successfully completed (e.g., poor accrual or lack of resources)
- New evidence from other sources that changes the risk–benefit ratio for participating in the research.

In conducting the deliberations of the TEMC, the sponsor or its designee (e.g., a coordinating center in the case of multicenter studies) provides the TEMC with information regarding the performance of the study and the treatment effects. In some circumstances, the sponsor or other interested parties may be present for the review of the performance data, but not for the interim treatment effects data.

Performance reports usually provide aggregate data (Table 13–2). The TEMC may specify what additional information should be incorporated into the performance report. Some performance information such as accrual and retention may be reviewed as grouped by treatment assignment in order to assess possible information bias. Although responsibility for adequate performance lies with the investigators, the role of the TEMC is to assure that the study is proceeding in a satisfactory manner. The TEMC needs to pay particular attention to the timeliness and accuracy of outcome measures that influence the interpretation of the study results. Specific quality assurance measures are often applied to key outcome measures such as central reading or review of data collection. In the end, the TEMC must use the performance data to offer recommendations to the study's sponsor on the following issues:

- Do the protocol or procedures need to be altered?
- Is the study progressing in a manner such that it can answer the primary research questions?
- Should the study continue to enroll and treat research subjects?
- Does the study need to add or delete participating sites?

The primary mission of the TEMC is monitoring of treatment effects, including an analysis of both efficacy and safety. In general, in therapeutic trials, both issues must be evaluated concurrently as the recommendations of the committee must balance both the risk and the benefit of participating in the study. Efficacy and safety monitoring are usually provided in a report that aggregates participants

by treatment assignment. In some circumstances, it may be important to review data further stratified by baseline demographic or clinical characteristics that are thought to influence treatment response. The main efficacy measures are usually defined at the outset of the study, although some early phase studies or exploratory research may not have a primary design variable. The TEMC should work with the sponsor or coordinating center to decide how best to present the efficacy data. Specific issues that need to be addressed are:

- Should the committee review all accumulating data or only that from participants who have completed the study?
- Should the committee review unadjusted data or should it be adjusted or stratified by baseline characteristics?
- Which secondary outcome measures should be reviewed?
- Does the committee have any preferred graphical or tabular displays?

Although these questions are often addressed at the initial meeting of the TEMC, it is common that a TEMC will want to modify the initial format of the report during the course of the study.

Safety monitoring data is usually presented to the committee in tabular form summarizing adverse events regardless of severity. Serious adverse events are usually presented in narrative form. The committee needs to decide whether it wishes to review all serious adverse events in detail or just those that are considered unexpected or attributable to participating in the study. In some cases, the TEMC may want to review all serious adverse events as they are reported, and in other cases, the TEMC may want to evaluate aggregate events at scheduled meetings. For the study of conditions that involve high rates of death and hospitalization, it is usually infeasible to review all such events in adequate detail, and therefore the TEMC must rely on tabular or summary information. Other adverse effects that include symptoms and laboratory abnormalities are typically presented in tabular format by treatment assignment and specified as mild, moderate, or severe. In some cases, it is necessary for the TEMC to work in conjunction with other committees such as a clinical endpoint or safety committee that is tasked with classification and causation of adverse events.

Based on review of treatment effects, the TEMC should address the following questions:

- Do the protocol or procedures need to be altered?
- Does the study need to modify or suspend a treatment regimen?

## TABLE 13–2

### Commonly Used Measures of Research Study Performance*

Number of patients screened

Number of patients enrolled

Rates of screening and enrollment

Causes for screening failures

Timeliness of visits

Completion rates of visits, specimen collection

Reasons for missed visits, loss of follow-up

Timeliness of data entry/transfer

Accuracy of data entry

Completeness of data entry

Quality measures of data and specimen acquisition

Baseline characteristics of study participants

Protocol deviations or violations

*Measures of research study performance are usually presented as aggregate data and for each performance site. Baseline pretreatment characteristics of participants may be presented by treatment assignment to evaluate balance between treatment groups. Key performance data should be presented over time to assess trends in study performance.

- Are there subgroups of patients who should be excluded from the research because of excessive risk or because of proof of treatment benefit?
- Are the potential benefits of the intervention and the acquisition of medical knowledge appropriately balanced against possible risk to research volunteers?
- Has the study answered the primary and secondary research questions with sufficient clarity and confidence to permit early termination?
- Should the study be terminated because it is unlikely to provide useful outcome information?
- Is there compelling evidence that the study should be extended or enlarged?
- Should the study continue to enroll and treat research subjects?

A number of statistical approaches to estimating whether adverse events are the result of experimental treatments have been developed for clinical trials, but there are no such formal approaches for small studies. Thus, those charged with monitoring human experiments must often rely on judgment and intuition.

## MONITORING AND REPORTING OF ADVERSE EVENTS

Along with the investigators, the sponsor, and the IRB, the TEMC is charged with monitoring adverse events. In general, all adverse events that occur should be reviewed by the committee in tabular format stratified by treatment assignment and severity of the events. Using the standards of Good Clinical Practice (see Chapter 14), *serious* adverse events are those that are life threatening, fatal, result in hospitalization or extension of hospitalization, cause significant disability, or a congenital defect. Other events that threaten the patient or require surgery may also be considered serious adverse events. Some adverse events are expected to occur as a result of the underlying condition that brings participants into a research study, while others are not expected. In general, an *unexpected* adverse event is one that is of such a type or severity that it is not ordinarily known to be associated with the underlying condition or treatment. An *unanticipated* adverse event is one that was not mentioned in the initial IRB-approved protocol review and consent form. An adverse event may be judged to be associated with the experimental intervention or research procedures if there is a possibility that it is caused by them. In the monitoring of medical devices, the FDA uses the terminology *adverse effect,* which implies both causality and an adverse condition or event that is associated with use of a medical device.

It is the responsibility of the investigators as well as sponsors to report adverse events to oversight bodies such as the IRB, FDA, or NIH. In many circumstances, it will be impossible for these bodies to evaluate the importance and meaning of the events because the data are not presented by treatment group. In masked studies, it is not unusual that the TEMC is the only body that has the competency to evaluate such adverse events with knowledge of the treatment assignment for the affected individual. In such cases, the responsibility for reporting as well as interpreting adverse events may be assigned by the sponsor or investigators to the TEMC (1). Because of the complexity of such reporting, the assumption of legal as well as moral responsibility, and the administrative effort that this entails, the TEMC members should have a clear understanding with the investigators and sponsors about the procedures for such reporting. The legal requirements for such reporting can be complex and the requirements for investigators and sponsors are different (Tables 13–3 and 13–4).

## CONSTITUTION AND OPERATION OF A TREATMENT EFFECTS MONITORING COMMITTEE

Selection of TEMC members is the initial step. In large, multicenter trials, voting members should reflect a range of expertise including medical scientists, basic scientists, statisticians, ethicists, and representatives of the public. (The typical size of such committees is four to six voting members and about an equal number of nonvoting members.) In smaller, single-center, investigator-initiated translational research studies, the composition of the TEMC will often be considerably simpler. In all cases, the primary consideration is that members possess adequate expertise in their respective field to address the subtle and complex issues posed by monitoring of research studies. There is an obvious advantage to having an odd number of voting members to avoid tie votes.

The chair of the TEMC is an individual who has previous experience with data monitoring, the ability to conduct effective meetings, and has expertise in the subject matter of the research. Nonvoting members of the TEMC may include individuals who represent the sponsor, the statistician who conducts the interim analyses, and representatives of the investigators. A written charter should be developed by the research sponsor to delineate the responsibilities and reporting structure. The charter should also outline the member's responsibilities for attendance at meetings and teleconferences,

## TABLE 13–3

### Adverse Event Reporting Requirements of Investigators

| Reporting to: | Type of Event | Time Frame | Regulatory Citation |
|---|---|---|---|
| IRB | Unanticipated problems involving risks to participants or others | "Promptly" | 45 CFR 46.103(b)(5); 21 CFR 56.108(b)(1) |
| IRB, NIH | Any serious adverse event in human gene transfer protocols | "Immediately" | NIH Guidelines on Recombinant DNA, Appendix M-VII-C. |
| IRB | Unanticipated adverse effect associated with a device | Within 10 working days after the investigator first is aware of the effect. | 21 CFR 812.150 |
| IRB | Unexpected serious adverse events associated with a drug | Within 15 calendar days of the investigator becoming aware of the event. | ICH Guidelines for Good Clinical Practice (GCP) 3.3.8 |
| Sponsor | Any adverse event that may reasonably be regarded as caused by or probably caused by the drug | "Promptly." If the event is "alarming," it should be reported "immediately." | 21 CFR.312.64(b) |
| Sponsor | Unanticipated adverse effect associated with a device | Within 10 working days after the investigator first is aware of the effect. | 21 CFR.812.150. |
| Sponsor | Serious adverse events, except for those specifically identified in the protocol as not needing immediate reporting | "Immediately" | ICH Guidelines for Good Clinical Practice (GCP) 4.11.1 |

the number of members necessary for a quorum, and voting status. Of particular importance is the specification of what happens with recommendations of the TEMC. The TEMC recommendations may be reported either to the investigators, the IRB, other regulatory bodies (such as a committee of an institution's general clinical research center for research conducted within a GCRC), the sponsor, or some combination (including all) of these parties. In any event, all major parties should be aware of major recommendations from the TEMC, as they all share inescapable responsibility for the safety of participants and the validity of the science.

Voting members of a TEMC should be free of financial conflict of interest in the treatments being tested and should not be actively involved in the research project or be employees of the sponsor. Other conflicts of interest, such as involvement with a competitive treatment, past experience with similar research, strongly held beliefs or positions relevant to the research project, and prior interactions with the sponsor should be disclosed.

Payments to members of the TEMC should reflect the expertise and effort involved in the consultative activities, but should not be so high as to be perceived to influence committee recommendations. Although practices vary, the TEMC should maintain regular communications with the major participating entities in the research enterprise including representatives of the investigators, the sponsor, and other key stakeholders. The goal of maintaining independence of the TEMC should not be carried to the point where their effectiveness in evaluating interim data is impaired by artificial separations between the monitor and the investigators. One effective means of improving the competency of the TEMC is to involve representatives of the investigators and those who collect and analyze the research data as nonvoting members in the monitoring process, which is the case in a majority of large clinical trials.

The initial meeting of the TEMC is often best conducted as a face-to-face meeting prior to the onset of the research so that the committee can

## TABLE 13-4

### Adverse Event Reporting Requirements of Sponsors

| Reporting to: | Type of Event | Time Frame | Regulatory Citation |
|---|---|---|---|
| FDA | Unexpected serious adverse event or experience associated with use of a drug or biological agent. | Within 15 calendar days of the sponsor's initial notification | 21 CFR.312.32(c) 21 CFR 314.80(c) 21 CFR 600.80(c) |
| FDA | Unexpected fatal or life-threatening experience associated with the use of a drug. | As soon as possible, within 7 calendar days after initial notification | 21 CFR 312.32(c) |
| FDA | Evaluation of unanticipated adverse device effects. | Within 10 working days of the sponsor's receipt of such evaluation | 21 CFR 812.150 |
| Other investigators | Unexpected serious adverse event or experience associated with use of a drug or biological agent. | Within 15 calendar days of the sponsor's initial notification | 21 CFR 312.32(c) |
| Other investigators | Unexpected fatal or life-threatening experience associated with the use of a drug. | As soon as possible, within 7 calendar days after initial notification | 21 CFR 312.32(c) |

understand and accept its charge. Potential outcomes, definitions of clinically important treatment effects, and the format and frequency of data review should be discussed. Often the committee has an open session that includes all of the committee members—voting and nonvoting. The committee may have a closed session for review of data that excludes nonvoting members or those with direct participant contact. Careful consideration needs to be given to the common practice of excluding participating investigators from review of interim data. The concern that investigators may lose their equipoise and influence the enrollment of participants if they review interim data needs to be balanced against the reality that investigators who participate in the research are often the people best equipped to explain anomalies or trends in the emerging data. The isolation of investigators from the data that they collect does not release them from their ultimate responsibility for the safety of the research participants. Moreover, there is little opportunity for bias to be introduced into the study when the treatment assignments are masked, when the major outcome measures are objective (such as mortality), or when the major outcome measures are collected by others.

Minutes of the TEMC, documenting the recommendations to the sponsor, to regulatory bodies, or to investigators, should be maintained and approved by all of the voting members. The minutes should include a declarative statement whether the committee has voted approval for the study to continue without alteration. A particularly sensitive issue is the disposition and confidentiality of TEMC minutes and interim data reports, particularly if they contain confidential information or pertain to critical phases of research when beneficial or harmful treatment effects are emerging but not considered definitive. To date, TEMCs have not been the object of litigation, but this is not a trivial concern (6,7).

### EXTENDED ROLES OF THE TEMC

The primary role of the TEMC is to monitor accumulating data for the purpose of ensuring patient safety as well as the continuing value of the research (8). However, TEMCs are often given other responsibilities:

- Approval of the research protocol and amendments
- Review of consent statements
- Recommendation of protocol amendments
- Approval of ancillary studies
- Shaping the statistical analysis and interpretation of data
- Review and comment on final manuscripts

- Publication of deliberations
- Review of current and interim scientific literature that bears on research risk and benefit
- Recommendations on how to disseminate results
- Review and adjudication of major clinical endpoints
- Review of serious adverse events for attribution to study treatments or procedures

## ACADEMIC IMPORTANCE OF RESEARCH STUDY MONITORING

Individuals who serve on TEMCs provide a role in the advancement of scientific knowledge that is equivalent to those who conduct research, review research grant proposals, and edit scientific journals. Indeed, the decisions faced by TEMC members can be among the most difficult and sensitive faced by any research scientist. They involve judgments about the strength of evidence, plausibility of outcomes, effect on medical knowledge and practice, and ethical constraints to research on other humans. Making such recommendations may require subtlety of thought, breadth of knowledge, and strong ethical purpose. Because such deliberations are often conducted in confidence and isolation from the investigators, those who serve on TEMCs often do not get the recognition that is warranted. Academic and commercial organizations should support and encourage their medical and scientific staff to participate in monitoring committees, and should recognize the importance of these efforts as a component of promotion. Sponsors and investigators should also encourage TEMC members to publish the analyses and thought processes that lead to important or difficult recommendations.

## SUMMARY

- Treatment effects monitoring is the process of reviewing accumulated outcome data by study group to determine whether the research study should continue as originally planned. The primary purpose of treatment effects monitoring is prevention of harm to current or future participants in the research project.
- Since 2000, all NIH applications for research involving human participants must be accompanied by a plan for data monitoring.
- Some form of treatment effects monitoring is required whenever there is some avoidable risk to research participants, either from participating in study procedures, from adverse experiences from an experimental treatment, or from withholding an effective treatment.
- Reasons for terminating a study prematurely may include evidence indicating that an experimental intervention may be harmful, low probability that continuing the study will provide valuable experimental data, or that the study can be successfully completed, or new evidence from other sources that changes the risk–benefit ratio to participating in the study.

## REFERENCES

1. Organization, review, and administration of cooperative studies (Greenberg report): a report from the Heart Special Project Committee to the National Advisory Heart Council, May 1967. Control Clin Trials. 1988;9:137–148.
2. http://grants1.nih.gov/grants/guide/historical/1979_06_05_Vol_08_No_08.pdf. Accessed March 13, 2005.
3. http://grants.nih.gov/grants/guide/notice-files/not98-084.html. Accessed March 13, 2005.
4. http://grants.nih.gov/grants/guide/notice-files/NOT-OD-00-038.html. Accessed March 13, 2005.
5. http://grants.nih.gov/grants/guide/notice-files/not98-084.html. Last accessed March 13, 2005.
6. Black B. Subpoenas and science—when lawyers force their way into the laboratory. N Engl J Med 1997; 336:725–727.
7. Hulka BS, Kerkvliet NL, Tugwell P. Experience of a scientific panel formed to advise the federal judiciary on silicone breast implants. N Engl J Med 2000;342:812–815.
8. Wilhelmsen L. Role of the data and safety monitoring committee (DSMC). Stat Med 2002;21:2823–2829.

# Special Topics

# CHAPTER 14

# Responsible Conduct
# of Research

Philip A. Ludbrook, Diane K. Clemens,
Ronald Munson, Patricia M. Scannell

Human Experimentation: a value conflict between freedom of scientific enquiry and the protection of individual inviolability.

—Jay Katz, 1972

The right to conduct research on an individual is a privilege granted to an investigator by an individual who chooses to participate in a research study. This privilege requires investigators to conduct their research responsibly. Research must be scientifically appropriate, the benefits maximized, and the risks to participants minimized to protect the safety of participants to the greatest possible extent.

A National Commission for the Protection of Human Subjects of Biomedical and Behavioral Research, established in 1974, provided investigators with an ethical framework to help them determine the "right" way to conduct clinical research. In its seminal *Belmont Report* (3), the Commission distinguished clinical research from medical practice. Levine defines research and practice as follows:

Research refers to a class of activities designed to develop or contribute to generalizable knowledge. Generalizable knowledge consists of theories, principles, or relationships (or the accumulation of data on which they may be based) that can be corroborated by accepted scientific observation and inference.

The practice of medicine or behavioral therapy refers to a class of activities designed solely to enhance the well-being of an individual patient or client. The purpose of medical or behavioral practice is to provide diagnosis, preventive

treatment, or therapy. The customary standard for routine and accepted practice is a reasonable expectation of success." (4)

It may be argued that physicians are always engaged in research, as when physicians treat patients, they are also trying to learn something to benefit some other patient or group of patients. This may be so, but finding out more about a disease or helping someone other than the individual patient is not the primary intent of physicians. The aim of research, by contrast, is to make new discoveries potentially helpful for the diagnosis and treatment of diseases. Thus, the goal of research activities is to acquire data relevant to previously established hypotheses and contributing to the development of general theories and principles of diseases, including prevention, therapies, and management. The concern is usually less with an individual patient than a population of patients.

Institutional Review Board (IRB) approval is generally necessary before initiating any clinical activity in which the investigator intends to report the findings within the medical or scientific community. If "research on existing data" might yield information worth sharing with the scientific community, IRB approval should be sought prior to the data collection. In general, all research involving human participants, including review of records, tissue, or other derived materials must receive IRB approval before the research is initiated. It is the intent of the activity at the time the study was initiated that is the criterion for IRB approval. Some research may qualify for certain exemptions, but most institutions require review by the IRB to ensure that the research qualifies

Note: Investigators are advised that every component of the federal regulations, as well as other applicable documented advisories, ethical codes, and federal and state law must be followed when preparing human participant research protocols. This chapter presents only selected aspects of each discipline—readers should refer to the DHHS and FDA regulations (1, 2) and Belmont Report (3) for details.

under the exemption categories (1,2). IRB approval must also be obtained before initiating any revision or amendment to the research protocol or the informed consent document.

The standards by which IRBs evaluate human participant research are documented by federal regulations promulgated by the Department of Health and Human Services (DHHS) at 45-CFR-46 of the Code of Federal Regulations, and by the Food and Drug Administration (FDA) at 21 CFR, Parts 50, 56, 312 (1,2). IRBs' deliberations are also influenced by certain documented codes of ethics, the *Belmont Report*, and other principles of moral ethics including utilitarian, deontologic, and rights-based ethics. Although sometimes less well identified, federal and state law also impact the IRB's review processes, as may IRB members' subjective impressions, anecdotal experiences, scientific curiosity, paternalism, personal interest, and personal advocacy for specific population groups or selected scientific endeavors. More recently, concerns regarding increasingly frequent litigation against investigators and IRBs have also inculcated an element of defensive review of research, much as "defensive medicine" has impacted medical practice. Although all of these considerations influence, to a greater or lesser extent, IRB review of human participant research, the federal regulations constitute the most tangible, consistent, and enforceable standards to which IRBs may be held accountable.

## A BRIEF HISTORY OF THE REGULATION OF HUMAN PARTICIPANT RESEARCH

As opposed to the ethics of medical practice, which date as far back as the Hippocratic Oath (circa 600 BC), research ethics are a relatively modern discipline. The ethics of human participant research are based to a large extent on the fundamental rights of the individual to choose what may or may not be done to his or her own body. As stated by Katz, "human experimentation is a value conflict between freedom of scientific enquiry and protection of individual inviolability" (5). The AMA Council on Ethical and Judicial Affairs (6) recently affirmed that "it is fundamental social policy that the advancement of scientific knowledge must always be secondary to the primary concern for the individual." Inherent in Katz's "value conflict" problem is the potentially conflicted role of the individual physician-investigator, who is obligated by professional standards to always act in the patient's best interest.

## Nuremberg Code

As a monument to the Nuremberg trials and the indictment of the Nazi doctors for their inescapable responsibility for the medical atrocities they conducted, the Nuremberg Code, published in 1949, has made a fundamentally important and lasting impact on research ethics (7). The code emphasizes first and foremost that the "voluntary consent of the human subject is absolutely essential, and requires the legal capacity, free choice, and sufficient knowledge and comprehension for the subject to make an informed decision, while excluding any force, fraud, deceit, duress, or coercion." Likewise, the code emphasizes the importance of weighing the risks of the research (specifically, that the "degree of risk should never exceed the humanitarian importance of the problem"), requires minimization of risks to participants, use of appropriately qualified investigators possessing the highest degree of skill and care, and demands that the research will be performed with due scientific rigor and is likely to be scientifically useful.

By its insistence that (1) the degree of risk of the research must be in proportion to the humanitarian importance of the problem, (2) that risks to human participants be minimized, and (3) the experiment be of scientific worth, the Nuremberg Code elevated the concept of the risk–benefit ratio as it applies to medical research to a level of fundamental importance for IRB approval of research in today's world.

## Helsinki Declaration

In 1964, the World Medical Association created the Declaration of Helsinki, embodying the Ethical Principles for Medical Research Involving Human Subjects. The declaration has since been amended five times, most recently in 2002. Helsinki reaffirms that "considerations related to the well-being of human subjects should take precedence over the interests of science and society." This requirement "upgrades" the priority implied by Nuremberg's reference to the "humanitarian importance of the problem" to the preeminent concern for the well-being of the individual human participant of research, which in turn trumps the interests of science and society.

Taken literally, the Helsinki standards might be interpreted as imposing a restriction on the conduct of nontherapeutic research, which explicitly lacks benefit for the individual participant. Earlier versions of the Helsinki code, if taken literally ("Helsinki fundamentalism") essentially proscribe placebo controlled studies by their assertion that "every patient—including those in a control group, if any, should be assured of the best proven diagnostic and therapeutic method." The 2002 revision of the Helsinki code softens that proscription slightly, stating that "the benefits, risks, burdens, and effectiveness of a new treatment or new method should be tested against those of the best current prophylactic, diagnostic and therapeutic method. This does not exclude the use of placebo, or no treatment, in studies where no proven prophylactic, diagnostic or therapeutic method exists."

Despite such controversy, the current revision of the Declaration of Helsinki embodies many widely accepted ethical standards intended to protect the rights and welfare of human participants, which underlie the criteria for approval of research by IRBs today.

### American Research Scandals of the 1950s and 1960s

In 1966, several egregious violations of existing ethical codes and standards of research were exposed in a landmark paper published in the *New England Journal of Medicine* by Henry Beecher (8). Beecher reported that 22 of 100 consecutive human research studies published in "an excellent journal" in 1964 involved "unethical or questionably ethical procedures." He stated that "many...patients...never had the risks satisfactorily explained to them [and many] had not known that they were the subjects of an experiment although grave consequences have been suffered as a direct result of [these] experiments." In addition to a lack of valid informed consent, many of these studies were blighted by a high risk–benefit ratio, and most exploited vulnerable or disadvantaged persons as research subjects. These studies flaunted the ethical principles of respect for persons in terms of lack of consent for participation, and of justice as a "fair sharing of the benefits and burdens of research" (8).

Public concern regarding unethical research, especially research funded by federal dollars, was further fueled by publication in the medical literature and lay press of several human research studies that transgressed existing ethical standards, particularly standards of justice or fairness. The most egregious of these were the Tuskegee Syphilis Study, in which 400 black men with syphilis were followed without effective therapy even after the introduction of efficacious antibiotics; the Willowbrook Studies, intended to elucidate the natural history of infectious hepatitis, in which mentally defective children were deliberately infected with the hepatitis virus; the Jewish Chronic Disease Hospital Studies in which

live cancer cells were injected into patients suffering from chronic illnesses in order to study human transplant rejection; and the San Antonio Contraception Study in which poor Mexican American women presenting for contraceptive advice were randomized to placebo or a contraceptive vaginal cream (summarized in reference 4, pp. 69–72). These studies were all designed with laudable intent to develop useful new knowledge, but disregarded the preeminent rights of human participants, whose interests were subordinated to the anticipated gains for science and society.

### DHHS/FDA Regulations

In response to these and similar developments, the U.S. Surgeon General, in 1966, established the requirement for local committee review of all human participant research funded by the United States Public Health Service (USPHS, which includes the National Institutes of Health), to ensure that the rights and welfare of human participants of research were duly protected.

In 1974, the policies and guidelines of the Department of Health and Human Services and the Food and Drug Administration were raised to the stature of federal regulations, requiring the establishment of institutional review boards in all institutions receiving federal funding for human participant research. Initially codified in 1974 and subsequently revised in 1983 (45 CFR-46, 21 CFR 50, 56, etc.) (1,2), the federal regulations established in detail the requirements for the composition of IRBs, and the regulatory structure under which they were to operate. In 1991, these regulations were formulated as the Common Rule by 15 federal departments and agencies as a common set of protections for all participants. The Common Rule has subsequently also been adopted by three other federal agencies.

### THE ETHICAL BASIS OF THE REGULATIONS
### The Role of Ethics

The federal regulations, like all legalistic documents, are wide in scope and broad in application. They were intended to "cover the waterfront." Ethics, on the other hand, are moral principles with individual, case by case, implications and imperatives. Ethical norms speak to what "should" or "ought" to be done in specific situations, sometimes even addressing what "must" or "must not" be done. And if a reason is needed, an ethical principle applies because "it's the right (or wrong) thing to do" (4). So for the physician-investigator committed to the *ideal*, or even *optimal* treatment of human research participants, the moral values and imperatives of ethics may demand higher standards of protection than do the regulations.

## The "Ideal" Investigator

Most investigators who undertake human participant research are highly motivated toward, and enthusiastic about, the research they are conducting. One might even question whether, lacking such interest, the investigator should be conducting the research at all. That said, perhaps the most reliable safeguard of the welfare and rights of research participants is provided by an intelligent, well-informed, conscientious investigator, whose primary motivation is altruistic, and who exercises his or her idealism in the design and conduct of human participant research, the selection of participants, and the efforts to recruit them in accordance with the participants' best interests and best judgment (8). For the ideal and idealistic investigator, then, adherence to the federal regulations and to applicable state and federal law should be the minimum standard for the protection of human research participants. The ethical principles of virtue, honesty, altruism, compassion, skill, and the unswerving commitment to act always in the research participant's best interest must be paramount.

The *Belmont Report* offers three basic principles as ethical foundations for evaluating the ethical legitimacy of research involving human participants. The principles are "generally accepted as being so uncontroversial as not to require argument." They comprise respect for persons, beneficence, and justice.

## Respect for Persons

The principle of respect for persons requires that investigators recognize that all people have inherent worth. They must be valued in themselves, not merely because they have some instrumental ("utilitarian") value. It would be wrong, for example, to deceive someone into thinking she has a disease in order to see what effect its therapy would have on a well person. Under the right circumstances, people may ethically be treated as a means to an end, but not as a means only. Thus, a participant in a randomized controlled trial is a means to achieving the "ends" (i.e., goals) of the trial, but respect for the participant as a person requires that he be an informed, consenting and comprehending volunteer.

### Autonomy

Showing respect for persons requires investigators to acknowledge that rational individuals are autonomous agents, that is, persons whose actions are self-determined. Autonomy is violated when an individual's behavior is deliberately coerced or manipulated—even if unintentionally. A timid person may be intimidated by a medical environment, while someone else may comply simply to please the physician-investigator. If autonomy is to be exercised genuinely, it must be protected and promoted—this is the purpose of informed consent.

### Informed Consent

The *Belmont Report* states "although the informed consent doctrine has substantial foundation in law, it is essentially an ethical imperative." Nevertheless, both legal and ethical prerogatives clearly impact the elements as well as the imperative of valid informed consent (Table 14–1). Although the federal regulations allow for waiver of informed consent for research participants under certain strictly defined criteria (Table 14–2), informed consent is ordinarily regarded by all as a fundamental right of the prospective research participant and a fundamental responsibility of every investigator.

Informed consent is a process intended to diminish the possibility that people will be coerced, manipulated, or otherwise treated in such a way that their autonomy is violated. Individuals cannot be said to be directing the course of their lives if their decisions are made in ignorance of relevant information presented in a comprehensible fashion. This means, in a research context, information about the purpose of the research, the procedure that will be followed, and the anticipated risks and benefits. Individuals also need to know about other options available to them, and that, if they decide to volunteer, they can later change their mind, and drop out of the study without suffering prejudice. The information provided must be understandable, relevant to the decision at hand, and sufficient to allow them to weigh the character and consequences of the options open to them.

Because the investigator is usually highly motivated to recruit participants, and his or her enthusiasm may be overtly or covertly conveyed to the prospective participant, an element of coercion may be (subtly or not so subtly) introduced into the consent process. Perhaps such an influence is unavoidable. And perhaps it is a reason for a qualified individual other than the investigator, for example, a research coordinator, to conduct the process of informed consent in certain instances.

The function of informed consent is not to protect people from the consequences of their actions, or from adverse consequences of their participation in research, but to protect their autonomy to make decisions regarding themselves, and

## TABLE 14–1a

### Basic Elements of Informed Consent [45-CFR-46.116(a)]

- A statement that the study involves research, an explanation of the purposes of the research and the expected duration of the patient's participation, a description of the procedures to be followed, and identification of any procedures which are experimental
- A description of any reasonably foreseeable risks or discomforts to the research participant
- A description of any benefits to the research participant or to others which may reasonably be expected from the research
- A disclosure of appropriate alternative procedures or courses of treatment, if any, that might be advantageous to the research participant
- A statement describing the extent, if any, to which confidentiality of records identifying the research participant will be maintained
- For research involving more than minimal risk, an explanation as to whether any compensation and an explanation as to whether any medical treatments are available if injury occurs and, if so, what they consist of, or where further information may be obtained
- An explanation of whom to contact for answers to pertinent questions about the research and research participant's rights, and whom to contact in the event of a research-related injury to the participant; and
- A statement that participation is voluntary, refusal to participate will involve no penalty or loss of benefits to which the participant is otherwise entitled and the participant may discontinue participation at any time without penalty or loss of benefits to which the participant is otherwise entitled

## TABLE 14–1b

### Additional Elements of Informed Consent [45-CFR-46.116(b)]

When appropriate, one or more of the following elements of information shall also be provided to each research participant:

- A statement that the particular treatment or procedure may involve risks to the research participant (or to the embryo or fetus, if the participant is or may become pregnant), which are currently unforeseeable
- Anticipated circumstances under which participation may be terminated by the investigators without regard to the participant's consent
- Any additional costs that may result from participation in the research
- The consequences of a participant's decision to withdraw from the research and procedures for orderly termination of participation
- A statement that significant new findings developed during the course of the research that may relate to the willingness to continue will be provided to the participant
- The approximate number of participants involved in the study

so acknowledge the investigator's respect for them as persons. Consent involves more than saying "yes." It requires that individuals have an opportunity to deliberate about their options, consider the information provided, ask questions, and then arrive at a decision. During this process, they must be protected from undue influences, situational and time pressures, or other factors that can infringe on their autonomy and thus compromise their decision-making power. To emphasize the importance of this requirement, consent should be "free and informed."

Thus, for consent to be legitimate in a research context, participants must be (1) competent to understand relevant information and capable of exercising judgment; (2) provided with information, appropriately presented, about the research and its potential benefits and risks; and (3) free to make a decision in circumstances in which there is no coercion or undue influence.

## TABLE 14–2

**Requirements for Approval of Waiver of Consent [45-CFR-46.116(d)]**

- The research involves no more than minimal risk to the participants.
- The waiver or alteration will not adversely affect the rights and welfare of the participants.
- The research could not practicably be carried out without the waiver or alteration.
- Whenever appropriate, the participants will be provided with additional pertinent information after participation.

Nevertheless, much study and experience indicates that, in practice, informed consent frequently fails to achieve its intended goals. All IRB members experienced in research review, and most thoughtful investigators, acknowledge the many limitations of the practice of informed consent, including limitations that apply to the investigator, to the research participant, or to the process or documentation of informed consent. Despite due diligence and careful attention to all of the requirements for optimal informed consent, some authorities argue that informed consent is an inherently flawed process. Their accusations appear to be supported by numerous published studies showing poor understanding and retention of informed consent material by many subjects following the consent process. Nevertheless, although valid informed consent is difficult to achieve, most agree that it is absolutely essential to strive for it.

### Vulnerable Populations

Autonomy is the capacity for self-determination; when this capacity is impaired or undeveloped, valid informed consent is not possible. An impairment may be temporary when it is due to shock, alcohol, medication, injury, or illness. It may be episodic when it involves, for example, temporarily uncontrolled schizophrenia or other psychosis or illness. Or, the impairment may be permanent when it results from mental retardation, some form of brain damage or a dementing illness. Whatever the cause, someone suffering from mental confusion, or lacking the ability to understand information relevant to becoming a research participant, lacks the capacity for legitimate consent. Special precautions must also be taken when recruiting volunteers from populations that are vulnerable.

Infants and very young children are not considered capable of legitimate consent. Older children may be able to understand the research they are invited to participate in, and their assent (agreement or acquiescence) should be sought, but they cannot give legally valid consent until they reach the age of mature judgment.

Each group of "vulnerable" people presents particular problems with respect to enrolling them in research protocols. Decisions affecting them, if they are allowed to become participants in human research, must be made on their behalf, by others. Typically, this means the parents, the courts, or whoever is legally responsible for their individual welfare. Individuals who are incompetent to consent, however, still have the moral status of persons and must be treated as possessing inherent worth. Those responsible for making decisions on behalf of an incompetent person must be committed to acting in the person's best interest. Some people may have the capacity to exercise their autonomy but may be in circumstances that compromise it. Employees, students, and members of the armed forces may fear incurring disfavor were they to refuse someone with the power to influence their career who asks them to consent to becoming a research participant. Those who are homeless or poor may be induced to become participants by the offer of what, for others, would be an inconsequential sum of money or trivial award. Prisoners may fear reprisals, or may be encouraged to become volunteers by invoking the favor of a parole board or the promise of some reward, such as a better diet or health care, that ought to be provided anyway as a matter of course.

### Beneficence

"As to diseases, make a habit of two things," states the famous Hippocratic dictum, "to help, or at least to do no harm." The rule is essentially equivalent to the principle of beneficence. The principle is interpreted in the *Belmont Report* as imposing on everyone a moral obligation to act in ways that avoid causing harm, maximize the benefit, and minimize the harm.

This principle has a straightforward application in the physician-patient relationship: The physician should not deliberately do anything that might make the patient's condition worse and should act in ways that promote the patient's medical welfare. Yet the application is far from straightforward in a research context, because application of the principle can extend from an individual patient to groups of patients in a particular research project, and even to the enterprise of human research itself.

### Risks and Benefits

"Risks" typically refer to the possibility that participants may suffer harm due to acts of either omission or commission. Harm may result from participants not receiving a treatment recognized as effective from which they could be expected to benefit, or from receiving an experimental treatment that may produce harm directly. The language of risk is often ambiguous, and various criteria have emerged for determining when risk is minimal or greater than minimal. Describing a procedure as posing small risk, when this reflects a low probability of great harm, is misleading and so violates the principle of informed consent.

A benefit is an outcome that has value with respect to the health and well-being of a participant. Thus, receipt by a participant who agrees to participate in research of a small sum of money intended only to compensate his time and inconvenience, should not be construed as a benefit. That a participant will be monitored closely for signs of progressive hearing loss may be a benefit, although offering it as a benefit to participation in research may be viewed as coercive.

Harms are the opposite of benefits. Thus, an outcome that has a negative effect on the health and well-being of a participant is a harm. In assessing risks and benefits, both the probabilities of the occurrence of particular harms and benefits, as well as their kinds and magnitude, must be considered. Methods for determining risks and their likelihood should be explicit, and estimates should be consonant with those of other investigators with recognized expertise in the area. Ultimately, however, researchers and IRBs must make their decisions by exercising their best judgment after considering the basic ethical principles and deliberating about them in light of all relevant information.

A variety of possible harms (physical, psychological, economic) and benefits (physical, psychological) should be considered. And while the risks and benefits for an individual research participant should receive special weight, the risks and benefits for others (participants' families, others with the same disease, society as a whole) should also be considered.

## Scientific Legitimacy

An essential condition for the ethical acceptability of research that involves putting humans at any risk is that it be grounded on good science. Scientific legitimacy is required of a study's hypothesis or content as well as its design. The success of a research proposal should be based on more than mere speculative possibility. The design of the research and the methods it proposes to employ must be in accordance with recognized and accepted practices of scientific inquiry. This requires that the study be designed in such a way that results can be obtained that either are significant in

themselves or can determine whether further study is warranted.

## Clinical Equipoise

"Equipoise" in general refers to an equal distribution of weight or forces so that they are in balance. Clinical equipoise exists when all available relevant data neither confirm nor refute the possibility that a particular experimental intervention carries greater risk or benefit than some alternative (10). The investigator may hope that the study will prove otherwise, but equipoise exists as long as the available data are not determinative in the judgment of similarly informed physicians or investigators. Only when a state of clinical equipoise exists is it legitimate for investigators to ask people to consent to becoming participants in a research protocol in which they will be assigned randomly to different groups.

Of course, the state of equipoise may change as new data accumulate or come to light. Should equipoise come to an end, investigators have a moral duty to terminate the study. After all, when the research participant consented, it was with the understanding that all options available to them were assumed to be of equal value.

## Placebo

Placebo-controlled studies are valuable because their results can provide compelling evidence to establish a causal connection between an intervention and its outcome. The use of a placebo control is ethical when the intervention is compared to currently accepted standard treatment; that is, the intervention is meant to add to the current standard, not replace it. The use of a placebo is much more controversial when it means that an acceptable treatment is withheld to allow comparison to the experimental intervention. For example, it would be wrong to approve a study comparing long-term treatment with a new antihypertensive to placebo in severe hypertensive patients when very effective alternatives are currently available. On the other hand, some hold that if the disorder under study is minor, or when the standard option is "wait and see," and the results of not receiving effective treatment are not likely to be serious, use of placebo is acceptable. Others maintain that when a treatment is only partially or sporadically effective, placebo use is permissible, because no serious harm is done. Ultimately, decisions by the investigator and IRB must be made on a case-by-case basis.

## Justice

The *Belmont Report* is concerned with "distributive justice"—that is, with the distribution of benefits and burdens. All theories of justice endorse the principle that "similar cases ought to be treated in a similar way," that is, fairly. The principle of fairness depends on having in place at least one substantive principle of justice, and the *Belmont Report* lists five substantive principles of justice that it describes as "widely accepted." They assert, in a general way, the rules for distribution. To give them their usual names, they are (1) Principle of Equality: an equal share should be given to each person; (2) Principle of Need: need should determine what each person is given; (3) Principle of Effort: individual effort should determine what each person is given; (4) Principle of Contribution: the social contribution of a person should determine what that person is given; (5) Principle of Merit: merit should determine what each person is given.

An attempt to apply all of these principles to individual research proposals could lead to irreconcilable contradictions; that is, someone with great need may have made little social contribution. The *Belmont Report* makes no effort to harmonize the principles; it leaves it up to IRBs to make decisions about which practices are just. Weighing all factors, they must decide, for example, whether it is just for a group of participants to take greater than minimal risks in research that promises to benefit them little or not at all, yet may benefit others considerably. No simple algorithm can solve such problems.

## Selection of Research Participants

Considerations of justice are especially important when selecting research participants. Fairness and the principle of equality demand that those who stand to benefit from the results of research should also share its risks. Thus, it would be unjust to single out a specific social group, say on the basis of race, education, economic, or social status, and allow that they alone bear the risks both for themselves and for the larger population.

Likewise, its equally important to ensure that various social groups are included, when scientifically appropriate, in clinical research studies. For instance, women and African Americans have traditionally been underrepresented in clinical trials; the lack of data from these groups leaves open whether research findings in such studies can be extended to these patients.

Issues related to patient recruitment are addressed in greater detail elsewhere.

## CONFLICTS OF INTEREST IN HUMAN PARTICIPANT RESEARCH

Reference has already been made to the physician-investigator's conflict of interest with regard to the research participant; that is, to the conflict between a physician's obligation to place the patient's best interests above all else and the investigator's obligation to conduct research with the greatest scientific integrity and with the greatest potential of advancing knowledge. Unbiased informed consent, secured in a manner that protects patients from undue influence (including the enthusiasm of an investigator) is the best way to disempower the conflict inherent in the physician-investigator role.

In the present day setting, the term *conflict of interest* most often refers to the risk of bias, or even the appearance of bias, which might predispose or motivate an improper decision, or wrongdoing by the investigator. In practical terms, conflict of interest may be defined as a "set of conditions in which an investigator's judgment concerning a primary interest (e.g., human participants' welfare) may be biased by a secondary interest (e.g., personal gain)." Even more stringently, Kassirer and Angell (12) refer to financial conflicts of interest as "an association that would cause an investigator to prefer one outcome . . . to another. . . . [The] conflict is a function of the situation, and not of the investigator's response to the situation. Thus, the opportunity *need not be acted upon* to represent a conflict of interest."

Conflicts of interest are often, but by no means always, financial. Personal self-interests, including success in research or its spin-offs (e.g., publications, reputation, career, promotion, grants, awards) may also be puritanically viewed as a potential or actual conflict. However, it is the appearance or the actuality of a conflict of interest based on *personal financial reward* that is perhaps the most damaging to research and even to the public perception of the credibility of the scientific enterprise.

For many such potential transgressions, the honesty, integrity, virtue, and good judgment of the investigator may be the only available protection and may well be all that is necessary. Most investigators are motivated by scientific and humanitarian good and the pursuit of new knowledge, albeit tempered by their awareness of the dire consequences that might result from the discovery of less than honorable research practices or overt scientific misconduct. Such consequences, of course, are of more grave concern should the potential conflict deteriorate into actual violations of scientific integrity such as plagiarism, fabrication, or alteration of the data, data trimming, selective reporting, or statistical manipulations of observed data (see Chapter 15). Recent history is regrettably replete with highly publicized examples of such transgressions that have brought disgrace on individual investigators, their mentors, institutions, granting agencies, and even science itself (4,8).

The USPHS and the National Science Foundation established in 1995 a requirement for disclosure of "significant financial interests" for investigators applying for federal funds (13). The guidelines require individual institutions receiving federal research grants to establish mechanisms (e.g., disclosure review committees) to which investigators are required to report financial interests (14). Many institutions have elected to accept the USPHS's threshold for significant financial interests; that is, $10,000 in income, $10,000 in equity, or 5% ownership in a company.

In addition to emphasizing the practical management of financial conflict by disclosure review committees, IRBs should also be vigilant to exclude financial inducements for physicians, investigators, and other health care professionals to refer their patients for enrollment in research activities. Such finder's fees are generally proscribed by many IRBs (15) on the grounds that the practice subverts the primary fiduciary obligations of the provider to the patient, prioritizing the provider's anticipation of personal gain over the interests of the prospective subjects.

## RIGHTS OF RESEARCH PARTICIPANTS

Individuals who choose to participate in research activities are afforded certain rights and protections. These rights have evolved in response to certain egregious research activities that were regarded as unacceptable by both the public and scientific communities.

As previously mentioned, the Nuremberg Code, which evolved from the war crimes trial against the Nazi medical researchers, is perhaps the most formidable example of this reactionary paradigm for establishing research participants' rights. The code identifies ten qualities that every study involving human participants should possess. Among these ten points are two fundamental rights: the right of an individual to voluntarily consent to the experiment and the right to bring the experiment to an end.

To understand how Nazi physicians were able to violate the rights of those they experimented on under the guise of "just following orders," Stanley Milgram embarked on a widely criticized study of obedience and authority in the late 1950s (16,17). Participants in this study were deliberately deceived about the purpose of the study. They were told that the experiment comprised a study of the relationship between learning and punishment. The participants were instructed to administer an electric shock to the "learner" for every wrong answer provided. The participants were not aware that the "learner" in the experiment was an actor who did not actually receive any shock at all. As the experiment progressed, the apparent voltage of the shock was progressively increased. Milgram hypothesized that most individuals would follow their conscience and refuse to harm the "learner." In fact, the study revealed that more than half of the participants continued through to the highest shock level, though often with much personal distress.

Twenty-five years after Nuremberg, the exposure of the egregious Tuskegee Syphilis Study ignited public demands to improve the rights of research participants in the United States. This culminated in the creation of the *Belmont Report* and ultimately the code of federal regulations that now protect human participants in research. The Tuskegee study brought to the forefront the rights of research participants to receive standard appropriate protections as well as applicable medical treatment.

Technological advancements in information systems in the 1980s and 1990s made access to data, including private information much easier. The ease of obtaining information gave rise to a high-level debate about the need to protect private information. In 1995, the *Washington Post* disclosed one of several incidents involving inappropriate use of private information. The story involved a 13-year-old daughter of a hospital employee who took a list of patients' names and phone numbers from the hospital when visiting her mother at work. As a prank, she contacted the patients and told them they had been diagnosed with HIV. The occurrence of such abuses of information caused concern for the rights and welfare of the public, and reemphasized the need to protect every individual's right to privacy.

### Right to Privacy: The Health Insurance Portability and Accountability Act (HIPAA)

Proposed in 1996, HIPAA was created to provide a national standard for the protection of health information. The Privacy Rule, the first of HIPAA's three components, regulates how health information may be used by covered entities. A covered entity is defined in the HIPAA regulations as a health plan, a health care provider, or a health care clearinghouse (e.g., a billing service). Thus, research is not a stated target of HIPAA. In fact, research activities are only regulated by HIPAA when conducted by a member of a covered entity. Therefore, it is important for researchers to consult with their institutional officials (HIPAA mandates that each covered entity have an appointed privacy officer) to evaluate how HIPAA affects their studies.

In fact, however, even before HIPAA, IRBs were required by federal regulations to ensure that every study has "adequate provisions to protect the privacy of subjects and to maintain the confidentiality of data" [45-CFR-46.111(a)]. "Protecting the subject's privacy" refers to the individual's right to decide if private information should be revealed.

Maintaining confidentiality of the data refers to the investigator's responsibility to protect that information after it has been provided to the investigator.

## Third-Party Rights

Any time a researcher intends to ask questions about a participant's family, the issue of whether third-party involvement in the research exists, and whether consent from the third party is necessary must be addressed. Federal regulations define a human participant as "a living individual about whom an investigator conducting research obtains (1) data through intervention or interaction with the individual, or (2) identifiable private information." Therefore, when an investigator obtains information about family members (for instance, when information is desired as part of a genetic study), those family members may come to be regarded as research participants, entitled to all the rights allocated to the primary participant.

When direct participation or consent is required of a third party, a secondary issue arises, namely, how to contact those individuals. Guidance by the National Human Research Protections Advisory Committee (NHRPAC) in 2002 indicated that it is not acceptable for an investigator to obtain names or addresses of family members from a research participant in order to contact them to obtain their consent to participate. Rather, the initial contact should always be made by the primary participant: the person familiar to the individual being contacted. A common method for contacting third-party participants is entrusting the primary participant with the responsibility of contacting and securing the permission of the third party to be contacted by the investigator. If direct participation is needed, a card with a self-addressed envelope should be provided for the third party to return, granting permission for the investigator to contact him.

## Right to Research Participation

In the 1980s, the research community faced two unfamiliar situations; the AIDS epidemic and a strong political lobby of AIDS activists. Historically, the development of new drugs has been a multiple-year process that involves several phases of study before the drug becomes approved for treatment purposes. However, the AIDS patient population suffered from a fatal disease, and treatments, even if experimental, were demanded (18, 19). The AIDS movement highlighted a component of research that has been, for the most part, overlooked; that is, the potential benefit of access to new treatments.

In addition to demanding access to new treatments, the activists challenged the customary practice of excluding minorities, women, and children from research studies. Investigators' reasons for excluding such populations particularly include the desire to reduce variability of biological data and the protection of vulnerable populations. For example, there may be variation of disease prevalence, progression, and response across different ethnicities. With regard to vulnerable populations, the unfortunate past history of some populations being exploited by certain research programs resulted in virtual exclusion of those populations from research. The hormonal and metabolic variations of women and children may introduce wide variability and therefore distort the study data. Likewise, the possibility of harm in women of childbearing capacity may be greater due to the possibility of pregnancy and potential for teratogenic effects.

## Right to Standard Medical Treatment

The right to standard medical treatment reflects all three principles of the *Belmont Report*: respect for persons, beneficence, and justice. The principle of respect for persons is violated if an individual is not offered the choice between participating in research and receiving a standard treatment. The principle of beneficence is violated if a research study does not provide a minimum standard of care and thereby places the individual at greater risk than necessary. The principle of justice is violated if a particular segment of the population disproportionately shoulders the burdens of research, without receiving the benefits. These issues are complicated by the fact that what constitutes standard care is itself highly variable and often disputed.

Standard medical care, as it relates to respect for persons, is often debated in the context of research in certain underprivileged populations. Medical care administered as part of a research study is often provided at no cost to the participant. For individuals with limited means for obtaining or paying for health care, research participation may offer a significant free benefit. The concern, then, is that the individual may participate in the research solely to obtain medical treatment that he or she could otherwise not afford, without properly considering the risks involved. The opportunity for "free health care" may coerce the individual to participate in a study he or she would not otherwise choose. In such an instance, the individual's autonomy is impaired. Investigators could attempt to protect such individuals by providing the choice of no-cost standard medical care without research participation to individuals. Or, when the research involves a substantive amount of risk to the individual with little possibility of benefit, financially vulnerable individuals might be excluded from participation.

## Right to Withdraw Without Loss of Benefits

The voluntary nature of participation in research should be guaranteed not only at the onset of the project, but throughout the length of participation. An individual cannot give truly voluntary consent if his or her welfare might be jeopardized by refusal to participate in a research study, or if an individual's decision regarding continuing consent to participation is influenced by the possibility of a loss of future benefits if he or she does not continue to participate. The participant should be assured that there will be no retaliation by the investigator, staff, or institution should the individual decide to end participation in a research project.

## The Right to Full Disclosure of Information About Research: Deception Research

In some cases, deception of participants may be the only means possible to obtain valid data. This is often the case in research that is meant to observe individuals in their natural state. The Milgram study discussed earlier is a classic example of deception research. Regardless of the type or level of deception involved with a study, researchers must still respect the individual's right to informed consent. The IRB may grant a waiver of consent to conduct the study, but that waiver may be temporary. The use of deception merely suspends the right to informed consent; it does not obviate it (20). At the earliest possible opportunity consistent with the conduct of the research, the true details of the study should be disclosed to the participant. Additionally, the participant should be allowed to exercise autonomy in deciding whether to allow his individual data to be used in the project (21). Doing so, shows respect for the principles of the *Belmont Report* without prohibiting the conduct of deception research altogether.

Furthermore, undergoing a "debriefing" process at the end of participation fulfills the fourth criterion of a waiver of informed consent: "the subjects will be provided with additional pertinent information after participation." Deception research covers a wide range of research activities, from observation of public activities to sham surgery. Obviously, the

spectrum of risks and benefits involved is just as varied.

### Tissue Ownership Rights

The development of genetic research and especially the use of stem cell lines has resulted in a claim by some that individuals have a right to ownership of their donated tissues. As of now, this is still an area of developing law and regulation.

## THE FEDERAL REGULATIONS

As noted earlier, the federal regulations, as articulated under 45-CFR-46 and 21 CFR 50 and 56 et al., govern clinical research sponsored by the federal government.

### Responsible Conduct of Research

Ideally, the responsible conduct of research should best be considered as human participant research that is conducted by appropriately qualified, skilled, knowledgeable, idealistic, altruistic, ethical, compassionate, just, and unbiased physician-investigators, for whom the rights and welfare of research participants supersede the interests of science and society, yet who are committed to research that is worthwhile from both the humanitarian and scientific perspectives, and to appropriate, honest, meticulous, unbiased interpretation of that research (4,8). *Responsible Conduct of Research* is also a specific USPHS policy promulgated by the Office of Research Integrity (ORI) in order to establish USPHS policies for education and the responsible conduct of research for staff engaged in investigation. Additional information about regulated aspects of clinical research are addressed elsewhere.

### Good Clinical Practice Guidelines

Government laws, regulations, and guidelines intended to protect the safety and rights of human research participants of research while ensuring the accuracy and validity of data, are collectively represented in the Guidelines for Good Clinical Practice (GCP). GCP guidelines apply to all parties involved in the research process, including pharmaceutical companies and other sponsors of research and their employees and agents, contract review organizations that manage the conduct of clinical trials, IRBs, investigators, research coordinators, research staff, and all others participating in the process of human participant research. GCP guidelines require adherence

> ### TABLE 14–3
>
> ### Criteria for IRB Approval, Based on Federal Regulations at 45-CFR-46 and 21 CFR 50 and 56 et al
>
> (1) Risks to research participants are minimized
> (2) Risks to research participants reasonable in relation to anticipated benefits
> (3) Selection of research participants equitable
> (4) Valid informed consent (unless properly waived)
> (5) Informed consent appropriately documented (unless properly waived)
> (6) When appropriate, data monitoring to ensure safety of research participants
> (7) Protection of privacy and confidentiality of research participants
> (8) Additional protections for vulnerable research participants

to the standards of many accepted, legal, regulatory, and ethical injunctions, and are congruent with the principles of the Declaration of Helsinki.

### Criteria for Approval of Research by IRB

To be approved by an IRB, a research proposal must meet all criteria specified by the Code of Federal Regulations 45-CFR-46.111, which reflect the ethical standards established by the *Belmont Report*. The criteria for approval of research by IRBs are given in Table 14–3. The historical and ethical bases for these regulations have been described in previous sections.

### SUMMARY

- The right to conduct research on an individual is a privilege granted to an investigator by an individual ("participant") who chooses to participate in a research study.
- IRB approval is generally necessary before initiating any clinical activity in which the investigator intends to report the findings to the medical scientific community.
- The standards by which IRBs evaluate human participant research are documented in the Code of Federal Regulations at 45-CFR-46 and 21 CFR, Parts 50, 56, et al.
- The Nuremberg Code, the Helsinki Declaration, and the *Belmont Report* were all important landmark publications that helped define the current ethical bases for conducting human participant research.
- The major ethical principles that permit and govern clinical research practice are respect for persons, beneficence, and justice.

- The principles and practices of autonomy, informed consent, and special protections for vulnerable populations are derived from the principle of the respect for persons.
- The risk–benefit ratio paradigm, the importance of scientific legitimacy of the research, the need for clinical equipoise, and the proper role for placebos in research design are principles derived from the principle of beneficence.
- Care about selection of participants is governed by the principle of justice.
- Conflicts of interest that pertain to clinical research include conflicts applying to the research participant financial, and other personal self-interest conflicts.
- Research participants are afforded certain rights, including a right to the privacy of their medical information, rights that apply to third-party relations to the research participant, the right to have the opportunity to participate in research, the right to expect standard medical treatment during the research study, the right to withdraw without loss of benefits, the right to full disclosure of information related to the research, and possibly to ownership rights related to donated tissues.

In addition to the federal regulations cited above, a set of guidelines known as Good Clinical Practice (see Chapter 15) are meant to ensure the accuracy and validity of data collected during the study.

### REFERENCES

1. Code of Federal Regulations. Title 45A–Department of Health and Human Services; Part 46–Protection of Human Subjects, Updated 1 Oct. 1997. Accessed March 13, 2005. http://www4.law.cornell.edu/cfr/45p46.htm.

2. Code of Federal Regulations. Title 21, Chapter 1-Food and Drug Administration, DHHS; Part 50-Protection of Human Subjects. Updated 1 Apr 1999. Accessed March 13, 2005. http://www4.law.cornell.edu/cfr/21p50htm.

3. National Commission for the Protection of Human Subjects of Biomedical and Behavioral Research. The Belmont Report: Ethical Principles and Guidelines for the Protection of Human Subjects of Research. (DHEW (OS) 78-0013 and (OS) 78-0014.4). Washington DC: U.S. Government Printing Office, April 18, 1979. Accessed March 22, 2001. http://ohsr.od.nih.gov/mpa/belmont.php3

4. Levine R. Ethics and Regulations of Clinical Research, 2nd Ed. 1988. New Haven: Yale University Press.

5. Katz_J. Experimentation with Human Beings. New York: Russell Sage Foundation, 1972.

6. American Medical Association, Council on Ethical and Judicial Affairs; 1992 Code of Medical Ethics-Current Opinions. Chicago: American Medical Association, 1992.

7. Trials of War Criminals before the Nuremberg Military Tribunals under Control Council Law No. 10, Vol. 2. Washington, DC: U.S. Government Printing Office, 1949:181–182.

8. Beecher HK. Ethics and Clinical Research. N Engl J Med 1966;274:1354–1360.

9. PHS Policy on Instruction in the Responsible Conduct of Research (RCR). Office of Research Integrity, U.S. Department of Health and Human Services, Dec. 1, 2000.

10. Freedman B. Equipoise and the ethics of clinical research. N Engl J Med 1987;317:141–145.

11. National Institutes of Health. Conference on Human Subject Protection and Financial Conflicts of Interest, August 15–16, 2000, Transcript.

12. Kassirer JP, Angell M. Financial conflicts of interest in biomedical research N Engl J M 1993;329:570–571.

13. Office for Human Research Protections. Draft interim guidance: Financial relationships in clinical research: issues for institutions, clinical investigators, and IRBs to consider when dealing with issues of financial interest and human subjects protection, January 24. 2001. Accessed April 20, 2001. http://www.hhs.gov/ohrp/nhrpac/mtg12-00/finguid.htm. Accessed March 13, 2005.

14. Code of Federal Regulations. Title 42, Chapter 1-Public Health Service, DHHS; Part 50-Policies of General Applicability. Updated 2001. http://www4.law.cornell.edu/cfr/42p50.htm.

15. Lind SE. Finder's fees for research subjects. N Engl J Med1990;323:192–195.

16. Baxter G. Psychology: Obedience. University of Otago. http://designweb.otago.ac.nz/grant/psyc/OBEDIANCE.HTML. Accessed March 13, 2005.

17. Blass T. www.stanleymilgram.com. Accessed March 13, 2005.

18. Elks ML. The Right to Participate in Research Studies. J Lab Clin Med 1993;122(2):130–136.

19. Epstein S. Impure Science: AIDS, Activism, and the Politics of Knowledge. Berkeley: University of California Press, 1996.

20. Research involving deception. NHMRC Human Research Ethics Handbook: A Research Ethics Collection. June 2001. Updated September 2003.

21. Protecting Human Research Subjects: Institutional Review Board Guidebook. NIH Guide. Edited by Robin Lerin Penslar, in consultation with OPRB and its advisors. Washington, D.C. 1993:22(29).

# CHAPTER 15

# Regulatory Oversight

Mickey Clarke, Denise A. McCartney, Barry A. Siegel

All research projects are subject to oversight at many different levels in the hierarchy of the investigator's institution or health system, as well as oversight by a private or governmental sponsor. Review of a research proposal by the investigator's IRB has been discussed in Chapter 14, so we will not dwell on this process except to say that the intent of the IRB review is to assess the risks and benefits of the proposed research and to ensure the adequacy of informed consent. A requirement for *continuing* review by the IRB is met through submission of periodic reports, annually or more often in some cases, detailing progress, enrollment, and any problems encountered since the last review. A movement to expand the post-IRB-approval review of open research protocols has surfaced in recent years, related to prominent media coverage of grave consequences for human participants in a variety of research projects around the country.

Oversight of a research study does not end, however, with IRB approval. The federal sponsor and the institution impose several additional ethical expectations of any investigator conducting human research. The researcher must conduct research that is free of bias and that generates independent results that are of high quality and are reproducible. The research must be conducted with integrity. There is a need to maintain the confidentiality of the research record to protect volunteer participants. The investigator and the institution should also provide a safe environment in which employees can conduct research and should protect the community in which the institution is located.

The investigator, in addition to protecting volunteers that participate in a research project, is also expected to be a good steward of the federal or private funds awarded to conduct the studies. The investigator's institution may impose policies, in addition to those of the agency or sponsor, which require careful accounting and stewardship of funds awarded for research.

The investigator is also expected to comply with any regulations or institutional policies related to either the conduct of the research or the outcomes of such research. Outcomes may include such arrangements as licensing agreements or patents where the institution may have a vested interest.

When the investigation involves the development of a new drug or device that will be administered to or used to treat humans, the Food and Drug Administration also has authority and oversight over the research through its programs for investigational new drugs and investigational devices. This authority also applies to existing drugs and devices when the researcher seeks to test a new dose regimen of the drug, or to test drug or device efficacy in a new disease state or a new population.

Many of these ethical principles are reinforced or regulated through myriad laws, federal or sponsoring agency regulations, and institutional policies that may seem confusing and daunting to a new clinical investigator (Figure 15–1). However, successful conduct of research requires the willingness of members of the community to volunteer and participate. To recruit sufficient numbers of research volunteers, both the institution and the principal investigator must exhibit standards that inspire the confidence and trust of the public. Adherence to the policies of sponsors and the federal and state regulators is one way to assure members of the public that their trust is well guarded by both the institution and its researchers, and that their rights and welfare will be protected by

The authors wish to thank Tina Tyson and Jane Ditch at Washington University for contributions to the section on Clinical Trials Billing.

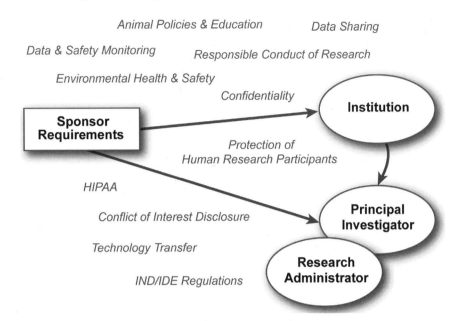

**FIGURE 15–1** ● Some of the many regulatory issues affecting and governing the conduct of clinical research.

both the institution and the individual investigator. Further, failure to adhere to these policies may negatively impact the individual or institution's ability to obtain future funding for research projects.

## REGULATIONS AND POLICIES RELATED TO ETHICAL RESEARCH PRACTICES

Just as the body of research knowledge continuously evolves and changes, so do the regulations and policies governing ethical research practices. All investigators must stay abreast of the changing regulations that apply to their research. Most universities or hospitals develop specific institutional policies that explain the application of regulations to an investigator; working closely with the institution's administration is key to successfully navigating the complex maze of regulations. Due to frequent changes in the regulations (and therefore, in institutional policy), the following sections are not intended to provide specific terms of the regulations but rather to instill a sense of the undertaking necessary to conduct research responsibly. Many sources of information about regulatory oversight are excellent tools to help maintain an awareness of the issues (Table 15–1). Clinical researchers are often involved in multiple research programs that are interrelated and are funded through a variety of federal, private, and institutional sources. An understanding of the regulatory environment is useful regardless of the type of clinical research conducted.

The Department of Health and Human Services (DHHS) is the oversight agency for both the Public Health Service (PHS) and the Food and Drug Administration (FDA). The National Institutes of Health (and its specific institutes) receive their funding through the PHS and in turn award grants and contracts for research of all types. DHHS policy is overarching, but each of the others, PHS, NIH, and FDA, promulgate regulations and guidance related to their specific programs and functions (Table 15–2). Nonfederal agencies and corporate sponsors have their own grant or contract language that informs the researcher of their particular requirements.

### Objectivity in Research

PHS, the FDA, and other federal agencies such as the National Science Foundation (NSF), have promulgated regulations applicable to grantees that are intended to promote objectivity in research (1). PHS explains that its conflict of interest program promotes "objectivity in research by establishing standards to ensure there is no reasonable expectation that the design, conduct, or reporting of research funded by PHS will be biased by any conflicting financial interest of an Investigator" (42 CFR Part 50, Subpart F). This program has come to be known as the "conflict of interest policy." Although the PHS and NSF policies are similar, the specific procedures and compliance requirements vary.

In general, institutions that receive funding from any source covered by the Public Health Service Act

**TABLE 15–1**

**Useful Resources**

| National Institutes of Health | NIH medical and behavioral research grant policies, guidelines, and funding opportunities | http://www.nih.gov |
|---|---|---|
| Food and Drug Administration | General FDA information and policies related to GCP, GMP, and IND/IDE use | http://www.fda.gov |
| National Science Foundation | Policies, guidelines, and funding opportunities through NSF | http://www.nsf.gov |
| Office for Human Research Protections | Oversight of IRBs and human research participant protection regulations | http://www.hhs.gov/ohrp/ |
| Office of Research Integrity | Oversight of mechanism for scientific misconduct investigation and reporting | http://ori.dhhs.gov/ |
| Office of Civil Rights | Oversight of HIPAA and Privacy Rule | http://www.hhs.gov/ocr/hipaa/ |
| Association for Accreditation of Human Research Protection Programs | Voluntary accreditation organization with total research protection program | http://www.aahrpp.org/www.aspx |
| National Committee for Quality Assurance | Organization with multiple quality assurance programs including human protections accreditation in the VA system | http://www.ncqa.org/ |

must have policies in place to determine whether any investigators have financial interests that could influence the direction or outcome of their research efforts. These policies most often describe a process in which investigators (faculty and staff) disclose to an institutional official their financial interests in excess of a prescribed dollar amount. The regulations clearly define the level of financial interest as follows: "anything of monetary value, including but not limited to, salary or other payments for services (e.g., consulting fees or honoraria); equity interests (e.g., stocks, stock options, or other ownership interests); and intellectual property rights (e.g., patents, copyrights, and royalties from such rights) in excess of $10,000." The institutional official then determines whether a conflict exists and outlines the process for managing, reducing, or eliminating the interests that might bias the investigator's research (http://grants2.nih.gov/grants/guide/notice-files/not95-179.html). In addition to the federal regulations, policies at state institutions may also need to reflect state law. Institutions may also develop policies and management strategies directed at reducing the *appearance* of conflict, as well as actual conflicts. These institutional policies, for instance, may extend the requirements

for disclosure of financial interest to all federally funded research or even to all research projects. Incidents where apparent financial conflicts of interests potentially affected the outcome of research and the safety of human research participants have heightened the sensitivity of many institutions to these issues. A case in point is the death of Jesse Gelsinger in 1999 after his participation in a gene therapy trial where the principal investigator had a financial interest in the company sponsoring the trial (see http://msnbc.msn.com/id/4962216/).

The PHS and NSF regulations describe their specific agency's requirements for reporting conflicts to their central grant management officers. Regulations also require continued reporting throughout the grant award period to assure PHS and NSF that the conflicts are being appropriately managed. Any new disclosures are to be reported to the agency within 60 days.

A chart outlining the sequence of events surrounding disclosure and management of a significant conflict is provided as Figure 15–2. As the chart indicates, conflicts can be managed in a variety of ways. It is important to note that the PHS policy extends to subcontractors and consortium

## TABLE 15-2

### Key Federal Regulations Affecting Clinical Research

| Regulation | Source | Requirement |
|---|---|---|
| Confidentiality | NIH Guidelines and Section 301(d) of the PHS Act | Protects the confidentiality of subjects participating in research. |
| Data Monitoring and Safety | 45 CRF 46:11(a)(6) | When appropriate, the research plan makes adequate provision for monitoring the data collected to ensure the safety of subjects. |
| Debarment and Suspension | 45CFR Part 76 | Investigators and key personnel must not be debarred or inelegible from covered federal transaction. This includes being convicted of or had a civil judgment for certain types of fraud, falsification, theft, or other crimes. |
| Education in the protection of Human Research Participants | NIH policy notice: NOT-OD-01-061 | All key personnel are required to complete training in the protection of human participants. |
| Radioactive Drug Use in Research | 21 CFR 361.1 | Requirements for radioactive drugs administered to human research subjects. |
| Research on Human Fetal Tissue | 45 CFR 46.208(a)(2) and subsection 498 (a) and (b) http://grants.nih.gov/grants/guide/notice-files/not93-235.html. State and local laws | Specific NIH guidelines describing compliance with federal requirements. |
| Research Using Human Embryonic Stem Cells | President's Policy Statement, August 9, 2001. NIH Notice: NOT-OD-02-005 | Federally funded research using human pluripotent stem cells is funded from federal sources only under specifically described circumstances. |
| Ban on Human Embryo Research and Cloning | P.L. 105-78 Section 513 | No NIH funds may be used to support human embryo research or for cloning of human beings. |

participants. The subcontract or consortium agreement must specify whether the subcontractor employees will be subject to the policies of the principal investigator's institution or those of their own institution.

Both the investigator and the institution have responsibilities to ensure appropriate protection of humans whenever a potential conflict of interest is identified. Research volunteers might not be aware that an investigator has a significant financial conflict of interest that might affect the research study unless specifically told through the informed consent process. In May 2004, the secretary of the Department of Health and Human Services issued a final guidance document called "Financial Relationships and Interests in Research Involving Human Subjects: Guidance for Human Subject Protection." Although the document is nonbinding and does not change any existing regulations or requirements, the guidance has important implications for institutions and investigators. The complete text of the guidance document may be found at: http://www.hhs.gov/ohrp/humansubjects/finreltn/fguid.pdf.

In addition to an individual investigator's conflicts of interest, the institution itself may also have conflicts of interest that potentially impact the safety of human research participants. Institutional conflicts of interests arise when the financial interests of

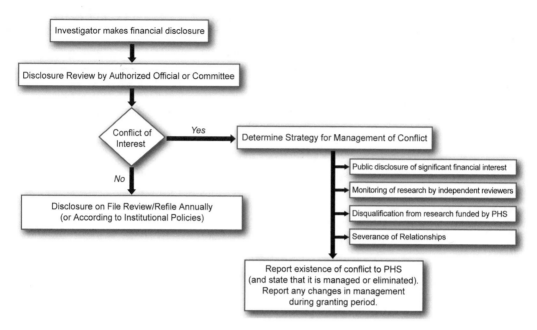

**FIGURE 15–2** ● A common scheme for managing conflicts of interest by investigators.

the institution or of an institutional official may affect or may appear to affect the oversight of human participant research. Although no regulations currently exist, guidelines have been published by a variety of professional associations to help institutions manage such conflicts. The associations include the American Association of Universities (see http://www.aau.edu/research/COI.01.pdf), and the Association of American Medical Colleges (http://www.aamc.org/members/coitf/start.htm). As with many issues affecting clinical research, the information, guidance and regulations may change in the future.

### Research Integrity

As recently as 2002, the Institute of Medicine's Committee on Assessing Integrity in Research Environments felt a need to publish its book, *Integrity in Scientific Research: Creating an Environment That Promotes Responsible Conduct*. This publication occurred despite the fact that institutions receiving federal research funding have been required since 1990 to provide assurances of processes for scientific misconduct investigation and management. Clearly, the process of ensuring integrity in research has not been a given.

The public expects that scientific investigations will be of high quality, verifiable, and reproducible. The grantee institution is responsible for fostering a culture of striving to meet that expectation.

Investigators are also responsible for fostering this culture in their laboratories and among their colleagues and trainees. Because ethical conduct is the expectation but sometimes not the reality, the federal government, on behalf of its granting agencies, enacted regulation in 1990 that requires institutions to have written policies and procedures surrounding allegations of scientific misconduct. At that time, DHHS and the NSF each issued definitions of scientific misconduct that include fabrication, falsification, and plagiarism. The NSF also included a prohibition of retaliation against any person who reports or provides information about alleged misconduct.

The definitions of both agencies were superseded in December 2000 by publication of the Federal Policy on Research Misconduct issued by the Office of Science and Technology Policy (OSTP) (Federal Register Vol. 65, No 235: 76260-76264). The new policy retained the fabrication, falsification, and plagiarism basics and defined each action. It also described the requirements for procedures necessary to reach a finding of scientific misconduct. PHS added a policy to prohibit retaliation against any person who reports allegations of misconduct.

The procedures involve an initial inquiry into the substance of the allegations, a formal investigation of allegations deemed substantive, and an adjudication process where recommendations for sanctions or corrective actions are imposed. If allegations are deemed substantive, they must be reported to any granting agency that has funded the investigator in question. When the institution has completed its investigation, the findings and actions are reported to the agency. Agencies may accept the institution findings and sanctions, but may also initiate an agency-level investigation and may impose additional sanctions if they are felt to be warranted.

The 2000 OSTP policy is subject to discussion and disagreement related to the definitions of misconduct and to the procedure outlined for reaching a finding of misconduct. Scientists differ in their interpretations of statements such as "significant departure from accepted practices of the scientific community." Many comments were received during the comment period after initial publication of the proposed policy. OSTP reviewed all comments, acted on some, and acknowledged shortcomings pointed out in others. Ultimately, federal agencies were asked to implement the policy within a year.

Research institutions receiving federal funds are required to adopt a formal policy (and procedures) regarding misconduct in science. Most follow the OSTP policy and adopt its definitions of fabrication, falsification, and plagiarism. Some institutions have expanded their policies related to the conduct of researchers. Such expansions include policies related to authorship, academic misconduct, or questionable research practices. Additional guidelines that may be imposed by research or academic institutions relate to data management, violation of generally accepted research practices, misappropriation of funds, abuse of confidentiality, publication and dissemination, maintenance of records, and investigators' roles and responsibilities.

## DATA SHARING

The continued advancement of scientific endeavors depends on researchers sharing data. The ability to reproduce results in additional laboratories raises the confidence level regarding original outcomes. To that end, major granting agencies have developed policies pertaining to the sharing of research data by those awarded funding. Both the NIH and the NSF have published their guidelines related to data sharing.

The NSF policy on the dissemination and sharing of research results is available on its website in section 734 of the Grants Policy Manual dated July 2002. The policy states that investigators are expected to publish results of their work promptly and with recognition of all those who participated in the project. It goes on to say that primary data, samples, physical collections, and other supporting materials should be made available to other researchers at no more than minimal cost. Although NSF investigators retain principal legal rights to their intellectual property, NSF states that this does not "reduce the responsibility that investigators and organizations have as members of the scientific and engineering community, to make results, data and collections available to other researchers" (NSF GPM 2002).

The final NIH "Statement On Sharing Research Data" was issued on February 26, 2003 and became effective on October 1, 2003 (http://grants.nih.gov/grants/guide/notice-files/NOT-OD-03-032.html). The NIH has adopted a policy similar to that of the NSF. Currently, an additional requirement of the NIH involves inclusion of a data-sharing plan in any grant submission that requests more than $500,000 in direct costs in any grant year. This requirement for a data-sharing plan may also be included in specific program announcements for applications that request fewer dollars.

The brochure entitled "NIH Data Sharing Policy" may be downloaded from the NIH website at http://grants1.nih.gov/grants/policy/data_sharing/. It contains information that will be helpful to investigators as they prepare applications that must include data-sharing plans. It also elaborates on the NIH position that data should be made available to the scientific community as well as methods for sharing data, addressing privacy concerns, and the time frame for making data available.

## Intellectual Property, Technology Transfer, and Licensing

The creation of new information as a result of the research endeavor may take a variety of forms including new processes or procedures, biomaterials (e.g., animals, plants, cell lines, DNA), or computer software. The legal definition of intellectual property includes patents, licenses, trademarks, and proprietary matters. As long ago as 1945, the foundations were being laid for transfer of intellectual property and technology from research and academic institutions to the public domain. The report, "Science: The Endless Frontier," by Vannevar Bush, Director of the Office of Scientific Research and Development, to President Franklin D. Roosevelt outlined the need for continuation of the knowledge development and transfer that had its roots in the search for medical and technologic superiority during the war years. Bush's report stimulated the founding and allocation of funds to the NIH, the NSF, and the Office of Naval Research.

This activity was codified, however, only in 1990 with the passage of the Bayh-Dole Act (P.L. 96-517, The Patent and Trademark Law Amendment Act).

This legislation is intended to provide incentives for the prompt transfer of new technology and new material to the public arena. Grantees must comply with regulations to ensure timely transfer of new technology; in return, the rights of the institution are protected as well as those of the federal government. Through a series of timed agreements and disclosures, institutions and their investigators tell the grantor of any new technology or patentable invention created using grant funds. Compliance with the timetable allows the institution the right to maintain patent rights and to set in place appropriate licenses for public dissemination of the material. Failure to comply with the timetable of disclosure results in the institution's loss of patent and licensing rights.

Clinical researchers may find that they are affected by regulations and policies governing intellectual property in a number of different ways. Examples include, but are not limited to, the following. (1) Conflicts of interests may arise if the investigator has a financial interest resulting from the commercialization of his intellectual property and is still conducting research involving human subjects. (2) Investigators are often asked and are willing to share biomaterial with collaborators at other institutions. Material transfer agreements govern the transfer of such materials and may involve intellectual property rights as well as other requirements for the use of the materials. (3) The investigator's right to publish may be restricted in certain contractual situations.

## HEALTH AND SAFETY ISSUES

Many of the previous comments have been directed toward regulations and ethical expectations that protect human subjects. This section explores the health and safety issues that might arise in certain types of clinical research. In addition to protecting human research participants, the investigator is also responsible for providing a working environment that minimizes the potential for injury or illness to other researchers, staff, and members of the community in which the institution is located.

In addition, many regulations exist that promote the safety of the environment, the appropriate use of hazardous materials, and the handling and transfer of radioactive materials. Many agencies are involved in overseeing these activities, including the Environmental Protection Agency (EPA), the Occupational Safety and Health Administration (OSHA), the NIH, and the Nuclear Regulatory Commission (NRC). These regulations are too numerous to cite but it is important to understand some of the key issues that affect clinical research (Table 15–2). It is also important to note that investigators are subject not only to federal laws and regulations but also to those of state and local agencies.

The possession and use of radioactive materials is carefully controlled by the NRC and comparable state agencies. Various FDA regulations additionally govern the administration to human research participants of radioactive drugs. Institutions are obligated to comply with the standards and regulations published by the NRC and to ensure the safety of human research participants and employees involved in the research. In addition to careful review of the research protocols using such materials by institutional committees and the IRB, the investigator and staff are carefully evaluated for the appropriate qualifications necessary for the use of such materials. Rigorous training requirements are also required for individuals using radioactive materials.

Following the events of September 11, 2001, laws and regulations governing the use of certain select agents and toxins were tightened. The Public Health Security and Bioterrorism Preparedness and Response Act was designed to provide protection against the misuse of select agents and toxins. The Centers for Disease Control and Prevention (CDC) plays an important role in the oversight of this law. Additionally, the US Patriot Act provides criminal penalties for the possession of biological agents or toxins not justifiably used in research or other peaceful purposes. Investigators must work closely with institutional officials when conducting research of this nature.

The NIH Guidelines for Research Involving Recombinant DNA Molecules apply to all research projects that involve recombinant DNA and are conducted at or sponsored by an organization that receives NIH support (http://www4.od.nih.gov/oba/rac/guidelines/guidelines.html). In addition to the NIH guidelines, DNA research is also subject to certain CDC and US Department of Agriculture (USDA) regulations. The NIH guidelines fully describe the compliance requirements for this type of research but two specific issues need the attention of clinical researchers. First, all research projects of this nature must be reviewed by an institutional biosafety committee (IBC) for compliance with the above guidelines. This review is in addition to the review conducted by the IRB. Secondly, all adverse events must be reported to the NIH's Office of Biotechnology Activities (OBA), and the IBC as well as the IRB.

Investigators also need to be aware of the regulations governing employee exposure to blood-borne pathogens, occupational exposure to hazardous chemicals in laboratories, and other occupational health safety standards.

## OVERSIGHT OF CERTAIN SPECIALIZED RESEARCH

The discussion of research oversight in this chapter has focused mainly on requirements that apply to all funded research. In addition to the general requirements, certain specialized types of research have their own unique oversight and regulatory requirements.

### Radioactive Drugs

FDA regulations at 21 CFR 361.1 entitled "Prescription Drugs For Human Use Generally Recognized as Safe and Effective and Not Misbranded: Drugs Used In Research" provide a mechanism that allows the use of radioactive drugs in human research under certain specific conditions. The use of radioactive drugs in human research that meet these specific conditions can be performed without an FDA-approved new drug application or an FDA-accepted investigational new drug (IND) exemption. Among the conditions specified at 21 CFR 361.1 is the requirement that each research project be approved and monitored by a radioactive drug research committee (RDRC) that is itself approved by the FDA.

When research involves the use of radioactive drugs, the RDRC as well as the IRB must review the protocol. The RDRC reviews the scientific merit of the proposed research, the methods of preparation and quality assurance of the radioactive drug, the potential for pharmacologic effects, and the estimated radiation dosimetry, as well as the consent form. The scientific merit is reviewed in light of the radiation exposure to the research participants; that is, does the knowledge gained as a result of the research outweigh the risks to the research participants from radiation exposure? The consent form must explain the radiation exposure to the research participant in terms that can be easily understood. The statistical nature of the risk of radiation exposure is not an easy concept to explain to a layperson; however, models can be used to attempt to explain exposure in terms that the participant population can understand (2).

In addition, the investigator using radioactive drugs must meet training requirements for handling and safety (both for the investigator and his or her staff, as well as for the participants) that can be specified by the RDRC or by the radiation safety committee of the institution.

### Centers for Specialized Research

Many institutes of the NIH and other granting agencies fund specialized centers of research. These centers may deal with a specific disease or organ system, or may support research in an institution by funding research activity in a generalized way. Two that are most well known are the Designated Cancer Centers of the National Cancer Institute and the General Clinical Research Center Program.

The NCI-designated cancer centers conduct multidisciplinary research to reduce the incidence of cancer, as well as the morbidity and mortality attributable to cancer. Cancer-related research at an NCI-designated cancer center is supported by a cancer center support grant and each cancer center has special characteristics and capabilities for research programs. Research funded by an NCI cancer center support grant must be conducted in accordance with the specific terms and conditions of its notice of grant award. One of these is the establishment of a protocol review and monitoring system for cancer-related clinical trials performed at the institution. There is often an additional level of research review, prior to or concurrent with the IRB review of a proposal. The cancer center may impose additional scientific review and requirements on an investigator. There also may be a monitoring program for all open cancer studies that reviews research records and results in ongoing trials.

The National Center for Research Resources states that it has a unique responsibility at the NIH to "develop critical research technologies and provide cost-effective, multi-disciplinary resources to biomedical investigators." The General Clinical Research Center (GCRC) program is a research resource program that is funded to provide "optimal settings for medical investigators to conduct safe, controlled, state-of-the-art, in-patient and outpatient studies of both children and adults." (See NCRR website at http://www.ncrr.nih.gov/.) Each GCRC is developed and based on the host institution's strengths and needs. The centers' resources include laboratories, research personnel, and inpatient/outpatient facilities. Investigators are eligible to apply for access to the GCRC facilities if they have research funding from the NIH or other peer-reviewed sources. As part of the program, their research protocols are reviewed by the board of the facility. In addition, monitoring of open protocols for adherence to regulations and patient safety is a mandated activity of the GCRC. All of the federal regulations discussed in this chapter apply to research conducted in the GCRC. The host institution's policies and procedures are also applicable. In addition, the GCRC requires the appointment of a research subject advocate whose purpose is to maximize patient safety as detailed in the approved IRB protocols.

## STEM CELL RESEARCH

On August 9, 2001, President George W. Bush announced that federal funds may be awarded for research using human embryonic stem cells if the following conditions are met:

- The derivation process was initiated prior to August 9, 2001.
- The stem cells were derived from an embryo created for reproductive purposes and are no longer needed.
- Informed consent for the donation of the embryo was obtained and no financial inducements were used.

If these conditions are not met, research conducted with direct or indirect federal funds is not allowed. The restriction on the use of indirect federal funds means that no equipment or facilities that are federally supported may be used for research on unapproved stem cell lines. For this reason, many institutions have developed internal policies and procedures to oversee and monitor the use of stem cells in research. An investigator using human embryonic stem cells is still required to comply with all other regulations, policies, and procedures pertinent to the specific research projects; examples of such other regulations are discussed throughout this chapter. If interested in conducting research using human embryonic research, the investigator is urged to review the relevant NIH website (http://stemcells.nih.gov/index.asp) which contains a great deal of information on this topic. This website includes the federal policy, the stem cell lines available for federal support, and a frequently asked questions section. As this chapter has frequently stated, the interested investigator is urged to consult with appropriate local university officials and offices.

## RIGHTS, WELFARE, AND PROTECTION OF HUMAN SUBJECTS

A number of regulations govern the rights, welfare, and protection of human research participants not described in the above sections. Frequently, these regulations apply only to investigators involved in some more specialized areas of research. These regulations have been developed to ensure that investigators who conduct certain types of research use specific precautions for the protection of human research participants. The NIH Grants Policy Statement has an excellent summary of these issues in the chapter titled "Public Policy Requirements and Objectives." In addition, several institutes of the NIH and other agencies have sets of regulations targeted to specific areas of research.

The institution is responsible for policies and procedures that ensure compliance with these policy requirements. Some of the key policies have been discussed in some depth. This list may no longer be complete by the time of publication of this textbook, so communication with the local IRB, sponsored research office, or institutional official is essential. It is also important to review the specific regulations and policies of any funding source. It is just as important to read the terms of the award, contract or research agreement to identify specific issues requiring investigator compliance. Much of the focus in this section has been on the NIH but other sponsors may have different policies. Published FDA regulations for research are more closely examined in a later section of this chapter.

## HIPAA

The Health Insurance Portability and Accountability Act of 1996 (HIPAA) and the regulations in the act related to the privacy of health information and its transmission caused great consternation in the medical research community. The act was passed in 1996 and the regulations related to the act were revealed slowly to the medical and research community, with the first regulations taking force only as of April 14, 2003.

These regulations, commonly known as the Privacy Rule, concern "protected health information" (PHI) and the care that must surround the use of this information. PHI includes information about patients that is transmitted by electronic media; maintained in any electronic media; or transmitted or maintained in any other form or medium. The Privacy Rule enumerates a list of 18 elements that are considered PHI. The elements include the expected name, address, date of birth, and social security number, but in addition includes such items as e-mail address, vehicle identification numbers, IP addresses, and telephone and fax numbers. The rule also established the conditions under which entities covered by the rule may disclose PHI to outside entities for any reason, including research.

Although some researchers will not be covered, most, in fact, will be subject to HIPAA and the Privacy Rule. The entities covered under the rule are defined as (1) health care plans; (2) health care clearinghouses; and (3) health are providers who electronically transmit any health care information in connection with transactions for which HHS has adopted standards. Thus, any researcher who works for a hospital or an academic medical center is subject to the Privacy Rule.

Obviously researchers will need access to, or may create, PHI during the course of a medical research project involving human research volunteers. Because the Privacy Rule supersedes any regulations in place related to health information (unless these are more stringent than the rule), researchers will need to be informed about the rule and how their particular institution has opted to handle this new layer of regulation in the research arena.

The second wave of HIPAA regulations became effective April 1, 2005. These regulations deal with the security of "electronic protected health information" or EPHI. The same diligence must be observed with electronic forms of data that is exercised with written records. The security of electronic data, however, is more problematic and specific policies and processes will need to be developed to meet the intent of these new regulations.

The NIH website provides information regarding how research may be affected by the Privacy Rule. It has frequently asked questions, and a useful booklet entitled "Protecting Personal Health Information in Research: Understanding the HIPAA Privacy Rule." Enforcement of the Privacy Rule is in the Office for Civil Rights in DHHS. More information will be found at that website (http://www.hhs.gov/ocr/hipaa/).

Finally, it should be noted that the HIPAA regulations may have similarities to the regulations governing the protection of research participants, but both sets of guidelines are in effect. Consultation with the institutional IRB about these complex issues is recommended prior to the submission of the first research protocol.

## FINANCIAL STEWARDSHIP

Investigators are often awarded large sums of public or industry funds to conduct research to develop new knowledge, develop new clinical procedures, or assess best practices. Appropriate stewardship of these funds is an investigator responsibility, a requirement of all institutions, and is regulated by a number of federal and sponsoring agency statements. The regulations regarding the appropriate use of federal funds are primarily designed to establish the "principles for determining costs applicable to grants, contracts and other agreements." Federal funds are regulated by the Office of Management and Budget (OMB) in accordance with OMB Circular A-21, which describes in detail the principles governing the budgeting and expenditure of federal funds. The principles in Circular A-21 are applicable to all costs necessary to conduct federal research, including but not limited to compensation and benefits of the investigator and key personnel designing, conducting, or reporting the research; the purchase of equipment, supplies, and material necessary for the research; the costs of clinical services; the administrative or overhead costs incurred during the conduct of the research; and much

more. In addition, the principles often require that the costs be reasonable, allocable to the project being charged, and allowable under the agency or circular guidelines (e.g., an expenditure for alcoholic beverages is not an allowable charge to a federal grant or contract). Particular attention should be paid to the salary and fringes charged to research funding in relation to the actual work expended on the project. Most institutions publish detailed policies describing the rules governing the expenditures of federal funds. Institutions may also publish policies for the acquisition of equipment, supplies, materials, or other resources necessary to conduct the research.

Regardless of the source of funds, the budget for the research program should appropriately reflect the program's scope (Chapter 17). The budget becomes an important tool in either the application for federal funds or the negotiation of a contract with industry sponsors. Once the investigator accepts the award or contract from the sponsoring agency, he or she is responsible for meeting the terms and conditions of the award. In addition to the appropriate expenditure of funds, investigators are obligated to demonstrate that the funds expended meet the goals and aims of the research project. This may include producing progress reports, financial expenditure reports, or other sponsor-specific requirements. Frequently, the institution has obligations as well, such as assuring the various agencies that compliance with the many regulations has been met during the research project period. Many institutions therefore, have implemented policies, procedures, and monitoring programs to assess compliance in the form of audits or reviews of the financial management of the research program funds.

## CLINICAL TRIALS BILLING

One of the unique aspects of conducting clinical trial research is the frequent overlap between research and patient care activities. This is clearly evident in the regulations and policies governing billing for services, tests, or other charges incurred during a clinical trial study. Increasingly, investigators conducting clinical trials research are asked by their potential sponsors to consider building into their budgets coverage for the costs of routine or standard-of-care items or services. This is in part due to a Medicare national coverage policy effective for items and services furnished on or after September 19, 2000. At that time, the Center for Medicare and Medicaid Services (CMS) issued a National Coverage Determination (NCD) on Medicare Coverage for Clinical Trials. The NCD essentially states that Medicare will cover the "routine costs" of qualifying clinical trials as well as reasonable and necessary items and services used to diagnose and treat complications arising from participation in all clinical trials. Although this sounds rather straightforward, in actuality an investigator should review important considerations when designing a clinical study with a budget that includes billing to any third-party payer.

First, any clinical trial receiving Medicare coverage of routine costs must meet the following three requirements:

1. The subject or purpose of the research must be the evaluation of an item or service that falls within a Medicare benefit category such as physician's service, diagnostic testing, or durable medical equipment and is not statutorily excluded from coverage (e.g., cosmetic surgery, hearing aids).
2. The research must have therapeutic intent and must not be designed exclusively to test toxicity or disease pathophysiology.
3. Studies must enroll patients with diagnosed disease rather than healthy volunteers although trials of diagnostic interventions may enroll healthy patients in order to have a proper control group.

In addition, the following desirable characteristics should also be included in order to qualify for Medicare coverage:

1. The principal purpose of the study is to test whether the intervention potentially improves the participants' health outcomes.
2. The study is well supported by available scientific and medical information or it is intended to clarify or establish the health outcomes of interventions already in common clinical use.
3. The study does not unjustifiably duplicate existing studies.
4. The study design is appropriate to answer the research question being asked.
5. The study is sponsored by a credible organization or individual capable of executing the trial successfully.
6. The study is in compliance with federal regulations relating to the protection of human research participants.
7. All aspects of the study are conducted according to the appropriate standards of scientific integrity.

Thus, in general, most translational research (which is the focus of this book) does *not* qualify for coverage under these requirements, and therefore Medicare can not and *should* not be billed for routine care costs. Because this subject is still evolving and, as yet, there is relatively little experience with compliance, investigators are urged to seek guidance from the local institution about their process for enrolling the trial in the Medicare clinical trials registry.

The above statements are applicable to Medicare charges. Investigators may also want to work with the billing offices at their institutions to understand the specific policies and practices of non-Medicare third-party payers. Investigators should understand that differentiation of standard-of-care costs and the investigational costs are critically important at the time of the budget preparation and during the research itself regardless of the payor. Failure to identify these costs appropriately could result in the institution inappropriately billing Medicare or other third-party payors for costs that should have been charged to the research project. These types of inappropriate billings may result in serious findings and penalties for both the institution and the investigator.

In addition, the investigator should be aware that some third-party payors may cover the routine costs of care for patients enrolled in clinical research while others may deny all claims as a matter of practice. The practices of various payors differ substantially from region to region and even between institutions in the same region. Understanding the billing procedures at the institution or institutions where the research is to be conducted is important. Denials may increase the patient's out-of-pocket expenses, such as deductibles or copays. The investigator should also consider the risks to a patient's confidentiality for participating in a research project that includes billings to a third-party payor. The investigator should disclose pertinent financial and confidentiality risks in the informed consent process.

Clearly, billing for items and services in clinical research is a complex activity requiring the cooperation, oversight, and monitoring of the investigator, the IRB, the institution's billing office, and billing compliance office. The investigator should communicate early and often with these and other offices described by the institution in order to best protect the research participant, the institution, and the investigator. If done well, appropriate billing requires careful attention to detail, policy, regulations, and documentation.

## INSTITUTIONAL POLICIES

The publication of federal or sponsoring agency regulations often requires the development of institutional policies that clarify the responsibilities of the investigator, key research staff, and the responsibilities of the organizational offices charged with oversight and monitoring of the compliance with the regulations and institutional policies. It is not unusual for the institutional policies to extend the applicability of federal or sponsoring agency regulations to other funding sources. Such practices, for instance, were cited earlier in this chapter for the conflict of interest policies; institutions often require human participant protection education for all researchers using human participants regardless of the source of funds. Accessing the institution's policies, procedures, forms, and educational opportunities provide essential help in complying with regulations and polices that impact the investigator's ability to conduct research ethically and responsibly at each institution.

## OVERSIGHT AND ENFORCEMENT

Investigators are entrusted by both their institutions and their sponsors to conduct their research ethically, protect their participants, and meet regulatory and sponsor obligations. However, because of the large sums of money funding research, the risks of research conducted using human participants and recent problems at academic institutions, significant oversight and enforcement mechanisms are now in place to ensure compliance. Some of these mechanisms are external, but frequently they are institutional. Several examples of these mechanisms are explored in this section.

### Institutional Oversight

One mechanism most institutions have in place to provide institutional oversight is the publication of policies and procedures. As mentioned throughout this chapter, an institution typically publishes policies and procedures that provide key information about how to meet the obligations of sponsors, regulations, and institutional polices but also to explain the roles and responsibilities of investigators, key research team members, and institutional officials or offices. Many of these policies also define the imposition of sanctions when these obligations are not met. Recently, many institutions developed and implemented compliance programs that provide educational programs about policies and regulations, conduct monitoring of research programs and documentation, publish codes of conduct, and investigate allegations of wrongdoing. In many cases, an institution may have an internal audit department that reviews financial expenditures or conducts other compliance reviews. These institutional compliance efforts are intended to help the investigator demonstrate that internal policies, sponsor regulations, and federal, state, and local laws are met during the execution of research programs.

### External Oversight

Federal granting agencies are required to audit grant transactions of the organization. Frequently conducted by an external auditor hired by the institution, these audits are focused primarily on financial information, and assess whether management and controls are appropriate and in compliance with federal laws and regulations. Audits of federal grants may also be conducted by each agency's inspector general, by the institution's cognizant audit agency (e.g., DHHS), or by the General Accounting Office (GAO), which functions as the audit, evaluation, and investigative arm of Congress. These groups may review and audit any aspect of the management of federal awards; a recent GAO review focused on how academic institutions were meeting the conflict of interest requirements cited in an earlier section of this chapter. The Office for Human Research Protections (OHRP) has a compliance oversight process that monitors the quality of review conducted by IRBs at institutions that hold a federal wide assurance.

The FDA also performs audits and on-site inspections of research conducted under the regulations regarding Good Clinical Practice and Clinical Trials. It has an extensive monitoring program and clearly defined mechanisms for handling and reporting instances of noncompliance. Careful review of the website outlining these issues (http://www.fda.gov/oc/gcp/regulations.html) is strongly recommended for anyone conducting FDA-regulated research. For those investigators conducting research sponsored by private industry, in-depth monitoring by the company is also standard operating procedure. The sponsor's responsibility to meet the FDA requirements may result in on-site visits and audits of documentation of the investigator's compliance with regulatory statutes. Any audit may result in the need to take corrective actions or the imposition of sanctions.

In addition to audits, agencies such as the NIH are now taking more proactive roles in reviewing and assessing the compliance of recipient institutions and investigators. These site visits may involve conversations with investigators on myriad compliance and regulatory issues. The Office for Human

Research Protections, in addition to their compliance oversight process, has a self-assessment process that an institution can use to measure its compliance with federal policies.

## Accreditation Programs

Investigators conducting research at hospitals may be familiar with the Joint Commission on the Accreditation of Healthcare Organizations (JCAHO). Although not involved directly in the research endeavor, JCAHO accreditation may impact the conduct of research on patients in an accredited health care organization. Two relatively new organizations now provide voluntary accreditation programs that recognize excellence in protecting human research volunteers. The Association for the Accreditation of Human Research Protection Programs (AAHRPP) and the National Committee for Quality Assurance (NCQA) for VA medical centers are now conducting accreditation reviews.

## Sanctions

An understanding of the oversight and enforcement activities associated with conducting clinical research is essential. Any audit may result in the need for corrective actions on the part of the institution or investigator. Demonstrated failures to comply with the regulations governing research can have serious consequences. Depending on the type and seriousness of the compliance failure, the institution and the individual may face serious sanctions and penalties. An investigator or member of the research staff might face termination of employment under specific circumstances. A sponsoring agency may decide to suspend research funds. An institution could see its right to review and approve human research protocols revoked, thereby eliminating all investigators' opportunity to conduct research involving human participants. In the worst scenario, monetary or criminal penalties may be imposed on either the institution or the individual investigator. Although not considered a sanction, the actions that led to a failure of compliance, the investigation of that failure and the sanctions and penalties may be discussed in the public news media. Universities, hospitals, and similar organizations obviously eschew such adverse publicity.

The best way to avoid such sanctions is to understand the regulations, the institutional policies, and procedures, and to work closely with agency and institutional officials to conduct research ethically, responsibly and in accordance with laws, regulations, and policies.

## SUMMARY

- The outcomes of clinical research may have significant impact on the body of clinical knowledge available to medical practitioners. For this reason, clinical investigators have an obligation and a responsibility to conduct research ethically in order to maintain the trust of the patient, the public, the sponsoring agencies, and the institution for which they work.
- Regulations change frequently and circumstances drive new regulations. It is thus incumbent on clinical investigators to adopt practices that will help maintain an awareness of the issues and regulations that impact their research programs, including the development of relationships with scientific and program staff from the institutions sponsoring the research.
- To maintain objectivity in research, conflicts of interest should be declared and avoided when possible.
- The key forms of scientific misconduct include fabrication, falsification, and plagiarism.
- NIH-sponsored projects requiring more than $500,000/yr in direct costs must specify a data-sharing plan.
- Intellectual property regulations may affect the sharing of biomaterials with investigators at other institutions; in other situations, a sponsor's right to intellectual property might restrict an investigator's right to publish.
- The investigator is responsible for providing a working environment that minimizes the potential for injury or illness to other researchers or staff.
- The investigator is responsible for safeguarding "protected health information" under the Health Insurance Portability and Accountability Act (HIPAA) that might be generated during a clinical research study.
- The investigator is responsible for financial stewardship of funds granted to perform clinical research by either government or private sponsors.

## REFERENCES

1. Task Force on Financial Conflicts of Interest in Clinical Research. Protecting Subjects, Preserving Trust, Promoting Progress II: Principles and Recommendations for Oversight of an Institution's Financial Interests in Human Subjects Research AAMC. October 22, 2002.
2. Castronovo FP Jr. An attempt to standardize the radiodiagnostic risk statement in an Institutional Review Board consent form. Invest Radiol 1993;28:533–538.

# CHAPTER 16

# Funding Clinical Research

Patricia J. Gregory, Theodore J. Cicero

Research costs money—to pay for investigator and staff salaries, for procedures and tests, and for various administrative costs (like IRB review). Thus, grant seeking is a critical skill for any clinical researcher. Although the vast majority of funding for investigator-initiated medical research comes from the NIH, investigators nevertheless have access to a wide array of grant opportunities from other sources, including disease-focused charities, private foundations, professional societies, and sometimes gifts and other sources within their own institutions. This chapter is designed to help the new clinical research scientist learn the steps involved in transitioning from training grant support to long-term research funding.

Fortunately, both federal and private funding opportunities for clinical research have expanded in recent years to encourage more physicians to undertake patient-oriented investigations. In addition to several new grant programs introduced in the mid-1990s, the NIH also offers attractive loan repayment programs, making it possible for physicians who have accumulated substantial educational debt to consider careers in patient-oriented research.

## HOW TO IDENTIFY FUNDING OPPORTUNITIES

A wealth of information about research funding opportunities is available today on the Web, making it easy to narrow a search for the best funding sources (1,2). The NIH maintains an extensive website (http://www.nih.gov) with detailed guidelines for all of its grant programs. Investigators can find competitive grant opportunities offered by all 26 federal grant-making agencies through a single website called Grants.Gov, which was introduced in 2004. Most private funding agencies also maintain websites that guide investigators in the submission of proposals.

Many universities subscribe to fund searching services, such as the Community of Science (COS) or the Sponsored Projects Information Network (SPIN), which allow faculty at a subscribing institution to create customized searches and receive targeted e-mail alerts of relevant funding opportunities.

Investigators working at institutions that do not subscribe to such services still have access to other searchable databases that are free. For example, GrantsNet (http://www.grantsnet.org), which is sponsored by the Howard Hughes Medical Institute and American Association for the Advancement of Science, provides information on funding opportunities in biomedical research and science education, including research funding for graduate and medical students, postdoctoral fellows, and junior faculty (3). Another free service is the Illinois Researcher Information Service (IRIS) (http://carousel.lis.uiuc.edu/~iris/databases.html), sponsored by the University of Illinois.

Finally, colleagues, mentors, and the staff of sponsored research and development offices can help the clinical researcher identify funding sources and get the most out of funding opportunity databases.

## TRAINING GRANTS AND INDIVIDUAL FELLOWSHIPS

For the past three decades, National Research Service Award (NRSA) training grants have been the major source of fellowship support for training in basic biomedical and clinical sciences. Physicians training for clinical research careers can be supported by either an institutional or individual NIH training grant. Institutional NRSA "T32" training grants are made to an institution based on its ability to provide high quality research training experiences and attract outstanding trainees, rather than on the qualifications of a particular trainee. These grants allow the director to select the trainees and to design and oversee their educational and research experience during the period of support.

In contrast to the institutional NRSA, individual NRSA "F32" fellowships support a single trainee. The trainee prepares the application outlining his or her proposed training experience, rather than the program director. Trainees are limited to a total number of three fellowship years on NRSA training grants, whether institutional, individual, or a combination of the two. Medical students and residents are not eligible for support under these two training grant mechanisms.

In both training grant award types, the fellowship recipient is required to pursue full-time research training. Only clinical duties that are directly related to the research training experience can be performed during the fellowship tenure.

## PRIVATELY FUNDED FELLOWSHIPS AND GRANTS

In addition to federal training grants, many private funding organizations offer fellowships for basic scientists, clinical researchers, or both (Table 16–2). Although institutions must expend substantial resources to cover some or all of the facilities and administrative costs that are often excluded or limited by private funders, grants from foundations, and public charities can be invaluable to researchers, especially new investigators who have not yet secured their first NIH grant or established investigators who embark on high-risk projects outside of their funded research programs.

The largest agencies have well-developed guidelines and application forms and employ a system of scientific peer review similar to the NIH. The same is true for professional societies in various subspecialties that offer grants to members. Proposals should follow the same general principles as proposals to the NIH, as outlined later in this chapter.

Although the largest private funders of medical research use scientific peer review in evaluating proposals, smaller organizations may not consult with experts when making funding decisions. In those cases, applications must be written in a way that allows a layperson to grasp the importance of the proposed work, but should also contain enough technical information to convince a scientist— who may not be working in the same field—that

the research plan is sound and the applicant is qualified to accomplish it. A foundation relations specialist at the investigator's institution can tell faculty which foundations use peer review, and which must be approached in the same way their institution's development staff solicit individual donors for support (see page 195).

Today, most private funding agencies maintain websites with guidelines for prospective applicants. Although funding databases such as COS, SPIN, and IRIS are excellent for staying abreast of funding opportunities, not all private foundations listed as medical research funders are viable prospects for funding. This is because the income tax returns of some foundations may be the primary source of information for fund-searching databases—and tax returns don't tell the whole story.

Another point to keep in mind is that although a foundation or corporation may have a lot of money, it does not have to distribute it "fairly" to the scientists that experts believe are the best. As long as its grant recipients are tax-exempt organizations, funding may be directed to a local institution, to developing countries, or to the alma mater of a board member. Funding programs for medical research may even be discontinued.

Although there are more than 60,000 U.S. private foundations, most of them have no staff, so they are unable to read and respond to unsolicited proposals. A foundation relations specialist can help guide an investigator to the foundations that are most likely to be receptive to a proposal. Otherwise, faculty may waste valuable time applying to the wrong sources.

## NATIONAL INSTITUTES OF HEALTH GRANTS

The NIH, which is part of the Public Health Service within the U.S. Department of Health and Human Services, funds more academic research than any other organization in the world. In fiscal year 2003, NIH awarded $18.5 billion in competing and noncompeting research grants.

The NIH website (http://www.nih.gov) provides links to current NIH funding opportunities and information about the application and award process. The Office of Extramural Research lists the postmarked receipt dates, review, and award cycles for all active programs.

NIH funding opportunities are announced throughout the year. Program announcements (PA) alert investigators to grants in areas of increased priority or to particular funding mechanisms, sometimes accepting proposals on several deadlines during the year. Requests for applications (RFA) have a more narrowly defined focus for which one or more NIH institutes have set aside funds. An RFA usually has a single receipt date. A request for proposal (RFP) solicits proposals for contracts, usually for one deadline.

Many investigators, however, successfully secure research grants from the NIH by submitting proposals without reference to a specific PA, RFA, or RFP. To identify the most appropriate institute or center within NIH for support of a particular research project, investigators can search the NIH Computer Retrieval of Information on Scientific Projects (CRISP), which lists projects that already have received funding.

NIH research funding is distributed by its component institutes and centers, each of which has its own mission and research agenda. The Center for Scientific Review (CSR) manages the receipt and referral of all grant applications to NIH (Figure 16–1). In fiscal year 2003, CSR received 64,187 applications. Approximately 70% of those applications were reviewed with the help of more than 11,000 scientific reviewers from various research institutions and 200 full-time staff.

To make a funding decision, the CSR assigns each application to an institute or center and to a scientific review group (commonly known as a "study section") to assess scientific and technical merit. The study sections are organized into integrated review groups (IRGs) according to scientific areas. An applicant can improve his or her chances of success by requesting that his or her proposal be assigned to a particular institute or study section and by communicating regularly with NIH staff during proposal preparation and review.

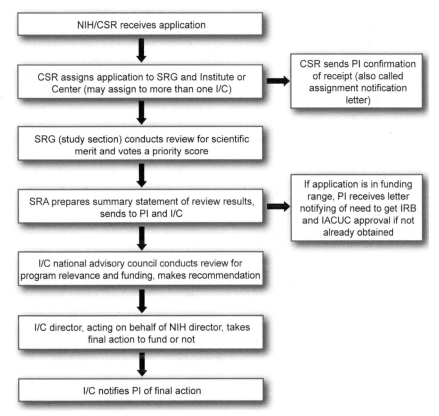

**FIGURE 16–1** ● Typical sequence of events from the time a grant application is submitted to the NIH until a funding decision is made.
CSR = Center for Scientific Review
IACUC = Institutional Animal Care and Use Committee
I/C = NIH Institute or Center
IRB = Institutional Review Board
PI = principal investigator
SRA = scientific review administrator
SRG = scientific review group.
Data from the Howard Hughes Medical Institute and Burroughs Wellcome Fund, Chevy Chase, MD.

## TABLE 16–1

### NIH Clinical Research Funding Mechanisms

- Mentored Medical Student Clinical Research Program (R25)
- NRSA Short-Term Institutional Research Training Grants (T35)
- NRSA Institutional Research Training Grants (T32)
- Ruth L. Kirschstein NRSA For Individual Postdoctoral Fellows (F32)
- NRSA Individual SENIOR Fellowships (F33)
- Mentored Clinical Scientist Development Award (K08)
- Mentored Patient-Oriented Research Career Development Award (K23)
- Clinical Research Curriculum Awards (K30)
- Clinical Research Loan Repayment Program
- Transition Career Development Award (K22)
- Investigator-Initiated Research Grant (R01)
- Midcareer Investigator Award in Patient-Oriented Research (K24)

Each study section reviewer assigns a rating or priority score to all applications. Applications in the lower half are "streamlined"—which means the reviewers read the proposals and prepare written critiques, but the applications are not discussed by the full study section or given a priority score. Scores range from 100, which is the highest possible score, to the lowest score of 500. All the reviewers' scores are averaged to create a final score, and NIH computes a percentile rank by using the following formula:

$$P = 100 \times (R - 1/2) / N$$

(P = percentile; R = rank or priority score; and N = total number of applicants)

Percentile ranking helps the NIH adjust for the different scoring approaches that naturally exist between study sections.

Once the study section review is complete, an application goes through a secondary review by the national advisory council of the institute or center. The advisory council is composed of established scientists, patient advocates, human volunteers participating in clinical studies, ethicists, and laypersons, all of whom are not otherwise affiliated with the institute. The council reviews the study section's scientific assessment and makes a recommendation on the funding of the application. Typically the institute director carries out the advisory council's recommendation. For more information about study sections, see the CSR website (http://www.csr.nih.gov).

Although any clinical, preclinical, or behavioral science investigator is eligible to apply for a research grant, the NIH has designed several funding opportunities specifically for clinical researchers (Table 16–1; Figure 16–2). The NIH defines this clinical research as

> *patient-oriented clinical research conducted with human subjects, or research on the causes and consequences of disease in human populations involving material of human origin (such as tissue specimens and cognitive phenomena) for which an*

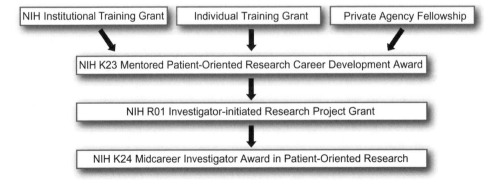

**FIGURE 16–2** ● Current typical pathway for career funding development in clinical research.

*investigator or colleague directly interacts with human subjects in an outpatient or inpatient setting to clarify a problem in human physiology, pathophysiology or disease, or epidemiologic or behavioral studies, outcomes research or health services research, or developing new technologies, therapeutic interventions, or clinical trials.(4)*

Mentored Patient-Oriented Research Career Development Awards (K23) support investigators who have made a commitment to clinical research (5). The K23 award provides investigators with three to five years of supervised study and research to develop independent research skills and to gain experience in the methods and experimental approaches needed to carry out patient-oriented research. In fiscal year 2003, 42% of the K23 applications reviewed by NIH were funded. To be eligible for this award, investigators must have a doctoral degree in a clinical discipline, must identify a mentor with extensive research experience, and must be willing to spend at least 75% of their professional effort conducting clinical research. They must also have status as a U.S. citizen, noncitizen national, or permanent resident. Ineligible individuals include current and former principal investigators on most other NIH-sponsored research grants.

To facilitate the transition from career development to independent researcher, NIH now encourages K23 recipients to seek funding as a principal investigator on a competing research grant award or a cooperative agreement, or as project leader on a competing multiproject award. If the research grant is awarded, the effort required on the career award may be reduced up to 50% and replaced by effort from the research award so that the total level of research commitment remains at 75% or more for the duration of the mentored career award. Investigators interested in applying for a K23 career development award should refer to the list of participating centers and institutes in the K23 program announcement on the NIH website, and contact the designated institute staff to discuss the proposed application.

For more advanced clinical researchers, the NIH offers Midcareer Investigator Awards in Patient-Oriented Research. This support, known as the K24 award, gives clinicians protected time to devote to clinical and patient-oriented research and to mentor beginning clinical investigators. The award is intended to relieve clinical investigators of patient care and administrative responsibilities for a period of three to five years to help them further develop patient-oriented research skills and pass those skills along to more junior investigators.

In fiscal year 2003, NIH funded 45% of the K24 applications it reviewed. Eligibility criteria for the award include a doctoral degree in a clinical discipline, completion of specialty training within 15 years of submitting the K24 application (some exceptions are granted), a record of conducting patient-oriented studies in a research environment, a publication record, successful competition for research grants, independent research support at the time of the K24 application, a record of supervising junior clinical researchers, and a demonstrated need for protected time to advance the applicant's clinical research and mentoring activities.

Recipients of K24 grants are required to spend between 25 and 50% of their time conducting patient-oriented research and mentoring and to devote the remaining time to other clinical, teaching, or research activities that relate to the overall objectives of the K24 program. To apply for a K24 award, investigators should contact the designated staff of the participating center or institute listed in the K24 program announcement.

In addition to research grant support, the NIH has several loan repayment programs that offer repayment of up to $35,000 of the principal and interest of educational loans for qualified health professionals who agree to conduct clinical research for at least two years (6). This mechanism also reimburses award recipients 39% of the repayment amount to cover federal income taxes and may also reimburse them for state income tax payments. The five NIH loan repayment programs open in 2004 included those focused on clinical research, pediatric research, health disparities research, contraception and infertility research, and a clinical research program for individuals from disadvantaged backgrounds.

More than half of applicants to NIH loan repayment programs are successful. Eligibility criteria include a doctoral degree; status as a U.S. citizen, national, or permanent resident; qualifying educational debt in excess of 20% of the applicant's annual income; and engagement in clinical research.

Of the grants awarded to individual investigators, the RO1 research project grant is the most common funding mechanism. In fiscal year 2003, NIH awarded 28,698 RO1 grants totaling $9.7 billion (7).

Most of the RO1 grants awarded by NIH are continuations of previous grants, attesting to the stability of this funding mechanism throughout an investigator's career. Still, NIH reports that 18,733 new RO1 grant proposals were reviewed in fiscal year 2003 and more than 4,500 were awarded, indicating that new investigators can find a foothold in the NIH grant system. Indeed, study sections give special consideration to applications from new investigators.

## TABLE 16–2

**Examples of Private Funders of Clinical Research**

| Funding Source | URL for Guidelines |
|---|---|
| American Cancer Society | http://www.cancer.org |
| American Diabetes Association | http://www.diabetes.org |
| American Heart Association | http://www.americanheart.org |
| Arthritis Foundation | http://www.arthritis.org |
| Burroughs Wellcome Fund | http://www.bwfund.org |
| Damon Runyon Cancer Research Foundation | http://www.cancerresearchfund.org |
| Doris Duke Charitable Foundation | http://www.ddcf.org |
| Juvenile Diabetes Research Foundation International | http://www.jdrf.org |
| Leukemia and Lymphoma Society | http://www.leukemia.org |
| Muscular Dystrophy Association | http://www.mdausa.org |
| National Alliance for Research on Schizophrenia and Depression | http://www.narsad.org |

## TIPS FOR NEW INVESTIGATORS SEEKING NIH FUNDING

1. Find a mentor. An experienced and supportive mentor can make all the difference in a new investigator's success, especially if the mentor is at the same institution, engaged in related research, and has served on a study section. Mentor relationships can evolve naturally as part of the faculty recruitment process, or a new investigator may find a mentor during fellowship training. If they are given enough lead time, mentors can help improve the clarity and focus of a proposal, spot weaknesses that could derail the application, and provide the kinds of comments reviewers are likely to make. Although criticism can be difficult to accept, mentors who challenge the proposal's ideas and provide a detailed critique are more useful that those who find little to criticize.

2. Keep it simple. In their earnest attempts to compete successfully for their first grant, new investigators may propose expansive projects that would be impossible to complete over the normal term of a research project grant. Study section reviewers, who want to fund proposals that will be successfully implemented and produce results, may conclude that the investigator lacks focus. The best strategy is a concise proposal with no more than five clearly defined aims that are achievable within the grant period.

3. Don't just go after the money. Although the availability of funding for a particular area can sometimes suggest new directions for investigations, changing the proposed research plan to match the stated agenda of a particular NIH institute can backfire if that agenda is not shared by the study section reviewers. Instead, investigators should pursue projects that interest them and avoid switching research directions entirely to compete for a slice of an unfamiliar pie.

4. Revise before resubmitting an application. Even though most new RO1 applications are not funded, unsuccessful applicants can learn a great deal from the comments provided by study section reviewers and use that advice to improve the proposal. Disregarding reviewers' comments because "they don't understand" the research is a mistake. Investigators should carefully consider the reviewers' comments and clearly explain the rationale if a reviewer's suggested changes are not incorporated in the revision. If the proposal's priority score does not improve after the second submission, a mentor may be able to suggest how the proposal could be improved.

5. Establish a track record and connect with other researchers. Scientists who have a successful record of securing NIH grants have a significant advantage over new investigators. Young investigators should focus on publishing their research in peer-reviewed journals to show that they can complete a research project. Attending scientific meetings not only allows investigators to stay abreast of research directions, but the scientists with whom they interact may serve as study section reviewers.

## OTHER FEDERAL AGENCY GRANTS

Although the NIH is the largest sponsor of medical research, clinical investigators should not overlook other federal agencies, such as the Centers for Disease Control and Prevention, the Health Resources and Services Administration, and the Department of Defense. The Grants.Gov website is an easy way to find other federal sources.

## INDUSTRY FUNDING

New drugs, medical devices, diagnostic tests, and screening tools must be tested in patients before they receive government approval for use. The pharmaceutical industry alone spent more than $33 billion on research and development in 2003, including clinical trials, a vital part of which was clinical research conducted by physicians (8,9,10).

There are many mechanisms for industry funding of academic researchers. Unlike NIH grants and private fellowships, however, industry funding of an unsolicited, investigator-initiated grant proposal is relatively unusual. Rather, by following the literature and attending scientific meetings, company scientists may approach academic partners with specific expertise to complement research conducted within the company or to gain access to patient populations or research technologies. Collaborations may involve consulting, sharing of research materials, licensing of technology developed by university scientists, performance of basic "discovery" research, specialized laboratory tests, and clinical studies that use a reagent, test, or procedure that has been developed by the academic investigator. Indeed, these latter types of studies are classic examples of translational clinical research. For the academic investigator, the value of such collaborations often comes from being able to use a new drug as a probe of a novel mechanistic pathway in a disease of interest.

## INSTITUTIONAL FUNDING

Institutional or departmental funds provided to newly recruited faculty as "start-up" funding can be used to begin a research project immediately while the investigator applies for grant support. Endowment funds and other gift support can also be used to support research. Other internal sources include institutional grants that contain funding for pilot projects, which is distributed to faculty at the grantee institution in response to internal proposals. Although this funding is substantially less than a research project grant would provide, it can help an investigator obtain preliminary data that will help demonstrate a project's feasibility when applying for a grant. Another mechanism that can be used to support physician-scientists in the early postgraduate years is support as a research associate on a grant made to an established investigator. Finally, faculty at institutions that have an NIH-funded General Clinical Research Center can receive funding through that mechanism (11).

## GIFTS FROM INDIVIDUAL DONORS

The United States has a remarkable tradition of philanthropy. More than $240 billion was given to charitable organizations in 2003, mostly by individual donors (12). Many institutions receive gifts from individual donors in support of medical research, but the way such funds are raised is often a mystery to faculty. In fact, the term *fund-raising* is misleading because it implies that the recipient institution is somehow extracting money from a donor.

Universities rarely receive substantial gifts through the techniques that are most familiar to the public—mass letter appeals, fund-raising dinners, walk-a-thons, and telephone solicitation. Rather, large gifts are cultivated over time. Faculty often have a pivotal role in the process, and they can benefit enormously from working closely with their development office to ensure that the amount, purpose, requestor, documentation, and timing of the gift are right.

Unlike other scientists, clinical researchers are in a special position to identify prospective donors because they care for patients and can thus identify people who have the inclination and the financial capacity to make a gift. Faculty who are uneasy asking for money may think that fund-raising is like begging, or that soliciting funds for their own research is selfish. People who are philanthropically inclined, however, give because they want to see progress in a field or disease that is personally important to them, or because they have faith in an institution or a particular scientist's ability to succeed. By listening to a donor's interests and exploring possible mechanisms of support, faculty and development officers can assist a donor in making a meaningful contribution.

Grateful patients may offer to make a gift. The size of the gift may not be apparent initially, but the development office can assist donors with both small and large contributions. Following up on a patient's expressed interest in making a gift can be handled by the development staff, who will guide faculty in engaging the donor, gauging his or her interest, planning a solicitation (if appropriate), thanking and recognizing the donor, and assisting with stewardship after the gift is made.

Modest contributions can lead to larger gifts. However, fund-raising is not an overnight process, nor are gifts mass produced. The number of prospective major donors is small, so faculty will not be required to expend an inordinate amount of time cultivating and soliciting gifts. Finally, university development offices often have specialized expertise in planned giving and other gift vehicles with tax advantages for the donor. They can also tell faculty whether the institution has already engaged the donor for another purpose so that faculty avoid embarrassment and the donor is protected from multiple solicitations.

## THE ROLE OF THE CLINICAL RESEARCHER IN ENHANCING PUBLIC UNDERSTANDING OF SCIENCE

No chapter on securing funding for medical research would be complete without emphasizing the vital role of physician-scientists in promoting public understanding of research (13,14). All funding, whether federal or private, ultimately depends on the public's recognition of the importance of research and the willingness of people to support it.

Most scientists understand intuitively that it is important to thank an individual donor for a gift, but writing a letter expressing appreciation to a foundation, health agency, or industry sponsor can also have a profound impact on promoting goodwill and encouraging continued support of research. People fund research because they believe that it will lead to improvements in health and treatments for disease. Yet the enormous expense of medical research and the inherently slow pace of advances can lead to disillusionment unless the meaning of incremental discoveries and their connection to ultimate breakthroughs are understood.

Nowhere is such advocacy as crucial as with elected officials. If Congress does not understand why medical research is important, the budget of the NIH will decline and research grants will be harder to obtain. Moreover, well-organized groups that condemn controversial techniques, such as stem cell research, will dominate the discussion if scientists don't assume responsibility for educating their senators and members of Congress about the unprecedented promise of such technologies.

The easiest way to share research news with the public is by working with university public information officers who write press releases, assist television crews in covering medical stories on campus, and develop feature articles in campus magazines and newspapers. Alerting them to upcoming publications of important findings or funding for new

projects can result in publicity that benefits the entire scientific community. Other ways to get involved are giving talks to high school classes or groups of alumni, writing a letter to a newspaper editor, setting out brochures about research for patients in clinic waiting rooms, judging science fair projects, participating in exhibits at local science museums, or simply engaging friends and neighbors in conversation at social events.

Advocacy groups, such as Research!America, work tirelessly to influence public policy, but they cannot do it alone. If the primary stakeholders—the researchers—sit on the sidelines and assume someone else is taking care of Congress, the funding climate can change drastically. In a January 2004 speech, former congressman John Porter urged researchers to get involved personally and assured them that their voices would be heard. If scientists do not take an active role in sustaining research momentum, Porter cautioned, they risk being perceived as ungrateful for the federal resources they receive, or dismissed as a weak and unorganized political force that can be ignored in the future.

Professional societies and advocacy organizations can help scientists get involved at the national level, including planning key conversation points in meetings with elected officials, writing letters on key issues, calling senators and members of Congress to urge their support for important bills, and thanking them for a vote in favor of medical research.

## SUMMARY

- The best source of long-term funding for clinical research is the National Institutes of Health, but investigators can tap into many other sources of funding, including private agencies, loan repayment programs, industry, other federal agencies, and sources within the investigator's own institution.
- Investigators can maximize their chances of success by working with a mentor, grant program officers, and staff at their home institution who specialize in funding opportunity searches, private funding, public relations, technology transfer, and clinical studies.
- For anyone planning to submit a first grant proposal, five pieces of good advice are (1) find a mentor, (2) keep the proposal simple, (3) focus on what is interesting, not just what is fundable, (4) revise before resubmitting an application that was not funded the first time, and (5) establish a track record and connect with other researchers.
- The K23 award from the NIH is specifically targeted toward entry-level clinical investigators.

## REFERENCES

1. Foundation Yearbook, 2004. New York: The Foundation Center.
2. FC Stats, Researching Philanthropy, The Foundation Center. http://fdncenter.org/fc_stats. Accessed March 16, 2005.
3. Guberman J, Shapiro B, Torchia M. Making the Right Moves: A Practical Guide to Scientific Management for Postdocs and New Faculty. Project Developers: Maryrose Franko, Ph.D., and Martin Ionescu-Pioggia, Ph.D. Editor: Laura Bonetta, Ph.D. The Howard Hughes Medical Institute and Burroughs Wellcome Fund, 2004.
4. Nathan D. Clinical research: perceptions, reality, and proposed solutions. NIH Director's Panel on Clinical Research. JAMA 1998;280:1427.
5. Clinical Research Career Development. National Center for Research Resources, National Institutes for Health, Department of Health and Human Services. March 2004. http://www.ncrr.nih.gov/clinical/crcdfact.pdf. Accessed March 16, 2005.
6. NIH Loan Repayment Programs. http://www.lrp.nih.gov
7. NIH Competing and Noncompeting Research Grant fiscal years 1998–2002, Office of Extramural Research, National Institutes of Health.
8. Pharmaceutical Research and Manufacturers of America (PhRMA). Pharmaceutical Industry Profile 2004, Washington, DC: PhRMA, 2004. http://www.phrma.org/publications/publications//2004-03-31.937.pdf. Accessed March 16, 2005.
9. ClinicalTrials.gov, A Service of the US National Institutes of Health, developed by the National Library of Medicine. http://www.clinicaltrials.govct.
10. Witkin KB. Using pilot studies to chart a course in clinical research. MD & DI June 1997;6:81. http://www.devicelink.com/mddi/archive/97/06/018.html Accessed March 16, 2005.
11. General Clinical Research Centers. National Center for Research Resources, National Institutes for Health, Department of Health and Human Services. December 2003. http://www.ncrr.nih.gov/clinical/crfact.pdf. Accessed March 16, 2005.
12. Center on Philanthropy at Indiana University. Giving USA, a publication of the AAFRC Trust for Philanthropy University, Indianapolis, IN: Author, 2003.
13. The Scientist 10[6]. March 18, 1996. http://www.the-scientist.com/yr1996/mar/comm_960318.htm
14. Porter JE. What's going on in Washington: we need to talk! Winter Conference on Brain Research, Copper Mountain, Co. January 25, 2004. http://www.researchamerica.org/advocacy/Porter. JAN04.pdf. Accessed March 16, 2005.

# CHAPTER 17

# Research Budgeting

Denise Canfield

A properly conducted clinical investigation often demands costly resources. Diagnostic exams and procedures, equipment, support resources, and knowledgeable, talented people are expensive. Accurately estimating the cost of a study prior to requesting funds from a sponsor (governmental or private) is imperative for a successful study. This chapter will describe the key elements common to almost all budgets for translational or experimental clinical research, and will suggest a systematic approach to generating these budgets.

## KEY ELEMENTS IN A CLINICAL RESEARCH BUDGET

Ideally, someone who is experienced and knowledgeable about the costs of clinical investigation should prepare the budget. To avoid wasting time and effort, the budget should be prepared only after the final protocol is produced (although preliminary estimates are often necessary). It may be necessary to create and maintain a set of budgetary "tools" to manage and monitor costs. Preferably, the same person preparing the budget would put these tools into place.

To properly develop an accurate budget (Table 17–1), the following items (at the very least) are needed: the completed protocol, data collection and case report forms, price lists from providers (e.g., IRB reviewing fees, radiology fees, diagnostic or central laboratory fees including sample processing costs, technical and professional fees associated with procedures, and lab sample shipping costs), costs related to data management or processing (which can be considerable, with imaging studies for instance), costs of secretarial support,

and personnel costs. It's important that each of these items be considered, and included as appropriate, in the budget justification that accompanies any grant application or other request for funding. Sufficient detail should be included to adequately justify each requested item. A common mistake of investigators is to assume that reviewers of a proposal will support budgetary requests based solely on the quality of the science, without adequate support for the funding requests themselves.

Accurate, detailed job descriptions can be useful when budgeting. Job descriptions that clearly describe the education and experience of research personnel will be needed to justify (for instance, in a grant application) the cost of hiring and retaining qualified people. Personnel costs must include salary and benefits, along with increases over the life of the investigation. Table 17–2 provides a worksheet for estimating (and justifying) the personnel costs associated with conducting a study.

## PREPARING THE BUDGET

The most important task in the budgeting process—meticulously reading and understanding the protocol—may seem evident but is often not pursued as rigorously as it should be. While reading the protocol, the ideal budgeter should note each task and estimate the amount of time needed to complete it. Time requirements are frequently underestimated, especially by budget preparers who have not actually conducted a clinical investigation previously. Notations should include protocol-driven tasks and procedures, the number of times each task and procedure is performed, the amount of time to perform each task and procedure, and whether or not a technical or professional fee

| **TABLE 17–1** |
| :--- |
| **Essential Components Needed to Estimate a Clinical Research Budget** |
| • The completed protocol<br>• Data collection and case report forms<br>• Price lists from providers for procedures and tests<br>• Costs of secretarial support<br>• Administrative costs for regulatory oversight<br>• Advertising costs, if any<br>• Data management/data processing<br>• Information technology costs<br>• Compensation to the participant and reimbursement for transportation, if any<br>• Research personnel costs (including time for screening, obtaining informed consent, time required to complete procedures, or to fill in case report forms) |

(e.g., obtaining chest radiographs as part of the research protocol) is associated with the task.

This last example raises a critically important point. Say, for instance, that a study involving hospitalized patients requires periodic chest radiography as part of the research protocol. These same radiographs may or may not have been necessary as part of routine clinical care. However, the budget preparer should (and must!) specifically budget only for those tests which are protocol prescribed and are not part of routine care (e.g., a screening radiograph performed hours prior to the investigational intervention, or a follow-up radiograph to be obtained at a specific time after the intervention). Technical fees charged for performing tests and professional fees charged for interpreting the results should be included when appropriate. It is mandatory, however, that the costs (and documentation) of research-driven testing and costs associated with standard or expected clinical care be kept clearly, even scrupulously, separate. Serious consequences may result from investigators seeking to cross-subsidize the cost of research testing by billing a funding agency (such as Medicare) for the test while accepting payment for the test from a sponsor (such as the National Institutes of Health). For more on this important topic, see Chapter 15.

It is common to underestimate the time required for a research coordinator to complete his or her tasks. It may be useful to "visualize" the process for actually conducting the study and to include time to arrange protocol-driven tasks, procedures, and visits (e.g., call and remind the participant, order the required exams for the visit, reserve space to conduct the visit), and collect and organize source documents noting results of the tasks, procedures, and visits (which may include procuring medical record releases from the subject to provide to health information management). Payments to providers of tests and procedures must be arranged. Significant time is necessary to transcribe or enter data from source documents to case report records, to respond to date queries, to file documentation, and to meet with third parties (monitors, auditors, statisticians) to review data. Time and funds are necessary to prepare and arrange data archiving once the investigation is complete.

The investigator's clinical brochure or research grant application (when these exist) are helpful in determining the skill level of those who must monitor for adverse events and to estimate the amount of time necessary for monitoring. The complexity of known adverse events also will usually be described in additional detail (compared to the protocol itself). Obviously, observing a research participant daily after an investigational intervention while in the hospital is more time consuming than, for example, weekly calls to an outpatient.

Data collection tools must be examined closely to accurately estimate the time required to gather and analyze source documents and to enter data into the fields. It is impossible to budget for any investigation without first knowing what data must be collected. Likewise, it is far less time consuming to determine at the outset exactly what data needs to be captured than to attempt to capture a participant's experience retrospectively after the investigation is complete.

Master price lists for all service providers should be prepared and updated regularly. When possible, it can be useful to establish a relationship with authorities in pricing departments—for instance, a research discount is commonly granted by providers. As with personnel costs, anticipate price increases over the life of the study.

Budgeting must be pursued systematically. One method is to follow the order of the protocol. (Note that, traditionally, a formal protocol is often not prepared for investigator-initiated, single-center studies—just a grant proposal or other materials required by the IRB. However, this omission can be a serious mistake, resulting in many problems. See Chapters 11 and 12.) The protocol objectives reveal the amount of time necessary to follow the subject: for example, a 28-day, all cause mortality study requires daily

## TABLE 17–2

### Staff Salary Worksheet

Position _____

| Procedure | Time per Activity/Procedure | No. of Times | X | No. of Subjects | No. of Hours |
|---|---|---|---|---|---|
| **Recruitment** | | | | | |
| **Screening** | | | | | |
| Consent (inc. explain study, answer questions) | | | | | |
| Procedures and labs | | | | | |
| **Per Visit Activities** | | | | | |
| Vital Signs | | | | | |
| Lab Processing | | | | | |
| Interview (AE screening/ concomitant meds/diary) | | | | | |
| Prep, assist, perform assessments and procedures | | | | | |
| Study article accounting | | | | | |
| Instructions and schedule next visit | | | | | |
| **CRF** | | | | | |
| Monitor visits and CRF corrections | | | | | |
| SAE forms | | | | | |
| IRB correspondence | | | | | |
| Miscellaneous communication sponsor/coordinator | | | | | |
| **Other** | | | | | |
| **Total Protocol Hours** | | | | | |

Salary Calculations:
Hourly salary X Total Protocol hours = Total Base Salary _____
Total Base Salary X Fringe = Project Salary _____
Project Salary / Number of Subjects = Per Subject Salary _____

monitoring for 28 days, but a study of weight loss might only require monthly visits over 6–12 months. The study population description and inclusion/exclusion criteria sections provide an overview of the amount of time needed to identify potential participants and to determine eligibility requirements. The study design describes to what extent other providers' services are needed. Are services of an investigational drug pharmacist, for example, necessary to receive, store, inventory, prepare, dispense, and account for a study drug? Or is this task less burdensome and able to be done by a study coordinator, as is often the case in an outpatient study? The protocol will clearly describe required study assessments and procedures and indicate required lab services. It's important to remember to include charges for processing of laboratory samples. Adverse events and serious adverse events are defined in the protocol along with reporting requirements. These descriptions allow for accurate estimates of time to monitor participants, arrange visits to examine participants, record the experiences described by research participants, perform diagnostic exams, collect results, and report to regulatory bodies and funding sponsors.

Outpatients may be recruited via advertising and the cost of advertising must be carefully assessed prior to participating, especially in the case of commercial advertising services (graphic designers, radio, television, print, billboards). Time to obtain permission from authorities to post print advertisements must be considered. Many medical centers use a centralized service that creates and maintains a database or repository of community members who are interested in participating in clinical research. The cost of this service must be assessed (Table 17–3). The subject of patient recruitment is considered in greater detail in Chapter 5.

Almost always, the most time-consuming (and therefore, costly) task in clinical investigation is identifying and consenting potential research participants. Ideally, engaged and cooperative colleagues assist in identifying potential volunteers. Around-the-clock availability (to respond to colleagues' calls regarding potential participants) is costly but at times necessary to meet enrollment goals. If the budget won't allow this expense, the practice should not be implemented, as the associated costs can quickly overwhelm the budget overall.

Daily screening in an acute care facility for potential participants is cumbersome and very time consuming. The actual process should be practiced and timed. In one hospital, it may be necessary, for instance, to physically walk from ward to ward to identify participants needed for a study and to read their medical charts (assuming, of course, the IRB has granted a HIPAA waiver of consent to do so for recruitment purposes; see Chapters 14 and 15).

## TABLE 17–3

### Procedure/Item Expenditure Worksheet

| Item | Cost/Item | Total No. of Procedures | Totals |
|------|-----------|-------------------------|--------|
| **Procedures, Tests, and Labs** | | | |
| Safety laboratory panel | | | |
| Urinalysis | | | |
| Other labs | | | |
| **Diagnostic Procedures** | | | |
| Other | | | |
| **Salary/Fee Charges Per Subject** | | | |
| Principal Investigator | | | |
| Subinvestigators | | | |
| Coordinator/Research Nurse | | | |
| Data Manager | | | |
| Pharmacy Fee | | | |
| Phlebotomist/Lab Technician | | | |
| Secretarial Support | | | |
| Other/Misc. | | | |
| **Administrative Costs Per Subject** | | | |
| Advertising and Recruitment Costs | | | |
| Subject Compensation | | | |
| Data Archiving | | | |
| Transportation | | | |
| **Other** | | | |
| **Total** | | | |

Table 17–2 provides one method for estimating the costs of screening. For example, assume that an experienced coordinator requires 2 hours daily (Monday through Friday) to review patients in each of five intensive care units. The coordinator, then, would spend 10 hours X 50 weeks screening for a study estimated to last for one year (omitting 2 weeks vacation). These 500 hours of labor are a fixed cost. If the coordinator is compensated at a rate of $30/hr, the total screening cost would be $15,000/yr, regardless whether a patient was actually enrolled or not.

If multiple clinical investigations in the same (or very similar) therapeutic or disease areas are being conducted concurrently, screening time may be equally distributed among several budgets. Additional time-consuming tasks include daily screen log maintenance, periodic analysis of the screening log, and responding to screen log queries from sponsors. The cost of this effort should also be included in the budget.

Obtaining informed consent can consume a considerable amount of time, often several hours. Many variables determine the amount of time required. The most important variable, of course, is the participant's (or participant's family's) ability to understand the purpose, value, and risks associated with participation in the research. On the one hand, a stressful situation (e.g., in an intensive care unit or emergency department) may hinder a participant's ordinary ability to understand the purposes and risks of the research. In contrast, someone with a disease like AIDS may already be very knowledgeable about the disease and clinical investigation process. Regardless, ample investigator and coordinator time must be budgeted to conduct this basic and most important requirement in human research.

Miscellaneous time-consuming tasks are often overlooked. Time should be allotted for meeting with others regarding the protocol itself or conducting the study. Likewise, time should be budgeted to prepare the submission (and annual reporting) to the IRB and other regulatory committees (radioactive drug committees, General Clinical Research Center committees, scientific review committees, data and safety monitoring committees, the FDA if a regulated biologic, drug, or device is involved) as well as to respond with additional documentation as requested. Include estimates of this time in the budget as a study start-up cost. Time should also be budgeted to "clean" data and to resolve discrepancies. Generally, if an investigator has collected and filed all source documentation during a volunteer's participation, the answers will be readily available but retrieval takes time.

Finally, the budget should be reviewed and approved by the various key members of the investigative team (including, obviously, the principal investigator), and revised as necessary. Regular budget reconciliation is necessary to know whether the investigation is being conducted within the budget's projected constraints. Although not common, it may be necessary to renegotiate the budget with the sponsor after the first few subjects are enrolled.

## SUMMARY

- Budgets are necessary to accurately estimate the cost of a study prior to requesting funds from a research sponsor.
- Key elements in any budget are salary expenses for personnel; costs of required procedures and tests; and administrative costs for regulatory oversight, advertising, and compensation to the participant.
- All research-associated costs must be kept separate from clinical care costs. Documentation should verify this separation.
- It is common to underestimate the time required to complete research tasks, such as time needed for screening, for obtaining informed consent, and for completing research procedures' case report forms, and other regulatory documentation. Working from a detailed research protocol to estimate the budget will reduce the likelihood of such mistakes.

# CHAPTER 18

# "Small" Clinical Experiments

Martin C. Weinrich, David J. Tollerud, Carlton A. Hornung,
Suzanne T. Ildstad

Every clinical study, especially one involving an experimental intervention, should adhere to three principal standards: (1) the study should ask an important biomedical research question (Chapter 1); (2) it must optimize potential benefit but minimize risk to the research participant (Chapter 14); and (3) it must be designed so that an answer to the research question can be obtained (Chapters 7 and 8).

Whenever possible, standard research designs (Chapters 7 and 8) should be used in clinical studies because they employ well-established principles to ensure that these standards are met. Advances in biomedical science, however, depend increasingly on cell- and gene-based treatments. For studies employing such interventions, standard research designs, which often require large numbers of research participants to achieve adequate statistical power, may not always be possible or appropriate.

As a result, new strategies for optimizing the design and analysis of "small" clinical studies have emerged that can help the investigator address these situations. In this chapter, we will first contrast such studies with their larger cousins, suggest several contexts in which small clinical experiments would be useful or necessary, and review several approaches to designing these studies.

## SMALL CLINICAL TRIALS—WHEN ARE THEY USEFUL OR NECESSARY?

Ideally, a clinical experiment can be conducted in a state of equipoise (Chapter 14), wherein a balance exists between, say, the benefits and risks of being subjected to a drug with a novel mechanism of action and undergoing no treatment, a placebo, or continuing standard therapy. In other words,

investigators face genuine uncertainty about the relative value of exposing the research participant to the proposed experimental intervention.

The standard approach to designing a clinical study that depends on using an experimental intervention requires investigators to formally specify the magnitude of a clinically meaningful effect (or difference of effects) they wish to detect (Chapter 9). In addition, the acceptable error rate for failing to detect an effect when one is actually present, and for falsely "detecting" a nonexistent effect purely through chance, must also be specified. These rates, denoted by $\beta$ and $\alpha$, respectively, define the statistical significance level ($\alpha$) and the power ($1 - \beta$) of the study (Chapter 23).

Unfortunately, unless the effects of the experimental intervention are substantial, a rather large sample size may be required to attain sufficiently small values for both types of error rates. Whenever this sample size is not feasible, the study will be underpowered. Indeed, one definition of a "small clinical experiment" could be "an underpowered clinical experiment to study a clinically important effect." Yet even if the traditional goal for power (80% probability of detecting the desired effect) cannot be met, the potential benefits of new knowledge obtained by conducting the study may still justify its performance.

Designing a clinical experiment with a small sample size—one that is known at the outset to be too small to achieve the desired statistical power—poses a number of challenges for the investigator. Meeting these challenges involves making trade-offs between various aspects of study design, data collection, data analysis, and statistical analytic approaches. The investigator, the epidemiologist, the biostatistician, the ethicist, and others on the research team must combine their diverse skills to work closely together to design the entire protocol. In particular, the statistician should have the clearest possible understanding of the clinical and general scientific context (Chapter 27), so that the data collected may provide the most useful information possible. Ethical considerations and the requirement for appropriate human studies (institutional review board, Chapter 14, and data safety monitoring board, Chapter 13) approvals are the same for both small and large clinical studies.

It is important to design the study protocol so that it is flexible and can be adapted as necessary. At the same time, investigators must consider how the study procedure will perform in practice (perhaps by simulating several plausible scenarios), in order to ensure that the welfare of the subjects is protected, and to evaluate the probability that the study's goals will be met.

Investigators should attempt to define multiple clinically important outcomes in broad terms, including the use of surrogate measures, and to identify a range of measurement approaches for each. This means using multiple indicators of each outcome and recording and storing the data in its most precise form (e.g., a ratio measurement). Data reduction can always be performed later, if needed. Using multiple indicators of multiple outcomes makes it easier to use more than one statistical approach to analyze the data, and to assess the consistency and robustness of the results. Circumstances where small clinical studies may be appropriate are shown in Table 18–1. Note that in many situations, several of these contexts may apply simultaneously.

## SELECTED EXAMPLES

### Case Study 1: Bone Mineral Density Loss During Space Missions

This example is discussed more fully in reference (1). During extended space travel, microgravity and radiation exposure may result in both muscular atrophy and skeletal mineral loss. Countermeasures (interventions such as different types of exercise or medications) to prevent these potentially life-threatening conditions must be explored if long missions in space are to be feasible. However, the number of missions (and therefore astronauts) available to test the multiple interventions before the launch of a long space mission are very limited. Here, it is imperative for the study to proceed despite the small number of participants.

### Case Study 2: Pilot Study to Induce Tolerance in Cardiac Allograft Recipients

The replacement of a defective heart with a functional one has become a clinical reality as a result of transplantation. However, at the present time, heart transplant recipients receive multiple medications each day to prevent rejection of their transplant. In addition to their high cost ($15,000 to $25,000 per year), these immunosuppressive agents have serious side effects. These drugs also often fail to prevent rejection and the eventual loss of the organ graft, even in highly compliant patients.

Total bone marrow transplantation (BMT) from the organ donor would be expected to induce a state of tolerance for the donated organ, but

---

## TABLE 18–1

### Appropriate Contexts in which to Consider a Small Clinical Study

- A new drug or procedure will be used for the first time in human research participants.
  **Example:** A traditional phase I study may be used to determine the maximum tolerated dose level for a new drug.
- The number of research participants available for study is extremely limited.
  **Example:** The investigator wishes to study changes in bone mineral density in astronauts during extended stays in space.
- The study population is small, isolated, or unique, or the disease is rare.
  **Example:** The investigator is studying health outcomes unique to a small isolated tribe or in a rare disease (e.g., spinal cord injury).
- Using a control group would be impractical or unethical.
  **Example:** The intervention is almost certain to do no harm but may greatly benefit the research participants.

often results in graft-versus-host disease (GVHD), thereby creating a need for the same immunosuppressive drugs that the procedure sought to avoid. Recently, it has been shown that "partial BMT," after special processing of the donor bone marrow, may confer tolerance with minimal toxicity. The single greatest potential toxicity for these transplants is still GVHD. GVHD will not occur without engraftment, and engraftment is more successful—but GVHD, more likely—if a larger bone marrow cell dose is given. Experimental evidence indicates that tolerance is an "all or none" phenomenon, and that it can be achieved without GVHD using appropriate bone marrow processing techniques.

Thus, the goal of this study would be to determine the optimal bone marrow dose to achieve engraftment and tolerance without causing life-threatening GVHD in—say—over 95% of candidates. The basic study design would involve increasing the bone marrow cell dose with each new transplant recipient until engraftment occurred without GVHD. Tolerance is such a rare phenomenon that a series of 5 to 10 successfully treated patients should provide convincing evidence to justify a larger pivotal trial.

## METHODOLOGY FOR DESIGN AND ANALYSIS

The list of designs shown in Table 18–2 is not meant to exclude traditional designs for larger clinical trials from consideration, but only to present some designs that may be particularly applicable for use in small clinical experiments. Each of these designs will be described briefly or illustrated with an example.

### "n-of-one" Trials (Subject Serves as his Own Control)

This approach would be useful to study a chronic condition, particularly when the disease exists in

---

**T A B L E  1 8 – 2**

### Study Designs for Small Clinical Experiments

- "n-of-one" Studies
- Sequential and Adaptive Designs
- Designs Using Decision Analysis
- Hierarchical Models
- Bayesian Designs

---

several forms, or when the clinical course can differ considerably among different patients. Many of the same considerations that apply to crossover designs (Chapter 8) also apply here, both for design and statistical analysis. For instance, period and carryover effects must be taken into account. In addition, depending on whether the intervention is designed to prevent disease progression or to slow it down once it begins to recur, timing of administration of the medication (or placebo) will be affected.

### Sequential and Adaptive Designs

In a classic clinical experiment, the probability of a research participant's being assigned to the active intervention or control arm are fixed at the beginning of the study and do not depend on the results obtained from previous participants. In addition, the sample size is fixed in advance, chosen to control the risks of Type I and Type II errors. Early "peeks" at the data are either not allowed or are severely limited to avoid inflating the risk of Type I error.

Modern clinical experimental design allows two modifications to this traditional scheme. In the first case, (sequential) analyses of the incomplete trial are allowed to determine whether the partial results allow early termination of the study, for example, when the intervention has demonstrably achieved its intended effect, or for futility, when it is clear that the final results are unlikely to show the desired effect with sufficient statistical certainty. In the second instance, the probability of being assigned to the intervention (or interventions if more than one dose of drug is being evaluated) or control arm, can be made to depend on the earlier results. The latter (adaptive) approach can be used even when there is no control group, as in a dose-finding study. Although dose-finding studies are part of therapeutic drug development programs, the question of what dose of drug should be used as a probe of biologic mechanism is a common and relevant problem in translational clinical research as well. In many such cases, a typical dose-finding protocol might impose unnecessary risks. For instance, investigators at the NIH recently reported a protocol to assess lung inflammation that depends on direct bronchial instillation of small amounts of endotoxin (an agent known to cause septic shock when it enters the blood stream in high concentrations) (2). What dose of endotoxin can be used safely to cause focal lung inflammation without causing septic shock?

The oldest and probably still the most commonly used strategy for dose level determination is the "three plus three" method including its variations, under which groups of three patients at a time are assigned the same dose level. The decision to increase, decrease, or keep the same dose level, as well as the decision whether to pool results from the current group of three with the next group of three patients, depends on the outcomes in the current group. Details vary from implementation to implementation, but it has now been shown that this class of methods "wastes" patients by escalating dose levels too slowly and is also likely to terminate the trial prematurely, before the correct dose level is reached. An excellent discussion of this issue can be found in reference (3).

In many small clinical experiments, it may be appropriate to consider patients singly. In the case of instilling endotoxin into the lungs to produce focal inflammation, for instance, it would be useful to adjust the dosage in new patients using information from previous patients. If each patient's dosage is based on results from the previous patients, a "one-at-a-time" sequential procedure results.

Performing a partial bone marrow transplant for cardiac transplantation tolerance, mentioned earlier as Case Study 2, provides another example of a one-at-a-time design and offers an ideal clinical setting for a simple and intuitive sequential procedure to determine an acceptable dose level. The outcome of each procedure (rejection, successful engraftment, or severe GVHD) will normally be available in time to help determine the dose level for the next procedure.

The study can be designed so that it begins conservatively, using a low bone marrow cell dose level for the first patient. For the second patient, and for each succeeding patient:

- If no durable engraftment was attained, the bone marrow cell dose is increased by one level for the next patient.
- If durable engraftment was obtained, the same dose level is maintained for the next patient.
- If severe (grade III or IV) GVHD occurs, the dose will be dropped one level lower for the next patient.

The study terminates when a certain number of consecutive durable engraftments has been observed, a number that could be determined based on experimental data or clinical relevance. In that case, the final cell dose level is declared to be the optimal dose level for moving to a definitive clinical trial. The study also terminates, but unsuccessfully, if severe GVHD is observed in two successive patients. In that case, the entire trial will be halted until the cause can be determined and adjustments made in the amount of total body radiation or the level of immunosuppression administered before the marrow is infused, or in the mix of cell types in the inoculum itself.

The study design in this example is simple, practical, and easy to implement. Excellent data are already available from a mouse model to describe the J-shaped profiles for risk of rejection and risk of GVHD. Therefore, it is not necessary to specify an arbitrary statistical model for the dose-response curves for rejection or GVHD. Statistical simulations can be carried out using both the mouse model risk profile data and other published hypothetical risk profiles for failure to engraft and GVHD to evaluate the probability that the procedure will find the appropriate dose level, as well as the mean number of subjects that will be needed, and their (low or even negligible) risk of developing GVHD. Such simulations are vital in evaluating these and other intuitively appealing designs, because seemingly reasonable rules can yield very unsatisfactory performance in practice (4).

Other approaches are possible. Dixon and Mood's "up-and-down design" was an early procedure that used results of treatment in pairs of patients to determine whether to increase or decrease the dosage, or leave it unchanged (5). Durham and Flournoy (6) introduced the biased coin method for dose finding, under which the decision whether to change the dose level is random with probabilities that depend on the outcomes of the preceding study(s) and that change as the study proceeds. The idea is to maximize the probability that the desired dose level is determined. Both of these approaches have undergone extensive development and generalization. These and other approaches are discussed in greater detail in reference (7).

## Designs Using Decision Analysis

This more formal approach may have limited utility for small clinical trials, because it requires that the researcher determine the cost (or utility) of each possible outcome (in terms of dollars, quality of life, or life expectancy) along with the probability that it occurs in the treatment group and in the control group. The possible decisions and possible outcomes may be arranged in a decision tree, which shows the outcome probabilities for each branch, and may be used to compute the expected utility for each decision strategy. The idea is to choose the branch that minimizes the expected cost (or equivalently, that maximizes the expected utility). More often than not, the exact values of the probabilities and the utilities are unclear; sensitivity analyses to determine how resilient the optimal decision scheme is to changes in the model assumptions are generally carried out. The decision-analytic approach also combines very naturally with a Bayesian approach to specify the uncertainty in the investigator's knowledge about the outcome probabilities (see below).

## Hierarchical Models

These flexible and powerful models are appropriate to use wherever clustering of observations occurs, as it does in longitudinal studies, where the cluster consists of all the observations on a single subject over the life of the study. They are known by many names—mixed model, randomly dispersed regression parameters, random coefficient models, multilevel models, random-effects regression models, variance component models, to name a few; specific details of their implementation and interpretation vary widely.

The statistical methods that can be employed in these cases can also be quite useful in small clinical experiments, because they model each subject as having his or her own unique response to the experimental intervention over time. Although participants who receive the same intervention have dose-response profiles (or profiles over time) that resemble one another, the shape of their individual responses is allowed to vary randomly within their group, and that random variation is explicitly included in the model. In addition, many of these techniques can handle missing observations far better than competing analytic techniques.

The astronaut bone mineral density case provides an excellent example, where each mission comprises the separate cluster to which its participating astronauts belong. The IOM (Institute of Medicine) monograph (1) provides an excellent discussion of this example, including a detailed calculation of statistical power, and of hierarchical models for small clinical studies in general.

## Bayesian Designs

Thall and his associates have shown how a purely Bayesian approach can be adopted from the very beginning to generate rules for dose escalation/reduction and study termination (8). This approach guarantees that the optimality criteria associated with Bayesian methodology are satisfied. The behavior of the Bayesian procedures (their operating characteristics) can then be simulated for various clinical parameters and loss functions, obtaining an entire set of scenarios to present to the clinical team. The clinician, working together with the biostatistician, can then select the design with the most desirable properties from a clinical point of view. The great strength of this approach is that it yields a

design that is optimal statistically, makes sense clinically, and is very unlikely to "misbehave." The primary drawback is the large amount of computation, even with modern computing technology, that is required to arrive at the final study design.

Note that even if fully Bayesian techniques are used to design the study, investigators still must consider the operating characteristics of the proposed design, particularly with respect to the Type I probability error $\alpha$ (risk of a false-positive finding). An excellent summary of the Bayesian approach to monitoring sequential clinical studies can be found in Spiegelhalter et al. (9). Another innovation includes defining several clinically relevant outcomes prospectively and then designing the study to address as many of them as possible.

More recently, a simpler Bayesian technique, the continual reassessment method (CRM), originally introduced by O'Quigley et al. (10) has been reported. The basic idea is to use a particular one-parameter model to represent the dose-response relationship, and then to use the results of all the previous procedures to choose the dose level for the next patient. User-friendly software is available to perform CRM (11). Various modified CRM designs have been compared to one another, as well as to the standard "three plus three" design (12).

## SUMMARY

- Although it is preferable whenever possible to use traditional, adequately powered clinical research study designs, new biomedical and genetic advances increasingly call for innovative approaches that permit small clinical experiments to be conducted and yet still allow meaningful results to be obtained.
- These studies require a very close collaboration between clinicians, study designers, statisticians, and ethicists to assure that the goals of the study can safely and effectively be carried out.

## REFERENCES

1. Evans CH Jr., Ildstad ST (eds). Small Clinical Trials: Issues and Challenges. Washington, D.C., National Academy Press, 2001.
2. O'Grady NP, Preas HL, Pugin J et al. Local inflammatory responses following bronchial endotoxin instillation in humans. Am J Respir Crit Care Med 2001;163:1591–1598.
3. Thall PF, Lee SJ. Practical model-based dose-finding in phase I clinical trials: methods based on toxicity. Int J Gynecol Cancer 2003;13:251–261.
4. Gooley TA, Martin PJ, Fisher LD et al. Simulation as a design tool for phase I/II clinical trials: an example from bone marrow transplantation. Control Clin Trials 1994;15:450–462.

5. Dixon WJ. Staircase bioassay: the up-and-down method. Neurosci Biobehav Rev 1991;15:47–50.

6. Durham SD, Flournoy N. Random walks for quantile estimation. In: Gupta SS, Berger JO, eds. Statistical Decision Theory and Related Topics V. New York: Springer-Verlag, 1994:467–476.

7. Stylianou M, Flournoy N. Dose finding using the biased coin up-and-down design and isotonic regression. Biometrics 2002;58:171–177.

8. Thall PF, Russell KE. A strategy for dose-finding and safety monitoring based on efficacy and adverse outcomes in phase I/II clinical trials. Biometrics 1998;54:251–264.

9. Spiegelhalter D, Abrams K, Myles J. Bayesian Approaches to Clinical Trials and Health-Care Evaluation. Chichester, West Sussex, England: John Wiley and Sons Ltd, 2004.

10. O'Quigley J, Pepe M, Fisher L. Continual reassessment method: a practical design for phase 1 clinical trials in cancer. Biometrics 1990;46:33–48.

11. Zohar S, Latouche A, Taconnet M et al. Software to compute and conduct sequential Bayesian phase I or II dose-ranging clinical trials with stopping rules. Comput Methods Programs Biomed 2003;72:117–125.

12. Ahn C. An evaluation of phase I cancer clinical trial designs. Stat Med 1998;17:1537–1549.

# CHAPTER 19

# Clinical Studies in Pediatric Minority Populations

Michael R. DeBaun, Allison King

As noted in the Introduction to this book, the overall purpose of biomedical research is to improve human health. This goal must extend to all sectors and segments of society. For children that belong to ethnic minority groups, parity in the improvement of medical care goes hand in hand with equal access to clinical studies. If children from ethnic minorities are not included in clinical studies, then it is unlikely that there will be parity in their overall medical care. Yet, as discussed in this chapter, achieving that parity requires proactive efforts on the part of the investigative team.

## INCLUSION OF MINORITIES IN CLINICAL STUDIES

To ensure adequate representation of minorities and other groups in its sponsored studies, the NIH has issued guidelines that address the inclusion of minorities, women, and children. The NIH Revitalization Act of 1993, PL 103-43, signed into law on June 10, 1993, directed the NIH to establish guidelines to include women and minorities in clinical research (1). These guidelines force the investigator to justify any exclusion of these populations that historically have been underrepresented in research.

In addition to both legal and ethical arguments for including ethnic minority children in clinical studies, there are sound scientific grounds as well. As discussed in Chapter 4, inferences about the generalizability of a study's results to a larger population (for instance, "children") depend on how well the study sample represents that larger population. Because differences in genetic makeup may at times affect outcome, it's important that the sample population appropriately represent the diversity of genotype within the population as a whole. For instance,

pharmacogenetic studies show that certain gene polymorphisms are associated with enhanced responses to antineoplastic drugs, providing a partial explanation for differences in survival from acute lymphoblastic leukemia between Asians, African Americans, and Whites. A fertile area for future translational clinical research studies would be to develop more refined associations between these genotypes and clinical outcomes. Ethnicity as a proxy for genetic heterogeneity may help identify select genotypes that are responsible for improved responses to chemotherapeutic agents. Still to be answered, however, is how many ethnic minority children must be studied to account for genetic heterogeneity that exists and may lead to a difference in clinical outcome.

## RECRUITMENT

Research addressing how best to recruit, enroll, and retain ethnic minority children in clinical investigation is limited. Experience with clinical research in asthma in children, however, provides some important clues. Asthma is the most common chronic illness in childhood and disproportionately affects African American children. Given the high prevalence of asthma among African American children, any clinical trial aimed at improving the clinical care of children with asthma should include African Americans. The Childhood Asthma Management Program (CAMP) trial, a multicenter trial to recruit a total of 960 children, had a target for minorities of 33%. Eight centers participated and the investigators were successful in recruiting 330 children who were from racial or ethnic minorities (2). A more detailed look at the participation rate revealed three of the eight centers recruited at or above the expected rate from the beginning and accounted for more than 50% of the enrollment, while the other five centers had significant delays.

The three sites that were successful in recruiting children from minority groups had common features. Possibly, the most important one was the existence of primary care within the same system where the research team recruited the patients. Other commonly cited factors for success were a cohesive staff, endorsement of the study by the child's primary care provider, and flexibility of the staff that assessed progress and the value of the recruiting methods being used. Other approaches to recruit children to CAMP included a parent education center that offered parents an information slide show, posters, and flyers; recommendations from the staff in the clinic; newspaper advertisements; mailings from the clinic; and staff interactions at grand rounds or dinner meetings with physicians. When the original recruitment methods failed at centers, an outside consulting firm built a team to reorganize and refocus recruitment efforts. Letters to parents of children who were already participating in CAMP solicited their help by word-of-mouth promotion of the program as well (2).

Another example is provided by a study of sickle cell disease, an illness that primarily affects African Americans in the United States. Accordingly, understanding the natural history of this disease requires enrollment predominantly of African Americans. The Cooperative Study of Sickle Cell Disease (CSSCD) was a multi-institutional investigation of the natural history of the clinical course of sickle cell disease from birth through adulthood. Twenty-three institutions participated in this project, and 3,800 patients were recruited. The original goal was to recruit the patients over a 24-month period, and 3,200 patients were recruited after 27 months (3). Some common features were likely to have been responsible for the successful recruitment of individuals with sickle cell disease to this study. Most of the staff members involved in recruitment were African American, and most of the patients recruited (80%) were seen in clinic within the previous year (3). Again, the ongoing relationship with a primary care provider carried influence in the recruitment of minorities. This record of success must be balanced against the conflict of interest concerns regarding research participant recruitment by primary caregivers, discussed in Chapter 14.

## STRATEGIES TO INCREASE COMPLIANCE AND RETENTION OF PEDIATRIC MINORITY POPULATIONS IN CLINICAL STUDIES—COMMUNITY SUPPORT

As with any study, success is linked with retention of the research participants. In pediatrics, very few studies have addressed strategies to improve compliance and retention. As demonstrated in the Fat Reduction Intervention Trial in African Americans (FRITAA) and the Hip for Health Program in Chicago, community understanding and support can not only increase study recruitment, but also increase study retention (4). Both programs were aimed at reducing dietary fat in African American youth. Two separate African American communities within Chicago were the setting for these studies. For the Hip for Health Program, interacting with parents and children at an after-school tutoring program was a more effective approach than recruiting from local health clinics. For the FRITAA program, increased community awareness was most effective. The investigators spoke at gatherings in churches, community centers, and schools. They also mailed flyers and recruited by telephone. The church was instrumental in educating its congregation and disseminating information in African American populations.

## BARRIERS TO RETENTION OF MINORITY CHILDREN IN CLINICAL STUDIES

At least two major barriers must be considered when designing studies for children within minority communities. The first major barrier is the disproportionate number of minority children that come from families with limited financial or social resources. For instance, it's important for research participants to comply with the research protocol, but in the case of children, compliance often requires the active participation of one or more guardian adults. This support may be lacking in a disproportionate number of minority families. Overall, however, the reasons why children and their families may drop out of studies is poorly understood and not well described. Obviously, the retention of research volunteers is important for the successful completion of any clinical study.

Ultimately, investigators must develop strategies to ensure children with limited financial and family support can participate in intensive clinical studies. A useful model may have been developed by Fisher and his colleagues when they applied the Precede-Proceed model to document (1) community acceptance of a program to engage peer support of asthma management and care; (2) program revision to emphasize greater attention to availability of care and promotional events as channels for education; (3) engagement of intended audiences in planning and implementation; (4) participation of parents in program activities; and (5) peer-based education and support to reach parents, including socially isolated parents whose children experience heightened morbidity (5). Although such strategies are innovative, their efficacy and cost effectiveness have yet to be established.

The second major barrier to retaining minority children in clinical studies is related to the cultural context of conducting research in minority populations. Although medical history is riddled with examples demonstrating the exploitation of minority populations in clinical studies, the study that is most often referred to is the Tuskegee Study (Chapter 14). This observation study occurred between 1932 and 1972 and was conducted by the U.S. Public Health Service (PHS) on 399 African American men in late stages of syphilis. Most men were illiterate and poor, living in remote and rural areas of Alabama. The men were never told what disease they were suffering from, that it was a serious illness, or that an effective treatment was available. The men were simply left to develop tertiary syphilis, including heart disease, paralysis, blindness, insanity, and death. "As I see it," one of the doctors involved explained, "we have no further interest in these patients until they die" (additional data were to be obtained at autopsy). The legacies of such studies, along with everyday life experiences, has resulted in a deepseated mistrust of the true value of clinical studies within minority communities, particularly African American communities.

## SUMMARY

- When given the opportunity, ethnic minority children and their families are willing to participate in clinical trials and longitudinal cohort studies.
- The recruitment, enrollment, and retention of minority children in clinical studies, can be

challenging. Unfortunately, no current evidence-based strategies have been developed to address how best to overcome problems associated with limited financial resources or culturally sensitive materials.

- Based on experience and existing literature, enrollment of minority children into clinical studies can be greatly enhanced by first establishing a solid physician-patient relationship that exists regardless of whether the patient participates in the study.
- Although not clearly demonstrated as effective, including parents in program activities and peerbased education are reasonable strategies to improve patient participation for all patients, but may be particularly effective for parents of children with limited resources, of which a disproportionate number are from minority families.

## REFERENCES

1. NIH Revitalization Act of 1993, PL 103-43. NIH Guide, 1993;2.
2. Strunk R, Sternberg A, Belt P et al. Recruitment of participants in the Childhood Asthma Management Program (CAMP) description of methods. J Asthma 1999; 36:217–237.
3. Gaston M, Smith J, Gallagher D et al. Recruitment in the Cooperative Study of Sickle Cell Disease (CSSCD). Control Clin Trials 1987;8:131S–140S.
4. Fitzgibbon ML, Prewitt TE, Blackman LR et al. Quantitative assessment of recruitment efforts for prevention trials in two diverse black populations. Prev Med 1998;27:838–845.
5. Fisher EB Jr, Strunk RC, Sussman LK, Arfken C, Sykes RK, Munro JM, Haywood S, Harrison D, Bascom S. Acceptability and feasibility of a community approach to asthma management: the Neighborhood Asthma Coalition (NAC). J Asthma. 1996;33(6):367–383.

# CHAPTER 20

# Pharmacokinetics and Pharmacodynamics

Karen L. Hardinger

*P**harmacokinetics* is the study of drug absorption, distribution, metabolism, and excretion within and from the body (1). Drugs can enter the body through various means including the intravenous, oral, transdermal, or rectal routes. Intravenous medications reach the vascular supply immediately, while oral medications pass through the gastrointestinal tract before being absorbed into the vascular system. Once the drug is intravascular, it must be distributed to its target sites. Then, drugs are metabolized, most commonly by the liver, and excreted in the bile or via the kidney. *Pharmacodynamics* is the study of the relationship between the pharmacokinetics of a drug and its tissue effects. The sum total of these tissue effects produces the drug's overall clinical response. Thus, in essence, pharmacokinetics is the study of what the body does to a drug while pharmacodynamics is the study of what the drug does to the body.

Understanding the basic principles of drug movement into, within, and out of the body is necessary to determine the drug's maximum efficacy and minimum toxicity (Figure 20–1). Although of obvious importance to the pharmaceutical industry for drug development, these topics are also important for the translational clinical investigator because many drugs are used as pharmacologic "probes" of physiologic and pathophysiologic mechanisms in translational and experimental clinical research. This chapter will review these principles of pharmacokinetics and pharmacodynamics. Summary tables of important abbreviations and equations are included in Tables 20–1 and 20–2.

## BIOAVAILABILITY

The body's total exposure to a drug is depicted by the area under the blood concentration versus time curve (AUC), which represents a balance between the amount of drug (D) that reaches the systemic circulation and its subsequent clearance (Cl).

$$AUC = F \times D/Cl \qquad (1)$$

The term *bioavailability (F),* quantifies absorption and relates the percentage of drug (D) that reaches the systemic circulation after extravascular (EV) administration compared to the drug's being administered intravascularly (IV) or intravenously.

$$F = D_{IV} (AUC_{EV}) / D_{EV} (AUC_{IV}) \qquad (2)$$

If a drug has a high bioavailability, then most of the drug reaches the systemic circulation in an unbound state. In contrast, drugs with low bioavailability are not well absorbed or are highly protein bound.

Among the various factors that affect bioavailability, *absorption* is perhaps the most important. Absorption is the process by which the free drug reaches the vascular system, whether it is via the skin, gastrointestinal tract, or after intramuscular injection. For instance, after a drug is ingested, dissolution or disintegration of the dosage form occurs. The rate of dissolution is determined by the drug size, coating, and solubility. Other terms that relate the extent and the rate of absorption are the maximum concentration ($C_{max}$) and the time to maximum concentration ($T_{max}$), which is exemplified in Figure 20–2. For instance, compared to an immediate release formulation, sustained released formulations (such as sustained release morphine) have a lower $C_{max}$ and a longer time to the $T_{max}$ (useful features for the treatment of chronic pain).

Concomitant drug administration may influence absorption. Dietary products, antacids, and phosphate binders may decrease absorption of other medications including digoxin, quinolone antibiotics, and

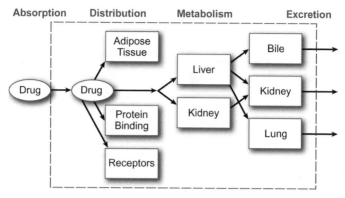

**FIGURE 20–1** ● Pharmacokinetics. The study of pharmacokinetics describes how the body absorbs, distributes, metabolizes, and excretes drugs.

tetracycline. When taken at the same time, chelation occurs and the drug cannot be absorbed. Therefore, it is recommended that administration of these drugs be separated by at least 2 hours.

Another example, cholestyramine, a medication given to lower cholesterol, forms a nonabsorbable complex with bile acids in the intestine. This complex inhibits enterohepatic reuptake of intestinal

## TABLE 20–1

### Important Abbreviations

| Abbreviation | Definition |
| --- | --- |
| AUC | Area under the time versus concentration curve |
| Cl | Clearance |
| $C_{max}$ | Maximum blood concentration |
| $C_{min}$ | Minimum blood concentration |
| $C_{ss}$ | Steady-state concentration |
| D | Dose |
| $E$ | Extraction ratio |
| EV | Extravascular |
| $F$ | Fraction of drug absorb into the circulation |
| k | Rate constant |
| $k_e$ | Elimination rate constant |
| $K_m$ | Affinity constant |
| IV | Intravascular |
| LD | Loading dose |
| MD | Maintenance dose |
| $Q$ | Blood flow |
| $t_{1/2}$ | Half-life |
| $T_{max}$ | Time for peak blood concentrations |
| $V_D$ | Volume of distribution |
| $V_{max}$ | Maximum rate of drug metabolism |
| $\tau$ | Dosing interval |

## TABLE 20-2

### Important Equations

**Equation**

$AUC = F \times D/Cl$

$Cl = Q \times E$

$Cl = (F \times Dose/f)/C_{ss}$

$Cl = Dose/AUC$

$Cl = kV_D$

$F = D_{IV} (AUC_{EV})/D_{EV} (AUC_{IV})$

$k = 0.693/t_{1/2}$

$t_{1/2} = 0.5 \, Css/k$

$V_D = D/Css$

bile salts, thereby increasing fecal loss of bile-bound cholesterol. Many drugs will not be absorbed when given with cholestryamine, because it also reduces the absorption of other molecules.

Many types of drug formulations are available, including solid, liquid, or gas molecules that may be given via various routes. Oral formulations include tablets, capsules, sustained and extended release products, solutions, or emulsions (2,3). Poor oral absorption occurs with large, insoluble, drug molecules and therefore other methods of drug delivery are necessary. For example, intravenous administration offers the most rapid onset of action for medications, while the duration of action may be limited. Intramuscular administration may provide a more delayed onset of action as the drug enters the muscle and surrounding tissue, then eventually the blood supply. Another route, sublingual administration, completely bypasses liver metabolism while rectal administration may only partially bypass the liver. Rectal administration is the preferred route for those who cannot tolerate oral administration. Likewise, research participants who cannot tolerate oral administration or are noncompliant, may also benefit form transdermal administration of drugs because the drug is released slowly over an extended time period. Last, local drug delivery can be achieved through nasal sprays, enemas, or topical administration of solutions, creams, lotions, or gels.

Changes to the gastrointestinal tract may influence absorption of medications. Gastrointestinal effects such as slow motility or emptying, low blood flow, and reduced surface area adversely affect absorption. In contrast, fluid intake such as an 8 ounce glass of water can increase absorption of medications. The effect of food intake on drug absorption can be unpredictable. At times, food can stimulate the production of acid and bile, which are needed to absorb medications, although other medications are best absorbed on an empty stomach, a basic environment. For instance, itraconazole tablets must be taken with food to enhance absorption, although itraconzole solution is recommended to be taken on an empty stomach. Medications that are taken on an

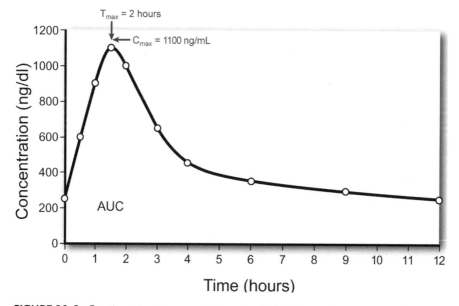

**FIGURE 20–2** ● Absorption. Measures of absorption include the maximum concentration ($C_{max}$), the time to maximum concentration ($T_{max}$) and the body's total exposure to drug or the area under the blood concentration versus time curve (AUC).

*One compartment*

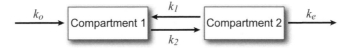

*Two compartment*

**FIGURE 20–3** ● Distribution. Models of distribution include one compartment, two compartment, and multicompartment models. In a one-compartment model, a drug is administered at a constant rate ($k_o$), immediately distributed to the target site ($V_D$), then eliminated from the body at a rate that is relative to the quantity of drug remaining ($k_e$). In a two-compartment model, the drug enters the central compartment, which includes blood and extracellular fluid (Compartment 1) and then moves to the peripheral compartment or the tissues (Compartment 2). The drug may be transferred between the compartments at varying rates ($k_1$ and $k_2$), then eliminated from the body.

empty stomach should be taken 1 hour before or 2 hours after a meal to prevent delays in absorption.

An important factor other than absorption that influences bioavailability is protein binding. Proteins such as α-1 acid glycoprotein, lipoprotein, or albumin bind to drug molecules in tissue and plasma, decreasing the rate and amount of drug that reaches the target site. Eventually, equilibrium between bound and unbound drugs is achieved and in most cases the free (or unbound drug) produces the physiological effect. Some conditions including liver disease, renal disease, malnutrition, advancing age, and severe burns may alter protein binding. When protein binding is decreased, more free drug is available. Thus, certain acidic drugs that bind avidly to albumin (e.g., furosemide, nonsteroidal anti-inflammatory drugs, penicillin, phenytoin, salicylates, and sulfonamides) will have increased bioavailability due to an increase in available free drug. Likewise, basic drugs bound to α-1-acid glycoprotein and albumin (e.g., lidocaine, phenothiazines, propranolol, quinidine, and tricyclic antidepressants) may display an increased free fraction of available drug. In contrast, in catabolic states, including times of stress such as surgery, the body produces more of these proteins, which can alter the degree of protein binding.

## DISTRIBUTION

After a drug is absorbed, it is distributed in varying degrees throughout the body. The body can be represented as a system of compartments that communicate with one another. In this case, the compartments do not have actual anatomic counterparts, but are simply sets of tissue that have comparable blood flow and drug affinity (Figure 20–3). (The topic of compartmental modeling is also germane to other techniques of translational clinical research. See Chapter 39.) An example of a one-compartment model is intravenous administration of a drug in which the drug is immediately distributed to the target site. In this model, the drug is rapidly distributed between the plasma and other body tissues, and then eliminated from the body at a rate that is relative to the quantity of drug remaining. In a two-compartment model, the drug enters the central compartment, which includes blood and extracellular fluid (Compartment 1) then moves to and from the peripheral compartment or the tissues (Compartment 2) before elimination.

*Distribution* is defined as the transfer of drugs between the vascular supply and peripheral tissues or compartments. The *volume of distribution* ($V_D$) is not a physiologic volume per se, but is the volume required to contain the entire drug in the body at the concentration found in the serum. Therefore, $V_D$ conveys the relationship between the amount of drug in the body in proportion to the serum concentration of the drug.

$$V_D = \text{Dose/Concentration} \qquad (3)$$

Drugs with a large $V_D$ are more concentrated in extravascular tissues and less concentrated intravascularly, while drugs with a small $V_D$ remain in the intravascular space. Drug distribution is determined by the drug's characteristics, including its molecular weight, protein and tissue binding, hydrophilicity or lipophilicity, and other more generalized characteristics, such as cardiac output. With peripheral edema, for instance, the total body water is increased and the volume of distribution for water soluble drugs will also be increased.

## METABOLISM

Even as drug absorption and distribution are taking place, drug elimination also begins. Before reaching the systemic circulation, orally administered medications pass through the liver via the portal circulation. The gastrointestinal tract or liver may contain enzymes that metabolize the drug before it reaches the systemic circulation. This process is termed *first pass* metabolism. Drugs administered rectally are absorbed into both the rectal and portal circulation, allowing a portion of the absorbed drug to avoid first pass metabolism through the liver. Medications administered via the intravenous or buccal route do not undergo first pass elimination.

Perhaps the most common measure of metabolism is drug *half-life* ($t_{1/2}$), defined as the time required for the serum drug concentration to decrease by one-half. Typically, researchers expect three to five half-lives (88 to 97% metabolized) before assuming a drug has effectively been eliminated from the body.

Reaction order refers to the effect the drug's concentration in blood has on its rate of metabolism. In a *zero-order reaction*, the amount of drug is decreasing at a constant time interval (k) and the drug concentration is proportional to the initial concentration. Zero-order elimination occurs when eliminating enzyme systems are saturated, most commonly in overdose or toxic exposures.

In a *first-order reaction*, the amount of drug decreases at a rate that is relative to the quantity of drug remaining. The half-life of a first-order drug reaction is constant; therefore, regardless of the drug concentration, the time required for the amount to decrease by one-half is constant. For example, if a drug concentration decreases from 50 ng/dL to 25 ng/dL over a time period of 8 hours, then in the next 8 hours the drug concentration will decrease again by half to 12.5 ng/dL.

A drug half-life depends on both its clearance (see following section) and its volume of distribution. The elimination rate constant (k) is the fraction of drug in the body eliminated per unit of time; it equals ln2 (0.693) divided by the half-life.

$$t_{1/2} = 0.693\ V_D/Cl \text{ or } k = 0.693/\ t_{1/2} \qquad (4)$$

Although there are many sites of metabolism, the liver is the most important location of oxidation, reduction, hydrolysis, and conjugation of drugs. Many metabolic reactions occur via the cytochrome P450 system, which is a group of heme-containing enzymes located in the membranes of the smooth endoplasmic reticulum in the liver, small intestines,

brain, lung, and kidney. Medications may inhibit, induce, or become a substrate for one or more of these isoenzymes. In humans, these include cytochrome P4503A4, 2C9, 2D6, 2A6, 2E1, and 1A2; cytochrome P450 3A4 is the most common (4). A list of common drugs metabolized by the cytochrome P450 system is shown in Table 20–3. These drug interactions can be very important to an investigator. For example, an investigator may wish to use tacrolimus (a substrate for cytochrome PA450 3A) in a study of immune tolerance. However, if the patient was recently started on ketoconazole, an inhibitor of this enzyme, an increase in tacrolimus bioavailability can occur altering the drug concentration and influencing the results (5).

*Pharmacogenetics* is a new, developing field that seeks to determine the genetic contribution to interindividual diversity in drug pharmacokinetics (see Chapter 21). Individuals may have more or less of an enzyme that is necessary to metabolize a drug. For example, subjects with multiple CYP2D6 gene copies may metabolize codeine, a prodrug, more rapidly to the active compound, morphine, whereas subjects that lack functional CYP2D6 genes do not metabolize codeine to morphine and do not experience the desired analgesic effect.

## ELIMINATION

*Elimination* is the last process involved in pharmacokinetics and involves how drugs are cleared from the body. Drug *clearance* (Cl) occurs primarily via the liver, kidneys, or lungs. The body's total drug clearance equals the sum of each organ system's clearance.

$$Cl_{total} = Cl_{hepatic} + Cl_{renal} + Cl_{lung} \qquad (5)$$

Total body drug clearance or the amount of drug removed from the body per unit of time, is the product of the drug's volume of distribution and its rate of elimination ($k_e$).

$$Cl = V_D \times k_e \qquad (6)$$

Drugs with a large volume of distribution and a low clearance will be eliminated more slowly. A large volume of distribution may be caused by drug lipophilicity, which generally promotes distribution within tissues; a low clearance may be due to a high amount of protein binding, which prevents clearance.

The extraction ratio (*E*) measures drug removal by an organ; in the case of drug clearance, the liver is primarily responsible for drug removal from the circulation after oral administration. Drugs with extraction ratios of one are completely removed from the bloodstream with one pass through the liver. If a drug has an extraction ratio of 0.80, only 20% of the

## TABLE 20–3

### Cytochrome Substrates by Family

| 1A2 | 2C9 | 2C19 | 2D6 | 2E1 | 3A4 |
|---|---|---|---|---|---|
| acetaminophen | diclofenac | diazepam | codeine | ethanol | alprazolam |
| caffeine | ibuprofen | omeprazole | fluxetine | isoniazid | astemizole |
| R-Warfarin | naproxen | | haloperidol | | carbamazepine |
| theophylline | phenytoin | | loratadine | | cisapride |
| | S-warfarin | | metoprolol | | cyclosporine |
| | | | paroxetine | | diltiazem |
| | | | propafenone | | erythromycin |
| | | | risperidone | | felodipine |
| | | | thioridazine | | fluconazole |
| | | | venlafaxine | | itraconazole |
| | | | | | ketoconazole |
| | | | | | lidocaine |
| | | | | | lovastatin |
| | | | | | midazolam |
| | | | | | nifedipine |
| | | | | | tacrolimus |

drug remains after one pass through the liver. For agents with high hepatic extraction ratios, a continuous intravenous administration may be necessary to maintain effective circulating levels of active drug. For example, lidocaine, propranolol, and morphine are highly dependent on organ blood flow for clearance. In contrast, drugs with low extraction ratios (including warfarin, phenobarbital, diazepam, and theophylline) are dependent on the levels of P450 enzyme activity and protein binding for clearance; as a result, these (and similar) drugs frequently interact with other drugs by protein binding, displacement, enzyme inhibition, or enzyme induction.

For drugs excreted by the liver, alterations in hepatic blood flow may significantly alter clearance. Medications such as hydralazine may increase blood flow while conditions such as shock or mechanical ventilation may decrease hepatic blood flow. The product of blood flow to the organ ($Q$) and the extraction ratio ($E$) equals clearance.

$$Cl = Q \times E \qquad (7)$$

For example, if the liver blood flow is 1 L/minute and the extraction ratio equals 0.25, then the liver clearance equals 0.25 L/minute.

Severe hepatic dysfunction or cholestasis will also affect drug metabolism and excretion. In severe liver disease, drugs may accumulate and dosing adjustments may be necessary.

Drugs that are excreted via the biliary route are typically high molecular weight compounds or polar molecules. These drugs may be recycled by the enterohepatic circulation, which occurs when a drug is excreted by the bile into the duodenum, metabolized by the normal flora of the gastrointestinal tract, and reabsorbed back into the portal circulation. This process can occur with digoxin, estrogens, nafcillin, testosterone, rifampin, and valproic acid.

Some drugs may be excreted in the kidney through glomerular filtration, the passive process by which the kidney filters molecules. Excretion of most renally eliminated drugs, like aminoglycosides and vancomycin, occurs through this process and therefore dosages are adjusted based on estimates of glomerular filtration or creatinine clearance (CrCl). A normal creatinine clearance ranges from 80 to 125 mL/min/m$^2$ and many factors can affect the production of creatinine, such as diet and muscle metabolism. The Cockroft and Gault equation estimates clearance by an adult subject's age, serum creatinine (SCr), and ideal body weight (IBW) (6). To determine creatinine clearance in females, the equation is multiplied by 0.85.

$$CrCl = (140 - age) \times IBW/ (SCr \times 72) \quad (8)$$

Given the relationships between dose and clearance to the final concentration of drug in the circulation (equations 3 and 4), equation 8 is commonly

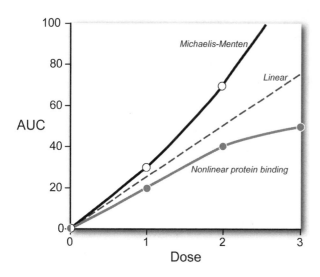

**FIGURE 20–4** ● Nonlinear pharmacokinetics. Types of nonlinear pharmacokinetic models include Michaelis-Menten and nonlinear protein binding. Some drugs that exhibit Michaelis-Menten pharmacokinetics reach their maximum rate of metabolism ($V_{max}$) when enzymes become saturated and therefore the concentration of drug increases more than expected with an increase in drug dose. With nonlinear protein binding, because proteins become saturated, the drug concentration and AUC increase less than expected after an increase in drug dose. Adapted from Bauer LA. Clincial pharmacokinetics and pharmacodynamics. In: DiPiro JT, Talbert RL, Yee GC, et al., eds. Pharmacotherapy: A Pathophysiologic Approach. 5th Ed. Stamford, CT: Appleton & Lange, 2002.

used to dose renally eliminated medications, including antibiotics and antiviral agents.

## NONLINEAR PHARMACOKINETICS

Unlike drugs with first-order (linear) pharmacokinetics, AUC, metabolism, elimination, and excretion are not proportional to the dosage for drugs with nonlinear pharmacokinetics. Accordingly, changes in the dosage of these drugs results in variable changes in plasma drug concentration. Drugs may exhibit nonlinear pharmacokinetics if their elimination pathways are saturated or are dose dependent (Figure 20–4). When enzymes become saturated, some drugs reach their maximum rate of metabolism ($V_{max}$); as a result, the half-life is constantly changing. This process is referred to as Michaelis-Menten pharmacokinetics and is exemplified in the equation below that involves the use of an affinity constant ($k_m$) or the serum concentration at which nonproportional changes in drug concentrations occur.

Rate of elimination = ($V_{max}$ × Drug concentration) / ($K_m$ + Drug concentration)

Phenytoin, a drug that displays these kinetic properties, has a $k_m$ of approximately 4 µg/mL. Therefore, above a concentration of 4 µg/mL, nonlinear increases in the serum concentration of this drug would be expected.

Nonlinear elimination can also occur if protein-binding sites are saturated. Typically, in this type of kinetic reaction, the drug concentration and AUC increase less than expected after an increase in drug dose. Because drug-binding sites are already occupied, a greater amount of free drug is available, resulting in increased clearance of the drug. Valproic acid exhibits saturable protein-binding pharmacokinetics.

## PHARMACODYNAMICS

Pharmacodynamics studies the relationship between the pharmacokinetics of a drug and the drug's tissue effects.

Drug + Receptor ➔ Drug-receptor complex ➔ Response

For example, the pharmacodynamic effects of an antihypertensive medication are monitored by the blood pressure rather than drug concentrations. It is possible that the pharmacokinetic analysis of a drug may reveal that the drug dosage is not within what is generally considered a "therapeutic" range (based on prior research) while the pharmacodynamic effects are still appropriate. For example, a digoxin concentration may be above this therapeutic range ("supratherapeutic"), while the research participant is effectively treated for congestive heart failure and shows no signs of toxicity. Alternatively, the individual might show signs of toxicity without any beneficial effect despite supratherapeutic blood concentrations of the drug.

Factors that may contribute to a drug's pharmacodynamic effects include the relationship between a drug and receptor, age, tolerance, and physiologic factors. The most important relationship between a drug and its receptor is termed *affinity*, which describes the level of attraction between two molecules. An *agonist* drug generates an effect, whether stimulatory or inhibitory, when bound to its receptor. Drugs can be partial or full agonists. An *antagonist* drug inhibits or prevents receptor mediated agonist effects by competing for the receptor. For example, a common antihypertensive, metoprolol is a β-antagonist that exerts its antihypertensive effect by blocking epinephrine binding to beta receptors.

Age also contributes to a drug's pharmacodynamic response. For instance, elderly individuals often have an increased dose response with many medications, and therefore elderly individuals must often start with lower doses. *Tolerance*, or tachyphylaxis, can develop over time; the result is that increasing amounts of drug are required to achieve an equivalent response. The most common example is cocaine or narcotic addiction. As time elapses, higher doses are needed for a person to experience previous responses. In some instances, the fading of a response to a drug over time is desirable, as for instance when sophisticated protocols are used to desensitize allergic responses to a drug. Lastly, pathophysiologic factors, including many disease states, including diabetes mellitus, thyroid disease, and hypertension, can alter receptor function, thereby changing a drug's pharmacodynamics.

Several terms are used to describe the interaction between a drug and its receptor. Synergy is defined as when the interaction of two or more agents combined is greater than the sum of their individual effects. For instance, if furosemide and metolazone are given together, they have a greater diuretic response than if given alone. Additive drug effects occur when the effects of two drugs combined form a sum effect. Lastly, potentiation occurs when one drug effect is enhanced or increased by the effect of another drug.

A dose response curve depicts the relationship between a drug and its clinical response. Many terms are used to describe a dose response curve. Efficacy describes the inherent capacity of a drug to produce a given response. The term *effective dose (ED)* is used to define the dose necessary to produce an effect in a percentage of individuals. For instance, the $ED_{50}$ will produce the desired effect in 50% of individuals. Potency is the amount of drug required to produce a response. Some drugs are more potent and produce an equivalent response with less drug. For example, fentanyl is more potent than morphine because a lower amount of drug (by weight) is required to produce an equivalent response.

## DRUG MONITORING

Therapeutic drug monitoring combines the principles of pharmacokinetics and pharmacodynamics, and validates the adequacy of a dosing regimen. For some drugs, a narrow therapeutic range defines the average plasma concentrations that differentiate drug toxicity and efficacy (7). Measurement of drug concentrations is most easily achieved in the blood, serum, or plasma, although drug concentrations may be obtained in tissues, urine, feces, or saliva.

Calculating the body's total exposure to drug, AUC, is the most sensitive method for monitoring medications, but it requires multiple blood samples, which is impractical and costly. Single time point monitoring is more convenient and cost effective in most cases. These points can include peaks, troughs, or random levels. Peak concentration reflects the highest exposure to drug, and a trough concentrations, obtained just prior to the next dose, reflects the lowest blood concentration. For many drugs, the timing of the sample collection is very important. Digoxin has a long distribution phase, and therefore drug concentrations should be measured at least 6 hours after the dose. Likewise, gentamicin peak concentration correlates with efficacy, while the trough concentration may correlate with toxicity. Drug concentrations, in conjunction with evaluation of the response to the drug, help when selecting an appropriate drug regimen. Research participant compliance should always be considered when evaluating a drug concentration.

Radioimmunoassay (RIA) is a common method of monitoring drug concentrations and is utilized in monitoring cyclosporine and digoxin concentrations. Enzyme-multiplied immunotechnique (EMIT), enzyme-linked immunosorbent assay (ELISA), and fluorescence immunoassay (FIA) are other available assays. High pressure liquid chromatography is less commonly utilized because of expense.

## PHARMACOKINETIC AND PHARMACODYNAMIC ISSUES IN TRANSLATIONAL AND EXPERIMENTAL RESEARCH

Before marketing a new drug, a company must seek a new drug application (NDA). Studies necessary for the NDA evaluate the pharmacokinetics, safety, and efficacy of the drug product. Likewise, for approval of generic products or new formulations of a drug with an active NDA, bioequivalency studies must be performed. The FDA provides a formulary of drug products that may be substituted or exchanged in the *Approved Drug Products with Therapeutic Equivalence Evaluations* ("The Orange Book"), which is published in the *United States Pharmacopeia*. If a drug product is coded "A," then the products are considered equivalent and may be exchanged. If a drug product is rated "B," it is not considered bioequivalent and may not be substituted with the established product.

In vitro and in vivo testing of drug products prior to drug marketing is required by the FDA to establish bioequivalence (8). To achieve *bioequivalence*, two products must have a similar rate and extent of

## TABLE 20–4

### Pharmacokinetic Study Design Example

| | Description | Pharmacokinetic Explanation |
|---|---|---|
| Background | Tacrolimus is a macrolide immunosuppressant routinely given in two equally divided doses every 12 hours. However, the time-dependent pharmacokinetics of tacrolimus suggest that once daily morning administration of tacrolimus may produce appropriate drug exposure. | Tacrolimus has superior absorption in the morning compared to evening administration because of time-dependent pharmacokinetics. |
| Hypothesis | Once daily administration of tacrolimus in kidney transplant recipients will have similar pharmacokinetics and safety as compared to twice daily administration. | Perhaps, because of the time-dependent pharmacokinetics, tacrolimus can be given once daily. The hypothesis encompasses pharmacokinetics and pharmacodynamics (safety and efficacy). |
| Study design | Open-label, two-period, crossover, sequential study: for twice daily dosing (phase I) and once daily dosing (phase II). | This crossover design accounts for intersubject variability in pharmacokinetic parameters. |
| Inclusion criteria | 1. Kidney transplant recipients (18 years or older) at taking tacrolimus-based immunosuppression. <br> 2. Stable kidney transplant recipients (>6 months post-transplantation, serum creatinine <2 mg/dL, no history of rejection). <br> 3. Stable immunosuppression (therapeutic tacrolimus concentrations, no change in tacrolimus dose within one month prior to the study). <br> 4. Patients must agree to abstain from alcohol and caffeine for 48 hours prior to the pharmacokinetic studies. | 1. The target population is adults because pediatric transplant patients metabolize tacrolimus at a quicker rate. <br> 2. Only stable patients will be included for safety reasons. <br> 3. Only stable patients will be included for safety reasons. <br> 4. Alcohol and caffeine may affect the pharmacokinetics of tacrolimus. |
| Exclusion criteria | 1. Pregnant women or nursing mothers <br> 2. Significant liver impairment (AST or ALT >2 x upper limit of normal, or total bilirubin > upper limit of normal) <br> 3. Anemia: Hematocrit <30% <br> 4. Use of concomitant P450 3A p-glycoprotein inducers or inhibitors <br> 5. Current smoking <br> 6. Patients with diabetes mellitus <br> 7. Patients unwilling or unable to comply with the protocol | 1. Pregnant patients have larger $V_D$ and nursing mothers were excluded for safety reasons <br> 2. Patients with liver impairment have impaired metabolism <br> 3. Tacrolimus is distributed to red bloods cells, therefore severe anemia may alter pharmacokinetics <br> 4. Tacrolimus is metabolized by cytochrome P450 3A and therefore drug interaction would be expected <br> 5. Smoking can influence metabolism of some medications <br> 6. Diabetic patients may not be able to fast overnight and are excluded for safety reasons <br> 7. Ensure adequate follow-up |

*(Continued)*

**TABLE 20–4 (Continued)**

| | | |
|---|---|---|
| Methods | Phase 1 (Study days 1–6) Patients will take their morning tacrolimus dose with 240 mL of water at approximately 0800 h and their evening dose 12 hours after the morning dose (at approximately 2000 h).<br><br>Period II (Study days 7–14) patients will be instructed to self-administer two-thirds of their total daily dose at 0800h with 240 mL of water.<br><br>On the last day of each period, serial blood samples will be collected from the indwelling catheter into EDTA-containing tubes. Phase I: at 0, 0.5, 1, 1.5, 2, 3, 4, 6, 9, and 12 hours after the morning dose and at 0.5, 1, 1.5, 2, 3, 4, 6, 9, and 12 hours after the evening dose. Phase II: 0, 0.5, 1, 1.5, 2, 3, 4, 6, 9, 12, 16, 20, and 24 hours after the dose. Aliquots of blood will be frozen and stored at –20°C. | The time of drug administration was strictly enforced to ensure adequate drug concentrations.<br><br>Fluid intake should be controlled because it can influence dissolution of medications. At least 6 days are allowed to reach steady state. ($t_{1/2}$ = 8–12 h, 8–12h x 5 half-lives = 40–60 hours).<br><br>The 24-hour study period was chosen to allow time for excretion and clearance of tacrolimus.<br><br>Blood sample collection times are more frequent surrounding the known $C_{max}$ of tacrolimus–approximately 1.5–2 hours after the dose.<br><br>Blood samples will be stored in a similar manner to prevent degradation of tacrolimus. |
| Diet | To control for the effects of food on tacrolimus pharmacokinetics, patients will be asked to fast from 2200 h and diet will be provided at the same times on both tacrolimus study days. Breakfast will be provided 2 hours after the morning dose of tacrolimus (at approximately 1000 h). For the evening dose on day 6, food will be allowed 2 hours before and 2 hours after the dose. | Tacrolimus absorption is delayed with food; therefore, patients were asked to fast before administration and at least two hours after dosing. Several studies have reported that the oral bioavailability of tacrolimus is altered after food consumption. An increase in $C_{max}$ (15–40%) and AUC (2–12%) have been reported in a fasting state versus a nonfasting state. |
| Outcomes | 1. Area under the tacrolimus blood concentration-time curve from time 0 to 24 hours following the morning dose ($AUC_{0-24}$).<br>2. Tacrolimus peak concentration ($C_{max}$), time to reach $C_{max}$ ($T_{max}$), tacrolimus trough concentration (12 hours after each dose on day 6; 24 hours after dose on day 14)<br>3. Allograft function (serum creatinine)<br>4. Adverse events | Pharmacokinetic ($AUC_{0-24}$, $C_{max}$, $T_{max}$) as well as pharmacodynamic effects (allograft function, adverse events) are primary events. |

absorption under experimental conditions. The two drugs must have statistically similar pharmacokinetic parameters including $C_{max}$, $T_{max}$, and AUC. These parameters must fall within a 90% confidence interval about the ratios of the means of the two drug products and must be within ±20%. When log-transformed data are used, the pharmacokinetic parameters must fall within 0.8 – 1.25 (80 – 125%) of the comparator drug.

Most bioequivalence studies compare a generic product to the innovator product and enroll adult, healthy individuals. Typical study designs are either single- or multiple-dose pharmacokinetic studies, although single-dose studies are generally more sensitive (8). A crossover study design is commonly used because it accounts for interindividual variability in absorption, metabolism, distribution, and excretion of the study drug.

Food effect studies are typically a single-dose, two-period, two-treatment, two-sequence crossover study in a fasting and nonfasting state. Typically, the test or reference product is administered with 240 mL of water (8). In general, research participants should be allowed water as desired except for 1 hour before and after drug administration, and participants should abstain from alcohol 24 hours before and during the study period. In a fasted study, volunteers should be allowed to eat at least 8–10 hours before drug administration. Additionally, food should not be allowed until 4 hours after drug administration. If a washout design is utilized, then the researcher should allow at least five half-lives for adequate removal of the drug.

Carefully consider pharmacokinetics and pharmacodynamics when designing translational and experimental research that depends on a drug as a mechanistic pharmacologic probe of a putative physiologic or pathophysiologic mechanism. The hypothesis to be tested should be appropriate for the pharmacokinetic and pharmacodynamic principles of the study drug and ensure that the study design will evaluate the desired endpoint. For inclusion and exclusion criteria, investigators should take into account the age and gender of the potential target population and try to include this type of volunteer in the study. Obviously, investigators should exclude research volunteers who are at high risk for a side effect of the study drug. The influence of food and water on drug absorption, metabolism, and clearance should be considered and the study protocol adjusted where necessary. Lastly, include pharmacokinetic as well as pharmacodynamic measures as secondary endpoints (when these are not the focus of the study itself). An example study and pharmacokinetic and pharmacodynamic considerations can be found in Table 20–4 (9).

## SUMMARY

- Absorption is the process by which a drug reaches the vascular system and depends on several factors, including drug formulation, concomitant drugs, and the tissue environment (e.g., gastrointestinal) in which the drug is delivered.
- Bioavailability quantifies absorption and relates the percentage of drug that reaches the systemic circulation after extravascular administration

compared to administering the drug. Intravascularly or intravenously. Protein and tissue binding also affect drug bioavailability.
- Metabolism is the breakdown of the drug to active or inactive metabolites.
- Distribution is defined as the transfer of drug from the vascular supply to peripheral tissues or compartments.
- Clearance is a measure of drug elimination from the body.
- Bioequivalence is defined as two drugs having a similar rate and extent of absorption under experimental conditions. They must have statistically similar pharmacokinetic parameters including $C_{max}$, $T_{max}$, and AUC.
- Pharmacodynamics is the study of the relationship between the pharmacokinetics of a drug and its tissue effects.
- Therapeutic drug monitoring combines the principles of pharmacokinetics and pharmacodynamics, and validates the adequacy of a dosing regimen.

## REFERENCES

1. Bauer LA. Clincial pharmacokinetics and pharmacodynamics. In: DiPiro JT, Talbert RL, Yee GC et al., eds. Pharmacotherapy: A Pathophysiologic Approach. 5th Ed. Stamford, CT: Appleton & Lange, 2002;33–54.
2. Nairn JG. Solutions, emulsions, suspensions and extracts. In: Gennaro AR, ed. Remington: The Science and Practice of Pharmacy. 20th Ed. Philadelphia: Lippincott, Williams & Wilkins, 2002;721–752.
3. Rudnic EM, Schwartz JD. Oral solid dosage forms. In: Gennaro AR, ed. Remington: The Science and Practice of Pharmacy. 20th Ed. Philadelphia: Lippincott, Williams & Wilkins, 2002;859–893.
4. Johnson MD, Newkirk G, White JR. Clinically significant drug interactions. Postgrad Med 1999;105:193–203.
5. Tuteja S, Alloway RR, Johnson JA et al. The effect of gut metabolism on tacrolimus bioavailability in renal transplant recipients. Transplantation 2001;71: 1303–1307.
6. Cockcroft DW, Gault MH. Prediction of creatinine clearance from serum creatinine. Nephron 1976;16:31–41.
7. Guidance for Industry: Bioavailability and Bioequivalence Studies for Orally Administered Drug Products—General Considerations. US Department of Health and Human Services, Food and Drug Administration, Center for Drug Evaluation and Research (CDER). March 2003. Retrieved from http:www.fda.gov/cder/guidance/index.htm. Accessed March 18–20.
8. Hardinger KL, Park JM, Schnitzler MA et al. Pharmacokinetics of tacrolimus in kidney transplant recipients: twice daily versus once daily dosing. Am J Transplant 2004;4:621–625.
9. Traub SL. Interpretation of serum drug concentrations. In: Traub SL, ed. Basic Skills in Interpreting Laboratory Data. 2nd Ed. Bethesda, MD: American Society of Health-System Pharmacists Special Projects Division, 1996;61–92.

# CHAPTER 21

# Gene Therapy and Pharmacogenomic Studies

Thomas Ferkol, Elliot Israel, Michael Wechsler

Beginning just 50 years ago, it became possible to determine how DNA encoded for proteins. The impact of this breakthrough on researchers' understanding of cellular and molecular physiology and pathophysiology has been nothing less than revolutionary. Now, and increasingly, biomedical research focuses on the structure and function of DNA, RNA, and proteins, in both health and disease. In the clinical arena, discoveries from this work have resulted in improved diagnostic tests and treatments. For example, pharmacogenetic studies can be performed to determine how genetic differences among individuals contribute to variability in responses to pharmacotherapy in these same individuals. Such information could be used to maximize the safety and efficacy of established drug therapies. Gene therapy, in contrast, involves new technologies designed to actually transfer genetic material (DNA or RNA) to diseased tissues as potentially powerful alternative treatments to standard drug therapy. Gene therapeutics could be used for diseases such as cancer, immunodeficiencies, cystic fibrosis, hemophilia, or inborn metabolic errors, among many others.

The use of genetic material or the study of individual genomic information raises many new problems for the design and conduct of clinical studies in areas such as pharmacogenetics and gene therapy. For instance, although it has been more than a decade since the first gene therapy trials were initiated, gene therapy has not yet become widespread because serious questions have developed about the safety of delivery systems ("vectors") used for gene transfer (1). Even so, results with some forms of gene therapy have been exciting and promising, and new studies continue to be designed and implemented. Accordingly, in this chapter, we briefly summarize the principles and basic concepts of gene therapy (including regulatory issues and processes required to initiate clinical trials). In addition, we summarize pharmacogenetic principles, discuss approaches to finding pharmacogenetic effects and confirming these effects prospectively, and finally, address the limitations and pitfalls of such approaches.

## GENERAL PRINCIPLES OF GENE THERAPY

The goal of gene therapy is the efficient introduction of functional, exogenous, genes into the somatic cells of patients, so that the transferred gene (the "transgene") will encode a sufficient amount of a therapeutic protein to ameliorate or even cure a disease. Several methods have been developed that can deliver genes to cells in tissue culture (in vitro) or to intact animals (in vivo), including recombinant viruses, liposomes, and molecular conjugates, each of which have unique advantages and disadvantages. Given the diverse conditions that could, potentially, be treated with gene therapy, it is unlikely that a single, universal vector will be applied to all situations. Undoubtedly, the best delivery system will differ for specific diseases, and the optimal method of gene transfer to be employed must be determined for each application.

In essence, gene therapy is simply a method of indirectly administering biologically relevant agents, that is, proteins, to specific cells or tissues. Instead of administering the protein directly as a drug ("biologic"), genes are administered with the goal of having them express sufficient amounts of the gene product to have a beneficial clinical effect. Thus, genes can be used as drugs in one sense, but the gene itself has no therapeutic effect; it must first be delivered to a target cell nucleus, transcribed into RNA, and ultimately expressed as a functional protein. The pharmacokinetics of the vectors and the efficacy of the therapeutics will vary (Figure 21–1) depending on the nature of the cells transduced, the tissue distribution of the vector, the efficiency and rate of DNA uptake, the rate of nuclear transport, the life span of both the transgene and the genetically modified cell, the rate of transcription and translation, post-translational processing, and the concentration, function, and duration of action of the transgene product (2–6).

A common misconception about gene therapy is that it leads to a permanent correction of a disease. Quite the opposite is true. Many of the vectors currently in use introduce foreign genes as episomes, and because the DNA is not integrated into the host genome, they will not persist. In these cases, transgene expression will be short-lived. Some viral vectors in fact insert, or integrate, the exogenous gene into the host cell's genome, but then the duration of expression depends on the survival of the transduced cell. Terminally differentiated cells have a finite life span, and genes delivered to these cells are lost when the cell dies. Progenitor or stem cells have become the "holy grail" for gene therapy, because their stable transduction could result in sustained or permanent correction of the host cell's phenotype. But even these cells may not produce a "cure" because foreign sequences can be unstable or transcription silenced by genetic and epigenetic mechanisms (7,8). Another concern is the development of neoplasia related to vector insertion. Recent reports have indicated that retrovirus and lentivirus vectors tend to integrate into transcriptional regulatory regions instead of randomly into the host genome as was previously thought (9).

The nature and characteristics of the targeted cell are important in determining the best approach for gene therapy. The first human gene transfer trials were performed using blood lymphocytes extracted from blood, genetically manipulated in culture, then reinfused into the patient (10). An advantage of an ex vivo approach is that the target cell population can be exposed to high concentrations of vector for greater periods of time to increase transfection efficiency. In addition, the phenotypic characteristics of the transfected cells can be studied before retransplantation, which should ensure that genetic correction has occurred (11, 12). Obviously, this technique is limited only to cells that are capable of reintegrating into the host, like circulating lymphocytes, bone marrow cells, and stem cells.

Conversely, other tissues, like those of the brain or lung, cannot be removed, treated, and reimplanted. They must be transfected *in vivo*, but direct gene delivery to these organs can have significant barriers. Anatomical obstacles can limit accessibility of target cells to the gene. There are also immunological barriers, because humoral and cell-mediated immunity can develop to the vector, gene product, or corrected cells (13–15). Indeed, immunogenicity of the gene transfer vector or gene product can be a limiting factor (16). In some cases, however, it can actually be the therapeutic goal. For recombinant vaccines and cancer therapy, immunogenic vectors that transiently express their transgene can be used (17–19). For other conditions that require long-term or permanent genetic correction, other vector systems will be needed.

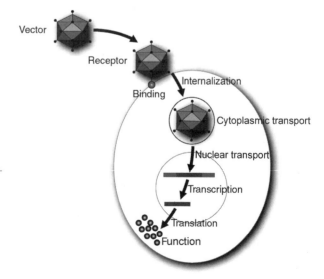

**FIGURE 21–1** ● Gene transfer vector packages the foreign DNA, binds to the cell surface, and undergoes internalization. Once inside the cell, the DNA escapes from the endosome and traffics to the nucleus, where it is transcribed into messenger RNA. The messenger RNA transcript is then transported to the cytoplasm, where it is translated into functional protein, which in turn affects the cellular physiology.

Gene therapy depends on the clinical goal and duration of transgene expression necessary to achieve the desired phenotypic change. Success depends on a thorough understanding of the genetic basis and pathogenesis of the disease. The timing and potential reversibility of the disease process related to mutant gene expression must be considered. For instance, gene therapy for many conditions, like metabolic diseases, must be applied before irreversible damage has occurred. Also, *all* gene therapy protocols to date have targeted somatic cells, and transfection of the germline has been consciously avoided. So far, germline transduction has not been shown in human clinical trials.

Thus, several factors must be considered when designing vehicles for gene delivery (Table 21–1). First, the vector must be able to effectively target genes to specific cell types. Although DNA can be nonselectively introduced into the cells ex vivo, vectors used for gene transfer in vivo require a targeting capability. Some systems rely on the presence of targeting moieties, for example, a ligand, or the natural tropism of the vector (as with some viral vectors) to direct genes to the affected cells. Alternatively, specificity can be achieved by the route of administration, producing localized delivery of the transgene, as in the case of intramuscular injection or aerosolized gene transfer *via* the respiratory tract. The vector should be able to package foreign genes of unlimited (or at least sufficient) size, thus permitting flexibility not only in the selection of the transgene but also its promoter regulatory elements. The choice of promoter is essential in determining the appropriate regulation of expression of the gene transferred into cells. The quantity and duration of transgene expression achieved by the candidate vector must be sufficient to correct the defect, because any vehicle used should have clear therapeutic benefits. If possible, the vector should be nonimmunogenic and nontoxic (Table 21–2). Finally,

## TABLE 21–1

### Considerations for Gene Therapy

- What organ systems should be targeted?
- What are the relevant cells to treat?
- What is the proportion of the affected cells and level of correction necessary to achieve a clinical benefit?
- Is overexpression of the transgene deleterious?
- What is the duration of expression of the transferred DNA?
- Will the gene transfer system or transgene product provoke an immune response?
- Can safety to the patient or others be assured?

treatment should not pose a risk to the patients or to their contacts, especially for viral vectors, where recombination is possible, which could result in infectious, replication-competent virus (20,21). And as noted previously, with some integrating vectors, investigators have increasing concerns about insertional mutagenesis leading to malignancy (22–24).

## CLINICAL TRIALS

Since 1989, more than 600 clinical trials involving human gene transfer have been approved. Many of the early studies were cell-marking trials, in which infiltrating cells were isolated from patients who had advanced tumors, transfected with a gene marker, then reinfused to examine the ability of genetically modified cells to home to tumors (10). Since then, the number of marker and therapeutic trials has rapidly expanded, with both ex vivo and in

## TABLE 21–2

### Immune or Pathologic Responses to Gene Transfer Vehicles

| Gene Transfer Vehicles | Cell-Mediated Response | Humoral Response | Cytotoxicity |
| --- | --- | --- | --- |
| Adenovirus | Yes | Yes | No |
| Adeno-associated virus | No | Yes | No |
| Retrovirus | No | No | No |
| Cationic liposomes | Rarely | Yes[a] | Yes |
| Molecular conjugates | No | Yes[a] | Yes |

[a]Dependent on ligand or other proteins incorporated into transfection complexes.

## TABLE 21–3

### Active or Completed Human Gene Therapy Protocols

**Infectious Diseases (40)**
Human immunodeficiency virus (37)
Other viral diseases (3)

**Monogenic Diseases (58)**
Alpha1-anti-trypsin deficiency (2)
Chronic granulomatous disease (3)
Cystic fibrosis (23)
Familial hypercholesterolemia (1)
Fanconi anemia (4)
Gaucher disease (3)
Hunter syndrome (1)
Ornithine transcarbamylase deficiency (1)
Purine nucleoside phosphorylase deficiency (1)
Severe combined immunodeficiency disease (6)
Leukocyte adhesion deficiency (1)
Canavan disease (3)
Hemophilia (5)
Muscular dystrophy (1)
Amyotrophic lateral sclerosis (1)
Junctional epidermolysis bullosa (1)
Neuronal ceroid lipofuscinosis (1)

**Cancer (405)**

**Other Diseases (66)**
Peripheral artery disease (24)
Arthritis (4)
Arterial restenosis (3)
Congestive heart failure (1)
Coronary artery disease (21)
Alzheimer disease (2)
Ulcer (3)
Bone fracture (1)
Peripheral neuropathy (1)
Parkinson disease (2)
Eye disorders (4)
Erectile dysfunction (1)
Intractable pain (1)

vivo approaches applied to a broad range of diseases (Table 21–3).

At first, gene therapy was considered most likely to be successful as therapy for monogenic diseases, primarily by reconstituting recessive genetic defects. Numerous clinical trials for autosomal and X-linked recessive diseases were initiated, including severe combined immunodeficiency, cystic fibrosis, hemophilia, Gaucher disease, Fanconi anemia, chronic granulomatous disease, familial hypercholesterolemia, and Hunter syndrome. The treatment goal in each case was to introduce a functional, normal gene into relevant somatic cell targets while avoiding the germline. Recipient cells for these diseases included circulating lymphocytes, peripheral blood stem cells, hepatocytes, myocytes, and respiratory epithelial cells. Some trials involved ex vivo gene transfection and reimplantation of genetically modified cells, but in many of these diseases, in vivo gene transfer was necessary.

More recently, acquired, nongenetic, or multifactorial diseases have been considered as potential targets for gene therapy. Cancer has by far been the most common clinical target in over 400

studies, but trials have been applied to AIDS, respiratory distress syndrome, rheumatoid arthritis, atherosclerosis, and peripheral vascular diseases. In many of these cases, the protocols have involved the introduction of "suicide" genes (18) or the expression of immunomodulatory cytokines in specific anatomic compartments.

Gene therapy successes have been few, and in most cases, therapeutic benefits have not been shown. One success story is the gene therapy protocol used for X-linked severe combined immunodeficiency. Results from these trials have been encouraging, though the recent development of T-cell malignancies in two patients has renewed concerns about safety.

## SAFETY AND REGULATION OF GENE THERAPY

The safety of gene therapy has become a matter of the highest priority, especially after the unfortunate death of one research volunteer and, as just noted, the development of malignancy in a few others. Gene therapy vectors can theoretically pose risks to the patients, their future children, and to the general population, all of which need to be minimized. Consequently, any gene therapy protocol that involves "deliberate transfer of recombinant DNA, or DNA or RNA derived from recombinant DNA, into human subjects" requires extensive review, and must be jointly appraised by each institution's IRB and IBC. Moreover, the NIH must review all protocols that are conducted at or sponsored by an institution that receives any support from the NIH (Table 21–4). The Office of Biotechnology Activities (OBA) is the office within the NIH that is responsible for reviewing and coordinating all activities relating to gene therapy, including certification of new vector systems. The OBA registers all human gene therapy experiments and maintains a complete database of such trials. Investigators must follow *NIH Guidelines* concerning recombinant DNA and gene transfer even if the trial sponsor has not received NIH funding support. A failure to do so jeopardizes *all* of the investigators' NIH funding, and not just that for the gene therapy protocol. The protocol review process is comprehensively discussed in the published *NIH Guidelines* (25) (http://www4.od.nih.gov/oba).

Once a gene therapy submission is received and reviewed by the NIH, the OBA determines whether submission to the Recombinant DNA Advisory Committee (RAC) is necessary. The RAC is the public advisory committee that advises the Department of Health and Human Services (DHHS) Secretary, the DHHS Assistant Secretary for Health, and the NIH Director concerning recombinant DNA research. The RAC examines clinical trials that involve the transfer of recombinant DNA to humans, and considers whether a proposed clinical gene transfer experiment presents characteristics that warrant public review, which is intended to foster the safe and ethical conduct of human gene transfer experiments.

The FDA can also be involved in the review process. The FDA, specifically the Center for Biologics Evaluation and Research (CBER), is the primary government agency dedicated to the review of new drug applications and regulation of human gene therapies (http://www.fda.gov/cber/infosheets/genezn.htm). Manufacturers or sponsors of new gene therapy vectors must meet FDA requirements before they can be sold in the United States. When a manufacturer is ready to study the gene therapy product in humans, it must obtain from the FDA an investigational new drug (IND) application, which describes study design, clinical benefits, possible risks, patient protection, and preclinical data that support the study. For more information about how to use preclinical data in support of a gene therapy study, see Chapter 22.

## TABLE 21–4

### Regulatory Documents for Human Gene Therapy

**Submission to Institutional Biosafety Committee (IBC)**

IBC Application Form

Human IRB Research Volunteer Panel Application Form

Human IRB Research Participants Consent Form

Investigational Brochure

Clinical Protocol

*NIH Guidelines* Appendix M

Proprietary information (if needed)

**Submission to Institutional Review Board (IRB)**

All items listed above, and IBC Approval Letter and Comments

**Submission to National Institutes of Health (NIH)**

*NIH Guidelines* Appendix M

Scientific abstract (1 page)

Nontechnical abstract (1 page)

Clinical Protocol

Appendices

IBC Approval Letter

IRB Approval Letter

Curriculum vitae for key personnel (2 page)

All human gene therapy trials must be approved by the IBC from each site participating in the study. The role of the IBC is to approve and oversee gene therapy projects in accordance with the responsibilities defined by the NIH. In forming their decision, the committee deliberates on the risks to research participants, anticipated benefits to participants, informed consent process, and importance of the knowledge to be gained from the trial. In particular, the IBC reviews the proposal to assess vector containment and potential for environmental release. Prior to the initiation of human gene therapy, the investigators must submit a registration document to the IBC that includes a description of (1) the gene and nature of the inserted DNA sequences; (2) the bacterial plasmid or phage vector; (3) the delivery vector to be used; (4) the protein that will be produced; and (5) the complete nucleotide sequence analysis or a detailed restriction enzyme analysis of the total construct.

The IBC must be informed which tissues or organs are to be the gene targets, and whether they will be characterized before and after treatment. For new in vivo gene transfer techniques, preclinical data describing efficacy of the proposed gene therapy system in cells or animal models may need to be provided, though for some approaches, results from animal gene transfer experiments have not predicted efficacy in humans (see Chapter 22). The investigators should indicate whether the transgene could be expressed in cells other than those targeted, especially whether germline transmission could occur. Reproductive hazards and possible risks to the fetus also need to be explained.

Vector toxicities must be described in the IBC application, including laboratory or clinical evidence of potential harmful effects of gene transfer, like neoplasia or immune response. The design of many existing vectors has minimized their pathogenicity, but investigators still must describe any potential hazards of the proposed vector to the patient and to persons other than those being treated. The IBC requires a clear description of containment conditions that will be implemented as specified in the *NIH Guidelines*. Containment depends on the gene transfer vector and how it will be used in the trial. Factors that should be considered in determining the level of containment include vector virulence, pathogenicity, infectious dose, environmental stability, route of spread, communicability, mode of administration, availability of treatment, and gene product effects such as toxicity and physiological activity. Any strain that is known to be more hazardous than the wild-type strain should be considered for handling at a higher containment level. Special care should be used in clinical trials that could potentially increase pathogenicity (e.g., insertion of a host oncogene) or broaden the host range of a viral vector. Also, the investigator must describe physical containment and laboratory procedures that are designed to prevent environmental spread, including special procedures and equipment that provide physical or biological barriers.

Any and all serious adverse events in response to the administration of a gene therapy vector must be reported *immediately* to the IRB, IBC, NIH Office for Protection from Research Risks, and FDA. A serious adverse event is any event occurring at any dose that results in death, a life-threatening event, in-patient hospitalization or prolongation of existing hospitalization, a persistent or significant disability, or birth defect. Important medical events that may not result in death, be life-threatening, or require hospitalization also may be considered a serious adverse event when, on the basis of appropriate medical judgment, they may jeopardize the human gene transfer research participant and could require medical or surgical intervention to prevent one of the outcomes listed in this definition. An adverse event is associated with the use of a gene transfer product when there is a reasonable possibility that the event may have been caused by the use of that product. Finally, the long-term safety of gene transfer needs to be monitored, and research volunteers require health surveillance *for years* beyond the treatment phase of the study.

## CYSTIC FIBROSIS AS A PARADIGM FOR A GENE THERAPY TRIAL

As mentioned previously, the design and implementation of clinical gene therapy studies depends greatly on the specific disease, the targeted tissue, and the chosen vector (for more about vectors themselves, see Chapter 22). Such trials are not generic. Preclinical mouse and primate studies showing efficacy, duration of clinical effect, and inflammatory or immune responses to the vector or corrected cells are useful, and data gathered from these investigations can provide general directions for clinical applications. However, not all diseases that could be amenable to gene therapy have animal models that recapitulate the human condition. Moreover, gene transfer into animals does not necessarily predict success or failure of the approach in patients, as was seen in initial gene therapy trials for cystic fibrosis (CF) (again, for more about the use of animal models for preclinical support of gene therapy, see Chapter 22).

CF is the most common inherited disease of Caucasians, occurring in 1:2,500–3,000 live births based on epidemiologic data from the United States (26). CF was once considered an ideal candidate for gene complementation because it is a monogenic, autosomal recessive defect. Only a small fraction of epithelial cells, roughly 6 to 10%, need to express the cystic fibrosis transmembrane conductance regulator (CFTR) for full correction of chloride transport (but not sodium hyperabsorption) of the epithelium, and low levels of functional CFTR, estimated at 10% of normal levels, could be sufficient to prevent lung disease (27,28). The most obvious target for gene therapy, the respiratory epithelial cell, is in contact with the environment, so airway application should direct the vector to the appropriate cells. Yet, despite promising cell and animal data, existing viral and nonviral vectors have only inefficiently delivered the CFTR gene to the patient's nasal or airway epithelium (29–32). This inefficiency is related to several different barriers (e.g., airway mucus) that exist in the diseased lung.

Despite these challenges, CF remains a highly attractive target for gene therapy. To conduct such a trial, approval is necessary, of course, from the investigator's IBC and IRB (and for new vectors, from the NIH and FDA). Phase I CF gene therapy studies are designed to first establish vector safety in affected, adult CF patients. These studies are not performed in non-CF volunteers. Safety markers depend on the vector, but usually include clinical and laboratory testing for local or systemic toxicity, pulmonary and radiographic evaluations, and measures of inflammation or immune responses directed against the vector.

For recombinant viruses, vector shedding, rescue, and germline transmission need to be assessed as well. Frequently, phase I clinical studies have a dose-escalation design, in which the first set of patients receives a low vector dose or titer, based on preclinical animal data. Once that vector dose is shown to be well tolerated and safe, the next set of research participants receives the next higher dose, and so on. For more on the design and analysis of studies involving small numbers of research participants, see Chapter 18.

In phase II studies, the highest, safest vector dose is used typically to obtain some evidence of efficacy of gene therapy at different times after treatment. The timetable for evaluating CFTR expression depends greatly on the selected vector and cells targeted. If successful, nonviral or adenoviral vectors typically have a brief duration of expression. Recombinant adeno-associated viral vectors, however, have the potential for prolonged transgene expression. Regardless of the vehicle chosen, long-term safety of gene transfer needs to be monitored, and research participants require health surveillance years beyond the treatment phase of the study.

A major challenge in any gene therapy trial is to decide on the most appropriate outcome markers. In CF, electrophysiological evidence of CFTR correction (i.e., cAMP-mediated chloride conductance across the nasal epithelium) and the "gold standard," CFTR transgene expression (i.e., mRNA or protein), are necessary to convincingly demonstrate that respiratory gene transfer has occurred successfully. One problem with these approaches is that CFTR gene expression or function can be measured in the nose or larger airways, but not at the most appropriate site for CF lung disease; that is, small-to-medium airways. The other problem, of course, is that mere expression of the transgene does not mean that a meaningful clinical effect has taken or will take effect. In CF, clinical outcome markers have included changes in pulmonary function and chest radiographs, but because CF is characterized by progressive, suppurative pulmonary disease that gradually produces irreversible airway obstruction, it is unlikely that any patient treated with gene therapy will have substantial *improvement* in pulmonary function (i.e., the goal at this early stage of development is to *prevent* additional lung dysfunction). Thus, truly relevant effects may take years to observe. Other proposed CF phenotypic markers, like a reduction in the hyperinflammatory response, are controversial. The absence of such clinically relevant measures has made it difficult to clearly judge

the success of CF gene transfer, a long-standing limitation to CF gene therapy. Similar problems plague many other gene therapy protocols.

## FUTURE DIRECTIONS

Although gene therapy holds promise for a number of diseases, and several approaches have been applied to patients, success has been limited so far. Complications have further reduced enthusiasm for some vector systems. Consequently, adaptations of existing technologies or the development of new vehicles are necessary to allow gene therapy to achieve its potential. The next generation of vectors will be critical for the future of gene therapy. Some of the more innovative approaches to gene therapy have focused on the genetic payload. The use of silencing RNA or antisense therapy has rapidly expanded, and such approaches are being examined in preclinical studies (33,34). Human artificial chromosomes, containing functional telomeres, centromeres, and origins of replication, are being designed to permit the regulated expression and independent replication of genes of unlimited size (35). Indeed, artificial chromosomes should be able to accommodate not only the transgene (cDNA or intact gene) but its promoter and enhancer elements as well. Although early results have been highly variable, homologous recombination (36), ribozyme technologies (37), and RNA-DNA chimeraplasty are being developed to "surgically" correct specific mutant alleles.

## GENERAL PRINCIPLES OF PHARMACOGENETICS

Pharmacogenetics is the term applied to the study of the contribution of genetic differences among individuals to the variability in the responses to pharmacotherapy among individuals. Pharmacogenetics uses genetic information to identify both the functional differences of various genes between individuals, as well as underlying mechanisms responsible for differences in therapeutic responses, with the potential for maximizing safety and efficacy of established drug therapies. While general associations between genetic variation and human diseases often require a large number of patients and a long period of time to assess for manifestation of a given disease, pharmacogenetic studies lend themselves to a true clinical trial paradigm where hypotheses can be tested relatively quickly with smaller populations.

To understand pharmacogenetics, one must first appreciate concepts concerning variability and repeatability of drug response. Within a population, all individuals with a given disease do not respond to the same extent to any one therapy. This "interindividual variability" reflects the fact that some individuals respond beneficially to a particular treatment, while others may experience no benefit, and still others may even experience an adverse effect. In addition to interindividual responses, each individual may respond variably to a given therapy on repeated occasions (repeatability or intraindividual variability). In general, interindividual variability of response to therapy exceeds intraindividual variability or repeatability.

Many potential explanations account for both interindividual as well as intraindividual variability, including severity of disease, environmental factors, medication compliance, interaction with other medications, and intercurrent illness. However, a substantial fraction of interindividual variability in response to drug treatments, as much as 70%, may be genetic in nature (38). If correct, this estimate suggests that a large proportion of the millions of medication-related adverse effects that occur annually in the United States (39) may have a genetic basis.

Genetic variation can produce variations in individual responses by three major mechanisms (Table 21–5). First, there may be genetic variants associated with altered distribution, metabolism, or uptake of a medication. These differences in pharmacokinetics (see Chapter 20) may lead to enhanced or impaired drug clearance or even drug inactivation. Second, genetic variations may result in a drug action that is outside of its intended therapeutic effect. For instance, women receiving hormone replacement therapy who harbor certain polymorphic alleles in the prothrombin gene are at increased risk of developing thromboembolism (40). The third major pharmacogenetic mechanism is the result of genetic variation within a drug target (such as an ion channel or a membrane receptor). Such variation may lead to altered drug efficacy or to differences in the expression of a physiological phenotype.

## TABLE 21–5

### Major Pharmacogenetic Mechanisms

1. Genetic variation associated with altered distribution, metabolism, or uptake of a given medication, leading to enhanced or impaired drug clearance or even inactivation of a drug.

2. Genetic variations resulting in an unintended action of a drug outside of its intended therapeutic effect.

3. Genetic variation in a drug target, leading to altered drug efficacy and differences in expression of a physiological phenotype.

To illustrate how genetic variability may lead to different responses to therapy, and how pharmacogenetics studies can help explain these different responses to therapy, consider the following two examples: gefitinib for lung cancer and pravastatin for cholesterol reduction.

### Example 1: Gefitinib

Gefitinib is an epidermal growth factor receptor (EGFR) inhibitor that is approved as a third-line therapy for the treatment of lung cancer. While antitumor activity is evident in vitro, fewer than 20% of lung cancer patients respond to this expensive and somewhat toxic therapy (41). To explore the possibility that a mutation in the EGFR gene accounts for the favorable response of some patients with lung cancer to gefitinib, the EGFR gene was sequenced in the tumors of those who did and those who did not respond to gefitinib (42) (for further discussion of using DNA sequencing in clinical research, see Chapters 31–34). Almost 90% of gefitinib responders, and none of the nonresponders, harbored a specific mutation within the tyrosine kinase domain of the EGFR gene. Although this mutation is rare, there was a clear beneficial response to those who harbored the mutation. Thus, pharmacogenetic information could be used in this instance to target therapy, maximize response, and minimize cost and toxicity.

### Example 2: Pravastatin

Pravastatin is a cholesterol-lowering therapy that inhibits the enzyme HMG-CoA reductase, and is effective in some but not all patients with high cholesterol. Retrospectively, it was determined that individuals heterozygous for a genetic variant in the HMG-CoA reductase gene experienced smaller reductions in cholesterol (up to 22% smaller reduction) when treated with pravastatin than individuals homozygous for the major allele of one of the gene's polymorphisms (43). This was the first study to demonstrate the impact of genetic variation on the efficacy of this popular and widely used class of drugs.

## APPROACHES TO FINDING PHARMACOGENETIC EFFECTS AND DESIGNING PHARMACOGENETIC TRIALS

Clearly, demonstrating a pharmacogenetic effect could have a major impact on the use of pharmacotherapy in general and on drug safety in particular. The impetus for a specific pharmacogenetic investigation may start with the desire to define the cause of a particular response, or alternatively, may stem from the discovery of a particular gene with

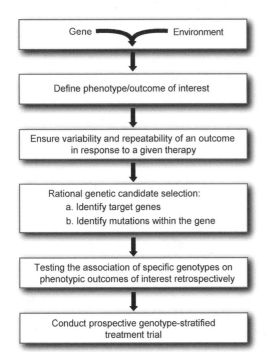

**FIGURE 21–2** ● Flowchart of how to approach undertaking a pharmacogenetics trial. Initial hypothesis may derive from an attempt to define the cause of a particular response, or alternatively, may derive from the discovery of a particular gene with functional properties or associations, which suggest that it may be involved in the response to a particular pharmacotherapy.

functional properties or associations that suggest it may be involved in the response to a particular pharmacotherapy. In either case, the strategy of pursuing a pharmacogenetic investigation should involve the following steps: (1) define the specific phenotypic response, (2) ascertain that the given outcome or response to therapy is variable within the population and repeatable within individuals, (3) identify a candidate gene and its variations, and then (4) ideally, test these associations retrospectively and, if possible, prospectively (Figure 21–2). These steps are considered in more detail below. In addition, all such studies must of course receive IRB approval, which requires special consideration and protections in these cases because genetic information about individuals will be acquired (see Chapter 14).

## DEFINING THE PHENOTYPE AND OUTCOMES OF INTEREST

Drugs typically have multiple effects, each of which, if associated with a particular genotype, could be considered a specific phenotype. Whether an investigator is searching for a gene to explain a pharmacogenetic response, or for a response to associate with a particular gene, only some of a drug's

possible phenotypic outcomes may be associated with a given genetic polymorphism. Thus, precisely defining both the phenotype and the outcomes of interest (e.g., symptoms, lab tests, functional assays) is crucially important when planning a pharmacogenetic study. Imprecise definitions can result in either false-positive or false-negative associations because a too narrow definition excludes participants that could have been identified with a broader phenotype definition, and a too broad definition dilutes the effects of genotype on research participants identified by a more narrowly defined phenotype. For example, in patients with asthma, a mutation may be associated with a response to a therapy that is only related to asthma exacerbations specifically but not to respiratory symptoms more generally or to objective changes in lung function. Thus, a failure to define the outcome of interest, in this case specifically as an asthma exacerbation, could result in a failure to identify the pharmacogenetic association.

Obviously, in cases where a particular genetic candidate is under investigation, the choice of outcome can be more informed if the functional effects of various polymorphisms in the gene are also understood. Thus, using the β-adrenergic receptor as an example of a candidate gene, initial investigations focused on outcomes reflecting the acute bronchodilator response to β-agonists. Later, an association with tachyphylactic responses to regular use of these agents was explored (44).

## DETERMINE VARIABILITY AND REPEATABILITY OF AN OUTCOME IN RESPONSE TO A GIVEN THERAPY

One of the most important aspects of choosing phenotypes and outcomes to study in pharmacogenetic studies is ensuring that the response to pharmacotherapy is variable among individuals within a population and that there is a degree of repeatability of response within each individual. With high levels of intraindividual variability, a pharmacogenetic effect will be difficult to detect (unless, in the case of gene-environment interactions, the environmental factor can be controlled). Alternatively, if there is little interindividual variability, it is unlikely that a strong pharmacogenetic effect is playing any role in determining responses to the drug.

## IDENTIFYING TARGET GENES AND THEIR VARIANTS

Although a detailed discussion of how to identify specific gene targets is beyond the scope of this chapter (see Chapters 32 and 33), it obviously becomes easier to identify a potential target gene as the mechanism responsible for a specific drug effect becomes better understood. For example, an investigator might wish to examine genes that are known to modulate a specific pathway that can influence a drug's metabolism or synthesis. A good example of such a case would be studies of polymorphisms of the HMG-CoA reductase gene and its association to responses to cholesterol lowering drugs (43).

In addition to this mechanism-based, heuristic model of gene selection, nonheuristic models of target gene identification, resulting from genome wide screens and expression profiling, are becoming more common. For a more detailed discussion of these techniques, see Chapter 34.

The choice of which variants to study within a gene may also have a significant effect on whether an association with a particular outcome will be identified. For any given gene, there may be multiple mutations within the gene that may be associated with a response to a given treatment. These mutations include, for instance, insertions, deletions, single nucleotide polymorphisms (SNPs), or variable nucleotide tandem repeats (VNTRs, or microsatellites). Each of these mutations may occur anywhere along the length of the gene, in both coding and noncoding regions of the gene or in the 5' and 3' untranslated regions. Not all of these mutations may cause changes in the amino acid sequence conferred by the genotype, and not all amino acid changes may cause changes in the function of the protein that is transcribed. Although variants that affect amino acid sequence are most likely to affect function, it should be noted that other variants may affect transcription or translation and produce clinical effects as well. In addition, combinations of variants along a chromosome (haplotypic combinations) may produce more significant effects than any single variant. Public databases (e.g., dbSNP) list many of the known mutations for each particular gene.

In choosing variants, be careful to choose mutations that occur with sufficient frequency in the population that further investigation is warranted. In general, focus on associations with combinations of mutant alleles that occur in at least 10% of the population. However, if there is a strong biological candidate with evidence for a large effect, investigators may consider SNPs occurring at lower frequencies.

## TESTING THE ASSOCIATION OF SPECIFIC GENOTYPES ON PHENOTYPIC OUTCOMES OF INTEREST

As the principal outcome in pharmacogenetic studies is the response to a given therapy, researchers must identify populations that have received the

therapy, and then assess the effect of each mutation on the response to that therapy. Having assembled a cohort, identified phenotypic responses of interest, and identified candidate genetic variations, a researcher can proceed to genotype the DNA of participants and then assess whether significant associations are present between different mutations and different phenotypes of interest. Genotyping technology is now widely available and its cost continues to drop (45). Although statistical approaches to genetic analysis and multiple comparisons are also widely available (see Chapter 26), it is prudent to confirm any apparent associations in a second population, if possible. Such replication increases the validity of the putative finding and, depending on the population examined, may address some of the most common caveats commonly raised regarding pharmacogenetic studies (discussed below). Further, to avoid associations related to population substructure, it is important to try to analyze specific effects in specific population subgroups (e.g., Caucasians, etc.).

## PERFORMING A GENOTYPE-STRATIFIED PROSPECTIVE TREATMENT TRIAL

Putative pharmacogenetic effects, because they involve administration of an intervention, lend themselves to potential confirmation in prospective, blinded studies with an experimental design (Chapter 8). Such pharmacogenetics studies are only now being conducted. Thus, if an association is identified and replicated in independent study populations, investigators should test the retrospective pharmacogenetic association in a prospective manner, especially before making clinical recommendations based on these findings. The most rigorous trials involve cohort studies by genotype, in which genotype identity is double-blinded and in which treatment is double-blinded (see example below). In these studies, when placebo controls are used, investigators can assess differences in response between genotype groups as well as the response to therapy within a given genotype. In developing such a trial, it is important to ensure that enough patients with the genotype of interest are studied and that the effect size will be large enough to be detected using the given sample size (see below).

## LIMITATIONS AND PITFALLS OF PHARMACOGENETIC TRIALS

Although pharmacogenetic investigations can potentially shed light on the relationship between genetic variability and differences among individuals in response to therapy, several caveats need to be considered. First, pharmacogenetic studies, by definition, are observational studies (Chapter 7) that can identify *associations* between genetic variants and responses to therapy but do not prove causation. As with all observational studies, careful consideration should be given to possible confounders, factors that in this case may confound the apparent relationship between genotype and drug response. For instance, the gene under investigation may not actually be causative itself but may be linked to another causative genetic variation. This linkage may be a result of the putative gene's proximity to the causative gene on the chromosome (linkage disequilibrium), due to a particular distribution of multiple variants in geographic proximity to each other (haplotype), or due to the distribution of susceptibility gene(s) in that particular population. For example, a particular SNP may be associated with a lack of response to a specific antihypertensive therapy in African Americans as compared to Caucasians but the SNP may also be over-represented in African Americans, who, for some other reason have a different response to this therapy. If the population under study contains both Caucasians and African Americans, then a pharmacogenetic effect may be falsely attributed to the SNP. Such confounding, due to stratification within the population examined, can be reduced by examining associations in genetically homogeneous subgroups. Further, genetic techniques that can examine the distribution of panels of SNPs across the entire genome allow investigators to detect substructure within a population.

Another possibility is that a particular polymorphism may be more prevalent in specific groups because of different environmental exposures. For example, if a certain ethnic group has a much higher rate of smoking, and smoking has been associated with resistance to corticosteroid therapy (46), then genes associated with that ethnicity might be incorrectly associated with diminished responsiveness to corticosteroid therapy. In addition, it is possible that epigenetic effects (interactions among different genes) with the variant of interest may be specific to a particular population and that subsequent associations may not hold up in other populations. Thus, the robustness of an association is best assessed if it can be replicated in a different population. Of course, a failure to replicate the original observation in a different ethnic population may not mean that the association was spurious, but rather may suggest that it requires an interaction with a genetic, or environmental, substrate not present in the population chosen for replication. In this regard, an examination of haplotypic structure (the pattern of variants in a gene

on a single chromosome) may yield clues as to which variants are indeed active.

A common and often major limitation of pharmacogenetic association studies is the sample size required in order to demonstrate a pharmacogenetic effect (see Chapter 9). Depending on the frequency of the allele, the relative effect size, and the degree to which the investigator corrects for Type I error probability, most association studies require large numbers of cases and controls, particularly as the investigator explores alleles that occur with lower frequency or that have less of an effect. Conversely, studying alleles that occur with greater frequency or larger effects reduces the necessary sample size. The problem of multiple comparisons when testing hypothetical links between multiple polymorphisms and multiple putative outcomes also needs to be considered. Such testing may lead to Type I errors, that is, where the association is accepted as real when it is in fact false. The fact that relatively few studies have replicated numerous reported associations suggests that this problem may confound many published studies. Replication of results in a separate population with strict correction for multiple comparisons makes such a result less likely.

As already mentioned, replication is important not only from a statistical point of view, but also from the viewpoint of overall scientific credibility. If the association persists in a replication population that is significantly different from the original population, then the chance that observed effects are related to gene-gene interactions or gene-environment interactions that are peculiar to the populations studied will be less.

## ASTHMA AS A PARADIGM FOR A PHARMACOGENETICS STUDY

Asthma is a disease that has been fruitful for studies of pharmacogenetic responses and serves as a model of how to undertake such investigations using the strategy outlined above (Figure 21–2).

### Step 1: Define Phenotype or Outcome of Interest

Asthma is a heterogeneous, complex syndrome characterized by recurrent bouts of airflow obstruction and bronchial hyper-responsiveness. Various inflammatory mediators and cytokines within the airways appear to produce a state of both chronic and acute airway narrowing. Potentially relevant outcomes that could be studied include physiologic measures (such as peak exploratory flow or forced expiratory volume over one second), clinical outcomes (such as respiratory symptoms, quality of life, number of clinical exacerbations), and measures of the concentrations of inflammatory markers within blood or airway secretions.

## Step 2: Ensure Variability and Repeatability of Response to a Given Therapy

Major modalities of asthma therapy include bronchodilating β-agonist therapy and anti-inflammatory agents (inhaled corticosteroids, or modifiers of leukotriene expression or effect). Although most asthmatics derive some benefit from these treatments, there is a wide spectrum of response (interindividual variability) to each of these agents. For instance, there is a large variability in the response to β-agonists within a group of mild asthmatics (47). Similarly, there is significant variability in the response to both inhaled corticosteroids and leukotriene modifiers (48,49). Nonetheless, for each of these agents, there is a repeatability of response to therapy, that is those who respond at some point, generally respond again.

## Step 3: Rational Target Gene Identification

β-agonists and leukotriene modifiers both have well-defined mechanisms of action for their salutary effects. The β-agonists work in asthma by binding the $β_2$-adrenergic receptor. Leukotriene modifiers work by interfering with the action or synthesis of the leukotrienes, for which the biosynthetic pathway has also been well defined. In the case of the $β_2$-adrenergic receptor, both synonymous and nonsynonymous SNPs in the coding and noncoding regions of the $β_2$-adrenergic receptor gene have been associated with functional changes in receptor biology (44). Similar work has been done with regard to the leukotriene modifiers in which the 5-lipoxygenase and LTC4 synthase genes have been identified along with variants within these genes (50,51).

## Step 4: Assess Effect of Specific Genotypes on Phenotypic Outcomes of Interest Retrospectively

Initial pharmacogenetic studies of β-agonists in asthma focused on nonsynonymous SNPs in the coding region with significant minor allele frequencies (e.g., the 16 and 27 amino acid position of the $β_2$-adrenergic receptor gene). Martinez et al. (52) studied the effects of $β_2$ receptor genotype on lung function in a group of 78 children with a history of wheezing. Of those individuals who were homozygous for arginine at position 16 of the β-2

receptor gene, 60% had a positive response to albuterol, compared with only 13% response in those individuals who were homozygous for glycine at that position (p = 0.05). Israel et al. showed that this arginine β-agonist receptor polymorphism was associated with apparent increased tachyphylaxis as indicated by a decline in peak expiratory flow with regular use of the β-agonist albuterol (47). Further, Taylor et al. demonstrated that patients with the Arg/Arg genotype had an increased frequency of asthma exacerbations during regular treatment with albuterol compared to treatment with placebo (53). These studies in different populations of different ages suggested that there was a true association between the polymorphisms under study and β-agonist response. Of note, recent studies examining patterns of synonymous and nonsynonymous SNPs (haplotypes) suggest that patterns of β-adrenergic receptor SNPs may also be useful in determining pharmacogenetic associations.

## Step 5: Conduct a Prospective Genotype-Stratified Treatment Trial

The retrospective findings of differential effects of regular albuterol use by genotype have recently been corroborated in a genotype-stratified prospective trial that stratified subjects based on genotype (Arg/Arg versus Gly/Gly) and examined outcomes in response to various asthma therapies. Israel et al. demonstrated that Arg/Arg homozygotes had improved peak expiratory flow when withdrawn from "as needed" β-agonist use with albuterol (54). Thus, multiple studies over the last several years have confirmed a pharmacogenetic association between β-adrenergic receptor genotype and response to albuterol. Again, it appears that patterns of different polymorphisms in nearby areas, or genetic haplotypes (the ordered arrangement of different alleles of a given gene), may also play a role in predicting individual responses (55).

## SUMMARY

- Gene therapy involves the transfer of genetic material (DNA or RNA) to diseased tissues as potentially powerful alternative treatments to standard drug therapy. This therapeutic strategy may be applicable to a broad range of monogenic and polygenic diseases. The goal of gene therapy is the efficient introduction of functional, exogenous, genes into the somatic cells of patients, so that the transferred gene (the "transgene") will encode a sufficient amount of a therapeutic protein to ameliorate or even cure a disease.

- Various viral and nonviral vectors can be used to effect gene transfer. The pharmacokinetics of the vectors and the efficacy of the therapeutics vary depending on the nature of the cells transduced, the tissue distribution of the vector, the efficiency and rate of DNA uptake, the rate of nuclear transport, the life span of both the transgene and the genetically modified cell, the rate of transcription and translation, posttranslational processing, and the concentration, function, and duration of action of the transgene product.

- Safety continues to be a major concern for gene therapy. Accordingly, in addition to approval by the institution's IRB, additional regulatory scrutiny by various NIH, FDA, and institutional review committees must be undertaken before beginning any gene therapy study in humans.

- A key decision in any gene therapy study is to decide on the most appropriate outcome and safety markers. The latter depends on the vector used, but usually includes clinical and laboratory testing for organ or systemic toxicity, measures of organ function, and measures of inflammation or immune responses directed against the vector.

- Pharmacogenetics is an emerging discipline that allows clinical investigators to determine whether associations exist between genetic variability and the response (both salutary and adverse) to various pharmacotherapies. These associations hold out the promise of being able to individualize pharmacotherapy by providing specific drug treatments to those most likely to respond, while avoiding therapy in those most likely to suffer adverse effects.

- The key elements of designing a pharmacogenetics study are (1) to define the specific phenotypic response, (2) to ascertain that the given outcome or response to therapy is variable within the population and repeatable within individuals, (3) to identify a candidate gene and its variations, and then ideally, (4) to test these associations retrospectively and, if possible, prospectively.

- Unless very large effects from a polymorphism are expected, polymorphisms with frequencies of 10% or greater in the population are usually required if the population study sample is to be of reasonable size.

- Initial investigations may benefit by studying populations that are relatively racially and ethnically homogeneous. Broader applicability of any initial findings requires additional testing in more diverse populations. It may also be important to consider pharmacogenetic associations with different haplotypes, which may indicate that an interaction among different genes accounts for a given phenotype.

## REFERENCES

1. Somia N, Verma IM. Gene therapy: trials and tribulations. Nat Rev Genet 2000;1:91–99.
2. Shapiro Ledley T, Ledley FD. Pharmacokinetic considerations in somatic gene therapy. Adv Drug Deliv Rev 1998;30:133–150.
3. Kamiya H, Akita H, Harashima H. Pharmacokinetic and pharmacodynamic considerations in gene therapy. Drug Discov Today 2003;8:990–996.
4. Flotte T, Ferkol TW. Genetic therapy. In: Koren G and Bailey B, eds. Clinical Pharmacology. Pediatr Clin North Am 1997;44:153–178.
5. Russell SJ, Peng KW. Primer on medical genomics: Part X: gene therapy. Mayo Clin Proc 2003;78:1370–83.
6. Papadakis ED, Nicklin SA, Baker AH et al. Promoters and control elements: designing expression cassettes for gene therapy. Curr Gene Ther 2004;4:89–113.
7. Jackson DA. Chromosome structure and nuclear architecture: implications for gene therapy. Curr Opin Mol Ther 2002;4:290–298.
8. Pannell D, Ellis J. Silencing of gene expression: implications for design of retrovirus vectors. Rev Med Virol 2001;11:205–217.
9. Laufs S, Gentner B, Nagy KZ et al. Retroviral vector integration occurs in preferred genomic targets of human bone marrow-repopulating cells. Blood 2003; 101:2191–2198.
10. Rosenberg SA, Aebersold P, Cornetta K et al. Gene transfer into humans—immunotherapy of patients with advanced melanoma, using tumor-infiltrating lymphocytes modified by retroviral gene transduction. N Engl J Med 1990;323:570–578.
11. Thomas CE, Ehrhardt A, Kay MA. Progress and problems with the use of viral vectors for gene therapy. Nat Rev Genet 2003;4:346–358.
12. Dunbar CE, Emmons RV. Gene transfer into hematopoietic progenitor and stem cells: progress and problems. Stem Cells 1994;12:563–576.
13. Gautam A, Waldrep JC, Densmore CL. Aerosol gene therapy. Mol Biotechnol 2003;23:51–60.
14. Rainov NG, Kramm CM. Vector delivery methods and targeting strategies for gene therapy of brain tumors. Curr Gene Ther 2001;1:367–383.
15. Aguilar LK, Aguilar-Cordova E. Evolution of a gene therapy clinical trial. From bench to bedside and back. J Neurooncol 2003;65:307–315.
16. Yang Y, Jooss KU, Su Q et al. Immune responses to viral antigens versus transgene product in the elimination of recombinant adenovirus-infected hepatocytes in vivo. Gene Ther 1996;3:137–144.
17. Ribas A, Butterfield LH, Glaspy JA et al. Current developments in cancer vaccines and cellular immunotherapy. J Clin Oncol 2003;21:2415–2432.
18. Dermime S, Armstrong A, Hawkins RE et al. Cancer vaccines and immunotherapy. Br Med Bull 2002;62: 149–162.
19. Niculescu-Duvaz I, Springer CJ. Introduction to the background, principles, and state of the art in suicide gene therapy. Methods Mol Med 2004;90:1–27.
20. Selden RF, Skoskiewicz MJ, Russell PS et al. Regulation of insulin-gene expression: Implications for gene therapy. N Engl J Med 1987;317:1067–1076.
21. Collins FS. Cystic fibrosis: molecular biology and therapeutic implications. Science 1992;256:774–779.
22. Hacein-Bey-Abina S, Le Deist F, Carlier F et al. Sustained correction of X-linked severe combined immunodeficiency by ex vivo gene therapy. N Engl J Med 2002;346:1185–1193.

23. Hacein-Bey-Abina S, von Kalle C, Schmidt M et al. A serious adverse event after successful gene therapy for X-linked severe combined immunodeficiency [letter]. N Engl J Med 2003;348:255–256.

24. Baum C, von Kalle C, Staal FJ et al. Chance or necessity? Insertional mutagenesis in gene therapy and its consequences. Mol Ther 2004;9:5–13.

25. Guidelines for Research Involving Recombinant DNA Molecules (NIH Guidelines). Department of Health and Human Services National Institutes of Health. April 2002 (http://www4.od.nih.gov/oba/rac/guidelines/guidelines.html)

26. FitzSimmons SC. The changing epidemiology of cystic fibrosis. J Pediatr 1993;122:1–9.

27. Johnson LG, Olsen JC, Sarkadi B et al. Efficiency of gene transfer for restoration of normal airway epithelial function in cystic fibrosis. Nat Genet 1992;2:21–25.

28. Chillon M, Casals T, Mercier B et al. Mutations in the cystic fibrosis gene in patients with congenital absence of the vas deferens. N Engl J Med 1995;332:1475–1480.

29. Knowles MR, Hohneker KW, Zhou Z et al. A controlled study of adenoviral-vector-mediated gene transfer in the nasal epithelium of patients with cystic fibrosis. N Engl J Med 1995;333:823–831.

30. Noone PG, Hohneker KW, Zhou Z et al. Safety and biological efficacy of a lipid-CFTR complex for gene transfer in the nasal epithelium of adult patients with cystic fibrosis. Mol Ther 2000;1:105–114.

31. Moss RB, Rodman D, Spencer LT et al. Repeated adeno-associated virus serotype 2 aerosol-mediated cystic fibrosis transmembrane regulator gene transfer to the lungs of patients with cystic fibrosis: a multicenter, double-blind, placebo-controlled trial. Chest 2004;125:509–521.

32. Wagner JA, Messner AH, Moran ML et al. Safety and biological efficacy of an adeno-associated virus vector-cystic fibrosis transmembrane regulator (AAV-CFTR) in the cystic fibrosis maxillary sinus. Laryngoscope 1999;109:266–274.

33. Devroe E, Silver PA. Therapeutic potential of retroviral RNAi vectors. Expert Opin Biol Ther 2004;4:319–327.

34. Shuey DJ, McCallus DE, Giordano T. RNAi: gene-silencing in therapeutic intervention. Drug Discov Today 2002;7:1040–1046.

35. Grimes BR, Warburton PE, Farr CJ. Chromosome engineering: prospects for gene therapy. Gene Ther 2002;9:713–718.

36. Yanez RJ, Porter AC. Therapeutic gene targeting. Gene Ther 1998;5:149–159.

37. Freelove AC, Zheng R. The power of ribozyme technologies: the logical way ahead for molecular medicine and gene therapy? Curr Opin Mol Ther 2002;4:419–422.

38. Drazen JM, Silverman EK, Lee TH. Heterogeneity of therapeutic responses in asthma. Br Med Bull 2000;56:1054–1070.

39. Johnson J, Bootman J. Drug-related morbidity and mortality. Arch Intern Med 1995;155:1949–1956.

40. Poort SR, Rosendaal FR, Reitsma PH et al. A common genetic variation in the 3'-untranslated region of the prothrombin gene is associated with elevated plasma prothrombin levels and an increase in venous thrombosis. Blood 1996;88:3698–3703.

41. Green M. Targeting targeted therapy. N Engl J Med 2004;350:2191–2193.

42. Lynch T, Bell DW, Sordella R et al. Activating mutations in the epidermal growth factor receptor underlying the responsiveness of non-small-cell lung cancer to gefitinib. N Engl J Med 2004;350:2129–2139.

43. Chasman D, Posada D, Subrahmanyan L et al. Pharmacogenetic study of statin therapy and cholesterol reduction. JAMA 2004;291:2821–2827.

44. Liggett SB. Polymorphisms of the $\beta_2$-adrenergic receptor and asthma. Am J Respir Crit Care Med 1997;156:S156–S162.

45. Haga SB, Burke W. Using pharmacogenetics to improve drug safety and efficacy. JAMA 2004;291(2):2869–2871.

46. Chalmers GW, Macleod KJ, Little SA et al. Influence of cigarette smoking on inhaled corticosteroid treatment in mild asthma. Thorax 2002;57:226–230.

47. Israel E, Drazen JM, Liggett SB et al. The effect of polymorphisms of the $\beta_2$-adrenergic receptor on the response to regular use of albuterol in asthma. Am J Respir Crit Care Med 2000;162:75–80.

48. Szefler SJ, Martin RJ, King TS et al. Significant variability in response to inhaled corticosteroids for persistent asthma. J Allergy Clin Immunol 2002;109:410–418.

49. Malmstrom K, Rodriguez-Gomez G, Guerra J et al. Oral montelukast, inhaled beclomethasone, and placebo for chronic asthma: a randomized, controlled trial. Ann Intern Med 1999;130:487–495.

50. Drazen JM, Yandava C, Dube L et al. Pharmacogenetic association between ALOX5 promoter genotype and the response to anti-asthma treatment. Nat Genet 1999;22:168–170.

51. Sampson AP, Siddiqui S, Buchanan D et al. Variant LTC$_4$ synthase allele modifies cysteinyl leukotriene synthesis in eosinophils and predicts clinical response to zafirlukast. Thorax 2000;55 Suppl 2:S28–S31.

52. Martinez FD, Graves PE, Baldini M et al. Association between genetic polymorphisms of the $\beta_2$-adrenoceptor and response to albuterol in children with and without a history of wheezing. J Clin Invest 1997;100:3184–3188.

53. Taylor DR, Drazen JM, Herbison GP et al. Asthma exacerbations during long term $\beta$-agonist use: influence of $\beta_2$ adrenoceptor polymorphism. Thorax 2000;55:762–767.

54. Israel E, Chinchilli VM, Ford JG et al. Use of regularly scheduled albuterol treatment in asthma: genotype-stratified, randomised, placebo-controlled cross-over trial. Lancet 2004;364:1505–1512.

55. Drysdale CM, McGraw DW, Stack CB et al. Complex promoter and coding region $\beta_2$-adrenergic receptor haplotypes alter receptor expression and predict in vivo responsiveness. Proc Natl Acad Sci USA 2000;97:10483–10488.

# CHAPTER 22

# Preparing for Gene Therapy Studies

Mark S. Sands, Jan A. Nolta, Gerhard Bauer, Thomas Ferkol

Gene therapy represents a conceptually simple and attractive form of therapy, especially for inherited monogenic diseases (1). Somatic gene therapy refers to the transfer of genetic material (usually a chimeric expression cassette containing cis-acting regulatory elements and an intact gene or cDNA) to nongermline cells. By targeting and limiting gene transfer to somatic cells, the genetic modification cannot be passed on to future generations. Nevertheless, if the gene transfer vector, either viral or nonviral, integrates into the somatic cell's genome, or remains as a stable episome, then this form of therapy has the potential to provide a lifelong source of the deficient or inactive protein. Although conceptually simple, the efficient transfer of genetic material into somatic cells has been technically challenging. In fact, although hundreds of gene therapy clinical trials have been performed, this seemingly simple approach has yielded little in the way of efficacy. This lack of success is the result of several factors. For one, DNA is a very large molecule and researchers still do not fully understand how to use cellular machinery to transfer intact DNA from the plasma membrane to the nucleus. Instead, mechanisms that viruses have evolved to transfer their genetic material to an infected cell's nucleus have been exploited for most in vivo gene therapy applications to date. Unfortunately, the understanding of viral life cycles and how viruses interact with the cellular machinery is also limited. Another factor contributing to the lack of clinical success is that the underlying pathogenesis for many complicated inherited diseases is just now beginning to be unraveled. Finally, the tools required to thoroughly study disease pathogenesis and to develop and test therapeutic strategies have

been lacking. Because of these limitations, gene therapy as a therapeutic field is still in its infancy. Once the tools become available to better understand gene expression, virology, cell biology, and disease pathogenesis, then gene transfer technology will hold extraordinary potential for the treatment of many inherited and noninherited diseases.

The goal of this chapter is to provide the conceptual framework needed to design a meaningful set of preclinical gene therapy experiments. This framework includes a discussion of the strengths and limitations of various gene transfer vectors and preclinical experimental approaches. This chapter will not provide a detailed overview of the technical aspects of the various gene transfer vectors. This information has been reviewed by a number of authors (2,3). This chapter does not discuss specific disease applications except to illustrate specific points.

## GENE TRANSFER VECTORS

Before initiating a preclinical gene therapy experiment, investigators should be familiar with the advantages and limitations of the various gene transfer technologies. Recombinant viral vectors have been the workhorses of human gene therapy and exploit the innate viral machinery that has evolved to efficiently deliver genetic materials into host cells. These vehicles are naturally occurring viruses that have been genetically engineered to encode the transgene and, in some cases, exogenous promoter elements while rendering them replication-incompetent. Many viral vectors have been developed but four have been used extensively in gene transfer studies: murine-based oncoretroviruses, lentiviruses, adenoviruses, and adeno-associated viruses (Table 22–1). These vectors possess characteristics particular to the native, wild-type virus, and the biology and tropism of these viruses predicts the potential use of a viral vector for gene transfer into target cells. However, genetic alterations of the virus can change the properties of the vector, so any newly developed gene transfer vehicle needs to be fully characterized before clinical use. Although generally less efficient, a variety of nonviral gene transfer techniques have been developed and will likely play a future role in human gene therapy protocols.

## Oncoretroviral Vectors

Recombinant murine-based oncoretroviral vectors established the paradigm for viral gene transfer vehicles (4–6). Moloney murine leukemia virus (MLV), a single-stranded RNA retrovirus, was the first gene transfer technology, and more clinical trials have been undertaken with MLV than with any other recombinant viral vector. These vectors represent important tools and have been used to transduce numerous cell types capable of proliferation in tissue

culture. Immortalized cell lines, hematopoietic cells, hepatocytes, and stem cells have all been successfully transduced in vitro using MLV vectors, delivering various marker and therapeutic genes (1). One advantage of MLV vectors is their stable integration into the host genome, which opens the possibility of persistent expression. Integration, however, can be a double-edged sword, and insertional mutagenesis leading to malignancy has been reported in one clinical trial (7). Unfortunately, all recombinant MLV vectors require host cell division for integration and expression. This requirement precludes the use of these vectors for cells that are quiescent or divide infrequently. Another limitation of MLV-based gene transfer vectors is that a high proportion of the proviral genomes become transcriptionally inactive in vivo (8–11). Although numerous hypotheses that could explain this phenomenon have been tested, this characteristic still remains a significant limitation in in vivo settings where strong selective pressure is not present.

## TABLE 22–1

### Gene Transfer Vectors

| Vector | Expression | Applications | Toxicity |
|---|---|---|---|
| Oncoretroviral | Yes/No[a] | - In vitro experiment<br>- Gene-marking studies<br>- Rodent gene therapy studies | No[b] |
| Lentiviral | Yes[c] | - In vitro experiment<br>- Ex vivo gene transfer<br>- Direct in vivo gene transfer | No |
| Adenoviral | Mo[d] | - In vitro experiment<br>- Proof-of-principle animal experiment<br>- Cancer gene therapy | Yes[d] |
| Adeno-associated virus | Yes[c] | - Direct in vivo gene transfer (CNS, intramuscular, hepatic, ocular, etc.) | No[e] |
| Nonviral | No | - In vitro experiment<br>- Cancer gene therapy | Yes |

[a]In most cases murine-based oncoretroviral gene transfer vectors shut down in vivo, however, a few reports demonstrate persistent in vivo expression in animal models.
[b]There was a single incident where retroviral insertion resulted in a leukemia-like phenotype in a human clinical trial.
[c]Stable in vivo expression has been demonstrated in animal models; however, the length of expression has not been determined in humans yet.
[d]Newly developed "gutless" adenoviral vectors may mediate persistent in vivo expression and have less toxicity compared to early generation vectors.
[e]No toxicity has been reported with adeno-associated viral vectors with the exception of a single study showing the development of malignancies in AAV-treated mice. The cause of the tumors has not yet been determined.

## Lentiviral Vectors

Lentiviruses are another class of retrovirus, which include human immunodeficiency virus, simian immunodeficiency virus, and feline leukemia virus. Recombinant forms of these viruses retain their ability to integrate into the host genome and have the added advantage of being able to transduce nondividing cells (12,13). Another advantage of lentiviral vectors is that they appear to be able to mediate persistent in vivo expression in a host of cell types (14–16). However, the duration of expression in the context of a human clinical trial has not yet been determined. Currently, the disadvantages of this vehicle include relatively low titers ($\leq 10^9$ infectious particles/mL) and the theoretical possibility of recombination and production of replication-competent, infectious virus within the patient. If lentiviral vectors can be engineered to ensure their safety, these vectors will likely play important roles in future ex vivo and direct in vivo human gene therapy clinical trials.

## Adenoviral Vectors

Adenoviruses are native human double-stranded DNA viruses that usually cause mild, self-limiting illnesses and have been modified for use as gene transfer vectors. Recombinant adenoviral vectors have been used to "correct" several genetic defects in different tissues (17–19). Advantages of adenoviral vectors include the ability to generate viral stocks with very high titers ($\geq 10^{13}$ particles/mL), and these vectors can mediate robust expression in some cells. One disadvantage of adenoviral vectors is that the expression is transient, due in part to the episomal nature of the vector but more related to the inflammation and cell-mediated immune response directed against the transduced cells (20). This severe limitation precludes the use of early generation adenoviral vectors for the treatment of inherited diseases where persistent expression is required. A dose-related inflammatory toxicity has been noted, and severe liver toxicity related to systemic inflammation following hepatic artery infusion of an adenoviral vector led to the death of a young man with a urea cycle defect (ornithine transcarbamylase deficiency) (21). Due to their inherent toxicity and transient expression, early generation adenoviral vectors were most useful for in vitro and in vivo proof-of-principle experiments. On the other hand, both the toxicity and transient expression could be viewed as advantages when considering adenoviral vectors for cancer gene therapy applications (22). Recent advances in the development of "gutless" (most of

the adenoviral genome is deleted) vectors made it possible to generate adenoviral vectors with lower toxicity and more persistent expression (23). However, these vectors are still in the early stages of development, and it will take a number of years before they become available for clinical application.

## Adeno-associated Virus Vectors

Adeno-associated virus (AAV) is a nonpathogenic, human single-stranded DNA parvovirus that infects the human respiratory and gastrointestinal tracts. AAV requires a helper virus, typically an adenovirus or herpes virus for its replication. Wild-type AAV establishes latent infection and integrates in a site-specific manner in human cells in the absence of helper functions. These vectors have been used to transduce a wide variety of cells in vivo, including myocytes, neurons, hepatocytes, and respiratory epithelial cells (24). Although the site-specific integration observed with wild-type AAV was considered a major advantage, recombinant AAV vectors integrate with low frequency and the site specificity is lost. However, recombinant AAV vectors persist as stable episomes and remain transcriptionally active in animal models for very long periods of time, up to years (25,26). Most of the initial work has been performed with a single serotype (AAV2), however, at least eight different AAV serotypes have unique capsid proteins. By pseudotyping AAV vectors with different capsids, the tropism and distribution in various tissues can be expanded greatly (27). It may be possible to custom design various AAV vectors for specific tissues or applications. Although wild-type AAV elicits an antibody response, it does not appear to affect transgene delivery or subsequent expression (28). The limitations of AAV vectors include the difficulty in producing large quantities of infectious particles and their small transgene packaging capacity ($\leq 4.5$ kb). In addition, AAV2 has been shown to be relatively ineffective for ex vivo gene transfer into hematopoietic cells due to the absence of the receptor required for internalization (29), and for other cells due to the episomal nature of the recombinant genome. Despite the limitations listed above, AAV may prove to be an effective gene transfer tool for human applications and several clinical trials are currently in progress.

## Nonviral Gene Transfer Vectors

Although viral gene transfer vectors are appealing, their applicability may be limited due to toxicity, packaging constraints, inappropriate tropism, and other factors. Functional genes have been delivered

## TABLE 22–2

### Nonviral Gene Transfer Methods

- Calcium phosphate coprecipitation
- DEAE-dextran
- Polybrene
- Electroporation
- Microinjection
- Direct injection of DNA [a]
- Gene-particle bombardment [a]
- Liposome-mediated [a]
- Receptor ligand-mediated [a]

[a]Methods used to transfer genes in vivo.

to eukaryotic cells in vitro by a variety of physical, noninfectious methods for decades (Table 22–2) (3). The advantages of nonviral gene transfer include having no theoretical limit to the amount of DNA that can be delivered and the possibility of unlimited repeat administrations. Unfortunately, many of these methods are impractical for gene therapy, because they involve membrane disruption and have substantial cytotoxicity. In addition, physical methods for gene transfer tend to be far less efficient than viral vectors, and transgene expression is generally transient and highly variable. However, a few techniques have been successfully adapted for in vivo DNA transfer and have delivered foreign genes into experimental animals, and in some cases into patients. These techniques include direct DNA injection, DNA-coated particle bombardment, liposome-mediated gene transfer, and receptor-mediated gene transfer. Although these approaches hold enormous promise, considerable research and development are required before nonviral gene transfer technologies will be routinely used in the clinic.

## IN VIVO GENE TRANSFER

Once a gene transfer vector or technology has been chosen, researchers must invest considerable thought to ensure that meaningful disease-specific preclinical efficacy studies are performed. For example, much of the early excitement surrounding gene therapy was based on experiments performed with gene transfer vectors in cultured cells using selectable marker genes (4–6). It is now widely believed that in vitro experiments in cultured cells or in vivo experiments using strong selective pressure are not predictive of clinical success. This is not to say that in vitro

gene transfer experiments are of no value; they often yield initial proof-of-principle data that allow an investigator to proceed with a strategy and are invaluable for testing novel gene transfer vectors. However, meaningful preclinical gene therapy experiments should be performed in a situation that mimics the human condition as closely as possible. This condition can best be accomplished by using either normal experimental animals or animal models of human disease (Table 22–3). In fact, gene therapy experiments in intact normal animals or in animal models of human disease are required before a clinical trial can be initiated. The development of authentic animal models of human disease can be a challenge. This is probably best illustrated in the cancer field. Gene therapy holds enormous promise for the treatment of primary and malignant tumors. However, the interpretation of preclinical experimental results obtained in animal models of carcinogenesis can be difficult and sometimes misleading. This is due to the fact that the biology of transplantable tumors is not the same as that of spontaneously forming tumors. Therefore, extreme care must be taken when devising an in vivo tumor model. The advantages and limitations of in vivo gene therapy experiments in various animal models will be discussed below.

## Small Animal Models

For the purposes of this overview, the discussion on small animal models will be limited to murine models. Due to the biochemical similarities to humans, mouse models with spontaneous genetic mutations have historically provided insights into many inherited disorders that are shared between mice and humans. From a practical point of view, the mouse also provides the opportunity to efficiently generate large numbers of genetically identical animals at a much lower cost than larger mammalian species. Over the last 10 to 15 years, the mouse has become even more important because researchers now have the technology to make very precise genetic changes to the mammalian genome by homologous recombination (30,31). The availability of totipotent murine embryonic stem cells (32,33) and the ability to select for homologous recombination events (34) has enabled investigators to create murine models of human disease. The impact that these spontaneous and induced murine models of human disease has had on biology and medicine can not be overstated. With respect to gene therapy, these models represent an important intermediary between in vitro vector development and clinical application.

## TABLE 22–3

### Model Systems for Preclinical Gene Therapy Studies

| Model System Applications | Advantages | Limitations |
| --- | --- | --- |
| In vitro | Vector development | Poor predictor of clinical success |
| | Proof-of-principle experiment | |
| Small animals | Efficacy studies | Short life span |
| | Toxicity studies | Biologic differences between mice and humans |
| | Genetic uniformity | |
| | Proof-of-principle experiment | |
| Large animals | Efficacy studies | Expensive |
| | Long-term studies | Genetic diversity |
| | Biology is closer to humans (nonhuman primates) | |
| Xenotransplant | In vivo experiment with human tissue | Complex biology (may not accurately mimic human environment) |
| | Proof-of-principle experiment | |

When considering a gene therapy experiment in a murine model, the investigator needs to determine whether an authentic model of human disease is required or whether a normal animal will suffice. For example, enormous progress has been made in the development of gene therapy approaches for the treatment of hemophilia B without the luxury of having a factor IX-deficient mouse (25,35,36). If the biology of a protein is well understood, if there is good evidence that simply replacing the missing protein will provide a therapeutic response (clinical evidence from administration of purified or recombinant factor IX), and if the levels of protein do not need to be precisely regulated, then an authentic disease model may not be necessary. This scenario probably exists for a number of secreted proteins.

For inherited diseases that (1) result in complex clinical phenotypes affecting multiple organ systems, (2) require cell-specific post-translational modification of the deficient protein, (3) require precise transcriptional regulation, or (4) involve the interaction of the deficient protein with other molecules, an authentic mouse model may be required to better understand the limitations of a gene therapy approach. One example where animal models have been invaluable for the development of gene therapy strategies is the lysosomal storage diseases. This class of inherited metabolic disease is composed of at least 40 distinct disorders usually caused by the lack of a specific lysosomal enzyme (37). Although

these are simple monogenic diseases, lysosomal enzymes are ubiquitously expressed and the lack of one of these enzymes often leads to a broad spectrum of clinical signs. Gene therapy studies in authentic mouse models of these disorders have revealed some surprising results that would not have been appreciated if a normal animal had been used. For example, it has been shown that transduction of a small percentage (1 to 10%) of cells in a particular organ or tissue can sometimes correct the disease throughout that tissue (38–40). In addition, the delivery of a gene therapy vector to localized regions of the brain in animal models of mucopolysaccharidosis type VII (MPS VII) and metachromatic leukodystrophy (MLD) can globally reduce the histologic evidence of disease and improve cognitive function (41–43).

The importance of animal models of specific diseases is further highlighted by the fact that the positive results generated in the above mentioned studies do not translate to other models of lysosomal storage disease. Due to the biochemical similarities of lysosomal enzymes, it was generally believed that most lysosomal storage diseases would respond similarly to a single form of therapy. However, the histologic and cognitive improvements observed in the mouse models of MPS VII and MLD following central nervous system (CNS)-directed gene therapy are not seen in mouse models of mucopolysaccharidosis type IIIB (MPS IIIB) or globoid-cell leukodystrophy (Krabbe disease) (44, 45). The studies discussed above effectively demonstrate how mouse models of specific diseases can uncover both surprising benefits and important limitations of gene therapy strategies.

Due to both the genetic and physiologic similarities of mice and humans, it is tempting to believe that a therapeutic response observed in a murine gene therapy study will translate directly to humans. This may or may not be the case. A major challenge when contemplating the translation of the gene therapy protocol from mice to humans is simply scale. Can a gene therapy approach be scaled up from a mouse (25–35 gm) to a human (65,000–75,000 gm)? Regardless of these limitations, the mouse is one of the most powerful in vivo tools an investigator can use during the initial stages of gene therapy development.

## Large Animal Models

Large animal models provide excellent systems to acquire preclinical data for human gene therapy trials (46). For example, preclinical studies of gene transfer to hematopoietic stem cells have been performed in nonhuman primates, dogs, pigs, sheep, rabbits, and cats (47). These models have relevance to human stem cell gene transfer because, in contrast to murine models, the larger animals have both more comparable life expectancies and hematopoietic demand from their stem cells. Large animal models thus mirror human physiology and stem cell biology more closely than rodent models. For instance, it has been shown that stem cells from larger mammals are far more difficult to transduce than stem cells from the mouse, when mitosis-dependent retroviral vectors are used (48,49). The low transduction efficiency obtained using stem cells from large animals is likely due to the fact that stem cells from larger mammals, including humans, do not cycle as rapidly and are not as easily prompted into cell cycle ex vivo as are stem cells from the mouse or rat. Therefore, with respect to hematopoietic-directed gene therapy, large animal models provide more meaningful data than can be achieved with small animal models.

By optimizing transduction conditions using standard Moloney murine leukemia virus-based retroviral vectors (the only type of retroviral vector currently approved for stem cell gene therapy trials), gene transfer efficiency to primitive repopulating cells in dogs and nonhuman primates has reached the range of 10 to 30% over the long term, out to several years in some studies (47). These transduction levels are clinically relevant for many diseases of the hematopoietic system, in particular if some myeloreduction of the diseased stem cells

can be done prior to infusion, or if in vivo expansion methods can be used.

In some of the studies discussed above, large animals that had received genetically modified HSC were followed for as long as 6 years and showed no evidence of adverse events such as insertional oncogenesis (47). Long-term follow-up studies after initiation of a gene therapy procedure is an extremely important and timely variable to follow, and can best be done in larger animals. This is because a larger number of stem cells (closer to what will be used in human clinical trials) can be infused, and large animal models have a longer life span than the mouse. Following the fate of transduced stem cells for more than 2 years (the life expectancy of a mouse) is beneficial in preclinical trials. The importance of long-term studies is highlighted by the adverse events that recently occurred in a human gene therapy trial more than 2 years after infusion of gene-modified cells (7). In this trial, unfortunately, vector-related leukemia developed in two out of ten human X-linked severe combined immunodeficiency (XSCID) patients who had received autologous stem cells transduced by a vector carrying the gene for the common gamma chain. It is widely believed that the strong selective pressure for the genetically "corrected" cells allowed the uncontrolled expansion of a subset of rare cells with a copy of the retroviral vector inserted near the LMO2 gene, a transcription factor involved in T-cell activation and growth. This adverse event dramatically heightened the sensitivity of regulatory agencies to the threat of insertional oncogenesis, and large animal models in which the transduced cells can be monitored for several years postinfusion are extremely useful for obtaining relevant preclinical data.

The use of large animal models can also support preclinical data generated in murine models and increase confidence that a gene therapy approach will be effective in humans. For example, both murine and canine models of the lysosomal storage disease MPS VII have been described. Extensive data generated in the mouse model of MPS VII demonstrated that early initiation with a gene therapy approach could prevent many of clinical signs associated with the disease (26). Similar studies performed in the canine model of MPS VII demonstrate comparable levels of correction (50). Therefore, it seems likely that similar gene therapy approaches performed in affected patients will also respond positively to the therapy.

## Xenotransplantation Models

Although both small and large animal models are powerful tools for gene therapy experimentation, there are circumstances where gene transfer technologies are best developed directly on human tissue. As mentioned earlier, the use of in vitro systems, even if using human-derived cells, can lead to erroneous results. In an attempt to accommodate this experimental need, investigators have developed xenotransplantation models where human cells can be transplanted and expanded in another species without those cells being rejected. The field of hematopoietic-directed gene therapy has exploited this technology more than any other. The fetal sheep model of human hematopoiesis has been used by several investigators (51). However, the level of human cell engraftment is low, and the model is expensive and technically difficult to work with. Models that have been more widely used are the murine xenotransplantation models (52). It was initially shown that mice with severe combined immunodeficiency (SCID) could support low levels of human hematopoietic engraftment with continued human cytokine support (53). It was then shown that by combining the nonobese diabetic (NOD) strain with the SCID mutation (54) higher levels of human engraftment (up to 80 to 90%) could be obtained. Since that time several additional mutations affecting immune function have been incorporated into these models to both increase radioresistance and enhance human engraftment (52). These immunodeficient mouse models are now the standard in the field for the in vivo study of human hematopoiesis and hematopoietic-directed gene therapy.

Considerable progress had been made in the development of efficient techniques for viral-mediated gene transfer into murine hematopoietic stem cells. However, the gene transfer techniques developed in murine models did not translate to clinical scenarios (55–57). It was clear that human hematopoietic stem cells differed significantly from murine HSCs and that novel approaches would be required for efficient gene transfer into human long-term repopulating cells. The development of lentiviral gene transfer vectors and their ability to transduce quiescent cells raised the possibility that pluripotent human hematopoietic stem cells could now be efficiently transduced. The best way to test this hypothesis was in an in vivo system. It was confirmed in murine xenotransplantation models that, in fact the lentiviral systems efficiently transduced primitive human hematopoietic stem cells that could give rise to fully differentiated, multilineage cells (58,59).

Although the availability of efficient and cost-effective xenotransplantation models has allowed investigators to develop gene transfer protocols directly in human cells and test them in vivo, these models generally do not have disease phenotypes beyond the immunodeficiencies that allow human cell engraftment. As discussed above, this can be an important attribute of a model system. Therefore,

a xenotransplantation model of human disease was recently created that exploited the ability of the NOD/SCID mouse to engraft human cells and harbored a mutation that results in the human lysosomal storage disease mucopolysaccharidosis type VII (60). This model was then used to determine the efficacy of human hematopoietic-directed, lentiviral-mediated gene therapy (61). This study demonstrated the utility of targeting human hematopoietic stem cells with a gene transfer vector for the treatment of this inherited metabolic disease.

The studies cited above demonstrate both the utility of murine xenotransplantation models and how unique combinations of mutations and strains can be used to design meaningful gene therapy experiments.

## REGULATORY CONSIDERATIONS

Before a clinical investigator in the United States can obtain approval for a gene therapy investigational new drug application (IND), several hurdles must be overcome. These hurdles include (1) protocol approval from the Recombinant DNA Advisory Committee (RAC), (2) approval from the NIH, if the institution utilizes any NIH funding, (3) approval from both the investigator's Institutional Biosafety Committee (IBC), and IRB, and (4) approval from the FDA. To convince these regulatory agencies that the proposed clinical trial approach is safe, well-designed studies in animal models should be presented. Without well-designed animal studies, gene therapy protocols have only a small chance of successfully navigating this regulatory maze. These issues are discussed in more detail at the following website (http://www.fda.gov/cber/ rules/bvactox.pdf).

The primary concern for regulatory agencies is safety, and a phase I human clinical study is always a safety study. It is expected that toxicities will be seen on dose escalation, and the demonstration of a safe dose range in the study of animals is imperative. For example, if an integrating vector system is used, a high copy number in the target cell genome may lead to insertional mutagenesis. Animals should be put on a tumor watch, and enough animals should be used to achieve statistically valid data. The principal investigator must report all results faithfully.

Where possible, the use of large animal models in preclinical gene therapy experiments is encouraged. However, the success of a clinical gene therapy trial does not depend on the use of such models. Most hematopoietic stem cell gene therapy trials in the past were approved using data generated in mouse models. Mouse models with specific disease phenotypes have been developed to show the efficacy of the particular gene therapy approach. Regulatory agencies encourage the use of such animal models.

New regulations for human clinical gene therapy trials also demand a possible clinical benefit for a patient (62). Mere marking studies in humans are strongly discouraged, because the risk–benefit ratio is being carefully scrutinized. If efficacy is demonstrated in an authentic animal model of human disease, the likelihood of approval for the human gene therapy protocol will increase (63).

To comply with FDA mandates, the principal investigator must use Good Laboratory Practice (GLP) methods to generate preclinical data. GLP is a method for generating reliable and reproducible data that can be traced back to the origin without a break in the chain of sequence. The following statement should be at the foundation of any GLP experiment: "If it isn't written down, it doesn't exist." A well-designed GLP grade experiment has everything documented. Items that should be recorded include (1) the origin of the animals, (2) how they were cared for, (3) what was done with them, (4) who took care of them, and (5) who performed the experiments. All reagents must be traced to their origin. The methods by which a plasmid was constructed, the sequence, where the starting reagents came from, and all certificates of analysis must be retained and documented. Obviously, GLP is the laboratory equivalent of Good Clinical Practice, the regulatory standards guiding the conduct of clinical trials discussed in Chapters 14 and 15.

To maintain Good Laboratory Practice, all source documents must be retained. A source document is the initial written documentation of a process. For example, if an investigator wrote a cell count from an animal study on a paper towel, the paper towel is the source document and must be kept, even after the numbers have been transferred into a lab book. This process minimizes human error, which can occur during transposition of numbers. Lab books must be retained for every experiment. A computerized record is not sufficient. A handwritten lab book, which is dated and cannot be altered or forged easily, is preferable to a computer file that can be changed at any time without the knowledge of a supervisor. The investigators must generate a "GLP sheet"—a document that is taken to the animal room whenever an animal experiment is performed. This sheet should contain (1) the date, (2) the type of animal used, (3) the cage number, (4) information about reagents or products used, (5) what exact experiment was performed, and (6) a brief summary of the outcome. This document is essential when tracking individual experiments and reagents possibly being used to summarize data for an IND. A sample sheet is available at the following website (www.jannoltalab.com).

## SUMMARY

- Animal models are essential to generate preclinical safety and efficacy data for later gene therapy experiments. A thorough set of statistically valid animal data obtained under Good Laboratory Practice will, in all likelihood, further the successful development and application of a human gene therapy clinical trial.
- Both viral and nonviral vectors can be used for gene transfer in humans.
- Although authentic animal models of human disease are relatively uncommon, when available they provide the best proof-of-principle preclinical data justifying translational clinical trials of gene transfer to patients.
- Regulatory endorsement of an initial gene therapy trial in humans requires approval from several federal government agencies, including the Recombinant Advisory Committee, the National Institutes of Health, the Food and Drug Administration, and the investigator's institutional biosafety committee and institutional review board.

## REFERENCES

1. Friedmann T, ed. The Development of Human Gene Therapy. Cold Spring Harbor, NY: Cold Spring Harbor Laboratory Press, 1999.
2. Wivel NA, Wilson JM. Methods of gene delivery. Hematol Oncol Clin North Am 1998;12:483–501.
3. Niidome T, Huang L. Gene therapy progress and prospects: nonviral vectors. Gene Ther 2002; 9:1647–1652.
4. Joyner A, Keller G, Phillips RA et al. Retrovirus transfer of a bacterial gene into mouse haematopoietic progenitor cells. Nature 1983;305:556–558.
5. Mann R, Mulligan RC, Baltimore D. Construction of a retrovirus packaging mutant and its use to produce helper-free defective retrovirus. Cell 1983;33:153–159.
6. Williams DA, Lemischka IR, Nathan DG et al. Introduction of new genetic material into pluripotent haematopoietic stem cells of the mouse. Nature 1984;310:476–480.
7. Hacein-Bey-Abina S, von Kalle C, Schmidt M et al. A serious adverse event after successful gene therapy for X-linked severe combined immunodeficiency. N Engl J Med 2003;348:255–256.
8. Guild B, Finer MH, Housman DE et al. Development of retrovirus vectors useful for expressing genes in cultured murine embryonal cells and hematopoietic cells in vivo. J Virol 1988;62:3795–3801.
9. Palmer TD, Rosman GJ, Osborne WRA et al. Genetically modified skin fibroblasts persist long after transplantation but gradually inactivate introduced genes. Proc Natl Acad Sci USA 1991;88:1330–1334.
10. Apperely JF, Luskey BD, Williams DA. Retroviral gene transfer of human adenosine deaminase in murine hematopoietic cells: effect of selectable marker sequences on long-term expression. Blood 1991;78:310–317.
11. Challita PM, Kohn DB. Lack of expression from a retroviral vector after transduction of murine hematopoietic

stem cells is associated with methylation in vivo. Proc Natl Acad Sci USA 1994;91:2567–2571.

12. Naldini L, Blömer U, Gallay P et al. In vivo gene delivery and stable transduction of nondividing cells by a lentiviral vector. Science 1996;272:263–267.

13. Poeschla EM, Wong-Staal F, Looney DJ. Efficient transduction of nondividing human cells by feline immunodeficiency virus lentiviral vectors. Nat Med 1998;4:354–357.

14. Blömer U, Naldini L, Kafri T et al. Highly efficient and sustained gene transfer in adult neurons with a lentivirus vector. J Virol 1997;71:6641–6649.

15. Kafri T, Blömer U, Peterson DA et al. Sustained expression of genes delivered directly into liver and muscle by lentiviral vectors. Nat Genet 1997;17:314–317.

16. Sutton RE, Wu HT, Rigg R et al. Human immunodeficiency virus type 1 vectors efficiently transduce human hematopoietic stem cells. J Virol 1998;72:5781–5788.

17. Smith TA, Mehaffey MG, Kayda DB et al. Adenovirus mediated expression of therapeutic plasma levels of human factor IX in mice. Nat Genet 1993;5:397–402.

18. Kay MA, Landen CN, Rothenberg SR et al. In vivo hepatic gene therapy: complete albeit transient correction of factor IX deficiency in hemophilia B dogs. Proc Natl Acad Sci USA 1994;91:2353–2357.

19. Stevenson SC, Marshall-Neff J, Teng B et al. Phenotypic correction of hypercholesterolemia in ApoE-deficient mice by adenovirus-mediated in vivo gene transfer. Arterioscler Thromb Vasc Biol 1995;15:479–484.

20. Yang Y, Ertl HCJ, Wilson JM. MHC class I-restricted cytotoxic t-lymphocytes to viral antigens destroy hepatocytes in mice infected with E1-deleted recombinant adenoviruses. Immunity 1994;1:433–442.

21. Marshall E. Gene therapy death prompts review of adenovirus vector. Science 1999;286:2244–2245.

22. Bischoff JR, Kirn DH, Williams A et al. An adenovirus mutant that replicates selectively in p53-deficient human tumor cells. Science 1996;274:373–376.

23. Schiedner G, Morral N, Parks RJ et al. Genomic DNA transfer with a high-capacity adenovirus vector results in improved in vivo gene expression and decreased toxicity. Nat Genet 1998;18:180–183.

24. Monahan PE, Samulski RJ. AAV vectors: is clinical success on the horizon? Gene Ther 2000;7:24–30.

25. Snyder RO, Miao CH, Patijn GA et al. Persistent and therapeutic concentrations of human factor IX in mice after hepatic gene transfer of recombinant AAV vectors. Nat Genet 1997;16:270–276.

26. Daly TM, Ohlemiller KK, Roberts MS et al. Prevention of systemic clinical disease in MPS VII mice following AAV-mediated neonatal gene transfer. Gene Ther 2001;8:1291–1298.

27. Davidson BL, Stein CS, Heth JA et al. Recombinant adeno-associated virus type 2, 4, and 5 vectors: transduction of variant cell types and regions in the mammalian central nervous system. Proc Natl Acad Sci USA 2000;97:3428–3432.

28. Chirmule N, Propert KJ, Magosin SA et al. Immune responses to adenovirus and adeno-associated virus in humans. Gene Ther 1999;6:1574–1583.

29. Summerford C, Samulski RJ. Membrane-associated heparin sulfate proteoglycan is a receptor for adeno-associated virus type 2 virions. J Virol 1998;72:1438–1445.

30. Smithies O, Gregg RG, Boggs SS et al. Insertion of DNA sequences into the human chromosome β-globin locus by homologous recombination. Nature 1985; 317:230–234.

31. Thomas KR, Capecchi MR. Introduction of homologous DNA sequences into mammalian cells induces mutations in the cognate gene. Nature 1986;324: 34–38.

32. Evans MJ, Kaufman MH. Establishment in culture of pluripotential cells from mouse embryos. Nature 1981; 292:154–156.

33. Martin G. Isolation of a pluripotent cell line from early mouse embryos cultured in medium conditioned by teratocarcinoma stem cells. Proc Natl Acad Sci USA 1981; 78:7634–7638.

34. Thomas KR, Folger KR, Capecchi MR. High frequency targeting of genes to specific sites in the mammalian genome. Cell 1986;44:419–428.

35. Scharfmann R, Axelrod JH, Verma IM. Long-term in vivo expression of retrovirus-mediated gene transfer in mouse fibroblast implants. Proc Natl Acad Sci USA 1991; 88:4626–4630.

36. Herzog RW, Hagstrom JN, Kung SH et al. Stable gene transfer and expression of human blood coagulation factor IX after intramuscular injection of recombinant adeno-associated virus. Proc Natl Acad Sci USA 1997; 94:5804–5809.

37. Scriver CR, Beaudet AL, Sly WS et al., eds. The Metabolic and Molecular Bases of Inherited Disease, 8th Ed. New York: McGraw-Hill, 2001.

38. Wolfe JH, Sands MS, Barker JE et al. Reversal of pathology in murine mucopolysaccharidosis type VII by somatic cell gene transfer. Nature 1992;360:749–753.

39. Watson GL, Sayles JN, Chen C et al. Treatment of lysosomal storage disease in MPS VII mice using a recombinant adeno-associated virus. Gene Ther 1998; 5:1642–1649.

40. Daly TM, Vogler CA, Levy B et al. Neonatal gene transfer leads to widespread correction of pathology in a murine model of lysosomal storage disease. Proc Natl Acad Sci 1999; 96:2296–2300.

41. Frisella WA, O'Connor LH, Vogler CA et al. Intracranial injection of recombinant adeno-associated virus improves cognitive function in a murine model of mucopolysaccharidosis type VII. Mol Ther 2001;3:351–358.

42. Consiglio A, Quattrini A, Martino S et al. In vivo gene therapy of metachromatic leukodystrophy by lentiviral vectors: correction of neuropathology and protection against learning impairments in affected mice. Nat Med 2001;7:310–316.

43. Brooks A, Stein CS, Hughes SM et al. Functional correction of established central nervous system deficits in an animal model of lysosomal storage disease with feline immunodeficiency virus-based vectors. Proc Natl Acad Sci USA 2002;99:6216–6221.

44. Fu H, Samulski RJ, McCown TJ et al. Neurological correction of lysosomal storage in a mucopolysaccharidosis IIIB mouse model by adeno-associated virus-mediated gene delivery. Mol Ther 2002;5:42–49.

45. Shen JS, Watabe K, Ohashi T et al. Intraventricular administration of recombinant adenovirus to neonatal twitcher mouse leads to clinicopathological improvements. Gene Ther 2001;8:1081–1087.

46. Donahue RE, Dunbar CE. Update on the use of nonhuman primate models for preclinical testing of gene therapy approaches targeting hematopoietic cells. Hum Gene Ther 2001;12:607–617.

47. Kohn DB, Sadelain M, Dunbar C et al. American Society of Gene Therapy (ASGT) ad hoc subcommittee on retroviral-mediated gene transfer to hematopoietic stem cells. Mol Ther 2003;8:180–187.

48. Miller DG, Adam MA, Miller AD. Gene transfer by retrovirus vectors occurs only in cells that are actively replicating at the time of infection. Mol Cell Biol 1990;10:4239–4242.

49. Shi PA, Hematti P, von Kalle C et al. Genetic marking as an approach to studying in vivo hematopoiesis: progress in the non-human primate model. Oncogene 2002; 21:3274–3283.

50. Ponder K, Melniczek JR, Xu L et al. Therapeutic neonatal hepatic gene therapy in mucopolysaccharidosis VII dogs. Proc Natl Acad Sci USA 2002;99:13102–13107.

51. Zanjani ED, Almeida-Porada G, Flake AW. Retention and multilineage expression of hematopoietic stem cells in human-sheep chimeras. Stem Cells 1995;13:101–111.

52. Dao MA, Nolta JA. Immunodeficient mice as models of human hematopoietic stem cell engraftment. Curr Opin Immunol 1999;11:532–537.

53. Kamel-Reid S, Dick JE. Engraftment of immune-deficient mice with human hematopoietic stem cells. Science 1988;242:1706–1709.

54. Cashman J, Bockhold K, Hogge DE et al. Sustained proliferation, multilineage differentiation and maintenance of primitive human hematopoietic cells in NOD/SCID mice transplanted with human cord blood. Br J Haematol 1997;98:1026–1036.

55. Brenner MK, Rill DR, Moen RC et al. Gene marking to trace origin of relapse after autologous bone-marrow transplantation. Lancet 1993;341:85–86.

56. Dunbar CE, Cottler-Fox M, O'Shaughnessy JA et al. Retrovirally marked CD34-enriched peripheral blood and bone marrow cells contribute to long-term engraftment after autologous transplantation. Blood 1995;85:3048–3057.

57. Hanania EG, Giles RE, Kavanagh J et al. Results of MDR-1 vector modification trial indicate that granulocyte/macrophage colony-forming unit cells do not contribute to posttransplant hematopoietic recovery following intensive systemic therapy. Proc Natl Acad Sci USA 1996;93:15346–15351 (Erratum appears in Proc Natl Acad Sci USA 1997;94:5495b).

58. Miyoshi H, Smith KA, Mosier DE et al. Transduction of human CD34+ cells that mediate long-term engraftment of NOD/SCID mice by HIV vectors. Science 1999; 283:682–686.

59. Woods NB, Fahlman C, Mikkola H et al. Lentiviral gene transfer into primary and secondary NOD/SCID repopulating cells. Blood 2000;96:3725–3733.

60. Hofling AA, Vogler CA, Creer MH et al. Engraftment of human CD34+ cells leads to widespread distribution of donor-derived cells and correction of tissue pathology in a novel murine xenotransplantation model of lysosomal storage disease. Blood 2003;2054–2063.

61. Hofling AA, Devine S, Vogler CA et al. Human CD34+ hematopoietic progenitor cell-directed lentiviral-mediated gene therapy in a xenotransplantation model of lysosomal storage disease. Mol Ther 2004;9:856–865.

62. Larson PJ, High KA. Gene therapy for hemophilia B: AAV-mediated transfer of the gene for coagulation factor IX to human muscle. Adv Exp Med Biol 2001;489:45–57.

63. Cheng SH, Smith AE. Gene therapy progress and prospects: Gene therapy of lysosomal storage disorders. Gene Ther 2003;10:1275–1281.

# Analyzing and Reporting Results

# CHAPTER 23

# Overview: Hypothesis Testing and Summary Statistics

Michael A. Province

C oncepts about using *probability* for decision making go back to the latter half of the 1600s, with DeMoivre and Bernoulli and their descriptions of how to improve the odds of winning at games of chance. In such cases, it's assumed that the games are "fair;" that is, the dice or cards behave with fixed and known probabilities. In today's language, we would say that the parameters of the underlying probability distributions are assumed to be known, and we just want to derive the corresponding probabilities of various events happening (flush versus full house, given cards already played). *Statistics* as a discipline, on the other hand, grew slowly from that time until it reached its golden age with Karl Pearson and his one time protégée and later lifelong enemy, R. A. Fisher, in the early 1900s. Statistics is the obverse of probability theory (much as subtraction is the obverse of addition, division is the obverse of multiplication and integral calculus is the obverse of differential calculus). In statistics, the underlying parameters that govern probability are not assumed, but instead they are inferred from experimental data. For example, if we flip a coin twice, and get heads both times, the probability of that happening is $(1/2)^2 = 1/4$. This is simple probability, assuming we are dealing with a fair coin with a 50:50 chance of heads each time. But what if we flip the coin 82 times and it still comes up heads each and every time? The probability of that happening by chance is $2.1 \times 10^{-25}$. At what point do we begin to "smell a rat" and start to wonder if the coin is really a fair 50:50 head:tail coin after all? Can we estimate how unfair the coin might be from the data? Can we formally test the hypothesis that "the coin is fair" versus "its really a fake" from the data? This is *statistical* thinking. In this chapter, we will set the basic statistical foundations for the analysis methods detailed in later chapters.

## HYPOTHESIS TESTING LOGIC

The logic by which hypotheses are formally tested in statistics usually seems overly complex and somewhat convoluted to most researchers who encounter it for the first time. Its subtleties are best illustrated by example.

Suppose a researcher wants to test whether a drug for AIDS has a particular effect. The researcher envisions two mutually exclusive *hypotheses* about the action of the drug, and decides how to measure that action; for example, average T-cell count, $\mu$, in two groups, treated and control. The researcher denotes the average T-cell count in the treated group by $\mu_1$, and the average T-cell count in the control group by $\mu_2$. Under the *null hypothesis*, $H_0$, the drug has no effect, whereas under the *alternative hypothesis*, $H_1$, the drug has some effect (for good or ill), so that the reality is either

$$H_0: \mu_1 = \mu_2 \quad \text{vs} \quad H_1: \mu_1 \neq \mu_2$$

The researcher does not know which hypothesis is true, so he does an experiment, putting one group of subjects on the drug with a control group off drug (say placebo controlled) and then measures the effect in T-cell count. Even if the null hypothesis were true (usually "under the null hypothesis") and the drug had no real biologic effect, the researcher would not be surprised (indeed, would probably expect) that the experiment would show *some* differences (presumably small) in mean T-cell counts between the groups, just because experiments are finite (i.e., data is only obtained on a *sample* of the population, not the entire population). A single sample does not always "run true" to the population from which it is drawn (even though many such samples tend to run true in the long run). But the researcher hopes that if the null hypothesis is true (i.e., no real biologic effect of the treatment), the differences between groups in the experiment would most likely be "small," and if the researcher redid the experiment over and over again, on average, there would be no group differences. On the other hand, if the alternative were true, the researcher might expect that an occasional experiment would show no differences between the treated and control groups but this should somehow be rare (i.e., would have a low probability of occurring). If the researcher could conduct the experiment many times, he or she would expect most often there would be differences between the two groups (if the alternative hypothesis were true). Even under the null hypothesis, it is *possible* to see huge differences between the treated and control groups, just by having picked an unusual group of patients (e.g., unusually hardy ones among the controls or unusually frail ones among the treated). How then can a researcher tell on the basis of a single experiment which hypothesis is true?

The key idea is that (assuming no "true" biologic action of the drug), any differences in the experiment between the treatment and control groups in mean T-cell count must have arisen *by chance*. Investigators can actually calculate the probability of such an unusual occurrence happening by making assumptions about how chance operates in collecting these data (e.g. sampling randomly from two normal distributions). This is called the *p-value*: the probability that *if the null hypothesis is true*, nevertheless data may appear that were extremely different from the null hypothesis by chance alone. Note that this is *not* the same as saying that the "p-value is the probability that the null hypothesis is true." Hypotheses do not have any probabilities associated with them (other than 0 or 1—for false or true). It is the *data* that have probabilities associated with them, not the hypotheses. In a very real sense, then, the p-value is a measure of how closely the data "fit" the null hypothesis. When the p-value is small (closer and closer to 0), the data would have to be a very unusual, perhaps from an "unlucky" sample, to have been as "non-null looking" as they are. When the p-value is large (closer to one), the data are quite compatible with the null hypothesis. So investigators use the p-value to decide whether the data come from the null or from the alternative.

The very first recorded use of the p-value was by Arbuthnott in 1711. Examining birth records in the previous 82 years, he observed that each year showed more male births than females (a phenomenon that persists today). He wondered if this was a statistical fluke or if there was some process behind it. Although he did not cast the problem exactly this way, his "null hypothesis" was that the proportion of males (denoted by $p_{Male}$) and females (denoted by $p_{Female}$) should be equal (i.e., $1/2$), whereas his alternative was that the proportions were different.

$$H_0: p_{Male} = p_{Female} \quad \text{vs.} \quad H_1: p_{Male} \neq p_{Female}$$

Because his data always showed imbalance for males in all 82 years, in Arbuthnott's mind, this was like flipping a coin 82 times and coming up with heads each time, which would occur with probability $(1/2)^{82}$, which he calculated as $P = 4.8 \times 10^{-24}$ (it is actually closer to $P = 2.1 \times 10^{-25}$ as noted earlier, but he can be forgiven not having access to modern calculators). This was the very first recorded p-value, although Arbuthnott did not call it that. Nonetheless, he used it exactly as it is today, arguing that because this was such a small probability ("From whence it follows, that it is Art, not Chance, that governs"), he rejected the null hypothesis, seeing instead the divine hand of providence in this sex imbalance.

Typically in science, the burden of proof is on those who want the alternative hypothesis to be true. The null hypothesis essentially represents the current state of scientific knowledge, the fallback position. For instance, for a new drug, as in the AIDS example, it is assumed the drug has no effect (null hypothesis) unless the data prove otherwise (alternative hypothesis). If evidence is unclear or equivocal, researchers revert to the null hypothesis by default. Only if the evidence is convincing is the alternative hypothesis accepted. In this sense, modern-day investigators are like the judge and jury in a criminal trial, where the "trial" is an experiment (in fact, this is where the term *clinical trial* comes from). Researchers decide between two possible verdicts: null (not guilty) or alternative (guilty). The null hypothesis is *assumed* and the alternative hypothesis is only accepted if the evidence is compelling, just as in the legal system the accused is presumed innocent until *proven* guilty beyond a reasonable doubt.

Obviously, researchers can make mistakes whenever deciding to accept either the null or alternative hypothesis. Type I error is when the null hypothesis is true (the reality) and the jury makes the mistake of

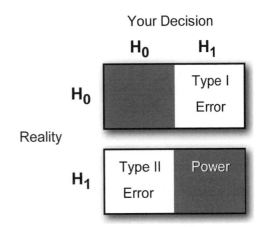

**FIGURE 23–1** ● Interrelations among the null hypothesis ($H_0$), the alternative hypothesis ($H_1$), Types I and II error, and power. Type I error occurs when the alternative hypothesis is accepted but the null hypothesis is actually true. The converse is true for Type II error. Power represents 1–Type II error.

deciding for the alternative based on experimental evidence (convicting an innocent man) (Figure 23–1). Whereas, Type II error is when the defendant is really guilty and he goes free. In Western thought generally, one kind of error is more egregious than the other. The classic standard in the law follows the dictum of Sir William Blackstone (1723–1780) that *"It is better ten guilty persons escape than one innocent suffer."* Typically, researchers are twice as fastidious as Blackstone in avoiding Type I error, and so the standard has been to set this at 1/20, so that researchers reject the null hypothesis whenever the p-value is $p < 0.05$.

Fixing the Type I error at 0.05 allows researchers to accept 1 in 20 false conclusions that the null is wrong (i.e., decide for the alternative) when in fact the null is the true case, then the size of the Type II error depends on the experimental data as well as the exact statistical test used. Usually, researchers think in terms of the *power*, which is (1–Type II error) or the probability of *correctly* deciding for the alternative hypothesis when it is true (in the trial analogy, finding the defendant guilty when he actually is so). In fact, statisticians judge whether one statistical test is better or worse for a particular kind of hypothesis test by comparing their powers (the t-test is the most powerful statistic to detect mean differences between two normal populations, for instance). The power to convict depends on the skill of the prosecutor (the power of the particular statistical test used), the total amount of evidence presented (sample size), as well as just how fantastically and openly guilty the defendant really is (how different the null really is from the alternative, because the alternative is that the means are "not equal," but does not specify whether they are just barely not equal or whether they are exceptionally different—the latter is much more easily and powerfully demonstrated than the former, just

as it is easier to convict an embezzler who has repeatedly stolen millions of dollars from multiple victims over many years compared to the defendant who slightly overcharged one client one time). Of course, these same considerations are at play when, instead of "power," researchers are interested in estimating the sample size required to demonstrate that the null hypothesis is not true, with a certain risk of making a Type I error, and given a certain size of the effect of the tested intervention (see Chapter 8).

## SUMMARY STATISTICS

An important first step in examining newly acquired data is to describe the distribution of values obtained for a measured variable using various statistics or numbers. The most basic set of descriptive statistics are those that quantify the center point around which most of the data lie, the so-called measures of *central tendency*. The most familiar of these is the *mean* or arithmetic average, which is simply the sum of all values, $x_i$, divided by the sample size, $n$ and is usually denoted by $\overline{x}$:

$$\overline{x} = \sum_{i=1}^{n} \frac{x_i}{n}$$

The *median* is the point that divides the data exactly in half, or the 50th percentile. At this point, 50% of the data lie above the median and 50% lie below. The *mode* (less often useful) is the single "most probable point." For instance, looking at income distribution in the United States, it is clear that a few individuals who are fantastically wealthy can pull the mean higher, so that "mean income" is not a very fair measure of the income of the great mass of people. There will be some salary that is exactly the same for more people than any other (e.g., the minimum wage), and that one will be the

Probability

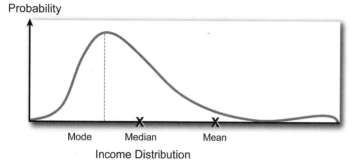

Income Distribution

*FIGURE 23–2* ● Schematic demonstration of a distribution of values (in this case, income) that is skewed to the right such that the mean > median > mode. In a normal distribution, all three measures of central tendency would be the same.

"most probable one" or the mode, but again, just because more people make exactly that salary than any other, does not mean that it is the one that best represents "most" people. In this case, the median salary would perhaps be a better measure of central tendency, since 50% of the people would have salaries below and 50% would have salaries above this level.

For a "normal" distribution (which has the shape of a bell-shaped curve when the data are graphed), the mean is the best measure of central tendency, but in that case, the median and mode will also be very close to the mean (see Figure 4–6, Chapter 4). For non-symmetric distributions ("non-normal"), the mean may not be the best way to quantify the center of the distribution (Figures 4–2 and 4–8 in Chapter 4).

After central tendency, the next thing to know about a distribution is its *dispersion* or how variable the data are. The most common measure of dispersion is the *standard deviation*, usually denoted by "*s*," the square of which is called the (Pearson) *variance*, and is given by the formula:

$$s^2 = \sum_{i=1}^{n} \frac{(x_i - \bar{x})^2}{n - 1}$$

The variance formula is nearly equal to the average square of the distance between each of the points and the mean [the only difference being it is divided by $(n - 1)$ instead of $n$]. The standard deviation is the best, most natural measure of dispersion for the normal distribution, but may not be a good way to characterize dispersion for other distributions, particularly nonsymmetrical ones (because the standard deviation is a symmetrical formula—i.e., values equally distant from the mean either above or below it contribute equally to the standard deviation). Another, more general measure of dispersion is the *interquartile range* (Figure 23–3). The data are divided into quartiles (four segments each containing one-fourth of the data points), which are denoted Q1, Q2, Q3, and Q4. The quartile Q2 is

exactly the median point (50% of the data falling on either side of Q2). The quartile Q1 is the point marking where the bottom 25% of the data fall, and Q3 is the point marking where the top 25% (or equivalently, the bottom 75%) of the data fall. The interquartile range is the distance (Q3–Q1), which captures the middle half of the data. For a normal distribution, the interquartile range is about 1.34 times the standard deviation.

The mean is often called a *first order moment*, because it involves sums of the variable (to the first power), while the standard deviation a *second order moment*, because it involves sums of squares of the variable (to the second power). There are third, fourth, and *higher order moments*, involving sums of the cubic power, fourth power, and so on. The third order moment is often called *skewness* (see Figure 23–2).

$$k = \frac{\sum_{i=1}^{n} (x_i - \bar{x})^3}{(n - 1)s^3}$$

It is a measure of asymmetry, because after subtracting the mean from each value, the cubic power will be positive for the positive numbers (above the mean) and negative for those points below the mean, and thus, the third order moment measures the imbalance between points above and below the mean. A symmetric distribution, such as the normal, has a skewness of 0.

The fourth order moment is often called *kurtosis* (see Figure 4–7, Chapter 4):

$$k = \frac{\sum_{i=1}^{n} (x_i - \bar{x})^4}{ns^4} - 3$$

It is a measure of whether the tails of the distribution are fatter than those of a normal distribution ("leptokurtic") or skinnier than those of a normal distribution ("platykurtic"). A normal distribution has kurtosis of 0.

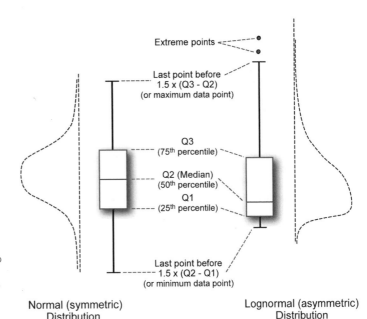

Extreme points

Last point before
1.5 x (Q3 - Q2)
(or maximum data point)

Q3
(75th percentile)

Q2 (Median)
(50th percentile)

Q1
(25th percentile)

Last point before
1.5 x (Q2 - Q1)
(or minimum data point)

Normal (symmetric)
Distribution

Lognormal (asymmetric)
Distribution

**FIGURE 23–3** ● Example of two box plots compared to two different distributions (normal and lognormal). The interquartile range usually refers to the range of values between Q1 and Q3.

## SAMPLING DISTRIBUTIONS

Even after deciding on the "best" statistic to characterize the distribution of data, researchers recognize that they have only drawn a *sample* from the underlying population and it may not reflect accurately that population (see Chapter 5). Much as a political pollster recognizes that any one sample of voters polled may, by chance alone, have too many respondents from one party affiliation or another, researchers acknowledge that the mean of the sample data may not represent the mean of the underlying population, even in the simple case when the overall population is normally distributed. Quantifying this uncertainty brings us to the idea of *sampling distributions*. (This topic was also considered in Chapter 9, in the context of estimating sample size for a study.) The sampling distribution is the distribution formed if a researcher repeats the sample from the same population. So when the pollster repeatedly surveys potential voters, each time tabulating the results, and looks at the distribution of those results, he or she is mapping out the sampling distribution. The theory of sampling distributions is key in statistics, because it is the way researchers quantify the uncertainty made in inferring what the "true" parameter value is in the whole population from a single statistic derived from a single random sample (much as a pollster tries to infer the way all voters will decide to vote based on the results from his or her sample survey).

The simplest example is the case where a researcher randomly samples from a population that

is *normally distributed*, and calculates (estimates) the mean. If the mean of the population is μ and its variance is $\sigma^2$ then the probability density for the overall normal population is given by:

$$f(x; \mu, \sigma) = \frac{1}{\sqrt{2\pi}\sigma} e^{-\frac{1}{2}\left(\frac{x-\mu}{\sigma}\right)^2}$$

where μ and σ are unknown, but they are inferred (i.e., the researcher wants to figure out, or estimate, what they might be). (Note that μ and $\sigma^2$ to denote the mean and variance of a *population*, while $\bar{x}$ and $s^2$ denote the mean and variance of a study *sample*.)

The researcher draws a random sample of size N from this population and takes the best estimate of the population's mean parameter, μ, which in this case is simply the mean estimate from the samples, $\bar{x}$. What is the sampling distribution of $\bar{x}$? It turns out that $\bar{x}$ is itself normally distributed, with mean μ and variance $\sigma^2/N$. It is not surprising that the mean estimator is distributed normally, nor that the mean of the mean estimator is μ. If the researcher takes the square root of this variance, he or she obtains the standard deviation of this mean, which is called the *standard error of the mean*. The researcher estimates the standard error of the mean from the sample, by substituting the best estimate of the variance, *s*, into the above formula, $s/\sqrt{N}$.

There is often great confusion about the difference between the standard deviation of the population, σ, (which is estimated by "*s*," the standard deviation of the study sample) and the standard error of the mean (which is estimated by $s/\sqrt{N}$).

The standard error of the mean is the standard deviation of $\bar{x}$, not $x$. It measures *the uncertainty in the estimate of the mean* when sampled with a fixed $N$ points, hence that uncertainty goes down whenever $N$ goes up (naturally a researcher is more confident in estimates given more data). The standard deviation estimate of the underlying population, $s$, (as taken from the data from the study sample) does not become smaller whenever there is a larger sample size, but the precision of that estimate does become smaller (better) (Figure 23–4).

Because the mean estimate from the sample is itself normally distributed, the researcher can form *confidence limits* around the estimate. A confidence limit is an *interval* (as opposed to a single point value, like the mean itself) that quantifies the uncertainty in the point estimate. Approximately ± two standard deviations encompass 95% of the probability in any normal distribution (in fact, the exact number is 1.96 standard deviations). Thus, the 95% confidence limit on the mean is given by $(\bar{x} \pm 1.96 \text{ stderr})$. This means we are 95% certain that the true population mean falls within the limits of this confidence interval around the estimate of the mean from the sample.

For example, if a researcher samples $N = 100$ individuals and measures their systolic blood pressures, and the mean for that sample is $\bar{x} = 121.6$ and its standard deviation is $s = 24.3$, then the standard error of the mean is $(24.3/10) = 2.43$ so that the 95% confidence limit for the mean is $(121.6 - 1.96 \times 2.43, 121.6 + 1.96 \times 2.43) = (116.84, 126.36)$. Thus, the researcher is 95% certain that the mean blood pressure in the population from which sample was drawn has a mean that is in this interval. Investigators can construct confidence

limits of sizes other than 95%, by picking the corresponding points off of the normal distribution that capture that amount of probability (e.g., a 99% confidence limit would use the value 2.58 instead of 1.96 in the above formulas). In fact, for any $\alpha$ level of "uncertainty" (e.g., $\alpha = 0.05$, $\alpha = 0.01$, etc.), investigators can construct a $100 \times (1 - \alpha)\%$ confidence limit (corresponding to 95%, 99%, and so on) by looking up the tabulated critical values of the normal distribution (or calculating them by computer) $z_{\alpha/2}$ and $z_{1-\alpha/2}$. These two points mark the upper and lower areas of the tails of the normal distribution containing half of the $\alpha$ uncertainty probability (so that the left over inner part of the density contains $(1 - \alpha)$ of the probability). The $100 \times (1 - \alpha)\%$ confidence limit would then be given by:

$$\left( \bar{x} + z_{\alpha/2}\frac{s}{\sqrt{n}}, \bar{x} + z_{1-\alpha/2}\frac{s}{\sqrt{n}} \right)$$

What is the sampling distribution of the variance estimate, $s^2$? This is the *chi-square distribution*, whose density is given by:

$$f(y; \eta) = \frac{1}{\Gamma(\eta/2)}\left(\frac{1}{2}\right)^{\eta/2} y^{(\eta/2)-1}e^{-\frac{1}{2}y}$$

where $\eta = (N - 1)$ are the "degrees of freedom." We can similarly construct a $100 \times (1 - \alpha)\%$ confidence limit on the variance estimate $s^2$ by using the critical points of the chi-square distribution $\chi^2_{\alpha/2}$ and $\chi^2_{1-\alpha/2}$ to obtain the confidence limits:

$$\left( \frac{(n - 1)s^2}{\chi^2_{1-\alpha/2}}, \frac{(n - 1)s^2}{\chi^2_{\alpha/2}} \right)$$

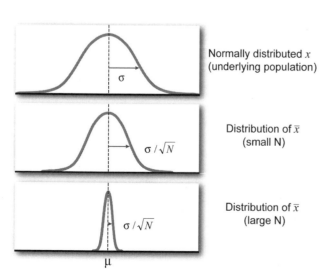

Normally distributed $x$
(underlying population)

Distribution of $\bar{x}$
(small N)

Distribution of $\bar{x}$
(large N)

**FIGURE 23–4** ● Schematic demonstration that as the number of measurements of a variable increase, the true mean does not change, simply the precision of the estimate of that mean.

In the previous blood pressure example, the variance estimate of the population from our sample is $s^2 = 24.3^2 = 590.49$, with 95% confidence limits (455.21, 796.86).

Another very common problem in statistics is how best to estimate a proportion (e.g., the pollster wanting to estimate the proportion of voters who will vote for one particular candidate, a geneticist wanting to estimate population allele frequencies, or a clinician wanting to estimate the prevalence of diabetes). Here, each sampled unit (voter, allele, research participant) is in one of two states, which are arbitrarily coded "1" and "0" (1 = for the candidate vs 0 = against; 1 = the target allele vs 0 = not the target allele; 1 = diabetic vs 0 = nondiabetic) Suppose each research participant has unknown probability, p, of being affected = "1." The probability of being unaffected = 0 is $(1 - p)$. If $n$ research participants are sampled, and k of them turn out to be affected (the other $[n - k]$ are unaffected = 0), then the best estimate of the unknown probability p is $\hat{p} = \dfrac{k}{n}$.

What is the sampling distribution of $\hat{p}$? Because $n$ is fixed and not a random variable, the sampling distribution is given by the *binomial distribution*:

$$f(k; p) = \binom{n}{k} p^k (1 - p)^{n-k}$$

where $\binom{n}{k} = \dfrac{n!}{k!(n - k)!}$ denotes the number of possible ways you can draw $k$ things from $n$. The mean of the estimator $\hat{p}$ is $p$ and its variance is $\dfrac{p(1 - p)}{n}$. When $n$ is large, the binomial distribution is nicely approximated by the normal distribution, so that these expressions for the mean and variance

of the estimator can be used to make simple $100 \times (1 - \alpha)\%$ confidence limits as before:

$$\left( \hat{p} \pm z_{a/2} \sqrt{\frac{\hat{p}(1 - \hat{p})}{n}} \right)$$

When $n$ is small, the expression is more complicated.

## BASIC GRAPHIC DISPLAYS

It can often be very useful to display data graphically because these "pictures" of the data can help identify problems (e.g., non-normal distributions; apparent group differences) much more readily than a simple look at number tables or summary statistics. One of the most basic graphic displays is the *bar chart*. For a discrete (categorical) distribution, there are only a finite number of possible values. A question that often comes up, then, is how frequently do these possible values occur (how probable are they)? In a bar chart, all possible values of the discrete variable are plotted on the x axis, with a bar whose height is the frequency (or proportion) for that value running along the y axis, as in Figure 23–5, in which 120 research participants are classified by their blood pressure status as hypotensive ($N = 23$), normotensive ($N = 65$), and hypertensive ($N = 32$).

The *histogram* is a display that generalizes the bar chart so that values of a continuous instead of a discrete variable are plotted along the x axis. For instance, using the actual measured (systolic) blood pressures instead of the three broad categories above produces finer detail about how probable are the various levels of blood pressure in the data (Figure 23–6).

Note that the histogram is highly dependent on how large or small the bar groupings are defined (to be a fair representation of the distribution, these must all be of a uniform size). In Figure 23–6, blood pressure levels have been grouped in 10 mmHg

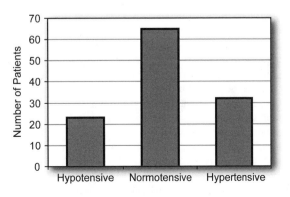

**FIGURE 23–5** ● Example of a simple bar chart.

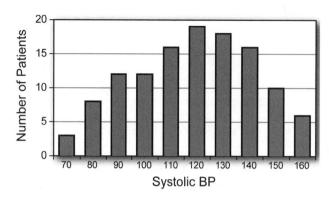

**FIGURE 23–6** ● Example of a simple histogram, using the same data used to generate Figure 23–5.

bins, so that all of those patients with blood pressures of 106 through 115 (inclusive) are counted as a single bar with midpoint value of 110. If bins that are either too fine or too large are used to group data points, the shape of the distribution can be lost, which is the whole point of the histogram in the first place. For example, if blood pressure was measured to hundredths of a mmHg, then, at the extreme, every group would have either exactly one or exactly zero data points, which would produce a histogram that looked like teeth on a pumpkin. Conversely, if a bin that is 500 mmHg wide was used, the histogram simply becomes a single bar representing the entire dataset. Neither of these extremes reveals much about the distribution of blood pressures in the study sample. Most good software for producing histograms allows the analyst to control the bin sizes to show the effect on the overall display.

An alternative method of visualizing the distribution is the *box-and-whisker plot* (Figure 23–3). In this stylized plot, the distribution of data is displayed along the *y* axis (unlike the histogram in which data traditionally are shown from side to side along the *x* axis). The box plot shows key percentile points, which mark large portions of the data, in particular the four quartiles discussed earlier: Q1, Q2, Q3, and Q4. A box is drawn around Q1 to Q3, with a line showing Q2 (the median). A whisker (line) is extended from the center of the box in each direction, below Q1 to either the minimum data point or the last point that is within 1.5 times the distance between Q2 and Q1 (whichever comes first). Likewise a whisker is drawn extending from Q3 above, to either the maximum data point or the last point that is within 1.5 times the distance between Q2 and Q3, whichever comes first. Individual points that lie beyond the whiskers represent more extreme data and are plotted as individual points. A symmetrical distribution will have a symmetrical box plot, with the upper (Q3–Q2) box equal in size to the lower (Q2–Q1) one, and the whiskers of approximately the same length. For a normal distribution, the box should

be symmetrical, skewed distributions can readily be identified in a box plot graph when asymmetry is present. Individual outlier points are also readily identified on the box plot. Some statistical methods (Chapter 22) are very sensitive to such outlier points. (It should be noted that some statistical programs use modifications of the box-and-whisker plot described here, such as using a star to denote the mean of the distribution; the reader should carefully review and describe in manuscripts the box-and-whisker plot produced by their program.)

Even more detail can be displayed using a *scattergram*. Here two variables are plotted in the $x - y$ plane, showing covariation between two variables. In Figure 23–7, age is plotted along the *x* axis and the systolic blood pressure along the *y* axis. The data for this plot were also used to construct Figures 23–5 and 23–6. Each data point is plotted individually, making the distribution of both age and blood pressure, as well as their covariation, readily apparent. In this example, there is a general trend for blood pressure to increase with increasing age. If there were no relationship between age and blood pressure, the points would be randomly scattered with no discernible pattern in either the *x* or *y* dimension.

## SUMMARY

- The standard experiment is a test to determine whether the null or alternative hypothesis is more likely to be "true" (i.e. whether the experimental intervention does not or does have an effect on some measured variable).

- The p-value is the probability that chance alone would produce data as non-null looking as actually measured if the null hypothesis is true. It is a measure of the extremeness of the data under the assumption of the null hypothesis.

- Type I error is the probability of accepting the alternative hypothesis (that the experimental intervention has an effect) as true when in fact it is not.

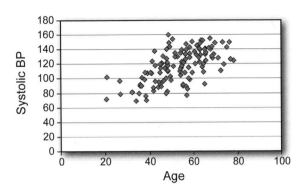

*FIGURE 23–7* ● Example of a simple scattergram, using the same data used to generate Figures 23–5 and 23–6.

- Type II error is the probability of accepting the null hypothesis (that the experimental intervention does not have an effect) as true when in fact it is not.
- Power is the probability of accepting the alternative hypothesis as true when it is in fact true (which is equal to 1–Type II error).
- There are different measures of the center point (measures of central tendency) around which most of the data in a study sample lie.
- In a normal distribution, the mean, median, and mode are all the same. When data are non-normal (e.g., skewed), these measures of central tendency are different.
- The most common measure of dispersion around a measure of central tendency (like the mean) is the standard deviation (SD). The square of the SD is referred to as the variance.
- The study sample represents only a portion of the total population of interest. The sampling distribution is the distribution of values obtained when a population is repeatedly sampled. This distribution can be normal, chi-square, or binomial, among others. The statistics used to analyze differences among sample groups depend on the known or assumed sample distribution.
- It is often useful to graph data to reveal features that are difficult to appreciate from reviewing individual values or summary statistics alone. Useful graphs include the bar chart, the histogram, the box-and-whisker plot, and the scattergram.

## ADDITIONAL READINGS

### Basic Statistics

1. Boniface DR. Experimental Design and Statistical Methods. Boca Raton, FL: Chapman & Hall CRC, 1999.
2. Grafen A, Hails R. Modern Statistics for the Life Sciences. New York: Oxford University Press, 2002.
3. Milton JS. Statistical Methods in the Biological and Health Sciences. Boston: McGraw-Hill, 1999.
4. Schork MA, Remington RD. Statistics with Applications to the Biological and Health Sciences, 3rd Ed. Englewood Cliffs, NJ: Prentice Hall, 2000.
5. Zolman JF. Biostatistics: Experimental Design and Statistical Inference. New York: Oxford University Press, 1993.

### History of Statistics

1. David HA, Edwards AWF. Annotated Readings in the History of Statistics. New York: Springer, 2001.
2. Salsburg D. The Lady Tasting Tea. New York: W.H. and Ce Freeman, 2001.
3. Stigler SM. The History of Statistics. Cambridge, MA: Belknap, 1986.
4. Stigler SM. Statistics on the Table. Cambridge, MA: Harvard University Press, 1999.

# CHAPTER 24

# Group Comparisons

Nancy L. Saccone

This chapter presents statistical tools that can be used to evaluate whether there are significant differences in outcomes between or among groups. These groups might be research volunteers studied repetitively on different occasions, subsets of patients with a particular disease compared to one another, or patients randomized to undergo different experimental interventions. Outcomes of interest for the statistical methods examined in this chapter will be continuous measures and might include a reduction in systolic blood pressure for patients studied on multiple occasions, a comparison of cardiac ejection fraction among subsets of patients with heart failure, or the serum levels of a putative inflammatory mediator after treatment with an inhibitory drug in one group of patients compared to a control group treated with a placebo.

## PARAMETRIC AND NONPARAMETRIC TESTS

As described in Chapter 23, statistical tests are designed to decide between a null and an alternative hypothesis. Classical parametric tests evaluate hypotheses by assuming that measurements made on the samples (e.g., research volunteers selected from a patient population) are drawn from a population that follows an assumed probability distribution. More often than not the data are assumed to come from a normal distribution, allowing researchers to use the t-test or analysis of variance (to be described below).

In contrast, nonparametric or "distribution-free" tests do not require data to be from a normal distribution. This chapter presents the nonparametric, rank-based tests of Mann-Whitney-Wilcoxon and Kruskal-Wallis.

Various factors should be considered when choosing between parametric and nonparametric tests for a particular data analysis. Nonparametric tests are more widely applicable because they are not restricted by the need to specify a particular distribution (e.g., normal). However, there is a potential cost to using nonparametric tests: if the data are in fact appropriately distributed for a parametric test (e.g., normal), resorting to a nonparametric test typically results in some loss of statistical power (i.e., the ability to detect a true difference between the groups). As a result, the nonparametric test may require more observations to achieve the same power as the parametric test, though in practice, in most instances the additional data required is relatively small, on the order of 2 to 10% additional data points needed. It is also useful to note that even if observed data do not appear to follow a normal distribution, often parametric tests may be applied after an appropriate transformation of the data to obtain an approximately normally distributed variable. For example, a log or square root transformation of skewed data can sometimes result in a more normally distributed set of values.

### Student's t-Test: Comparing the Mean of One Group to a Specified Value and Comparing the Means of Two Groups to Each Other

Many experiments in medicine involve sampling a set of numbers from one or two groups and asking

We thank William Shannon for helpful comments on an earlier draft of this chapter and Mary Akin for assistance in preparing the figures.

whether the means of the samples are equal to some specified value (one sample t-test) or are equal to each other (two sample t-test). In these situations, once the Z- or t-statistic has been computed, the null hypothesis can be accepted or rejected based on the statistic's value compared to a *critical value*, determined by the boundary of the critical region of the sampling distribution for the desired test (see both Chapters 9 and 21), keeping in mind whether a one- or two-tailed test is appropriate. The t-test is often called "Student's t-test" to acknowledge W. S. Gosset, who determined the sampling distributions of the t-statistic (refer to Chapter 23 for sampling distribution) and published his findings under the pseudonym "Student" (1).

## Comparing a Sample Mean to an Overall Population Mean

The one-sample t-test is perhaps the easiest statistical test to perform and describe, and the issues raised here apply to almost all other statistical tests to be discussed in this and other chapters of this book.

The one-sample t-test allows researchers to test whether the observed sample mean, $\mu_1$, of a group is equal to a given value, $\mu$. Most commonly, an investigator wishes to determine whether the sample accurately represents (comes from) a given population, in which case $\mu$ is chosen to be the known population mean. Under the null hypothesis, $H_0$, the sample belongs to that population, whereas under the alternative hypothesis, $H_1$, it does not, so that the reality is either:

$$H_0: \mu_1 = \mu \quad \text{vs} \quad H_1: \mu_1 \neq \mu$$

This case specified a two-sided t-test by defining the alternative hypothesis as $H_1: \mu_1 \neq \mu$, which allows for $\mu_1$ to be either greater or less than $\mu$. Alternatively, a one-sided test may be used if the researcher wishes to test only a directional hypothesis; that is, whether the sample mean is greater than the population mean ($\mu_1 > \mu$), or smaller than the population mean ($\mu_1 < \mu$), but not both. The effect of defining a one-sided or two-sided alternative hypothesis is to change the critical values used as criteria to determine whether the sample distribution is similar to the population distribution (see Chapter 21). Given the same data, a one-sided test results in a lower (more significant) p-value than a two-sided test, but should be used only if the investigator truly and justifiably is concerned with only a directional hypothesis.

After specifying the null and alternative hypotheses for the one-sample t-test, it is performed as follows. A random sample of $n$ independent observations $x_i$ ($i = 1, \ldots, n$) is collected from which

the sample mean $\bar{x} = (x_1 + x_2 + \cdots + x_n)/n$ and sample variance $s^2 = \sum_{i=1}^{n}((x_j - \bar{x})^2/(n-1))$ are computed. From these values the t-statistic is computed as:

$$t = \frac{\bar{x} - \mu}{s/\sqrt{n}}$$

Here $s$ is the standard deviation of the observations and is computed as the square root of the variance $s^2$.

Determining the p-value for the t-statistic requires knowing the degrees of freedom (*df*) for the experiment. In general, the degrees of freedom indicate the number of values that are free to vary under given restrictions on the data, and in some sense represents the amount of information contained in the experiment. Put another way, the degrees of freedom can be thought of as the number of independent values (observations) in the data, minus the number of independent parameters (restrictions) that are estimated from the observations to calculate the statistic. For the t-test calculated on a sample size of $n$ and a known sample mean, the $df = n - 1$ because the first $n - 1$ data points can take on any values, but once these data points are specified, the remaining observation is determined because there will be only one value it can take to produce the observed sample mean. Once the sample mean is determined from the data, the sample variance and thus the t-statistic can then be computed.

The degrees of freedom variable is used to decide the p-value for the computed t-statistic. Specifically, its role is to define the sampling distribution from which the t-statistic comes (see Chapter 21). In practice, these calculations are performed using statistical software that returns the appropriate p-value for the analysis. From an experimental design point of view, an increase in the degrees of freedom for the t-test, obtained by increasing the sample size, results in a smaller p-value, assuming the sample mean and standard deviation remain constant.

A final note about the one-sample t-test concerns the sample variance. If the population variance $\sigma^2$ is known, there is no need to estimate it from the sample. In this case, the t-statistic can be replaced by the z-statistic $Z = \frac{(x - \mu)}{\sigma/\sqrt{N}}$, which follows a standard normal sampling distribution, and is equivalent to specifying the degrees of freedom to be infinite (making the p-value smaller). In practice, however, there is little effect for moderately sized experiments. Additionally it can be argued that the population variance is in fact rarely known and thus, to be conservative, the sample variance should be used.

### Example 1

Suppose that the relationship between maternal DHA (docosahexaenoic acid) level and infant development is being studied in a randomly selected sample of 30 full-term infants born to women who were measured as having high DHA levels in the last trimester. Suppose a continuous developmental score was measured in these infants at 4 months of age, and assume that this score is normally distributed in the general population. The mean score in the 30 high-DHA exposed infants was 15, with a standard deviation of 4.2, while the mean score in the general population of full-term 4-month-olds is known to be 12. Is this difference significant at the 0.05 level?

### Solution

The problem states that we are testing for a significant difference, so we are making a nondirectional hypothesis and thus we should use a two-tailed test.

We compute $t = \dfrac{\bar{x} - \mu}{s/\sqrt{n}} = \dfrac{15 - 12}{4.2/\sqrt{30}} = 3.91$.

For a two-tailed t-test with df $= 30 - 1 = 29$, the critical value for $\alpha = 0.05$ is $t_{\text{crit}} = 2.045$. Because $t > t_{\text{crit}}$, we conclude that the difference is significant at the 0.05 level. (Note that in practice, the critical value, $t_{\text{crit}}$, is usually obtained using a statistical computer program (Chapter 28); tables of these values are also available in introductory statistics textbooks.)

### Comparing Means for Two Samples: Unpaired Observations

Suppose a researcher has two samples, $S_1$ and $S_2$, which are potentially from two different populations of unknown variances. The researcher can compute the two sample means $\bar{X}_1$ and $\bar{X}_2$ and ask whether the two population means $\mu_1$ and $\mu_2$ appear to be equal. There are two cases for performing the analysis, depending on whether or not the variances, $\sigma_1$ and $\sigma_2$, of the two populations can be assumed to be equal. Given the same data, assuming equality of variances results in a more significant p-value than if equality is not assumed. Later in this chapter we will discuss ways to determine when such an assumption is appropriate.

#### Variances Assumed to Be Equal

Let the number of observations in the $i$th sample be denoted by $N_i$, $i = 1, 2$, and let $s_i^2$ be the sample variance of the $i$th sample, computed in the usual way as in the previous section. To calculate the t-statistic here, use a pooled estimate of the common variance of the two populations, given by

$$s^2 = \frac{(N_1 - 1)s_1^2 + (N_2 - 1)s_2^2}{N_1 + N_2 - 2}.$$ The t-statistic is

then $t = \dfrac{(\bar{X}_1 - \bar{X}_2)}{s\sqrt{1/N_1 + 1/N_2}}$, with $df = N_1 + N_2 - 2$

degrees of freedom. Descriptively, this statistic is the ratio of the difference between the two means and the standard error of this difference.

### Example 2

An experiment is conducted to determine whether an experimental drug increases the activity level of an enzyme. (Note that in this case we purposely specify a directional hypothesis: our interest is *only* whether the drug *increases* the activity level of the enzyme and we choose to ignore the possibility that the drug might unexpectedly *decrease* the activity level. Such a decision should be based on the relevant science and requires sufficient information, for example, from previous published research or pilot studies, to justify such a choice.) The drug was administered to 22 research volunteers, while 10 research volunteers were given placebos. Suppose the mean activity level in the treatment group was 7.6 nmol/mg protein/hr, with a sample standard deviation of 1.2. The mean level in the placebo group was 6.1 nmol/mg protein/hr, with a sample standard deviation of 1.8. Suppose we wish to use a significance level of $\alpha = 0.01$ and to assume equal variances. Then,

$$t = \frac{7.6 - 6.1}{\sqrt{\dfrac{21(1.2)^2 + 9(1.8)^2}{30}}\sqrt{\dfrac{1}{22} + \dfrac{1}{10}}} = 2.795,$$

and $df = 30$. The hypothesis is directional so the test is one-tailed. Use of a t-distribution table (or statistical software) for $df = 30$ and $\alpha = 0.01$ gives a critical value of 2.457, which is less than the value of $t$, so the null hypothesis should be rejected. We conclude that the evidence indicates that the experimental drug does indeed increase the activity level.

#### Variances Not Assumed to Be Equal

In this case, let the number of observations in the $i$th sample be denoted by $N_i$, $i = 1, 2$, and let $s_i^2$ be the sample variance of the $i$th sample. Because we are not assuming equal variances, we do not use a pooled estimate of the variance, but instead

calculate $t' = \dfrac{(\bar{X}_1 - \bar{X}_2)}{\sqrt{s_1^2/N_1 + s_2^2/N_2}}$. However, this

statistic does not follow the t-distribution with $N_1 + N_2 - 2$ degrees of freedom. Instead, the Satterthwaite approximation (2) is commonly used to adjust the degrees of freedom. After this adjustment, $t'$ may be compared to the usual t-distribution with the adjusted degrees of freedom. The adjusted degrees of freedom are given by

$$df' = \frac{\left(\dfrac{s_1^2}{N_1} + \dfrac{s_2^2}{N_2}\right)^2}{\dfrac{s_1^4}{N_1^2(N_1 - 1)} + \dfrac{s_2^4}{N_2^2(N_2 - 1)}}; \text{ rounding}$$

$df'$ down to the nearest integer is the more conservative choice and will allow use of standard t-distribution tables. As a general rule, the adjusted $df$ will be less than the usual $df$, resulting in a less significant p-value than if variances are assumed equal.

**Example 3**

Consider Example 2 above, but suppose the researcher decides not to assume that the variances of the two groups are equal. Then:

$$t' = \frac{(7.6 - 6.1)}{\sqrt{(1.2)^2/22 + (1.8)^2/10}} = 2.4036, \text{ and}$$

$$df' = \frac{\left(\dfrac{1.2^2}{22} + \dfrac{1.8^2}{10}\right)^2}{\dfrac{1.2^4}{22^2(22 - 1)} + \dfrac{1.8^4}{10^2(10 - 1)}} = 12.78.$$

Rounding the adjusted degrees of freedom $df'$ down to 12, we would find that the critical value corresponding to $\alpha = 0.01$ is 2.68; rounding up to 13 gives a critical value of 2.65. In either case, $t'$ is less than the critical value: the test is not significant and we retain the null hypothesis and conclude there is no significant difference between the means for the two groups.

## Testing for the Equality of Two Variances

In the two examples above, the final conclusion about whether the two groups are "different" depends on whether or not equal variances are assumed. In some situations, there may be biological or scientific justifications for assuming equal variances; in other situations, investigators may wish to formally test for equality of the variances of the two groups, using the two samples of observations. Such a test is called an F-test in honor of R. A. Fisher, who derived the distribution of the F-statistic. The F-statistic is the ratio of the estimates of the two variances in question: $F = \dfrac{s_1^2}{s_2^2}$, with the smaller of the two variance estimates in the denominator, and with two degrees of freedom parameters, $df_1$ and $df_2$, corresponding to the numerator and the denominator respectively (these conventions must be followed if an investigator wishes to correctly look up critical values in standard F-distribution tables instead of relying on computer software).

**Example 4**

Consider the data in Examples 2 and 3. Suppose we want to test for equality of variances at a significance level of 0.05. Then, $F = 1.8^2/1.2^2 = 2.25$ with $df_1 = 9$ and $df_2 = 21$. Then for $\alpha = 0.05$ (i.e. cumulative area $1 - \alpha = 0.95$), the corresponding critical value turns out to be 2.37, which is greater than 2.25, so we retain the null hypothesis and conclude that the evidence indicates the two variances are equal. This means that an investigator may carry out the t-test analysis as in Example 2, assuming equal variances, and thus the conclusions of that example are justified.

Although the F-test provides a formal test for comparing variances of two populations, it is helpful to realize that, in fact, the t-test is robust with respect to moderate violations of the assumption of equal population variances. Sometimes rules of thumb are used to determine if the two-sample t-test can be applied *with* the assumption of equal variances, even if this assumption is untested or mildly violated. We will not present specific rules of thumb here, as it is arguable which are most appropriate and a full discussion is beyond the scope of this chapter. However, many of these rules of thumb involve checking whether the sample sizes are approximately equal or whether the sample variances are similar even if unequal, and it is useful to keep in mind that these considerations may allow application of the t-test with the equal variance assumption. Readers should consider consulting an experienced biostatistician when attempting to answer specific questions of this type (Chapter 27).

## Comparing Means for Two Samples: Paired Observations

Pairing of similar individuals or objects can be an important part of a study's design. Many translational clinical research studies are designed so that multiple measurements are made on the same person at different times. In the simplest case, a measurement is made on each person before and after an experimental intervention, and these measurements are naturally paired. In other designs, pairing of similar individuals offer the advantage that members of the pair can be chosen to be as alike as possible except with respect to the specific experimental intervention or variable under study. Ideally, the observed differences would then be due to that variable rather than to extraneous factors. When observations are paired, tests for group differences should take these pairings into account.

Suppose, then, that the investigator has N pairs of observed values, represented by $(x_i, y_i), i = 1, \ldots, N$. In the paired analysis, the investigator forms the differences $D_i = x_i - y_i$ between pairs and tests the hypothesis that the population of differences has a mean of zero. Thus, the analysis follows the same steps as a comparison of a sample mean to the fixed value of the "population mean" (in this case, zero) when the population variance is unknown, as discussed previously. That is, the investigator computes the statistic $t = \dfrac{(\overline{D})}{s/\sqrt{N}}$, where $\overline{D}$ is the mean of the differences and s is the standard deviation of the differences, and compare it to a t-distribution with $N - 1$ degrees of freedom.

**Example 5**

A study was conducted to measure characteristics of eight female smokers who attended a smoking cessation program and subsequently quit smoking for at least one year. The researchers were interested in whether significant weight gain for these women would be observed one year after the program. Preliminary data indicated that it would be appropriate to make a directional hypothesis and to assume that the distribution of weight differences is normal. The weight changes for each of the eight women before and one year after the program are given in Table 24–1. To determine whether there was a significant increase in the patients' weight at the $\alpha = 0.05$ level, we note that this is a naturally paired experiment, as weight is measured twice within each patient. We compute

$$t = \frac{(\overline{D})}{s/\sqrt{N}} = \frac{4.5}{6.9/\sqrt{8}} = 1.84.$$ The critical value at $\alpha = 0.05$ for the t-statistic with $df = 7$ is 1.895 for this one-sided test. Thus, we retain the

null hypothesis and conclude that no significant weight gain was observed.

## ANALYSIS OF VARIANCE (ANOVA): COMPARING MEANS FOR MORE THAN TWO GROUPS

Although the t-test is appropriate when comparing two groups only, a more general study design includes the need to make comparisons among more than two groups. For example, if four groups are to be compared, applying Student's t-test to the six possible pairs of comparisons is inefficient, requires correction of the critical value for multiple testing, and uses only part of the data for each pair-wise test. It would be preferable to analyze the data with a test that can consider all four groups simultaneously.

The appropriate approach is to use an analysis of variance (ANOVA). An ANOVA provides a test for equality of means across more than two groups. ANOVA methods analyze data in which an outcome (also called "response" or "dependent") variable is observed under several conditions that define different groups and correspond to sources of variation. For example, the outcome could be total cholesterol level, and the different conditions could correspond to smoking status—current smoker, ex-smoker, or never-smoker—giving rise to three groups. The relationship between the outcome and the sources of variation is then modeled linearly; thus, this technique can be thought of as a form of linear regression. Often in applications, at least one source of variation is a specific experimental intervention (sometimes called a "treatment" in

## TABLE 24–1

**Data for Example 5: Weight Changes in Eight Individuals After Participating in a Smoking Cessation Program**

| Subject | Weight Before Program | Weight One Year After Program | Weight Differences |
|---|---|---|---|
| 1 | 147 | 153 | +6 |
| 2 | 182 | 190 | +8 |
| 3 | 155 | 161 | +6 |
| 4 | 200 | 210 | +10 |
| 5 | 159 | 155 | −4 |
| 6 | 130 | 142 | +12 |
| 7 | 169 | 175 | +6 |
| 8 | 155 | 147 | −8 |
| Mean | | | 4.5 |
| Standard deviation | | | 6.9 |

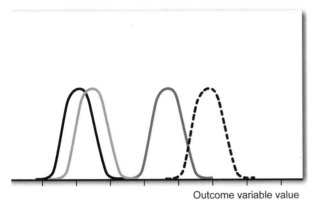

**FIGURE 24–1** ● Distributions of an outcome variable (e.g., cholesterol level) for four groups. In an analysis of variance (ANOVA), the total variation measured in a study can be divided into between-groups and within-group components. When the between-groups variance is sufficiently greater than the within-group variance, we can conclude that the groups are different (although this analysis alone does not indicate *which* groups are different from one another). In this example, the between-groups variance appears significantly larger than the within-group variance, suggesting that the groups are different.

Outcome variable value

the sense of experimental treatment and not necessarily a therapeutic treatment).

The key idea for testing for differences in group means by ANOVA is based on variances: if the means of the various groups differ significantly from one another, the overall variance of the combined groups will be noticeably larger than the variances of the individual groups (Figure 24–1). ANOVA provides simultaneous testing for multiple groups by separating the overall variance of all the observations into parts attributable to different sources of variability, and comparing the between-groups variance and the within-groups variance. The analysis assumes that the groups have a common variance.

Data for an ANOVA are typically cross-classified; that is, each source of variation is represented by a discrete classification variable. One-way or single classification analysis is the simplest setting for ANOVA and consists of testing for differences in the means of $K$ populations described by a single classification variable with $K$ categories. Thus, the differences in mean total cholesterol for current smokers, ex-smokers, and never-smokers would be tested using a one-way ANOVA where $K = 3$. When $K = 2$, the method essentially reduces to the t-test already discussed in the previous section. In a two-way ANOVA, observations are classified on two characteristics, each of which is represented by a discrete classification variable. For example, suppose we have total cholesterol levels measured for patients being treated for a particular disease, and also have these patients described by the following two classification variables: "family history of disease" divided into two categories (yes/no), and "treatment regimen" divided into four categories. The total cholesterol level would be the outcome variable of interest, and the family history and treatment categories would naturally create $2 \times 4 = 8$ groups of patients, according to the patients' status with respect to these two variables, as Table 24–2 shows. Many experimental study designs in translational clinical research can be analyzed by a one- or two-way ANOVA.

## TABLE 24–2

### Example of Cross-Classified Data: Patients Classified by Family History of Disease and Treatment Regimen, Resulting in Eight Groups

| Classification Variable 1: Family History | Classification Variable 2: Treatment Regimen | | | |
|---|---|---|---|---|
| | Class 1: Treatment 1 | Class 2: Treatment 2 | Class 3: Treatment 3 | Class 4: Treatment 4 |
| Class 1: No | $\overline{X}_{11}$ | $\overline{X}_{12}$ | $\overline{X}_{13}$ | $\overline{X}_{14}$ |
| Class 2: Yes | $\overline{X}_{21}$ | $\overline{X}_{22}$ | $\overline{X}_{23}$ | $\overline{X}_{24}$ |

Note: Table entries are mean outcome values (here, total cholesterol levels) for patients in that two-way category

## One-Way ANOVA

### Testing for Equality Across Means of Two or More Groups

Suppose researchers are studying $K$ populations (groups) where $K \geq 2$. The null hypothesis is that there is no difference in means among the $K$ groups, with all the observed values coming from a single distribution with a common mean and variance. To test this hypothesis, ANOVA estimates the overall variance in two ways and uses the F-test to test whether these two estimates are significantly different from one another.

The first estimate is based on the within-groups variance and is called the within-groups mean square, $s_w^2$; this mean square represents the variability within each of the groups. In fact, $s_w^2$ is a pooled estimate of the overall population variance $\sigma^2$, and in the case of $K = 2$, reduces to the pooled estimate used for the t-test when the variances are assumed to be equal. The second estimate of the variance is based on the between-groups variance and is called the between-groups mean square, $s_b^2$; this mean square represents the variability due to effects of group membership (sources of variability) as well as to experimental variability within each group.

In general, a mean square is computed as a sum of squares divided by the associated degrees of freedom. Thus, two sums of squares and their associated degrees of freedom are computed to obtain the two desired estimates of the variance. Then, the overall population variance $\sigma^2$ is estimated by the following: (1) $s_w^2 = \dfrac{S_w}{N - K}$, the sum of squares within groups divided by the associated degrees of freedom, and (2) $s_b^2 = \dfrac{S_b}{K - 1}$, the sum of squares between groups divided by the associated degrees of freedom ($N$ is the total number of observations across all the groups). Full formulas for these sums of squares are given in the appendix of this chapter. In practice, these quantities are computed using statistical software or other tools; the important steps for the investigator will be to define the variables and set up the analysis, and to appropriately interpret the results.

After $s_w^2$ and $s_b^2$ have been computed, under the null hypothesis, $F = \dfrac{s_b^2}{s_w^2}$ follows the F-distribution with $K - 1$ and $N - K$ degrees of freedom, and the F-distribution is used to determine whether to accept or reject the null hypothesis. Thus, if the computed $F$ exceeds the chosen critical value, we conclude that the group means are not all equal.

### Example 6

Consider a sample of 8 current smokers, 12 ex-smokers, and 13 never-smokers. The mean total cholesterol level in each group is 210, 188, and 200 respectively. A computer program to calculate the mean squares reports that the between-groups mean square is 175 and the within-groups mean square is 490. At the 0.01 significance level, is there evidence that the group means differ significantly?

**Solution**

The F-statistic is $F = \left( \dfrac{175/(3 - 1)}{490/(33 - 3)} \right) = 5.357$. With 2 and 30 degrees of freedom, the critical value at the 0.01 level is 5.18. $F$ exceeds the critical value, so we conclude that the two estimates of the variance are unequal, and hence that there is a significant difference among the group means.

### Testing Specific Comparisons Between Means

The above discussion describes an overall test to detect whether there are significant differences among the group means; however, this test does not indicate *where* these differences occur. The next step is to make specific comparisons between the means of the $K$ groups. Note that the appropriateness of a particular approach can depend on whether the comparison in question was selected for study pre- or postanalysis! If a specific comparison was selected beforehand (a priori) as being of interest, a basic t-test can be appropriate. However, in many cases, the goal of ANOVA is to identify what comparisons would be of interest for further study, and specific comparisons are chosen after ANOVA (post hoc). In this case, simple t-tests are generally not appropriate, and more advanced methods are needed. There are many post hoc tests available. Among the most commonly used are Tukey's honestly significant difference (HSD) test, the Newman-Keuls test, the Dunnett test, the Scheffé test, and the Bonferroni t-test, also known as Dunn's multiple-testing procedure. Also seen are the least significant difference (LSD) test and the Duncan multiple range test, but their use is not recommended because they tend to inappropriately declare significance too often when many tests are carried out. In general, for most straightforward analyses of one- or two-way ANOVA, we favor Scheffé's method because it is more general (has fewer restrictions) than the alternatives and is also more conservative. However, in certain circumstances other methods are more appropriate. Readers are urged to discuss specific uses with an experienced biostatistician, as a discussion of which method is most appropriate for a given application is beyond the scope of this chapter.

Although this chapter does not give a complete treatment of the various post hoc analysis methods, we will describe the key ideas behind them. In a post hoc analysis, a comparison between two means amounts to testing hypotheses about the difference, $\mu_i - \mu_j$ ($i \neq j$), between the means. More generally, investigators can test hypotheses about any linear combination of the means, $C = \sum_{i=1}^{K} c_i \mu_i$, where $\sum_{i=1}^{K} c_i = 0$; these expressions are called contrasts among the means. The contrast expression must be estimated using the estimates $\overline{X}_i$ of the true means $\mu_i$. The common way to evaluate hypotheses about these contrasts is to estimate the variance of the contrast expression and then form the $1 - \alpha$ confidence interval about the contrast expression. (See Chapter 23 for more on confidence intervals.) There are several specific methods for constructing the confidence interval for the contrast expression; some of them have certain restrictions (such as requiring equal numbers of observations in all cells) or apply only to special cases. However, the key underlying idea is that the resulting confidence interval indicates that the true value of the contrast expression lies within the confidence interval with "$1 - \alpha$ certainty." For example, if we are studying the contrast expression $\mu_i - \mu_j$, and 0 is *not* contained in the 95% confidence interval, we can then conclude that with 95% certainty, the true value of $\mu_i - \mu_j$ lies in the confidence interval and thus is not 0. Hence, with 95% certainty, $\mu_i \neq \mu_j$.

## Two-Way ANOVA

Although we will now focus on the analysis of two-way cross-classified data, the case for $N > 2$ is a natural generalization. For two-way data, there are two categorical variables (also called factors) that describe the data and can form the headings for the rows and columns of a table, as illustrated previously in Table 24–2.

The formulas and calculations for two-way ANOVA analysis are somewhat complex, but the logic of the analysis can be described without stating these formulas. (Readers interested in more details can consult references listed at the end of the chapter.) When performing a two-way ANOVA, investigators are interested in whether there are significant effects due to *either* of the classification variables. The question translates into testing two null hypotheses: first, that the row means are equal, and second, that the column means are equal (see Table 24–2). Investigators can again use

the F-statistic for a formal test. Hypothesis 1 is tested using the statistic formed from the ratio of the mean square for the column means over the residual mean square, and Hypothesis 2 is tested using the ratio of the mean square for the row means over the residual mean square. Analogous to the one-way ANOVA case, each of these mean squares is formed from a ratio of the relevant sum of squares over the associated degrees of freedom.

The overall effect of a single categorical variable alone is called a main effect, and the above discussion describes testing for the two main effects. A third question can also be asked: are there significant effects due not just to the first variable or the second variable alone, but due to the *combination* of variables? If so, we would say that there is an *interaction* between the variables. To test for an interaction effect, an interaction term must be included in the overall model. Figures 24–2 and 24–3 illustrate examples of two-way classifications for which the interactions are nonsignificant and significant, respectively.

## Design Issues for ANOVA

An important concept in ANOVA is that of blocking. Block designs are useful to control for possible confounding variables that may contribute to the observed variation in outcomes. Generally speaking, a block can be defined as a set of samples (e.g., research volunteers) that are homogeneous with respect to the possible confounder. Similarly, a block can be defined to be a set of samples whose observations are expected to be correlated, rather than independent. For example, when studying the effect of inhibiting a new putative mediator of a particular disease, blocks defined by age group would help control for possible age-related differences in the effect of the drug inhibitor. Alternatively, in another study, patients might be grouped together into blocks based on genotype patterns to help control for genetic variability at particular loci of importance. To define a block, an additional variable (blocking factor) is included in the ANOVA model.

In a repeated-measures design, just as the name suggests, repeated measures are taken on each research volunteer in the study. The repeated measurements may correspond to different levels of an experimental intervention (say, different doses of a drug), or to the same level of the intervention but measured at different times, or some combination thereof. Another way of thinking of this design is as a special case of a block design, where each block is defined to be a single individual to control

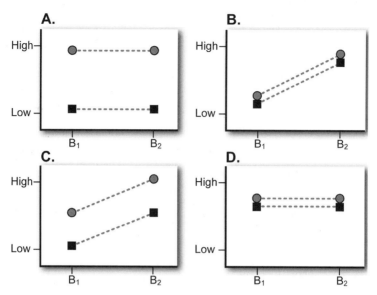

**FIGURE 24–2** ● Examples of *nonsignificant* A × B interaction effects. Effect A has two levels indicated by the circle and square respectively, and effect B has two levels indicated by $B_1$ and $B_2$ plotted along the *x* axis. The outcome variable is plotted on the *y* axis. Panel A: Variable A has significant main effect and variable B does not. Panel B: Variable B has a significant main effect and variable A does not. Panel C: Both variables A and B have significant main effects. Panel D: Neither variable A nor B has a significant main effect.

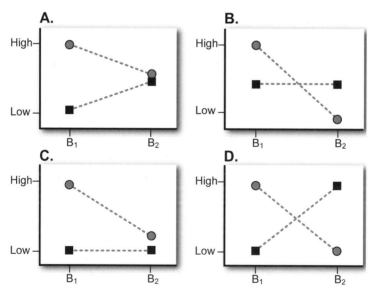

**FIGURE 24–3** ● Examples of *significant* A × B interaction effects. Effect A has two levels indicated by the circle and square respectively, and effect B has two levels indicated by $B_1$ and $B_2$ plotted along the *x* axis. The outcome variable is plotted on the *y* axis. Panel A: Variable A has significant main effect and variable B does not. Panel B: Variable B has a significant main effect and variable A does not. Panel C: Both variables A and B have significant main effects. Panel D: Neither variable A nor B has a significant main effect. Thus, although in each case, there is a significant A × B interaction, the interpretation (i.e., significance vs nonsignificance) of *main* effects for each panel is the same as Figure 24–2.

for interindividual variability. Such a design can be useful when the costs of the study are high (because such designs can be carried out using fewer research participants), or for a study in which the confounding variables are unclear. Note that if there are only two repeated measures, the repeated-measures ANOVA design essentially reduces to the paired t-test, with the natural pairing of the two measures within the same research participant.

As discussed in Chapter 8, once confounding variables have been identified and used to define blocks, there are different ways to assign the experimental intervention to block members. In a randomized block design, for each block, one or more members are randomly assigned to each of the different possible experimental interventions. The Latin square design is a particularly efficient blocking design that controls for two confounding variables having the same number of levels, $N$. The levels of the first confounding variable form the rows of a square table and the levels of the second variable form the columns. Then, $N$ levels of the intervention may be assessed by assigning them to the cells so that each level appears once in each row and once in each column. The advantage of this design is that the minimum number of individuals needed is $N^2$ (one per cell in the $N \times N$ table); this is an improvement on the minimum of $N^3$ persons that would be needed if we assigned each of the $N$ treatment levels to each of the cells (blocks) defined by the blocking factors, as would occur with a randomized block design.

The calculations for an $N$-way ANOVA are simplified if there are equal numbers of observations in each cell; such a design is called balanced, and some software routines that perform ANOVA are intended for analysis of balanced designs only. However, there can be good reasons for choosing an unbalanced design. For example, as just shown, a Latin square design has advantageous properties; however, it is in fact unbalanced because in the full $N \times N \times N$ table formed by the two confounding variables and the experimental intervention, some cell counts are zero. A related issue is missing data, a concern that is not specific to ANOVA of course. In general, consultation with an experienced statistician can help an investigator choose among the varied methods for handling missing data; such methods can range from deleting samples with missing data to imputing data when possible, using appropriate assumptions.

The terminology of ANOVA includes references to fixed and random effects. A classification variable (such as one representing various levels of experimental intervention) represents a fixed effect in an ANOVA statistical model if all its categories are considered to be all the possible categories of interest. On the other hand, it is referred to as a random effect if all its categories are a subset of a larger number of categories about which an investigator wishes to make inferences. An ANOVA that involves both fixed and random effects is called a mixed model ANOVA. For instance, a common study design that would be analyzed by a mixed model ANOVA would be a therapeutic clinical trial being administered via multiple hospitals: the treatment variable would in most cases be regarded as fixed, because the different treatments (e.g., drugs) are usually exactly the treatments of interest, although the hospital effect could be considered a random effect because the hospitals in the study are only a sample of possible hospitals that might deliver care. The discussion in this section has focused on fixed effects; readers interested in modeling random effects should consult a statistician for more information and guidance.

As shown, ANOVA provides a tool for comparing means among groups defined by *qualitative* (that is, categorical) explanatory variables representing sources of variation affecting a *single* quantitative outcome measure. If instead an investigator wishes to study the effect of *quantitative* (e.g., age) as well as qualitative explanatory variables on a single quantitative outcome, then an analysis of covariance (ANCOVA) would be the appropriate tool, and is implemented using multiple regression with dummy variables to represent qualitative variables (see Chapter 25 for more on regression). If, however, an investigator wishes to study *two or more* quantitative outcome measures, multivariate analysis of variance (MANOVA) allows an integrated analysis that can take the place of multiple ANOVAs. With MANOVA, a researcher can answer the overall question of whether there are any differences among groups in these multiple outcomes of interest (for more on MANOVA analyses, see Chapter 26). Finally, just as ANCOVA provides an extension to ANOVA, multivariate analysis of covariance (MANCOVA) provides an extension of MANOVA that can include quantitative as well as qualitative explanatory variables.

## NONPARAMETRIC TESTS

In an ANOVA, statistical inferences are based on a statistic (the F-statistic) that is expected to follow a theoretical distribution under the null hypothesis. The properties of this family of distributions are derived when observations are assumed to be randomly drawn from normally distributed populations, with equal variances. As an alternative, inference can be made based on an empirical distribution function, without assuming underlying normality; such an approach is called a nonparametric test. Nonparametric tests are also known as distribution-free tests, alluding to the fact that the tests are free from assumptions about the form of the distribution followed by the observations. Thus, the advantage of a nonparametric approach is clear: there is protection from possible deviations from the normality assumptions underlying a classical ANOVA; however, the trade-off is that resorting to a nonparametric method can lead to a loss of statistical power (i.e., the ability to detect true differences between or among groups) if the theoretical assumptions of normality are in fact reasonably satisfied.

### The Mann-Whitney-Wilcoxon Rank Test: Comparing Two Groups.

Suppose researchers have a one-way classification with two groups; that is, they have observations that are classified by a categorical variable with two levels. Note that intuitively, if the values in one group tend to be higher than those in the other group, the distributions of observations in the two groups would appear offset when plotted on the same axes, even if those distributions do not appear to follow a normal distribution. The Mann-Whitney-Wilcoxon rank test (3,4) capitalizes on this observation by replacing the actual observations by their ranks, and testing whether lower ranks tend to occur in one group and higher ranks tend to occur in the other group.

Suppose for the $i$th level ($i = 1$ or $2$), the investigator has $N_i$ observations, with $N = N_1 + N_2$. This test is carried out by computing the Wilcoxon score, also called, more descriptively, the rank sum, for each group: the actual observed values are replaced by their ranks (from 1 to $N$) in the full sample, and

for each of the two groups, the total of the ranks is computed. It is then assumed that each possible grouping of ranks into two groups of these sizes is equally likely. Then, the total number of ways of grouping the ranks into the two groups of size $N_1$ and $N_2$ respectively is $N$ choose $N_1$; that is,

$$\binom{N}{N_1} = \binom{N}{N_2} = \frac{N!}{N_1!N_2!}.$$ An empirical p-value is then obtained by counting how many of the possible occurrences of ranks in the two groups give a rank sum as extreme or more extreme than that which is actually observed.

If ties in ranks occur, the common practice is to give the tied observations the mean of the distinct ranks they would have if not tied; then, the sum of the ranks over all the observations remains constant. For example, if there is a four-way tie for rank 1, the researchers would give each of the four observations the rank of $\frac{1 + 2 + 3 + 4}{4} = 2.5$.

**Example 7**

Suppose we have data for two groups as described in Table 24–3, with values and ranks (from lowest to highest) as given. Here, $N_1 = 4$ and $N_2 = 5$. Let us focus on Group 1. The only ways to obtain a rank sum less than or equal to 13 for a group of 4 observations are with the following choices of ranks:

$$1 + 2 + 3 + 4 = 10$$
$$1 + 2 + 3 + 5 = 11$$
$$1 + 2 + 3 + 6 = 12$$
$$1 + 2 + 3 + 7 = 13$$
$$1 + 2 + 4 + 5 = 12$$
$$1 + 2 + 4 + 6 = 13$$
$$1 + 3 + 4 + 5 = 13.$$

### TABLE 24–3

**Data for Example 7**

| Group 1 | | Group 2 | |
|---|---|---|---|
| Observed Value | Overall Rank | Observed Value | Overall Rank |
| 10.2 | 4 | 16.5 | 6 |
| 9.4 | 3 | 18.2 | 7 |
| 8.0 | 1 | 8.8 | 2 |
| 16.0 | 5 | 20.1 | 9 |
| | | 20.0 | 8 |
| Rank Sum | 13 | Rank Sum | 32 |

Thus, there are seven ways of obtaining a rank sum as extreme or more extreme than that given by the data. Now, the total number of possible ways of placing ranks into the two groups is: $\binom{N}{N_1} = \binom{9}{4} = 126$, so the empirical p-value is $7/126 = 0.055$, which is not significant at the $\alpha = 0.05$ level.

For large samples, there is a useful approximate test based on the fact that asymptotically, the mean of the ranks of a sample is approximately normally distributed. The exact p-value can always be calculated but may be inconvenient for larger samples. In practice, computer software is used to calculate the p-values, so it can be useful to be aware of whether a given package allows both exact and approximate calculation.

### The Kruskal-Wallis Test: Comparing More than Two Groups

The Kruskal-Wallis test is the natural extension of the Wilcoxon test to the setting of $K$ groups, $K > 2$ (so that the one-way classification variable has $K$ levels). Suppose for the $i$th level, investigators have $N_i$ observations, with $N$ being the sum of all the $N_i, i = 1, \ldots, K$. As in the Mann-Whitney-Wilcoxon test, the actual observed values are replaced by their ranks in the overall, full sample, and the rank sum and mean rank sum $\overline{R}_i$ for each of the $i = 1, \ldots, K$ groups is computed. Kruskal and Wallis (5) derived a statistic based on these ranks that approximately follows an $\chi^2$ distribution with $K - 1$ degrees of freedom. Again, ties are handled as in the Wilcoxon test, with the mean of the involved ranks being assigned to the tied observations; however, then an additional adjustment of the statistic must be applied for each group of ties that occurs.

### FURTHER READING

Suggested sources for further reading (6,7) provide expanded coverage of ANOVA methods. Reference (7) also gives a readable and detailed discussion of nonparametric methods, including some methods not covered here.

### SUMMARY

- The t-test is used to compare the mean of one group to a specified value, or to compare the means of two groups to each other. It assumes that observations are drawn from a normally distributed population. If two groups are being compared, the t-test is carried out differently depending on whether or not the variances of the two groups may be assumed to be equal. If observations in the two groups are paired, a paired t-test is used.
- The F-test is used to compare two variances. It also provides the key statistic for ANOVA tests of equality of means.
- ANOVA is used to compare means across two or more groups. It does so by comparing within-group and between-group variances via the F-test, and indicates whether there is a significant difference among the means, overall, without identifying which means differ from each other. Additional comparisons of means for specific groups may then be carried out.
- Nonparametric tests include rank-based tests that replace observations with their overall rank in the dataset and assess how these ranks are distributed across the groups. The Mann-Whitney-Wilcoxon rank test compares two groups, and the Kruskal-Wallis test generalizes the approach to more than two groups.

### REFERENCES

1. Student. On the probable error of a mean. Biometrika 1908;6:1–25.
2. Satterthwaite, FE. An approximate distribution of estimates of variance components. Biometrics Bulletin 1946;2:110–114.
3. Wilcoxon, F. Individual comparisons by ranking methods. Biometrics Bulletin 1945;1:80–83.
4. Mann HB and Whitney DR. On a test of whether one or two random variables is stochastically larger than the other. Ann Math Stat 1947;18:50–60.
5. Kruskal WH, Wallis WA. Use of ranks in one-criterion analysis of variance. J Am Stat Assoc 1952;47:583–621.
6. Snedecor GW, Cochran WG. Statistical Methods. Ames, IA: Iowa State University Press.
7. Brownlee, KA. Statistical Theory and Methodology in Science and Engineering. John Wiley and Sons.

## ONE-WAY ANOVA

Typically, three sums of squares, and associated degrees of freedom, are computed to carry out the ANOVA analysis. The total sum of squares of deviations from the sample mean is computed from the formula

$$S = \sum_{i=1}^{K}\sum_{j=1}^{N_i} X_{ij}^2 - \frac{\left(\sum_{i=1}^{K}\sum_{j=1}^{N_i} X_{ij}\right)^2}{N},$$

and there are $N-1$ associated degrees of freedom; note that the ratio of $S$ over the degrees of freedom is a formula for the overall variance of all the observations. The sum of squares (of deviations) between groups is

$$S_b = \sum_{i=1}^{K} N_i(\overline{X}_i - \overline{X})^2$$

$$= \sum_{i=1}^{K}\left(\frac{\left(\sum_{j=1}^{N_i} X_{ij}^2\right)}{N_i}\right) - \frac{\left(\sum_{i=1}^{K}\sum_{j=1}^{N_i} X_{ij}\right)^2}{N},$$

and there are $K-1$ associated degrees of freedom. The sum of squares (of deviations) within groups is

$$S_w = \sum_{i=1}^{K}\left(\sum_{j=1}^{N_i}(X_{ij} - \overline{X}_i)^2\right)$$

$$= \sum_{i=1}^{K}\sum_{j=1}^{N_i} X_{ij}^2 - \sum_{i=1}^{K}\left(\frac{\left(\sum_{j=1}^{N_i} X_{ij}\right)^2}{N_i}\right),$$

but can be obtained from the above two quantities by the formula $S_w = S - S_b$; the associated degrees of freedom is:

$$\sum_{i=1}^{K}(N_i - 1) = N - K.$$

Then the overall population variance $\sigma^2$ is estimated by the following (1):

$$s_w^2 = \frac{S_w}{N - K},$$

the sum of squares within groups divided by the associated degrees of freedom, and (2):

$$s_b^2 = \frac{S_b}{K - 1},$$

the sum of squares between groups divided by the associated degrees of freedom.

# CHAPTER 25

# Regression

Rob Culverhouse

egression is used for two purposes: predicting outcomes and investigating the importance of predictors of outcomes. This chapter focuses on the method of linear regression. Two other regression methods, logistic regression and Cox regression, will be discussed briefly. The use of these methods involves finding, for the given type of regression, the model that fits the data "best" according to some predefined criteria. Which of the various approaches to regression is most appropriate depends on the type of data being analyzed. Linear regression is typically appropriate when the outcome variable is a measured quantity that can take on any value in a continuous range (e.g., height, blood pressure, cholesterol level). Logistic regression depends on binary outcomes (e.g., lived/died, response/nonresponse, toxic/nontoxic). Cox regression is used to analyze survival (time to event) data (time to death, time to relapse, time on therapy).

## LINEAR REGRESSION

Linear regression is the basic method from which the other methods developed, and it is still the most popular. The method is called linear because its models can be represented graphically by a straight line (or by a plane if there is more than one predictor variable). Although linear regression models can be constructed for data with any number of variables, we can illustrate many of the key concepts by first looking at how the method works for data with only two variables (bivariate data). Linear regression on data consisting of only two variables is often known as simple linear regression.

## Simple Linear Regression

A linear relationship between two variables is usually described by two numbers: the slope and the intercept. For instance, if there is a linear relationship between the variables $y$ and $x$, the relationship could be represented by the formula

$$Y = \alpha + \beta X$$

where $\alpha$ represents the intercept (i.e., the value of $Y$ when $X = 0$) and $\beta$ represents the slope (i.e., the amount $Y$ changes for each unit change in $X$).

This is the simplest kind of relationship between $Y$ and $X$, so researchers typically assume relationships are linear unless there is good reason to consider something more complicated. Real observations almost never fit a linear model perfectly, so the statistical model assumed is that for each individual $i$

$$y_i = \alpha + \beta x_i + \varepsilon_i$$

where $\varepsilon_i$ represents an unaccounted for deviation from the linear model. These deviations in the data may be due to simple measurement errors or to important predictive factors that were not measured for the experiment.

To see how a linear model might work, consider the relationship between the adult heights of fathers and their sons. If researchers collected data on many fathers and their sons, they could build the best fitting linear regression model predicting a son's height, $y_i$, from his father's height, $x_i$. They could then compare this model to the data that generated it to test the hypothesis that the height of the father has an influence on the height of the son (i.e., testing the hypothesis that $\beta \neq 0$). Alternatively, the same approach could be used as a method to guess the adult height of a baby boy from the height of his father.

## The Best Fitting Line

Among the variety of ways to define the best line, the most common is *ordinary least squares*. To see how the least squares line is found, consider the example of heights of fathers and their adult sons. Suppose researchers have measured 100 fathers and sons and let $\{(x_1, y_1), (x_2, y_2), \ldots, (x_{100}, y_{100})\}$ represent the pairs of heights, with $x_i$ representing the height of the $i$th father and $y_i$ representing the height of his son. Then, for any choice of $\alpha$ and $\beta$, the *predicted value* of $y_i$ can be defined to be the value obtained by plugging $x_i$ into the equation of the line [i.e., pred $(y_i) = \hat{y}_i = \alpha + \beta x_i$].

The observed height of the $i$th son is unlikely to be exactly what is predicted by the formula for the line, and the *prediction error* is defined for the $i$th point to be $\varepsilon_i = \hat{y}_i - y_i$ (i.e., $\varepsilon_i = \alpha + \beta x_i - y_i$). The researchers want to find the line that corresponds to the least overall prediction error, where overall prediction error is defined to be the sum of the squares of the prediction errors for all the points in the dataset. The prediction errors are squared so they will all be non-negative. Otherwise, predicted values that were way too high for some individuals and way too low for others could cancel out in the sum, possibly giving a poor-fitting line a low score.

The least squares regression line is the line with $\alpha$ and $\beta$ chosen so that the sum of the squares of the prediction errors is as small as possible. The formulas from which $\alpha$ and $\beta$ can be computed are easily derived from elementary calculus, but do not add much intuitive insight, so they are omitted here.

Any statistical package will quickly produce the line that minimizes the sum of the squared error. However, before computing the best predictive line for a dataset, one important step needs to be taken: checking the data to see whether or not a linear regression is appropriate. Typically, at least two checks should be performed. One is a statistical check performed by calculating a quantity called the *correlation*. The other is to make a visual inspection of the data, typically using a scatterplot.

## Correlation

The correlation is a measure of how closely the data comes to falling on a straight line. The most common measure of correlation, Pearson's correlation coefficient, can take on any value from $+1$ to $-1$. A correlation of $+1$ means that there is a single line with positive slope that passes through all the points in the data. More generally, any positive correlation means that as the predictor (height of the father) increases, the outcome (height of the son) tends to increase as well. Figure 25–1 depicts such a relationship.

The tendency of taller fathers to have taller sons is something that holds "on average," but not for every pair of points. It is not difficult to find pairs of points in Figure 25–1 where the son of a taller father is shorter than the son of a shorter father. Nonetheless, the tendency for the sons of the taller fathers to be taller than the sons of the shorter fathers is readily observable in the scatterplot.

A correlation of $-1$ also means that all the data points lie along a single line, but that the slope of the line is negative. In general, a negative correlation means that as the predictor value (cost of a copay) increases, the outcome variable (percentage of diabetics filling their metformin scripts) tends to decrease. Figure 25–2 depicts simulated data from a relationship like this.

A correlation of 0 indicates no linear relationship between the predictor and the outcome variable, as seen in Figure 25–3. However, as shown in

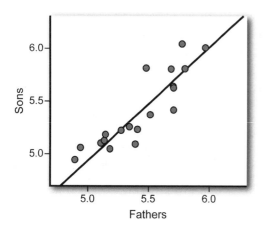

**FIGURE 25–1** ● Scatterplot of adult height of sons versus adult height of fathers. The heights are positively correlated. In this dataset, the correlation is high ($r = 0.898$). Also included is the regression line providing the best prediction of the height of a son from the height of his father.

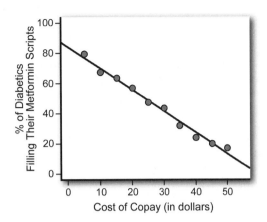

**FIGURE 25–2** ● Fictional example of data with a negative correlation. As the predictor variable (copay) increases, the outcome (percent filling their scripts) decreases, indicating a negative correlation. Also included is the regression line corresponding to the smallest sum of squares error. Because the correlation is negative, the regression line has a negative slope.

the next section, it does not mean that there is no relationship between the variables.

Correlations of $+1, 0,$ or $-1$ are very unusual, so values for $|r|$ are typically somewhere between 0 and 1. As a rule of thumb, if $0 < |r| < 0.5$ the linear association between the predictor and the outcome is considered to be weak. If $0.5 < |r| < 0.8,$ there is said to be a moderate association between the variables. If $|r| > 0.8,$ the variables are considered to be strongly associated.

$R^2,$ another measure of how well the dependent variable can be predicted from the regression line, has the nice property that it can be interpreted in terms of the sum of the squared prediction error. Let *SSE (regression)* be the sum of the squared prediction errors between the regression line and the observed data. In contrast, if we had not used the x-values to build the regression line, the best prediction for each of the y-values would be the average y-value, $\bar{y}.$ Let *SSE (mean)* be the sum of the squares of the differences between $\bar{y}$ and the

observed y-values. Then we define $R^2$ as follows:

$$R^2 = 1 - \left( \frac{SSE\ (regression)}{SSE\ (mean)} \right).$$

$R^2$ is the proportion of the variation in the outcome "explained" by the independent variables $[R^2 = 1 -$ (unexplained variation/total variation)]. Because the regression line corresponds to the smallest least squared error, even if $x$ is really not an important predictor of $y,$ *SSE (regression)* $\leq$ *SSE (mean).* On the other hand, because all the terms in the sum defining *SSE (regression)* are squares, the smallest *SSE (regression)* can be is 0 (achieved only if all the points in the dataset lie on a straight line). From this, $0 \leq R^2 \leq 1,$ and when $R^2 = 0,$ the value of $X$ does not say anything about $Y,$ and when $R^2 = 1,$ $Y$ can be perfectly predicted from $X.$

The fact that this sounds very much like the information we would get from $(r)^2$ is no accident. Surprisingly, it turns out that $R^2 = (r)^2$ (1).

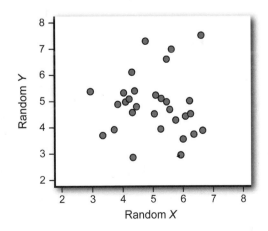

**FIGURE 25–3** ● Example of data with linear correlation = 0. This is very unusual in real data, but real data may often correspond to very small correlation coefficients.

## Scatterplots

Although $r$ and $R^2$ are measures of how well the data fit a line, no single number can adequately summarize the shape of a distribution. The datasets illustrated in Figures 25–1, 25–2, and 25–3 are what researchers usually imagine when presented with a correlation coefficient. However, raw data are rarely distributed so nicely. For this reason, it is always a good idea to get a visual impression of a dataset. One of the best tools for doing this is a scatterplot. Scatterplots are an excellent tool for discovering anomalies in a dataset that could lead to misleading results. Below are two classic examples of how investigators might be misled if they assume they can tell what the data distribution looks like simply by knowing the Pearson correlation coefficient value.

The first example serves as a reminder that $r$ and $R^2$ are measures of *linear* association. Investigators cannot conclude from a small (linear) correlation coefficient that the variables are not associated. The data plotted in Figure 25–4 has a linear correlation = 0. This is because high values of $Y$ are associated both with high values of $X$ and low values of $X$. However, after looking at the plot, few people would think that $x$ and $y$ are unrelated. In fact, $Y$ can be perfectly predicted from $X$, since $Y$ is the square of $X$.

The second illustration shows that even if the dataset has good correlation, a linear regression may not be appropriate. Each of the datasets illustrated in Figure 25–5 have $r = 0.7$. However, only the dataset illustrated in Figure 25–5A is appropriate for a linear regression analysis.

In Figure 25–5B, the data contain an obvious outlier. If the outlier is removed, the remaining data have $r = 0.0$. The point is probably due to an error of

some kind, but even if it is not, statistical conclusions cannot be reliably based on a single outlier point.

Figure 25–5C, like Figure 25–4, illustrates data for which $X$ is a useful predictor of $Y$, but in which the relationship between the variables is not linear. However, because of the relatively high linear correlation in Figure 25–5C, a naïve regression user who did not check the scatterplot would be tempted to use the poorly fitting least squares regression line, not realizing that the data called for a transformation before fitting a linear regression model. The issue of data transformation is discussed in a later section of this chapter.

For many other examples of nonlinear datasets with $r = 0.7$, see discussions in reference (2).

## Interpreting the Least Squares Line

Once the data have been cleaned of any unwanted outliers and it has been decided that no further transformations of the data are required, almost any statistical package quickly provides the least squares regression line fit to such data.

The least squares line regressing $Y$ on $X$ (i.e., predicting $Y$ from $X$) has several interesting properties. First, it passes through the mean point of the data [i.e., $(\bar{x}, \bar{y})$]. However, it is not the line that would normally be thought of as going down the center of the data. The center line would be the line passing through $(\bar{x}, \bar{y})$ and having slope equal to $s_Y/s_X$, (where $s_Y$ is the standard deviation of $Y$ and $s_X$ is the standard deviation of $X$). To find slope of the regression line, multiply the slope of the "center" line by the correlation, $r$.

The effect of this change in slope is illustrated in Figure 25–6. The slanted ellipse represents a cloud of data points. The dot at its center represents the mean of the data. The center line (also known as the

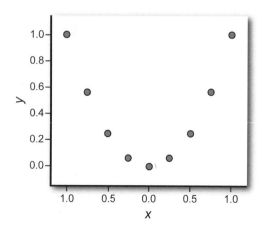

**FIGURE 25–4** ● Data with zero linear correlation even though $y$ can be exactly predicted from $x$ ($y = x^2$).

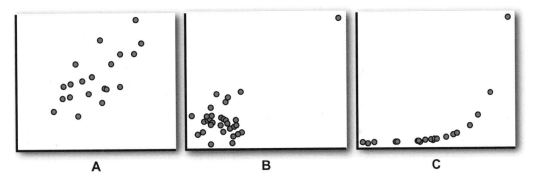

**FIGURE 25–5** ● Three datasets with $r = 0.7$. Dataset A is what researchers usually imagine when told that $r = 0.7$. Dataset B consists of an outlier and a mass of points with $r = 0$. Dataset C consists of data that should be log transformed before attempting to fit a line.

*sd* line) is the dotted line lying along the main axis of the ellipse. This line minimizes the sum of the squares of the *perpendicular* distance from the data points to the line. The line regressing $Y$ on $X$ is labeled "Reg." It also passes through the center of the data, but is slightly less steep. The reason for this can be seen if the rectangle above $x_1$ in the figure is examined. The goal of the regression line is to find the best prediction for $y_i$ for any given $x_i$. The center line does not pass through the center of the data in the strip above $x_1$; it is too high. In contrast, the regression line passes much nearer to the center of this slice of the data, so it is a much better predictor of the average value of $Y$ for that value of $X$.

This figure also helps illustrate why the regression predicting $X$ from $Y$ (i.e., instead of predicting the converse, as discussed) would produce a different line. To predict $X$ from $Y$, the line would still pass through $(\bar{x}, \bar{y})$, but would be designed to pass close to the centers of horizontal slices through the data.

## Interpreting the Coefficients from a Regression

The intercept, $\alpha$, is generally of little interest in a regression analysis attempting to explain the relationship between $X$ and $Y$. On the other hand, the slope of the regression line, $\beta$, is an estimate of the ratio of the change in $X$ to a change in $Y$ (assumed to be constant in a linear model). To illustrate, suppose a regression for the heights of sons from the heights of their fathers produced $\hat{\beta} = 0.9$. Then if a son's father is 5.0 cm taller than the average father, the best guess would be that the son would grow up to be $(0.9)(5.0) = 4.5$ cm taller than the average son.

However, not all regression estimates are equally good. Investigators would like to have some estimate of the accuracy of $\hat{\beta}$, their estimate of the true slope, $\beta$. In particular, they would like to know how confident they can be that $\beta \neq 0$ (i.e., that $X$ really is an important predictor for $Y$). Statistically, this is the question of whether to reject the null hypothesis that $\beta = 0$.

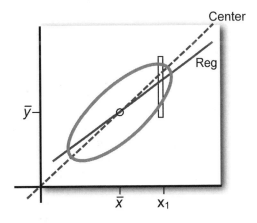

**FIGURE 25–6** ● Comparison of the line through the center of the data with the line regressing $y$ on $x$. The box above $x_1$ shows that, when the data is restricted to a single $x$-value, the regression line is closer to the mean than the center line is.

## Testing If $\beta = 0$

Under the null hypothesis, it turns out that the statistic obtained by dividing the least squares estimate of the slope, $\hat{\beta}$, by the standard error in that approximation will have a t-distribution with $n - 2$ degrees of freedom, where $n$ is the number of points in the dataset. The standard error for $\beta$ is given by the following formula:

$$s.e.(\beta) = \frac{s_y}{s_x} \sqrt{\frac{1 - R^2}{n - 2}}$$

where $R^2$ is the square of the correlation between $X$ and $Y$. This formula implies, as expected, that better estimates (i.e., smaller standard errors) can be obtained with larger samples (because a factor of $n - 2$ appears in the denominator of the radical) and higher correlation between the independent and predicted variable (because $R^2$ is subtracted from 1 in the numerator). A less commonly known fact is that better estimates can also be obtained if the spread of the independent variable is large (because the standard deviation of the independent variable is in the denominator). For this reason, when planning an experiment, it is generally good practice to try to design the study so that as wide a range of values of the independent variable are observed as possible.

To test the null hypothesis that $\beta = 0$, one simply compares the test statistic

$$s = \frac{\hat{\beta}}{s.e.(\beta)}$$

to the two-sided critical value for a t-distribution with $n - 2$ degrees of freedom, $t_{crit}$. (For large $n$, the standard normal distribution is a very good approximation for the t-distribution.)

Just because the null hypothesis that $\beta = 0$ can be rejected does not mean that the estimate $\hat{\beta}$ is particularly accurate. The standard assessment for the accuracy of a parameter estimate is to build a confidence interval.

### Building a Confidence Interval for $\beta$

Typically, the output from regression software includes the estimate of the model parameters (e.g., $\hat{\beta}$), the degrees of freedom, the standard error, and the probability that $\hat{\beta}$ would be as large as it was if the null hypothesis (i.e. $\beta = 0$) were true.

To build a $1 - \alpha$ confidence interval for $\beta$, first find the critical value for a significance of $\alpha/2$, denoted $t_{\alpha/2}$, in a t-distribution table. Then, the $1 - \alpha$ confidence interval for $\beta$ will be:

$$[\hat{\beta} - t_{\alpha/2}\,(s.e.(\beta)),\ \hat{\beta} + t_{\alpha/2}\,(s.e.(\beta))]$$

As an example, consider the case when $n$ is large enough that the t-distribution can be approximated by the normal distribution. The critical value of the standard normal distribution for $\alpha = (0.05)/2 = 0.025$ is 1.96. In such a case, the limits of the 95% confidence interval for $\beta$ would be $\hat{\beta} \pm 1.96\,(s.e.(\beta))$.

As a general rule of thumb, if $n > 60$, $\beta$ will be significantly different from zero ($\alpha = 0.05$) if $\beta > (2)(s.e.(\beta))$ and the 95% confidence interval for $\beta$ will be approximately $\hat{\beta} \pm 2(s.e.(\beta))$. Although the multiplying factor for smaller values of $n$ can be found in a t-distribution table (e.g., when $n = 10$, $\beta$ will be significantly different from zero ($\alpha = 0.05$) if $\beta > (2.228)(s.e.(\beta))$), confidence intervals for the coefficients are usually provided by statistical software and will not need to be computed by hand.

Note: The confidence interval for $\beta$ is a measure of the accuracy of the estimate $\hat{\beta}$. It is not an assessment of the explanatory power of the model. As stated earlier, $R^2$ is commonly used as a measure of how well the model fits the data.

## Multiple Regression

With multiple regression, more than one independent variable is incorporated into a single analysis. This method has two advantages. First, multiple regression provides more realistic models for prediction because outcomes are usually dependent on multiple factors. Second, multiple regression allows more sophisticated tests of the relationships between the variables. In particular, if the effects of the independent variables are linear, multiple regression allows the researcher to control for the effect of one independent variable when analyzing the effect of another. This process often makes a complex situation much easier to understand.

A note on terminology: Some people use the term *multivariate regression* as another name for *multiple regression* (one dependent variable, multiple independent variables). Others reserve the term *multivariate regression* to refer to regressions involving multiple dependent variables. The discussion in this chapter is confined to the former definition. For more on analyses of situations with more than one dependent variable of interest, see Chapter 26.

### Similarities Between Multiple Regression and Simple Linear Regression

The basic concepts of multiple regression are very similar to those of simple linear regression. For instance, if there is a linear relationship between the dependent (outcome) variable $Y$ and independent variables $X_1$ and $X_2$, observed data from this relationship could be represented by the formula:

$$Y = \alpha + \beta_1 X_1 + \beta_2 X_2 + \varepsilon$$

In this case, a least squares regression would find the values of $\alpha$, $\beta_1$, and $\beta_2$ that minimized the sum of the squares of the prediction errors. One difference is that now, instead of being able to represent the least squares model as a line fitted to a two-dimensional scatterplot, it must be imagined as a plane passing through a three-dimensional cloud of points. Dealing with more than two dimensions also makes regression diagnostics (such as identifying outliers) more difficult. Box plots of the individual variables (particularly the dependent variable) may be helpful in spotting some outliers and suggesting that a log transform may be called for. Suggestions for addressing this problem can be found elsewhere (3–4).

In multiple regression, $R^2$ is computed as it was for simple linear regression [i.e., $R^2 = 1 - SSE\ (regression)/SSE\ (mean)$].

The coefficients $\beta_1$ and $\beta_2$, of course, represent the rates of change of $Y$ with respect to independent changes in $X_1$ and $X_2$ respectively. In other words, in a multiple regression containing any number of independent predictor variables, $\beta_i$ will represent the average change in $Y$ for a unit change in $X_i$ while all other independent variables are held constant. In this way, multiple regression procedure provides a *statistical control* for the varying values of $X_2$ in the dataset. To determine the effect of $X_1$ on $Y$ independent of $X_2$ using *experimental control*, a researcher would first need to gather a dataset where all the $X_2$ values were the same. Then, a regression of $Y$ on $X_1$ would provide an approximate value for $\beta_1$. To determine $\beta_2$ using experimental control, a second dataset would need to be gathered in which all of the $X_1$ values were identical. Such a program would be difficult for two independent variables and be completely impractical with many independent variables.

Statistical control, although not as accurate as experimental control, has the great advantage of requiring only a single dataset. To understand how the influence of $X_2$ could be statistically removed from an analysis of the relationship between $Y$ and $X_1$, consider the following scenario:

If $r_{X_1,\,X_2} \neq 0$, some of the variation in $X_1$ can be accounted for by $X_2$. The linear influence of $X_2$ on $X_1$ can be written as $X_1 = a + bX_2 + \breve{X}_1$, where $\breve{X}_1$ denotes the part of $X_1$ which is not

explained by $X_2$. Similarly, the part of $Y$ that is separate from $X_2$ can be denoted $\breve{Y}$. Then, the slope of the regression line of $\breve{Y}$ on $\breve{X}_1$ should express the linear effect of $X_1$ on $Y$ independent of a linear effect from $X_2$. This slope is what a least squares regression of $Y$ on $X_1$ and $X_2$ produces for the value of $\beta_1$.

A similar procedure would determine the effect of $X_2$ on $Y$ independent of $X_1$ and would produce $\beta_2$.

As an example of how this concept might be useful, consider a study of the influence of age on the degree of coronary artery calcification in people with a family history of coronary artery disease (i.e., $Y$ = calcification, $X_1$ = age). If a regression were performed without taking the low-density lipoprotein (LDL) levels into account, the results would be questionable because people who have higher LDL levels typically have more coronary artery disease calcification. By including LDL level as a second independent variable, investigators can control for its effect on coronary artery disease callification, resulting in a clearer picture of the effect of age (the goal of the study) on coronary artery calcification among patients who have a family history of coronary artery disease.

Hypothesis tests and the construction of confidence intervals also parallel that of the simple regression model, but with a change in the degrees of freedom. In general, the degrees of freedom will be $n - (\text{\# of estimated coefficients})$. (Recall: the \# of coefficients is one more than the number of predictor variables.) The number of degrees of freedom is used both in the calculation of the standard errors and in the determination of the critical values used in finding the limits of confidence intervals.

## Multicollinearity

Although it is seldom the case that the independent variables in a dataset are completely uncorrelated, problems occur when the correlation is too high. This is known as the problem of *multicollinearity*.

*Perfect multicollinearity* occurs when one independent variable is *exactly* a linear function of one or more of the other variables. For example, if $X_1$ is the temperature measured on the Fahrenheit scale and $X_2$ is the same temperature measured on the Centigrade scale, then $X_1 = 32 + 1.8\,X_2$. When perfect multicollinearity occurs, unique solutions for the least squares coefficients do not exist, and a computer program will fail to reach a solution. For this reason, perfect multicollinearity is easy to detect. The solution is simply to remove a variable that can be written as a linear function of the others.

*High multicollinearity* occurs when one independent variable is highly, but not perfectly, correlated to a linear combination of others. When this happens, the standard error estimates for the slopes may become very large, leading to statistical insignificance for the coefficients.

How can investigators distinguish between high multicollinearity and a model whose independent variables are just not good predictors for the dependent variable? One strong indication of high multicollinearity is a regression model with a high $R^2$ but with nonsignificant coefficients. A weaker indication is if the regression coefficients change greatly when other independent variables are added or dropped from the regression. A third factor possibly indicating high multicollinearity is coefficients that seem unreasonably large or small, or even have the "wrong" sign. This last indication is particularly weak because it relies on assumptions of the researcher that may not be correct.

If there is reason to suspect high multicollinearity, it can be investigated by regressing each independent variable on all the other independent variables together. Unfortunately, it is not sufficient simply to look at the pair-wise correlations between the variables.

Consider the following scenario:

Researchers obtained the following model from least squares regression of $Y$ on $X_1$, $X_2$, $X_3$, and $X_4$:

$$\hat{y} = 5.7 + 2.4x_1 + 1.6x_2 - 4.6x_3 - 3.1x_4$$

For this model $R^2 = 0.43$, $n = 215$, and the standard errors of $X_1$, $X_2$, $X_3$, and $X_4$ were 8.2, 6.3, 4.5, and 1.1 respectively.

Because $n > 60$, they knew that coefficients more than two times their standard error would be statistically significant. This was only true for the coefficient of $X_4$. From what they knew about the experiment, this outcome seemed unlikely, so further investigation was in order. Regressing each independent variable on the other three, models were obtained with the following $R^2$ values: $R_{X1}^2 = 0.75$, $R_{X2}^2 = 0.98$, $R_{X3}^2 = 0.99$,

$R_{X4}^2 = 0.24$. Clearly, there was high collinearity.

When high collinearity occurs, there is not a universally satisfactory solution. If it makes sense, an investigator might combine the independent variables that are highly intercorrelated into a single variable. For instance, if it turns out that hours spent watching TV, hours spent exercising, and the amount of snack food consumed are highly correlated, it might be possible to make a combined "fitness" variable that would summarize these variables.

However, if the variables cannot be plausibly combined and if it is important to be able to have an interpretable model (i.e., a biologically plausible model, not just a model that predicts well), it will probably be necessary to remove one or more of the variables. This option poses the danger of eliminating a true explanatory variable and retaining surrogates, so the choice of which variable to remove should be given much thought.

Let's say that the researchers decided it was not reasonable to combine any of the independent variables. Because the goal of the study was interpretation, not prediction, they decided to remove a variable. The regression of $X_3$ on the other variables produced the highest $R^2$ value and $X_3$ did not, a priori, have better explanatory value than the other variables, so it was eliminated.

Repeating the regression on of $Y$ on $X_3$, $X_3$, and $X_3$ resulted in the following new regression model:

$$\hat{y} = 3.2 + 1.7x_1 + 2.8x_2 - 4.2x_4$$

For this model $R^2 = 0.41$, $n = 215$, and the standard errors of $X_1$, $X_2$, and $X_4$ were 0.6, 0.2, and 0.5 respectively. Under this model, all of the slopes were significant and the new model had almost as much explanatory power as the original (the $R^2$ value only decreased from 0.43 to 0.41 when $X_3$ was eliminated).

To confirm that they had dealt with the multicollinearity problem, they regressed each of the remaining independent variables on the others, finding that $R_{x1}^2 = 0.29$, $R_{x2}^2 = 0.34$, and $R_{x4}^2 = 0.13$. None of these was near 1.0, so multicollinearity was no longer a problem.

## Dummy Variables

The independent variables in a regression analysis typically represent quantitative measurements, such as dollars or grams, for which it is meaningful, for instance, to order them from least to greatest, or to say one is twice as large as another. However, in some cases it is useful to include a *qualitative* (or *categorical*) variable in a regression analysis.

### Dichotomous Variables

Qualitative variables that only have two possible values are called dichotomous variables, for example, sex (female/male) or response to treatment (yes/no). To use such a variable in a regression analysis, it is represented by a binary (0/1) dummy variable.

To see how this method would work, consider a situation where the dependent variable incidence of coronary artery disease ($Y$ = incidence) is being modeled as a linear function of age ($X_1$) and gender ($X_2 = 0$ if the individual is female, $X_2 = 1$

if the individual is male). The values of $X_2$ (0 and 1) are not measured and could have been assigned in the opposite manner. However, the choice of using 0 and 1 for the two values was not arbitrary, but has a particular desired effect. In the resulting regression model,

$$\hat{y} = \hat{\alpha} + \hat{\beta}_1 x_1 + \hat{\beta}_2 x_2$$

the predicted incidence of coronary disease for a woman of X age will be $\hat{y} = \hat{\alpha} + \hat{\beta}_1 X$ because $X_2 = 0$. For a man with the same age, the predicted incidence of coronary disease will be $\hat{y} = \hat{\alpha} + \hat{\beta}_1 X + \hat{\beta}_2$ because $X_2 = 1$. The effect of including the dummy variable for sex in the analysis is to produce parallel regression lines for women and men separated by a distance of $\beta_2$. The value of $\beta_2$ will reflect the average difference in the incidence of coronary artery disease between women and men after the effect of age has been taken into account.

Qualitative Variables with More than Two Values

If a qualitative variable can take $n > 2$ values, it is in general not legitimate to code the additional categories with 2, 3, 4, and so on. That would make the assumption that the categories are ordered and have additive effects (i.e., the difference between group 3 and group 0 is three times as great as the difference between group 1 and group 0). Instead, a categorical variable with $n$ categories should be coded with $n - 1$ dummy variables.

To do this, one of the categories is chosen as the reference category. For each of the remaining categories, a dummy variable is created that takes on the value 1 if the individual is in that category and 0 if the subject is not. To illustrate this idea, consider the problem of modeling incidence of coronary artery disease on age and ethnicity (where the possible values for the ethnicity variable were Caucasian, African American, Hispanic, Asian, and other). Once again, $X_1$ would represent years of age, but four dummy variables would be created to collectively represent the five ethnic categories. Caucasians were the largest group in the dataset, so they were chosen as the reference category: $X_2 = 1$ if the person was African American (0 otherwise), $X_3 = 1$ if the person was Hispanic (0 otherwise), $X_4 = 1$ if the person was Asian (0 otherwise), and $X_5 = 1$ if the person's ethnicity was "other" (0 otherwise). This coding scheme results in the following prediction model:

$$\hat{y} = \hat{\alpha} + \hat{\beta}_1 x_1 + \hat{\beta}_2 x_2 + \hat{\beta}_3 x_3 + \hat{\beta}_4 x_4 + \hat{\beta}_5 x_5$$

Although this equation looks complicated, it is much simpler when looked at from the point of view of each ethnic group. From that viewpoint, the model looks like the following:

$$\hat{y} = \hat{\alpha} + \hat{\beta}_1 x_1 + \begin{cases} 0 & \text{if Caucasian} \\ \hat{\beta}_2 & \text{if African Am} \\ \hat{\beta}_3 & \text{if Hispanic} \\ \hat{\beta}_4 & \text{if Asian} \\ \hat{\beta}_5 & \text{if other} \end{cases}$$

In this way, the deviation from the reference point for each ethnic group is independent of the others. Which ethnic group is used as the reference is arbitrary. Changing the reference group from Caucasian to African American would not change any of the predicted values; it would merely add $\beta_2$ to the intercept and subtract $\beta_2$ from each of the ethnicity constants.

**Assumptions of Linear Regression**

The statistical foundations of linear regression are based on five assumptions. Although regression may still be useful if some of these assumptions are not exactly true, the farther the data are from satisfying these conditions, the less trust one can have in the resulting models.

The five assumptions are:

1. Linearity: The dependent variable can be written as a linear combination of the independent variables plus a random error term.
2. Mean independence: For any values of $x_i$, the mean value of the error term is 0 (i.e. $E(\varepsilon) = 0$).
3. Homoscedasticity: The variance of the error is the same for all values of $x_i$.
4. Uncorrelated disturbances: The value of the error term for one individual is uncorrelated to the value for any other individual.
5. Normal disturbance: The error terms come from a normal distribution.

These five assumptions were chosen for the following reasons:

- Assumptions (1) and (2) guarantee that the least squares estimates of the $\beta_i$ are *unbiased* estimators, meaning that if the same study could be performed many times, the averages of the estimates of the coefficients in the model would be correct.
- Assumptions (3) and (4) guarantee that the least squares estimates of the coefficients have standard errors as small as any other unbiased, linear estimation method. On average, this method

produces the most accurate estimates possible for the coefficients.

- Assumption (5), combined with the others, implies that a t-table is a valid way to calculate the p-values for whether or not the coefficients are 0 and for calculating the confidence intervals on the coefficients.

## Data Transformation

In the data illustrated in Figure 25–5C, the data are clearly not linear. However, replacing the values of the dependent variable ($Y$) with their logarithms, would produce a scatterplot looking more like Figure 25–5A and the transformed data would have correlation = 0.9 (up from a correlation = 0.7 in the untransformed data). In this case, the transformation was able to change data that did not satisfy the five assumptions of linear regression very well into data that fit the assumptions much better. In fact, the logarithmic transformation is by far the most common transformation used to prepare data for regression analysis.

This case is very clearly one where the log transformation is appropriate. However, in addition to clear visual evidence, several clues may suggest that a log transformation of the data may be appropriate. These factors are related to the properties of exponentiation, because replacing the dependent variable with its log is equivalent to replacing the basic linear model $y = \beta_0 + \beta_1 x + \varepsilon$ (where $\varepsilon$ is an error term) with the model $y = \exp(\beta_0 + \beta_1 x + \varepsilon)$.

One of the most basic differences between the two models is that the untransformed model assumes that changing $x$ from 100 to 101 will result in the same absolute change in $y$ as changing $x$ from 1 to 2 [i.e., $y(2) - y(1) = y(101) - y(100)$]. The exponential model, in contrast, assumes that a unit change in $x$ will produce a fixed percentage change in $y$ [i.e., $y(2)/y(1) = y(101)/y(100)$]. As an example of where the exponential model might be the more appropriate model, consider the gender differences in mammals. It is probably a more reasonable thesis that, across species, male mammals weigh 15% more than the females than is the thesis that, across species, male mammals weigh 30 pounds more than the females.

In addition to an obvious curve in the data, the pattern of the scattering may suggest that a log transformation might be appropriate. If the y-values appear more spread out as the x-values get larger, it indicates a failure of homoscedasticity. If a log transform of the y-values makes the spread more even along the range of the observed x-values and improves the model $R^2$, there is good evidence that the transformation was appropriate.

Another basic difference between the linear and exponential models is that in the exponential model, the dependent variable is always positive. Thus, the exponential model may be appropriate when dealing with weights, ages, or time spent performing an activity. On the other hand, the log transform will not exist if any of the original y-values are less than or equal to zero.

Much more could be said about nonlinear distributions of data, but the key is to be on the lookout for nonlinearity and realize that there are methods to address this problem (such as removing outliers or performing a data transformation) before deciding that regression is inappropriate for the analysis. A brief discussion of some methods for dealing with nonlinear relationships can be found in Chapter 8 of reference (5).

## LOGISTIC REGRESSION

### The Logistic Model

When the dependent variable is dichotomous, a linear regression is generally not appropriate. Instead, a *logistic regression analysis* is typically used to estimate the probability that an individual is in one of the groups. Suppose the two possible values of the dependent variable Y are coded 0 and 1. Because there are only two possibilities, if you know the probability that $Y = 1$, $P(Y = 1)$, then you also know the probability that $Y = 0$, because $P(Y = 0) = 1 - P(Y = 1)$. Using linear regression directly to model probabilities would be problematic because a linear combination of independent variables can potentially take on any positive or negative value while probabilities always lie between 0 and 1. Instead, it is now common to use a linear combination of the independent variables to model the logarithm of the *odds* that $Y = 1$, denoted logit ($P(Y = 1)$). Thus, if there are two independent variables and $p = P(Y = 1)$, the logistic regression model will be:

$$\text{logit}(p) = \log\left(\frac{p}{1 - p}\right)$$
$$= \alpha + \beta_1 X_1 + \beta_2 X_2 + \varepsilon.$$

Because the true y-value for each of the points in the dataset is known, for each of them $P(Y = 1) = 0$ or $P(Y = 1) = 1$. Because logit is not defined for $p = 0$ or $p = 1$, the sum of squared errors between observed and predicted values cannot be computed, and thus, the least squares method cannot be used to find the best values of the model coefficients. Instead, the coefficients are determined by a more general method called *maximum likelihood estimation*. This method finds the values of the coefficients so that the observed data are more likely under the best model than they would have been under a model based on any other set of coefficients. Unlike least squares, maximum likelihood estimation is performed through an iterative process of repeated estimation, testing, and reestimation until the change in estimates from one cycle to the next are very small.

Although the logit is not a function that is particularly intuitive, it is equivalent to modeling $P(Y = 1)$ by:

$$P(Y = 1) = 1/(1 + \exp(-\alpha - \beta_1 X_1 - \beta_2 X_2 + \varepsilon))$$

If $X = \alpha + \beta_1 X_1 + \beta_2 X_2$, a plot of $X$ versus $P(Y = 1)$, illustrated in Figure 25–7, shows how the probability changes as a function of the independent variables. As $X$ becomes large, $P(Y = 1)$ approaches 1, indicating a high probability that $Y = 1$. When $X = 0$, indicating that we are getting no information about the value of $Y$ from the independent variables, $P(Y = 1) = 1/2 = P(Y = 0)$. If $X$ is highly negative, $P(Y = 1)$ is very close to 0, indicating that $Y = 0$.

To illustrate, consider a model attempting to explain why some medical intensive care unit (MICU) patients live while others die. The dependent variable could equal 1 for individuals who died and equal 0 for those who lived. Important independent variables might include $X_1$ = age and $X_2$ = a severity of illness score (obviously, many other potential variables could be evaluated as well). In this case the model would be:

$$logit(P(Y = 1)) = \alpha + \beta_1 X_1 + \beta_2 X_2 + \varepsilon$$

Under this model, we would expect that $\beta_1 > 0$ because older patients generally do less well than younger patients when confronted with almost any illness. Similarly, we would also expect that $\beta_2 > 0$ because the likelihood of dying should reasonably increase as the severity of illness increases.

A note of caution: When using computer software for logistic regression, make sure which value of the dependent variable the program is modeling, because switching the value being modeled changes the sign of the model coefficients. Some programs automatically model the lower of the two values for $Y$. So, for the coding in the example just described, the output would correspond to a model for $logit(P(Y = 0))$, resulting in $\beta_1 < 0$ and $\beta_2 < 0$.

## Significance of the Model

In a logistic regression, the analog for the $R^2$ measure of goodness of fit is the ratio of the likelihoods of the data under the regression model including the independent variables to the likelihood of the data under the best model without the independent variables (i.e., using just the intercept term). This is called the likelihood ratio (LR). The significance of the model is evaluated using the test statistic $2log(LR)$, which has a $\chi^2$ distribution under the null hypothesis. Output from regression software typically includes the degrees of freedom, the chi-square value, and the p-value from this test.

## Significance of the Coefficients

Similar to what is done for linear regression, the significance of an individual logistic regression coefficient is determined using the ratio of the estimated coefficient to its standard error. Under the null hypothesis, this ratio has a normal distribution and the square has a $\chi^2$ distribution. Output from statistical software includes estimates of the coefficients, their standard errors, the chi-square test statistics for each of the coefficients, and the corresponding p-values.

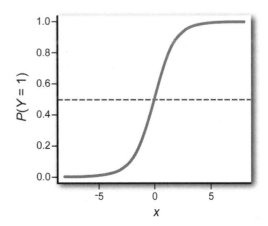

**FIGURE 25–7** ● Under the logistic model, the probability that $Y = 1$ is an S-shaped function of a weighted sum of independent variables. If the sum is large and positive, the probability that $Y = 1$ is close to 1. If the sum is negative, the probability is small, indicating that it is more likely that $Y = 0$.

## Categorical Dependent Variables with More than Two Values

Logistic regression analysis can be extended to the analysis of dependent variables with more categories. Readers who are interested can find a discussion of this in Chapter 5 of reference (6).

## COX REGRESSION

Survival analysis is used to explain or predict the timing of events. The name comes from the fact that the original developers wanted to model the survival times of cancer patients. Two main features of this area of research are censoring and time-dependent values for the independent variables.

To illustrate the problem of censoring, consider a 5-year study of predictors of cancer recurrence after surgery. A third of the patients had a recurrence during the 5 years and their time to recurrence was included in the data. A third of the patients left the study before the 5 years was over even though they had not had a recurrence, while the final third completed the 5 years without a recurrence. Because two-thirds of the patients do not have specific times to recurrence, the researchers cannot reasonably drop these patients from the analysis. Similarly, to treat patients as if they had a recurrence at the moment they left the study would substantially bias the recurrence time downward.

Time-dependent independent covariates have values that may change over the course of the study. For instance, in a cancer study the chemotherapy agent or the dosage might change over time due to toxicity.

The most popular method for dealing with both of these problems is Cox regression, or Cox proportional hazards regression, named after its inventor, Sir David Cox (1972). The Cox model for dealing with these situations is:

$$\log(h(t)) = \alpha(t) + \beta_1 X_1 + \beta_2 X_2(t) + \varepsilon$$

In this model, $h(t)$ is the *hazard function* representing the instantaneous risk of the event happening at time $= t$, $\alpha(t)$ is the log of a baseline hazard (i.e., the average hazard at time $= t$ for a person with all covariates equal to zero), $X_1$ is a covariate whose value cannot change over the course of the study (e.g., sex or size of tumor at initial surgery), and $X_2(t)$ is a covariate whose value might change over the course of the study.

Cox's two important innovations were the proposal of this model and the invention of a method to estimate the coefficients called *maximum partial likelihood*.

Similar to the logistic regression, the overall goodness of fit for a Cox model is evaluated using a likelihood ratio test, while the square of the ratio of a parameter estimate to its standard error can be used to test the significance of an independent variable.

Cox regression in particular, and survival analysis in general, are rich subject areas that cannot be fully covered in this chapter. Excellent overviews can be found in references (7–8).

## SUMMARY

- Regression is used for two purposes: predicting outcomes and investigating the importance of predictors of outcomes.
- Linear regression is typically appropriate when the outcome variable is a continuous, measured quantity; logistic regression is used for binary outcomes; Cox regression is used to analyze survival (time-to-event) outcomes.
- Data should be examined for anomalies before running a regression analysis. Outliers may need to be removed or the data may need to be transformed (e.g., using a log transform).
- Correlation measures the degree of scatter around a regression line, but does not fully describe the distribution of the data. $R^2$ represents the proportion of the variation in the outcome "explained" by the regression variables.
- Multiple regression allows investigators to statistically control for one independent variable when evaluating the effect of another on the outcome. This control is not as good as a randomized experiment, but allows one dataset to be used for multiple purposes.
- Highly correlated independent variables give rise to unreliable regression coefficient estimates. If interpretation of the model (not just predictive power) is the goal, the correlated variables need to be combined or pruned.
- Least squares linear regression finds the line (or plane) through the data that minimizes the sum of the squared prediction errors.
- Logistic regression specifies one of the two outcomes as the target and models the probability that an individual will be in the target group. The model is made linear using the logit function.
- Cox regression models *time-to-event* data (also known as *survival* data). The model is made linear using the logarithm of the hazard function. Cox regression is specifically designed to address the problems of censored data and independent variables whose values change over time.
- Estimates of the regression coefficients are usually evaluated using confidence intervals and hypothesis tests.

- For more in-depth discussions of regression, the reader is referred to material in references (9–11).

## REFERENCES

1. DeGroot MH. Probability and Statistics, 2nd Ed. Reading, MA: Addison-Wesley,1986:644.
2. Chambers J, Cleveland W, Kleiner B et al. Graphical Methods for Data Analysis. Boston: Duxbury, 1983.
3. Ryan TP. Modern Regression Methods. New York: John Wiley and Sons, 1997.
4. Cook RD. Regression Graphics: Ideas for Studying Regression through Graphics. New York: John Wiley and Sons, 1998.
5. Allison PD. Multiple Regression: A Primer. Thousand Oaks, CA: Pine Forge Press, 1999.
6. Menard S. Applied Logistic Regression Analysis. Thousand Oaks, CA: Sage, 1995.
7. Lee ET. Statistical Methods for Survival Data Analysis, 2nd Ed. New York: John Wiley and Sons, 1992.
8. Allison PD. Survival Analysis Using the SAS System: A Practical Guide. Cary, NC: The SAS Institute, 1995.
9. Freedman D, Pisani R, Purves R. Statistics. New York: W.W. Norton and Company, 1978.
10. Lewis-Beck MS. Applied Regression: An Introduction. Thousand Oaks, CA: Sage, 1980.
11. Schroeder LD, Sjoquist DL, Stephan PE. Understanding Regression Analysis: An Introductory Guide. Newbury Park, CA: Sage. 1986.

# CHAPTER 26

# Multivariate Analysis

## William Shannon, Xiao Yang

The focus of Chapter 24 (Group Comparisons) was on detecting statistically significant differences in a single outcome (or dependent variable) between or among groups. On the other hand, in Chapter 25, the focus was on modeling the relationship of a single outcome to one or more independent variables. It is rare, however, for a study to be conducted in which the investigator is truly interested in only one outcome (response) variable. Usually, the investigator has chosen one *primary* outcome of interest, but many *secondary* outcomes. Even more problematic are clinical studies that depend on the analysis of microarray (gene chip) data (Chapter 34), in which thousands of possible response variables (literally, the response of each gene represented on the chip), are possible. Although an investigator could perform a series of single (or univariate) tests for each response variable (e.g., run a separate t-test or ANOVA on each dependent variable), the risk of identifying a "significant" difference by chance alone increases as the number of tests increases (often referred to as "the multiple comparison problem"). In such cases, more appropriate statistical methods of analysis can and should be applied in which all the outcomes are tested in a single step. These statistical strategies include two classical methods—multivariate analysis of variance (MANOVA) and principal components analysis (PCA)—as well as a more recent method referred to as mixed models. In the last few years, mixed models have become the analytic method of choice in many clinical studies, and we expect that clinical researchers will incorporate this type of analysis into their studies with increasing frequency. For gene chip studies, a new approach

known as cluster analysis is often used. This chapter provides an introduction to these novel statistical strategies. More detailed information about these methods can be found elsewhere (1–6).

## MULTIVARIATE ANALYSIS OF VARIANCE (MANOVA) AND PRINCIPAL COMPONENTS ANALYSIS (PCA)

MANOVA extends the analysis of variance (ANOVA) method from testing the effect of independent variables on one outcome or dependent variable, to testing the effect of independent variables on more than one outcome or dependent variable simultaneously in a single statistical test. The use of MANOVA results in a significant increase in power when the dependent variables are correlated and avoids the problem of multiple testing that would arise by testing each dependent variable individually.

To illustrate MANOVA, consider a study that produced a dataset in which four measurements were made on patients who had heart attacks: age at the time of the heart attack and three echocardiographic measures of left ventricular function, including fractional shortening (a measure of contractility), E-point septal separation (another measure of contractility), and left ventricular end-diastolic dimension (LVDD, a measure of heart size at end-diastole). The principal question to be answered is whether these measures differ in the patients who survived versus those who did not survive.

In the standard univariate ANOVA approach to this problem, one variable, say age at the time of heart attack, would be evaluated at a time. Thus, the null hypothesis would be that the mean ages of patients who did not survive, $\mu_0$, and those who did survive, $\mu_1$, were equal:

$$H_0: \mu_0 = \mu_1$$

Instead, in a MANOVA framework, a vector of means is compared. In this hypothetical study of myocardial infarction, all four outcome variables would be compared between patients who survived and those who did not survive (age at the time of the heart attack, the fractional shortening, etc.) The null hypothesis, then, becomes a comparison of the vector of four mean values:

$$H_0: \begin{bmatrix} \mu_0^{age} \\ \mu_0^{fs} \\ \mu_0^{epss} \\ \mu_0^{lvdd} \end{bmatrix} = \begin{bmatrix} \mu_1^{age} \\ \mu_1^{fs} \\ \mu_1^{epss} \\ \mu_1^{lvdd} \end{bmatrix}$$

Here, the first column includes the means of the patients who did not survive and the second column includes the means of the patients who did survive.

Many investigators might approach this analytic problem by simply performing four separate t-tests, comparing each variable across the two groups. As shown in Figure 26–1, each variable does appear to be an important determinant of survival one year after the heart attack. This impression is confirmed by the p-values for each variable separately: age ($p = 0.023$), fractional shortening ($p = 0.0014$), E-point septal separation ($p = 0.0122$,) and LVDD ($p = 0.0026$). However, we must confront the multiple testing problem. Thus, after calculating the various p-values for the four different outcome variables, the p-values should be adjusted upwards by some method to ensure that there is truly a 5% chance or less of finding a statistically significant result by chance alone. One approach, the Bonferroni adjustment, operates by multiplying each p-value by the number of tests, four in this case, resulting in corrected p-values of about 0.08, 0.004, 0.04, and 0.008. These adjustments obviously mean that there has been some decrease in power (as seen by the larger p-values), and indeed, age is now no longer "significantly" different between the two groups.

Another problem with performing multiple univariate tests is that any interpretation of these tests should assume that the different outcomes were independent of one another. But in this case, this assumption would be false as only age had no correlation to the other variables. Because the remaining variables are derived from the same echocardiographic examinations, they are likely to be correlated with one another. Failing to take such correlations into account results in a serious inflation in the false-positive rate.

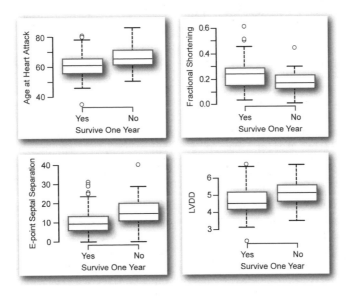

**FIGURE 26–1** ● Boxplots showing the univariate distributions of four variables comparing groups of patients in a hypothetical study of myocardial infarction, defined according to survival or nonsurvival at year one. LVDD = left ventricular end-diastolic dimension.

For instance, suppose only fractional shortening had been measured and there was truly no difference in this variable between the two groups. Even so, it is possible that a t-test (or other group comparison test) would declare this variable different (falsely positive) due to chance alone. Now suppose that in addition to the fractional shortening, EPSS and LVDD were also measured. Because these are correlated to, not independent of, fractional shortening, they are also likely to be declared falsely positive, and the overall likelihood of finding one of these or similar tests to be positive (but falsely so) increases as the number of tests increases, rendering the individual t-test approach statistically useless.

An alternative approach to multiple individual variable t-testing is to employ MANOVA, which accommodates the testing of all the outcome variables (age, fractional shortening, E-point septal separation, and LVDD) simultaneously assuming correlation among the variables. As it turns out, the resulting test for the null hypothesis from MANOVA for these data is significant, with $p < 0.0001$.

Note that the goal of this analysis is a test of equality of the *mean vectors* across groups. In other words, the researcher can evaluate how all the variables change simultaneously, but not differences for individual variables. Although additional steps, analogous to methods such as Tukey's multiple comparisons after an ANOVA (Chapter 24), can be taken to identify such differences, these methods require advanced linear algebra and are beyond the scope of this book. More to the point, MANOVA is not the best method to use if the investigator is interested in individual variable differences. Instead, if that is the goal of the analysis, individual tests, such as t-tests must be done, an adjustment for multiple testing (e.g., Bonferroni correction) must be incorporated, and the investigator will have to simply accept a loss in overall power. In the example described above, then, one appropriate approach would be to perform a separate t-test for the age variable, and to use MANOVA to analyze the echocardiographic data, especially if the investigator is more interested in whether *any* of the echocardiographic variables are different between the two groups, rather than specifically which one.

Another approach to the multivariate analysis problem is principal components analysis (PCA). The purpose of PCA is to reduce the number of variables that need to be analyzed to a smaller number that contain the same information as the entire set of variables. This data reduction is done by forming new variables that are linear combinations of the original variables. Technically sets of weights, $w_i$,

are found for each variable, $x_i, I = 1, 2, \ldots, p$, so that a linear combination can be formed, such as:

$$x' = w_1 x_1 + w_2 x_2 + \cdots + w_p x_p \quad (1)$$

where $x'$ represents a new variable in the data set. With $p$ variables, $p$ sets of weights would be developed (using matrix algebra). Each set of weights would be used to calculate a new variable in the dataset, $(x'_1, x'_2, \ldots, x'_p)$, which are called principal components.

A particularly valuable feature of PCA is that the set of weights, and therefore each new principal component, are independent of one another. Also, the principal components can be ordered according to the amount of variation in the original data explained by each principal component. Hopefully, as a result, the number of original variables can be reduced to a smaller set of two or three principal components that explain a large percentage of the variation in the original data, usually at least 80%.

To illustrate PCA, consider a hypothetical example of a nutrition study in which protein consumption in 25 European countries was measured from various food groups: red meat, white meat, eggs, milk, fish, cereals, starchy foods, nuts and oil-seeds, and fruits and vegetables. With PCA, groupings of countries that consume similar foods can be combined, reducing the number of variables to be analyzed. These combinations are created by a weighting of the various variables, as shown in the Table 26–1.

The value of the principal components is in their ability to describe the characteristics of subgroups. For example, in Component 1, a high protein percentage is obtained from cereals, nuts, and fruits and vegetables groups (positive scores) with a low contribution from the red and white meat, milk and fish groups. Missing components correspond to a weight of 0. Alternatively, Component 2 downplays the importance of cereals (weight = $-0.406$ versus 0.861 in Component 1 and places a positive importance on fish and fruits and vegetables. Component 3 describes yet a different weighting scheme where milk, fish, and nuts are positive and white meat very unimportant.

Mathematically, each component is used to calculate a new score for each data point based on the measured data—in this case the European countries based on each country's protein source measurement. Countries with a large value for a particular component are said to be influenced by that component. For example, in Table 26–1, countries with a large first principal component value have a high protein percentage obtained from cereals, nuts, and fruits and vegetables (positive scores) and low contribution from red and white meat, milk and fish, as

## TABLE 26–1

### The First Three Principal Components of Nutritional Data Indicating the Various Weights Applied to Each Protein Source

|            | Component 1 | Component 2 | Component 3 |
|------------|-------------|-------------|-------------|
| Red Meat   | −0.151      | −0.133      |             |
| White Meat | −0.129      |             | −0.798      |
| Eggs       |             |             |             |
| Milk       | −0.425      | −0.831      | 0.220       |
| Fish       | −0.127      | 0.292       | 0.522       |
| Cereals    | 0.861       | −0.406      |             |
| Starch     |             |             |             |
| Nuts       | 0.114       |             | 0.166       |
| Fr. Veg    |             | 0.169       |             |

Fr. Veg = fruits and vegetables

previously described. Similarly, countries with a small first principal component value do not have a high protein percentage obtained from cereals, nuts, and fruits and vegetables (positive scores) or low contribution from red and white meat, milk and fish.

Because the principal components are independent of one another, variables (in this case, countries) can be described in terms of the properties of each component. For example, a country might have a high first principal component (high contribution to protein from cereals, nuts, and fruits and vegetables) as well as a high second principal component (high contribution to protein from fish and fruits and vegetables).

Although the weightings may be interpreted directly, as in the preceding discussion, various graphical methods are also routinely used to understand how the data separate into subgroups. To identify groups, a *biplot display* is used, which in this example would be a plot of the country and food groups simultaneously (Figure 26–2). The biplot shows the first principal component (*x* axis) separates countries that depend on cereals, nuts, and fruits and vegetables (e.g., Albania, Hungary, Romania, Yugoslavia, Bulgaria on the right) from countries that depend on red and white meat, milk, and fish (e.g., W. Germany, Netherlands, Denmark, Belgium on the left). The second principal component (*y* axis) separates countries by fish and fruits and vegetables (top of the graph) versus red meat, milk and cereals (bottom of the graph).

## MIXED EFFECTS MODELS AND ANALYSIS OF REPEATED MEASURES EXPERIMENTS

Chapter 24 gave a general overview of ANOVA methods, where the different levels of the factors were chosen intentionally. In general, there are three types of ANOVA models: fixed effects models, random effects models, and mixed effects models. Among them, the mixed effects, or multilevel, model has been widely applied to many areas of biomedical research, especially in the area of longitudinal studies or repeated measures experiments.

### Fixed Effects versus Random Effects

The question of choosing a fixed effects model or a random effects model is dictated more or less by the objective of a particular study. In statistical analysis, each of these models is handled in a completely different manner. Therefore, a clear understanding of the difference between fixed and random effects is needed.

Traditionally, one criterion used to distinguish fixed and random effects was the type of statistical inference researchers were interested in. In many studies, where a specific set of interventions are included or purposely selected, the effects (corresponding to "factors"—see Chapters 8 and 24) are called *fixed effects* in the statistical models. For example, a clinical study might be set up to determine

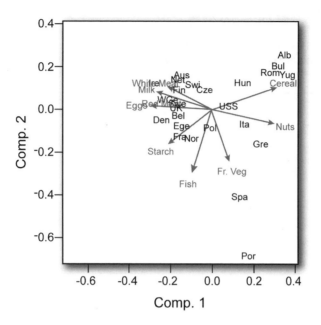

**FIGURE 26–2** ● Biplot display of the first two principal components (Comp.) for a hypothetical set of nutritional data, showing the separation of countries (dark grey) according to type of protein intake (light grey). The axis labels and coordinates are arbitrary and the interpretation of this plot is based on the relative positions of the countries and food groups, and not on their absolute values.

whether the inhibition of a newly identified membrane receptor with a particular drug affected some organ function of interest compared to a placebo control. However, what if preclinical data suggested that the drug's effects might also depend on gender? An investigator might propose a two-factor between-subjects study (Chapter 8) to address this question, which would be analyzed by a fixed effects model in which "drug" and "gender" were the two fixed factors, as follows:

$$y_i = \beta_0 + \beta_1\,Drug + \beta_2\,Gender + error \quad (2)$$

In this model, each factor has two levels: factor "drug" has the levels "active drug" and "placebo drug"; and factor "gender" has "female" and "male" as levels. In this example, both factors "gender" and "drug" are treated as fixed factors, because levels of each factor are deliberately chosen and statistical inference is confined to those levels.

On the other hand, many studies use factors in which the levels are merely representative of a larger population. For instance, an investigator might be interested in using blocking factors (e.g., hospitals or days) to provide replication over a selection of different conditions. In such cases, investigators are primarily interested in the average performance of the intervention across the various blocks. For example, in a pharmacogenomics study using microarrays, the experiments might use a sample of chips from different batches of production, or mRNA samples taken from different patients. Such factors in these cases (time, batches, patients) are called *random* effects. If all factors in the model have this interpretation, the ANOVA model is labeled a *random effects* model. Not surprisingly, then, if some factors are fixed and other factors are random, the ANOVA model is termed a *mixed effects* model. (Note that "time" can be either a fixed or random factor in the sense that the effects of an intervention at very specific times may be important while in other cases, the times selected are only meant to be representative of a given span of time.)

In practice, a rule of thumb for distinguishing random effects from fixed effects is as follows: for different levels of a given factor in a study (e.g., patients, hospitals), suppose the same study is to be repeated at a later time. If the same levels of that factor were chosen in the repeated study, then this factor should be treated as fixed; on the other hand, if any level chosen for the second study was different from the previous one, then this factor should be treated as random. This rule of thumb is roughly consistent with the previous discussion, as in a repeated sampling setting, the chance of choosing the same set of levels for a given factor is quite low, if samples were derived from a large population for that factor.

To demonstrate these differences, consider a multicenter trial example. A new drug has been tested and shown to be an effective antihypertensive in a small study. In a follow-up study, the drug has been tested on a larger scale. Twelve hospitals have taken part in the trial. For each hospital, a group of eligible individuals were chosen to either take the new drug or the placebo. The response variable is the difference in blood pressure (DBP) before and after treatment. The main objective of the second trial is to determine if the results from the small-scale study can be validated. A possible statistical model for this experiment is the following mixed effects model:

$$DBP_i = \beta_0 + \beta_1 \, Hospital + \beta_2 \, Drug$$
$$+ \, \beta_3 \, Hospital(Drug) + error \quad (3)$$

In this model, the factor "hospital" is a random factor, because the set of all hospitals (the "population" of hospitals) is actually quite large, and the true value of performing the second study will only be realized if the hospitals in this study are a valid representative sample from that population. On the other hand, factor "Drug" should be treated as a fixed factor with two levels (drug, placebo), as these are the only two levels of interest in this efficacy study. The factor Hospital (Drug) indicates the nested effect of the drug within a hospital. There is a vast amount of literature on differences between random and fixed effects models, and interested readers are referred elsewhere (7) for more details.

Note that the mathematical notation for the fixed and mixed models (equations 2 and 3) are similar but the algorithm for fitting the models and how to calculate the statistical tests are very different. In a simple fixed model, the fixed factor is tested based on a comparison to the error term. Specifically, the F-statistic (Chapter 24) is computed as the ratio of the fixed effects variance over the error term; the smaller the error term, the more likely the F-statistic will become statistically significant. In a mixed model, the error term is divided or partitioned into various components, each of which might be used as the denominator in the F-statistic. Therefore, an appropriately defined and fit mixed model generally uses a smaller error term to test the fixed effects, providing an increase, and often a significant increase, in the power of the test. Given the complexity of creating the appropriate models, the reader is

advised to obtain appropriate statistical support before employing a mixed model analytic strategy.

## Analysis of the Repeated Measures Experiment

One area in which mixed effects models have been applied frequently is in the area of longitudinal studies, or repeated measures experiments. The defining characteristic of longitudinal data is repeated measures over time on the same set of individuals. These repeated measurements may be obtained in a few minutes or over many years of observation. An example is growth curve data, such as monthly weight measurements of participants in a diet program. Another example is the effects of a drug over time after its administration.

A critical issue with the analysis of a repeated measures experiment is that the measurements tend to be correlated with one another because the repeated observations are made on the same individual. Therefore, appropriate statistical analysis must take this correlation into account since, as mentioned above, the effect of the correlation may be an unacceptable increase in the false-positive rate.

Typically, there are at least two goals to a repeated measures experiment. One goal is to identify whether there is a *general* response of research participants to the experimental interventions; that is, whether a change develops over time among different experimental groups. A second goal is to characterize how the response changes over time in the different groups; that is, whether subgroup profiles of change are different from the groups as a whole. For example, in a study of some experimental intervention that included male and female patients, both the profile of change for each gender might be of interest, as well as for the intervention itself with respect to all patients.

## Statistical Analysis of Repeated Measures Experiments

The analysis of a repeated measures experiment can be quite challenging, because, as mentioned earlier, repeated observations on the same individual tend to be correlated. This correlation structure needs to be taken into account if both the magnitude and pattern of change in the response variable is to be measured with acceptable statistical power. In general, there are three approaches for analyzing these experiments: univariate ANOVA (discussed in Chapter 24), multivariate ANOVA (MANOVA) (described in the previous section), and the mixed model approach.

These approaches and the process for analyzing them can be illustrated with an example of a simple hypothetical study that employed a drug with a novel mechanism to lower serum cholesterol. Assume, then, that the effects of a drug (Drug A) were compared to placebo in two groups of five patients each. Low density lipoprotein (LDL) cholesterol levels were measured at four time intervals after Drug A or placebo administration: 3 days, 6 days, 9 days, and 12 days. The study sought to answer two questions: Did Drug A have any effect on LDL cholesterol over time? And did Drug A have any effect compared to placebo? By its nature, this is a typical mixed factorial repeated measures experiment (Chapter 8).

The first step of the analysis should be to plot observed individual values of LDL over time (Figure 26–3). This step is very useful, because it helps to identify general temporal trends within individuals, including potentially nonlinear trends. In addition, these plots may provide some information about the magnitude of interindividual variability. When preparing such plots, it's often useful to identify subgroups on the same graph differently, which may help explain the source of any interindividual variability. So, in Figure 26–3, some variability is seen across individual patients, even within the same experimental group. However, the *mean* profile for each experimental group (Figure 26–4) shows an apparent difference developing over time, indicating that Drug A is having its intended effect.

The next step in the analysis is to choose an appropriate statistical model. In studies of this type, researchers are often tempted to ignore that the factors might be fixed or random. Although the data can often be successfully entered into many readily available computing programs, yielding the desired output of statistical results, the *interpretation* of this output may be flawed unless the model has appropriately taken into account whether the factors analyzed were of the fixed, random, or mixed

type. Once again, the beginning investigator will likely benefit from a discussion of these issues with an experienced biostatistician.

The statistical analysis of this experiment can be represented symbolically as:

$$LDL_i = \beta_0 + \beta_1\,Drug + \beta_2\,Patient(Drug)$$
$$+ \beta_3\,Time + \beta_4\,Drug * Time$$
$$+ error \tag{4}$$

In this model, factors Drug, Time, and (Drug*Time) are fixed factors, because only the performance of Drug A at these four time points is of interest. Note (Drug*Time) is an interaction term between Drug and Time, which can be used to test if the drug's effect changes over time. Factor Patient (Drug), by contrast, is a random factor, which is used to account for variation between patients, because we assume that these 10 patients are a random sample from the larger target population of patients (those with elevated cholesterol levels).

A common approach to implementing the model shown in equation 4 would be to use the univariate ANOVA method described more completely in Chapter 24. Although the univariate ANOVA strategy is frequently used to analyze mixed factorial experiments, it can be criticized for at least two reasons: first, an underlying assumption of the ANOVA model is that the levels of the within-subjects factor (e.g., time in our example) are randomly assigned. Secondly, observations are assumed to be independent from one other as in a fixed effects model, which is not valid for the repeated measures experiment where the values are not independent.

An alternative approach for analyzing repeated measures is a MANOVA model. In this model,

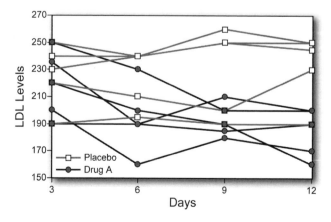

**FIGURE 26–3** ● Low density lipoprotein (LDL) levels for individual patients in a hypothetical study of a new drug (Drug A) to lower cholesterol, plotted over four time points.

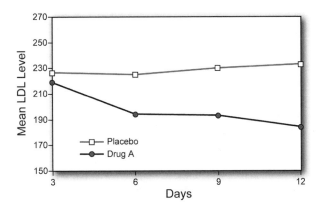

**FIGURE 26–4** ● LDL levels plotted by treatment group. A non-linear trend appears to be present for Drug A.

correlation among repeated observations can be addressed explicitly. For example, should adjacent time points be treated as correlated or more correlated than nonadjacent time points (in other words, perhaps the effect at time 2 is related to the effect at time 1, but the effect at time 3 is independent or less correlated to that of time 1)? Taking such possibilities into account increases the power of the test. The MANOVA model can also assume that the true correlation structure is not known or can allow the data to specify what the correlation structure is. Because correlation is included in the modeling, MANOVA is an improvement over the univariate ANOVA method. For our example, the MANOVA model can be represented as follows:

$$(Day1LDL_i, Day2LDL_i, Day3LDL_i,$$

$$Day4LDL_i) = \beta_0 + \beta_1 Drug + error \quad (5)$$

In this model, the response variable has a multivariate nature; namely, it is the LDL level at four time points, which is presented in a vector format. The right side of the model only has the Drug term.

Despite the advantage of increased power when employing MANOVA, this strategy requires that the data must be *balanced;* namely, there must be no missing data—a requirement that is difficult to achieve in many clinical research settings. Secondly, MANOVA assumes that the levels of the within-subjects factor (time points, in this case) are equally spaced, another stringent requirement that is often violated in practice. Lastly, MANOVA models do not produce a parameter that estimates rate of change over time for different treatment groups, which is often a practical question researchers want to address. Therefore, it can be difficult to analyze repeated measures experiments with MANOVA.

The third approach to analyzing a repeated measures experiment is to use a mixed effects model. Mixed models have several advantages over traditional univariate ANOVA and MANOVA approaches. Mixed models handle experiments with missing data or unequally spaced time points, and also take into account the correlation of repeated measures. Additionally, other covariates (e.g., patient's age) can be readily included in the analysis. Another advantage is that mixed models emphasize both whole group and subgroup components; therefore, it's possible to estimate individual-level and population-level nonlinear relationships between variables. In Figure 26–4, the mean profile for the Drug A group reveals a quadratic trend related to the drug's effects (i.e., the drug's effects on cholesterol levels are substantial initially but then seem to level off over time). To see if this trend is statistically significant, a quadratic term can be included in the mixed model:

$$LDL_i = \beta_0 + \beta_1 Drug + \beta_2 Patient(Drug)$$
$$+ \beta_3 Time * Drug$$
$$+ \beta_4 Time^2 * Drug + error \quad (6)$$

In this model, note that Time is no longer a factor but rather a regression variable. In carrying out the mixed model computations, it is possible to explicitly specify how the repeated measures are correlated, to test whether the data support how the correlation was identified, and to include the correlation in the model to increase the power of the analysis.

As with MANOVA, there are no established methods for post hoc testing of individual differences between or among groups after implementing the mixed models method (for instance, in this case, to test if the groups were different at a specific time). To identify such differences, the investigator would have to perform multiple t-tests (or comparable statistic) and adjust for multiple testing.

## Computational Issues

The literature on how to analyze repeated measures experiments using mixed effects models is substantial. Interested readers are referred elsewhere (8,9) for more detailed discussions. One issue to be noted is that normality is often assumed for the responses of variables analyzed in mixed models. However, in many practical applications, the response of interest may not have a normal distribution. For studies with other types of responses, such as count data (e.g., number of blood cells) or categorical responses (Yes or No), a generalized mixed model may be used. Examples include logistic regression for binary responses, or Poisson regression for count data. Another complication arises when the relationship between fixed and random effects is not linear (e.g., many applications in pharmacokinetics where dose effects over time are not linear). In such cases, a nonlinear mixed effects model may be used.

Computationally, there are many commercial, as well as free, software packages, such as SAS, S-Plus, SPSS, and R, which can be used to analyze such experiments. However, researchers are again encouraged to consult an experienced biostatistician to discuss which program, and more importantly, which statistical strategy is most appropriate for their particular set of experiments.

## CLUSTER ANALYSIS

As mentioned earlier, the advent of high throughput genomics has created a need for novel methods of performing multivariate analyses. The multivariate methods of cluster and classification analysis are two new tools for biomedical researchers to use (10). These methods differ significantly from the multivariate methods described above, where formal approaches for testing group differences are made. In the case of cluster analysis, the goal is to *identify subgroups* of data, such as genes, microarray chips, or patients that differ from one another. In the case of classification analysis, the goal is to develop methods to *predict subgroup membership* of data such as genes, microarray chips, or patients.

Predicting subgroup membership through classification, often called discrimination or supervised learning, requires data on covariates and group membership to create a so-called "training data set" (i.e., the data that are made available to fit a statistical model). For example, to decide if genotype can be used to predict whether a patient will respond to a drug (the goal of most pharmacogenomics studies), the training data would require genotype data from the participating patients (at those loci thought to be related to response) as well as drug response data. Once these data are used to find a good mathematical formula for classification, future patients can be predicted to respond or not respond based solely on their genotype, even before they are given the treatment.

We will not discuss classification analysis in detail in this chapter because high throughput genomics generally requires an investigator to use the clustering methods described below. However, several points about classification analysis should be noted.

First, researchers will often incorrectly use logistic regression (Chapter 25) as a classification method. Logistic regression is a modeling tool designed to uncover relationships between covariates and categorical outcome variables. Using threshold cutoff values of the log (odd) values from logistic regression to classify an observation into one of two classes is very inaccurate. The logistic model is fit using criteria not specifically designed to classify objects, but rather to maximize a partial likelihood measure. The use of logistic regression to achieve classification should therefore be avoided. Second, classification methods cannot overcome the problem of overdetermination where significantly more covariates are included in the analysis than the number of observations themselves. This is the case with microarray data where thousands of genes (covariates) are measured on a small number of samples coming from several groups, such as tumor versus normal tissue comparisons. When there are more covariates than observations, any model that is fit to the data is likely to produce spurious results and be useless for future predictions.

The reason for this phenomenon is as follows. Any statistical model is eventually selected after some criteria are optimized, such as fitting a linear regression model with minimum least-squares error. In overdetermined situations, an infinite number of models may produce acceptable fits to the data, and a computer program selects one based on the data provided and some measure of optimality. For example, for a simple linear regression, the optimal model selected has the minimum mean square error. In overdetermined situations, there can be an infinite number of distinct models with the same optimal minimum squared error making each equally good at describing the data. Also, changing the value of a single variable, or adding or deleting one observation, can result in an equally well fit model that is completely different from the first model; variables may be significant in one model and not significant in another.

Finally, besides logistic regression, there are many other ways of potentially fitting classification models, including linear discriminant analysis, classification trees or recursive partitioning, support vector machines, and artificial neural networks. Unfortunately, each of these alternative approaches is also subject to the problem of overdetermination. If a classification approach is to be used, we recommend getting the advice of an experienced biostatistician before deciding on a specific strategy.

Instead of a classification strategy, the analysis of genomics data often makes use of cluster analysis to identify subgroups of interest. For instance, cluster analysis is often used to analyze microarray data obtained from a set of tissue samples (Chapter 34). In contrast to classification methods, cluster analysis only requires access to the genomic expression data themselves; any information on the tissue type (e.g., tumor or normal) or gene type (e.g., gene function class) is not needed for the analysis.

The first goal of a cluster analysis is to find subgroups of observations that are more *similar* to one another in some sense than to members of other subgroups. To identify these subgroups, a "similarity" measure is calculated, based on "distance" (described next). In this way, then, subgroups consist of members that are "near" one another. For instance, say that in a hypothetical microarray study, 8 gene chips have been analyzed and the expression values of 20 genes measured on each one (Figure 26–5). The data in this figure appear to fall into two subgroups according to the expression level

of genes in the samples. In one subgroup of genes, there is high expression in samples 1–4 and low expression in samples 5–8, while in the second subgroup of genes, this pattern is reversed.

The second goal of cluster analysis is to reduce the amount of data (similar to the goals of principal components analysis) by finding an average or typical pattern in the subgroup. The dark lines on the plot are the average gene expression patterns, where the averages are calculated over the genes belonging to the subgroup. The genes in each subgroup can then be characterized by that subgroup's average expression value.

Similarity measures, or distances, have one serious drawback in statistical data analysis; namely that there is no well-defined probability model structure from which p-values can be estimated. In other words, cluster analyses do not provide statistical tests of hypotheses. Therefore, cluster analysis must be viewed as a data reduction and data summarization technique only; the use of these methods should be limited to generating hypotheses to be tested in future studies (for example, verifying increased expression of newly identified genes by alternative molecular biology techniques). In spite of this limitation, the power and need for cluster analysis is evident by their common use in modern genomic and proteomic research, and the large amount of ongoing statistical research for developing and refining these methods.

Several different approaches to cluster analysis have already emerged, including hierarchical and

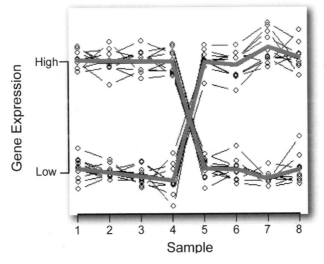

**FIGURE 26–5** ● Hypothetical gene expression data (*y* axis) showing two groups of genes measured across eight samples or chips (*x* axis). The dark thick lines represent the average expression level of the genes within a group.

## TABLE 26–2

### Gene Expression Data for 20 Samples or Chips Measured on 12,000 Genes

| | Sample | Gene1 | Gene2 | Gene3 | . . . | Gene12000 |
|---|---|---|---|---|---|---|
| | 1 | $x_{1,1}$ | $x_{1,2}$ | $x_{1,3}$ | . . . | $x_{1,12000}$ |
| $X =$ | 2 | $x_{2,1}$ | $x_{2,2}$ | $x_{2,3}$ | . . . | $x_{2,12000}$ |
| | ⋮ | ⋮ | ⋮ | ⋮ | ⋮ | ⋮ |
| | 20 | $x_{20,1}$ | $x_{20,2}$ | $x_{20,3}$ | . . . | $x_{20,12000}$ |

Each entry in the table corresponds to the expression of a specific gene (column) on a specific chip (row).

k-means clustering (developed by researchers within the statistics community), and self-organizing maps and artificial neural networks (developed by computer scientists). In the field of data mining (of which genomic and proteomic analysis is one example), cluster analysis is currently the most commonly used method. We focus on hierarchical clustering because this strategy is particularly useful for clustering patients or samples when there are relatively few samples (say, < 50), which is commonly the case in translational research.

Consider, then, an experiment where 20 tissue samples have been arrayed on gene chips that measure 12,000 genes. The raw expression data are illustrated in Table 26–2, where each row represents one of the samples and each column represents one of the genes. The table entries, $x_{i,j}$, represent the $i$th sample and $j$th gene, such as $x_{1,1}$ is the expression of gene 1 in sample 1, $x_{1,2}$ is the expression of gene 2 in sample 1, and so on.

We can define the "distance" between two samples by comparing their gene expression values (row vectors), using one of several different formulas. The Euclidean distance is one, commonly employed, formula. For samples 1 and 2, the Euclidean distance would be defined as:

$$d(s1, s2) = \sqrt{\begin{array}{l}(x_{1,1} - x_{2,1})^2 + (x_{1,2} - x_{2,2})^2 \\ + \cdots + (x_{1,12000} - x_{2,12000})^2\end{array}} \quad (7)$$

In hierarchical clustering, these pair-wise distances are used to find subgroups by sequentially merging the closest samples or subgroups of samples. To demonstrate, consider a hierarchical clustering of four genes, A, B, C, and D, using the expression value on two chips shown in Table 26–3. An average linkage algorithm can be used to form

the clustering, although many alternative clustering methods are available for this type of data. Details on these algorithms can be found elsewhere (5, 10). The average linkage algorithm is used for illustration only; other algorithms can also be used.

Using a Euclidean distance measure, the gene distances are displayed in a pair-wise distance matrix, Table 26–4, where each entry corresponds to the distance between two genes. For example, the distance between samples A and B is 1.58, and between A and D is 4.74. This implies that samples A and B are more similar to each other than samples A and D.

The genes are displayed graphically in the upper left plot of Figure 26–6, where the axes correspond to the two chips and the labeled points correspond to the four genes. Overlying this plot are the pair-wise distances. In the first iteration of the average linkage algorithm, genes A and B are merged into a subgroup because they are the closest pair (i.e., smallest

## TABLE 26–3

### Hypothetical Expression Data on Four Genes Measured on Two Chips

| Gene | Chip 1 | Chip 2 |
|---|---|---|
| A | –2.0 | 1.0 |
| B | –1.5 | –0.5 |
| C | 1.0 | 0.25 |
| D | 2.5 | 2.5 |

Values are in arbitrary units of expression

## TABLE 26-4

### Pair-wise Euclidean Distances Calculated for the Four Genes from Table 26-3

|   | A | B | C | D |
|---|---|---|---|---|
| A | 0.00 | 1.58 | 3.09 | 4.74 |
| B | 1.58 | 0.00 | 2.61 | 5.00 |
| C | 3.09 | 2.61 | 0.00 | 2.70 |
| D | 4.74 | 5.00 | 2.70 | 0.00 |

distance between them). After this merge, the distance from the AB subgroup is recalculated to gene C and D and the closest pair again merged—in this case genes C and D. The AB and CD subgroups have their distance recalculated and merged because they are the only remaining genes not merged. The

dendrogram in the bottom right corner displays this clustering process. Genes are merged at the height of the dendrogram at which they first become joined, and this height corresponds to the distance as displayed in the first three plots. The dendrogram therefore provides a visual display of how genes have been joined.

A serious caution must be given to the reader. The human eye has an amazing ability to identify clusters in data, like identifying subgroups in dendrograms. Thus, many people would say the data in Figure 26–6 show two clusters. The researcher must remember that even with random data where no clusters exist by definition, it is very easy to convince oneself that a dendrogram in fact appears to display distinct clusters. In practice, the results of a dendrogram should be validated with external criteria not used in constructing the dendrogram, such as whether tissue types appear in different frequencies in the different clusters, such as tumors in one subgroup and normal tissue in another subgroup.

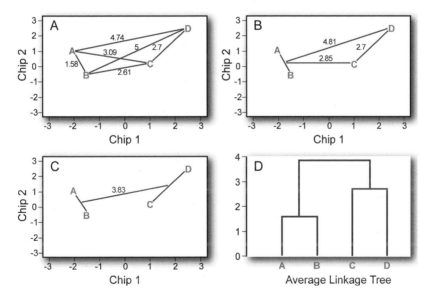

**FIGURE 26–6** ● Graphical representation of the average linkage clustering grouping the four simulated genes in Table 26–3. **A.** The genes are displayed graphically where the axes correspond to the expression levels of the genes on the two chips and the labeled points correspond to the four genes. The lines connecting the genes are the pair-wise distances. **B.** In the first iteration of the average linkage algorithm, genes A and B are merged into a subgroup because they are the closest pair (i.e., smallest distance between them). **C.** After this merge, the distance from the AB subgroup is recalculated to gene C and D and the closest pair again merged—in this case genes C and D. The AB and CD subgroups have their distance recalculated and merged because they are the only remaining genes not merged. **D.** The dendrogram displays this clustering process. Genes are merged at the height of the dendrogram at which they first become joined, and this height corresponds to the distance as displayed in the first three plots. The dendrogram therefore provides a visual display of how genes have been joined.

## SUMMARY

- Multivariate analysis is concerned with analyzing more than one outcome variable simultaneously, and generally results in a significant increase in power to test hypotheses.
- Multivariate analysis of variance (MANOVA) is an extension of analysis of variance (ANOVA) to the case of testing two or more groups for differences in more than one outcome
- Principal components analysis (PCA) is one of a class of statistical methods designed to reduce the complexity of multivariate data to a smaller set that can be used to identify patterns within the data.
- Mixed effects models represent state of the art analytic approaches for analyzing multivariate data, and solve many of the analytic challenges posed by classical methods, such as MANOVA, when confronted with real data.
- Cluster analysis is a powerful class of multivariate methods designed exclusively to find subgroups within data, and represent the class of statistical methods most often currently used in microarray data analysis.

## REFERENCES

1. Dunteman G. Principal Components Analysis. Thousand Oaks, CA: Sage, Quantitative Applications in the Social Sciences, 1989.
2. Bray J, Maxwell S. Multivariate Analysis of Variance. Thousand Oaks, CA: Sage, Quantitative Applications in the Social Sciences, 1986.
3. Girden, E. ANOVA: Repeated Measures. Thousand Oaks, CA: Sage, Quantitative Applications in the Social Sciences, 1992.
4. Luke D. Multilevel Modeling, 2004. Thousand Oaks, CA: Sage, Quantitative Applications in the Social Sciences, 2004.
5. Aldenderfer M, Blashfield R. Cluster Analysis. Thousand Oaks, CA: Sage, Quantitative Applications in the Social Sciences, 1984.
6. Timm, N. Applied Multivariate Analysis. New York: Springer-Verlag, 2002.
7. Searle SR, Casella G, McCulloch CE. Variance Components. New York: John Wiley and Sons, 1992.
8. Singer J, Willett JB. Applied Longitudinal Data Analysis: Modeling Change and Event Occurrence. New York: Oxford University Press, 2003.
9. Verbeke G, Molenberghs G. Linear Mixed Models for Longitudinal Data. New York: Springer, 2000.
10. Shannon W, Culverhouse R, Duncan J. Analyzing microarray data using cluster analysis. Pharmacogenomics 2003;4(1):41–52.

# CHAPTER 27

# Biostatistical Consulting

Kenneth B. Schechtman, Paul A. Thompson

An all-too-common view is that the role of the statistician is limited to providing p-values and determining sample size. Sometimes, statistician involvement in the research process begins at the end, long after the study has been designed, with a request for assistance with the analysis of study data. Alternatively, statistician involvement may be the mandate of reviewers who have rejected a grant application or manuscript because of data analytic, sample size, or design-related problems.

In this chapter, we suggest that the value of early consultation with a biostatistician is often overlooked during the planning phase of translational and experimental clinical research studies. We offer the view that the consulting relationship with a statistician should be an ongoing process that begins when scientific hypotheses are generated, that progresses through the development of a protocol or a grant application, that focuses on the quality control and scientific concerns that are critical as the study progresses, and finally, that concludes with the statistical analyses that precede and continue through the actual reporting of the study's data (Table 27–1). Many of the issues to be identified in the following sections have been discussed in greater detail in other chapters of this book. The orientation here is what should constitute a "complete" statistical review for a proposed study, providing insight into the potential benefits of a proactive—not retroactive—statistical consultation.

## ESTABLISHING THE CONSULTING RELATIONSHIP

Although most of the literature on statistical consulting is concerned with the technical and scientific features of the consultation, procedural and interpersonal issues can have a major impact on the ultimate success of the consulting relationship (1–6). Commonly, short-term goals are the focus of this initial encounter: data analysis in anticipation of an abstract deadline, a response to a specific analytic request for a manuscript, and a sample size computation for a grant application. However, experience often shows a large difference between what the investigator requests and what may actually be required, especially for less experienced investigators. For example, requests for a "quick" sample size computation are often made within the context of an application for research funding. From a purely quantitative perspective, the statistician could perform the computation in a mechanical fashion using general information about the design configuration of the study and using relevant data that include projected between-group differences, estimated standard deviations, and anticipated dropout rates (as discussed in detail in Chapter 9). But if science is to be best served, the computations should be accompanied by a discussion of the specific aims and hypotheses, the availability of eligible research participants, the priorities among the aims, the possible multiple comparison problems related to multiple endpoints, and the quality of the pilot data that may guide the power computations. If it turns out that the expected power is inadequate, more elaborate discussions of alternative designs, alternative endpoints, or modified eligibility criteria may be necessary.

## PLANNING THE STUDY

The biostatistician is often consulted when a study is first being planned (for instance, during preparation of a grant application for research funding). Issues of sample size, data management, and data

> ### TABLE 27–1
>
> ## Topics for a Biostatistics Consultation
>
> - Study design, including methods of randomization and masking
> - Strategies to reduce bias
> - Sample size estimates and power analyses
> - Strategies for data management
> - Strategies for data analysis, including multicomparison and "early look" problems

analysis are the obvious areas in which statistical input is critical, but the statistician can also provide guidance about other issues, such as how best to define the questions and hypotheses of interest (Chapter 1), how best to develop and defend the proposed design configuration (Chapters 7 and 8), how best to address major sources of potential bias and potential approaches to minimizing that bias (Chapter 6), and how to be involved in quality control activities as the study progresses (Chapter 12).

## Defining the Questions of Interest

Critical to the success of any study (and certainly any grant application) are specific aims and hypotheses that are precisely defined and achievable, and questions that are scientifically important (Chapter 1). The importance of specific aims that contain a precise description of scientifically significant research problems is highlighted by a study of 256 disapproved or poorly rated grant applications (7), which found that 47% received a poor rating, at least in part, for reasons related to how the hypotheses were presented, while 30% had problems associated with the apparent significance of the research questions. A proper biostatistical review of a grant application can help avoid an unsuccessful outcome by addressing the following standards:

1. Aims that are unambiguously worded and clearly associated with experimentally testable hypotheses. Appropriate discussion of the anticipated associations or differences in the data should be included.
2. Aims that are appropriate in number, with the most important aims identified separately from the secondary objectives of the study. More statistically inclined reviewers may be particularly concerned with multiple comparisons if there are too many apparently prime hypotheses to be tested. Ideally, the aims should describe a small number of primary hypotheses, with the remainder of the study's goals being clearly separated out as secondary or exploratory.

3. Sample size estimates and data analysis strategies that are precisely keyed to the specific aims and that precisely reflect the associated hypotheses.

## Developing the Study's Design

Even in the modern era, medical history is replete with therapies that were once "known" to be effective, only to be found subsequently to be either useless or harmful. Examples include routine tonsillectomies for children with recurrent sore throats, routine radical mastectomy for patients with breast cancer (8), back surgery for radiographically diagnosed vertebral disc abnormalities associated with back pain (9), and the recently charged controversy over the routine use of hormone replacement therapy in postmenopausal women. In each of these cases, carefully designed but uncontrolled observational studies suggested a benefit to the proposed therapy. Accordingly, a complete statistical review of a proposed study affords appropriate attention to the all-important issue of controls: which types of research participants might constitute an appropriate control group, how many control groups should be included, and why and how these groups will be compared to the target population.

Of course, proper controls don't ensure an unbiased result. Statistical review should also focus on issues related to masking (Chapter 6), assignment of the experimental intervention, and sample size estimates, among other issues. For instance, in one controlled study comparing two methods of assessing the gestational age of newborn babies, one observer was responsible for all assessments with one method and a second observer was responsible for all assessments with the second method (10). As a result, it was impossible to determine whether conclusions reflected differences between methods or differences between assessors.

In another example, Chalmers and colleagues (11) evaluated the importance of how the experimental intervention was assigned to each research participant in 145 controlled studies that used blinded randomization (N = 57), unblinded randomization (N = 45), and nonrandom assignment (N = 43). They found that the nonrandom assignment studies were the most likely to yield significant results, that the blinded studies were least likely, and that the unblinded randomized studies were in the middle. These examples illustrate that even in settings where it may be impossible to mask the assignment of the experimental intervention after randomization (e.g., in an exercise study), different levels of masking (such as the masking of the randomization process before participants are assigned and the masking of assessors) may be critical if unbiased conclusions are to be reached.

Other studies have shown repeatedly that close attention should be paid to sample size estimates because an inadequate sample size commonly yields spurious negative results (12–15) (Chapter 9). A related potential pitfall concerns protocol adherence and the assessment of outcome measures because poor adherence (16–18) and poor reproducibility of assessments (19) (Chapter 3) can substantially compromise the power of a study.

A complete statistical review should address the above issues and should discuss such details of study design as the strengths and weaknesses of one design format over another (e.g. a between-group versus a crossover design), the method and strategy for randomization (e.g. blocked and stratified randomization), and the methods to be employed for identifying the study population, because the estimate of risk associated with a putative risk factor will often be a biased overestimate if it results from a clinic-based as opposed to a more appropriate population-based study (20) (Chapter 4).

### Discussing Contingencies and Avoiding Bias

The responsibilities of an involved statistician include a thorough consideration and discussion of potential sources of bias. In such a discussion, it is important to not only address why certain options have been chosen, but also why others were rejected. For instance, a crossover study design (Chapter 8) might have many important advantages over other simpler designs, but in a given setting, substantial bias might result when many research participants who are doing well in a particular study group refuse to crossover to the other group. Likewise, it might be reasonable to reject the gold standard approach to measuring a particular outcome, but it is not enough to simply say that this has been done. It must also be argued, for example, that this decision has been made because there is an appropriate alternative to the gold standard and because the

gold standard might generate unacceptable burdens for the research volunteers, contributing to excessive dropout. Additional examples might include the need for the statistician to consider why potential volunteer or referral bias would not have unacceptable effects on the representativeness of a study sample; why a nonstandardized assessment technique with potential bias in the evaluation of some outcome measures could still be a reasonable choice; why a possible placebo effect could still cause little bias because prior experience has shown that the effect on between-group efficacy differences will be small, or why physician learning effects and investigator fatigue will only cause acceptably small temporal bias in a particular research setting.

### Sample Size, Statistical Power, and the Selection of Outcome Measures

No study will be funded if reviewers believe that the target sample size is inadequate or have substantial doubt that the target number of participants can be successfully recruited. Thus, the application should contain a discussion of sample size and availability that establishes adequacy for each primary specific aim.

In a standard comparative clinical study, power computations require preliminary estimates of anticipated between-group differences, of standard deviations when there are continuous outcome measures, and of expected dropout rates (Chapter 9). Ideally, such estimates will be generated for at least one primary outcome measure for each primary specific aim. If at all possible, the estimates should be based on research conducted by the investigator and a detailed review of the literature. The relevant prior studies should involve research participants and interventions that are similar to those proposed in the planned research. For each outcome measure, we recommend generating tables that contain information about different combinations of effect sizes, standard deviations, and dropout rates that have been observed in similar settings. Using these tables, and because it is better to overestimate than to underestimate sample size requirements, it is often best to use a conservative approach in which power computations assume smaller between-group differences and larger standard deviations and dropout rates than what the tabulated data might suggest is most likely. Also, if interim efficacy analyses are to be conducted, the Type I error rate used in the computations should reflect the necessary adjustment for these added analyses. In the event that the power for a particular outcome is unacceptably low, alternative outcome measures should be considered if they are scientifically important and can be reliably measured.

A discussion of sample size should include detailed consideration of the availability of enough eligible research participants, including the number of eligible individuals who can be expected to be available per unit of time and of the proportion of these individuals who are likely to enroll. If the available number does not exceed the target sample size, it may be necessary to change some endpoints, to seek additional clinics or institutions as sources of research volunteers, or even to remove a specific aim from the application.

## Analytic Strategies

It is important that the proposed analytic strategy precisely reflect the study design, the assessment schedule, and the outcome measures. Equally important, covariates that may impact outcome variables and the distributional properties of both the covariates, and the outcomes should be addressed. If the data from some variables are likely to be skewed, attention should be paid to how the data might be transformed so that certain analytic approaches can be legitimately adopted (Chapter 24).

The data analysis strategy should consider the need for interim analyses where applicable. In addition to considering the specific statistical methods that will be used in the interim analyses, such issues as the rationale for the analyses, the timing of the analyses, whether and why it may be necessary to blind investigators to the results of the analyses, and the specific group sequential adjustment that will be used when performing the analyses should all be addressed. Of particular interest are any modifications in study design that might result from these interim analyses, especially if they indicate that a study should be stopped early because efficacy has already been established, because the possibility of obtaining positive results is likely to be futile (and to continue would expose research participants to potential experimental side effects without a reasonable chance of benefit to themselves or society), or because a positive result is likely only if the target sample size can be modified. It is important to consider what factors will govern the decision-making process and who will be responsible for recommending and making such decisions (discussed in greater detail in Chapter 13).

## Quality Control

Quality control is a multifaceted process that includes a wide variety of activities (Chapter 12). A well-designed study (and a well-prepared grant application) should include quality control considerations such as the following.

1. *Quality control of the data.* In many instances, a biostatistician can perform quality control activities such as overseeing the development of data entry screens, facilitating double data entry, preparing datasets for statistical analysis and report writing, performing range checks on computerized data, initiating remedial procedures when there are erroneous or inappropriately missing data, and helping with the design of data forms that are user-friendly from the perspective of the data entry person.

2. *Evaluating the reproducibility of assessments.* The descriptions of standard measurement instruments are always strengthened if they contain relevant reliability data. If new instruments are to be developed or if existing instruments will be used in a new population, reproducibility is a fundamental but frequently ignored quality control issue. To assist in the assessment of reproducibility, a biostatistician can help in the design of the appropriate reliability studies and can compute the relevant reliability coefficients. If reliability is poor, alternative approaches, such as using the mean of repeat assessments at each time point to reduce variability and sample size requirements, should be evaluated.

3. *Maximizing subject adherence.* It has been repeatedly demonstrated (21–23) that adherence to medications and behavioral interventions can be extremely poor. It has also been shown that poor adherence can reduce the effectiveness of an intervention and, as a result, can reduce between-group differences and increase sample size requirements (16–18). Thus, a well-designed study (and an appropriately prepared grant application) should consider some or all of the following questions: What does the literature say about the adherence rate that can be anticipated? How large an impact might poor adherence have on sample size requirements? What will be done to enhance adherence? How will adherence be measured? How will participants who do not adhere be handled when the data are analyzed? Will there be a prerandomization run-in strategy designed to exclude participants who are likely to be poor adherers? What are the implications with respect to sample size and subject availability if a run-in strategy (Chapter 8) is implemented?

4. *Documenting investigator adherence.* Investigator adherence to the research protocol is another crucial component of quality control, particularly during a lengthy longitudinal study. Especially in multicenter studies, the biostatistician

may be called on to document and maintain a list of personnel who have been certified as competent to perform study procedures. In smaller translational studies conducted at a single center, the operational responsibilities of the consulting statistician may be limited to ensuring the quality control of computerized data.

## CONDUCTING, ANALYZING, AND REPORTING THE STUDY

While a study is ongoing, the biostatistician may or may not be involved in actual data entry and quality control measures such as those just discussed, depending on the size of the study and the resources of the investigator. After the study, the biostatistician will likely be directly involved with carrying out the prospectively determined analytic plan, unless the statistical methods are simple, straightforward, and within the competencies of the study's principal investigator. The biostatistician can be especially helpful with post hoc, unanticipated analyses that arise because of the study's results. Obviously, following the analysis, the biostatistician should take an active role in reporting the results for publication. Less well appreciated is the role that the biostatistician can play at times in ensuring the scientific integrity of the study.

### Ensuring Scientific Integrity

Even behaviors that have an innocent etiology may at times raise questions about scientific integrity, even in the absence of deliberate fraud. Frequently, such behaviors are mundane reflections of methodological naiveté or of an excessive but nonvenal investigator commitment to demonstrating efficacy or effectiveness of the proposed experimental intervention. Every statistician has been faced with the investigator who is disappointed by the borderline significance of his or her results and then returns with a few more experiments and discovers that the "borderline" result remains operative, by the investigator who is convinced—despite the absence of a control group—that the experimental intervention is effective because returning patients "feel better" than they did before the intervention, and by the investigator who may introduce—unintentionally—bias into an unblinded interpretation of some outcome measure. In each of these instances, the biostatistician may be the first person to identify the problem.

### Writing and Reviewing Manuscripts

At a minimum, as part of the consulting relationship, the biostatistician can be expected to describe the statistical methods used in the collaborative study. In other instances, when more substantive analyses are required, the biostatistician may not only describe the methods used but also generate tables for the paper, write relevant portions of the results section, and describe the results in abstract form.

## SUMMARY

- The most productive biostatistics consultative relationship is initiated early in the study planning process, with involvement in the precise statement of the experimental and study hypotheses, study design format, strategies to reduce bias, sample size estimates, data management, quality control, data analysis, and reporting of the study results.
- A complete biostatistics consultation can be expected to address such issues as the nature and number of control groups, methods of defining and identifying the appropriate study population, methods of randomization, methods and alternatives to masking, assessments of measurement reproducibility and validity, protocol adherence, and how to handle multiple comparison problems.
- During the conduct of a study, the biostatistician may or may not be involved in actual data entry and will have widely varying quality control responsibilities. Likewise, after the study is completed, the biostatistician may or may not participate in the preplanned data analysis, perform additional ad hoc unanticipated analyses (depending on the study's results), and contribute to manuscript preparation for publication. The scope of statistician involvement in these activities depends on the details of the study design and the complexity of the required data analyses.

## REFERENCES

1. Boen JR, Zahn DA. The human side of statistical consulting. Belmont, CA: Lifetime Learning, 1982.
2. Zahn DA, Isenberg DJ. Nonstatistical aspects of statistical consulting. Amer Stat 1983;37:297–302.
3. Froberg DG, Holloway RL, Bland CJ. A continuity model for research consultation in family medicine. J Fam Prac 1984;19:221–224.
4. Stegman CE. Statistical consulting in the university: a faculty member's perspective. J Edu Stat 1985;36:69–89.
5. Arndt S, Woolson RF. Establishing a biostatistical core unit in a clinical research center. Amer Stat 1991; 45:22–27.
6. Kirk RE. Statistical consulting in a university: dealing with people and other challenges. Amer Stat 1991; 45:28–34.
7. Cuca JM. NIH grant applications for clinical research: reasons for poor ratings or disapproval. Clin Res 1983;31:453–461.

8. Fisher B, Bauer M, Margolese R et al. Five-year results of a randomized clinical trial comparing total mastectomy and segmental mastectomy with or without radiation in the treatment of breast cancer. N Engl J Med 1985;312:665–673.

9. Jensen MC, Brant-Zawadzki MN, Obuchowski N et al. Magnetic resonance imaging of the lumbar spine in people without back pain. N Engl J Med 1994; 331:69–73.

10. Serfontein GL, Jaroszewicz AM. Estimation of gestational age at birth. Arch Dis Child 1978;53:509–511.

11. Chalmers TC, Celano P, Sacks HS, Smith Jr. H. Bias in treatment assignment in controlled clinical trials. N Engl J Med1983;309:1358–1361.

12. Freiman JA, Chalmers TC, Smith Jr. H et al. The importance of beta, the type II error and sample size in the design and interpretation of the randomized control trial: Survey of 71 "negative" trials. N Engl J Med 1978; 299:690–694.

13. Williams HC, Seed P. Inadequate size of "negative" clinical trials in dermatology. B J Dermatol 1993;128: 317–326.

14. Schechtman KB, Sher AE, Piccirillo JF. Methodological and statistical problems in sleep apnea research: the literature on uvulopalatopharyngoplasty. Sleep 1995; 18:659–666.

15. Fleming DM, Knox JDE, Crombie DL. Debendox in early pregnancy and fetal malformation. Br Med J 1981;283:99–101.

16. Palta M, McHugh R. Planning the size of a cohort study in the presence of both losses to follow-up and non-compliance. J Chronic Dis 1980;33:501–512.

17. Lachin JM, Foulkes MA. Evaluation of sample size and power for analyses of survival with allowance for nonuniform patient entry, losses to follow-up, noncompliance, and stratification. Biometrics 1986;42: 507–519.

18. Schechtman KB, Gordon MO. The effect of poor compliance and treatment side effects on sample size requirements in randomized clinical trials. J Biopharm Stat 1994;4:223–232.

19. Gordon MO, Schechtman KB, Davis LJ et al. Visual acuity repeatability in keratoconus: impact on sample size. Optom Vis Sci 1998;75:249–257.

20. Ellenberg JH, Nelson KB. Sample selection and the natural history of disease. JAMA 1980;243:1337–1340.

21. Cramer JA, Mattson RH, Prevey ML et al. How often is medication taken as prescribed? A novel assessment technique. JAMA 1989;261:3273–3277.

22. Glanz K, Fiel SB, Swartz MA et al. Compliance with an experimental drug regimen for treatment for asthma: its magnitude, importance, and correlates. J Chronic Dis 1984;37:815–824.

23. Kass MA, Meltzer DW, Gordon ME et al. Compliance with topical pilocarpine treatment. Am J Ophthalmol 1986;101:515–523.

# CHAPTER 28

# Statistical Computing

J. Philip Miller

With the advent of microcomputers, the use of software to perform statistics is now pervasive. Unfortunately, investigators often simply choose statistical software that they previously used in a course or that is already available in their setting. As a result, investigators may be disappointed when the software fails to meet their specific research needs. Although it is not our intent in this chapter to review features of specific software packages, we do raise issues to be considered before making an investment when obtaining and/or learning statistical software. A listing of software options, vendors, and websites cited in this chapter is given in Table 28–1.

## WHY IS STATISTICAL SOFTWARE NEEDED?

The days of computing statistics by hand, a time-consuming and error-prone task, are now long gone. Instead, using a computer to make the necessary computations is the standard alternative, but the question still remains: what software should be used? Is a spreadsheet program sufficient? And if not, which choice among a wide variety of high quality statistical software is the best choice? Or does it matter?

Probably the first consideration when making a software selection is whether the investigator will function alone or as a member of a team that includes a professional statistician or a database manager. If the latter, it is wisest to investigate which software the statistician normally uses. Most statisticians are likely to use SAS, SPSS, S-Plus, R, or STATA. If the investigator uses the same software as that used by the statistician, communication and data sharing between them will obviously be facilitated.

If the software programs are not the same, it is critical that the data can be easily transferred between the programs they use. Optimally, the statistician should also be familiar with the software chosen by the investigator.

Another consideration concerns the purpose of the statistical package to the investigator—is it to explore the dataset in order to assure its quality and to look for interesting relationships among the variables or is it to produce an analysis for publication in a manuscript? In the former case, ease of use and the ability to display patterns graphically in the data are salient characteristics. In the latter, it is the completeness and appropriateness of the statistical models supported that should dominate.

Almost all modern statistical packages now support both a graphical user interface (GUI, allowing, for instance, point-and-click functionality or drop-down menus) and a specialized programming language. Some packages are stronger in one interface than the other. The GUI used in JMP is particularly attractive to new users and users accessing unfamiliar operations. However, the GUI may not provide ready access to some features or options that may be necessary in a particular case. It should not be assumed that if the option is not present in the GUI, it is not available in the program altogether. Only a search through the program's documentation can establish whether a particular option is available.

Another problem with the use of a GUI is being able to document the precise steps and options that were chosen for a particular analysis. This problem presents a challenge when composing a manuscript or in replicating the analyses in the future (e.g., when requested by the reviewer of a manuscript). In addition, the GUI can be relatively inefficient when the same statistical model is used

**TABLE 28-1**

**Software Mentioned in this Chapter**

| Software | Vendor | URL |
|---|---|---|
| SAS | SAS Institute, Inc. | www.sas.com |
| SPSS | SPSS, Inc. | www.spss.com |
| S-Plus | Insightful | www.insightful.com |
| STATA | StataCorp | www.stata.com |
| R | The R Project | www.r-project.org |
| JMP | SAS Institute, Inc. | www.sas.com/jmp |
| Oracle | Oracle Corporation | www.oracle.com |
| Sybase | Sybase Inc. | www.sybase.com |
| SQL Server | Microsoft | www.microsoft.com/sql |
| PostgreSQL | PostgreSQL Global Development Group | www.postgresql.org |

repeatedly for different variables or subsets of the data (e.g., multiple point-and-click steps to achieve each separate analysis).

The programming languages implemented by many statistical packages are versatile enough that they can be used for many tasks in addition to those involved for statistical analyses per se. The same statistical software can often do studies involving large amounts of electronic data (e.g., physiologic monitoring, output of automated laboratory equipment, results of image analysis software), data manipulation, and the extraction of appropriate parameters for analysis. Automating clerical tasks for the management of the study (e.g. tracking appointments, generating progress reports) is another area that can frequently be implemented with the same statistical software tools. Mature systems also often contain modules that assist in conducting sample size estimates, power analyses, simulations, and randomization schemes. There is an obvious advantage to being able to use a single package for multiple tasks.

Although a large majority of users may be comfortable in working on a Microsoft Windows platform, others may be more comfortable using an alternative system such as an Apple or Linux. For technical, security, or licensing cost reasons, it may be desirable to work on a server-based computer rather than on a local system. These considerations may dictate the choice of computer software. If an investigator (or group of investigators) anticipates using multiple platforms, then software that runs on each of the platforms is obviously desirable. Most of the major packages do so, but some more specialized packages are limited to a single platform.

## DATA MANAGEMENT

Clinical studies frequently require the storage and manipulation of substantial amounts of data. Most statistical packages have a specialized, proprietary format so that the software easily manipulates the data. Large research organizations often use specialized database management software (DBMS), such as Oracle, Sybase, Microsoft SQL Server, Post-GreSQL, for storing and manipulating the data. Individual investigators and other organizations may choose to use the database management tools within the statistical software for merging data from multiple sources or from data gathered at different time points. Fortunately, with the power of current desktop systems, many of the statistical packages are quite capable of providing the necessary data management resources. Generating ad hoc reports is frequently a major effort during data cleaning activities.

Data cleaning is an important component of any statistical analysis, and the statistical software must have facilities to assist in supporting these activities. If the software supports a data-entry module, it should also provide capabilities for validating the data during data entry; for example, range checks, lists of valid values, valid dates/times as well as capabilities for cross-field checks (e.g., a pregnancy history by a man). The software should also support checking double data entry (keying the data twice) and raising an alert if the two versions are not identical. Some software supports a spreadsheet type interface for data entry. Although this is often convenient when entering only a small amount of data (that will be carefully examined by the investigators themselves), it is an inadequate method when others will enter the data unless appropriate data validation rules can be executed at the time the data are being entered.

If the data for a study are to be extracted from other electronic sources, then an important issue is how the data are going to be imported into the statistical software. Many systems are quite facile in having the capacity to import data in a variety of formats. Because the software creating the data may be able to export data in a variety of formats, finding a common format is often possible. Otherwise, programs need to be written to reformat the data so that the statistical software can read it.

Independent of how the data are entered, it is essential that the software provide easy facilities for identifying and correcting invalid data values. This process may involve procedures in the software system to display summary statistics, extreme values, histograms, scatterplots and other methods of summarizing the values of one or more variables. The investigator who understands the measured variables may be superior to a statistician in identifying problems with the accumulating data.

The topic of database development and management is considered in more detail in Chapter 10.

## NUMERICAL ACCURACY

Most investigators do not have the necessary training or time to write programs to implement statistical models for the analysis of their data. Surprisingly, even computers cannot always exactly represent something as simple as a written number exactly. Calculations performed for routine statistical procedures can break down by compounding small errors, producing completely wrong results. For example, in computing the mean and standard deviation of a set of numbers, the simple textbook formulas call for forming the sum of all of the numbers and the sums of the squares of the numbers. In some instances, such as the numbers having a wide range, this procedure can easily produce incorrect values. Most professional packages will use either a two-pass algorithm or other complex computing strategies to manage the accumulating errors. Starting with Longley (1) and continuing into more recent times (McCullough (2)), various reviewers have identified problems even in well-known statistical packages. In the case of specialized statistical packages, the danger of encountering this kind of problem is even greater as the necessary numerical analysis resources may not have been available to adequately address these issues.

Although substantial research has resulted in the development of many good numerical algorithms for different statistical methods, most methods will still fail for particular datasets. An important aspect of quality statistical software is that the numerical computations attempt to detect those cases where the numerical results are suspect and provide appropriate messages to the user. The display of such alerts is ample reason for most investigators to consult with a biostatistician (see Chapter 27).

Many of the statistical techniques that have become standard models in clinical research, such as logistic regression and proportional hazard survival models, require iterative maximization routines that are even more demanding in needing robust numerical methods. Virtually all these methods may fail to converge to an appropriate solution for particular datasets. Quality software both provides appropriate diagnostics when the models will not converge and may offer alternative maximization algorithms and the ability to specify particular starting values and convergence criteria.

## BREADTH OF ANALYTIC MODELS

A critical component for the selection of any statistical software is whether it will support the type of statistical models that are appropriate for the investigator's particular area of research. It should support other models as well, because in some cases the research may progress to needing other models (for instance, requested by reviewers or as suggested by other investigators in the area). It is obviously frustrating to use one package for routine descriptive and simple analytic statistics, only to find out that it does not provide sample size estimates or life table analyses.

Implementing and supporting new statistical models is an expensive undertaking by a software vendor. Thus, all packages are limited in the breadth of models that can be supported in a particular release of the software. In addition, all vendors continually add functionality with newer releases of the software. Therefore, while at one moment a particular package may be inferior to another in terms of the support of certain procedures, at the next release, their order may be reversed.

Most packages provide methods by which users may implement new features and share them between users. In some cases the vendor set up the system, and in other cases public libraries of such code may exist.

Most full-featured software systems also have capabilities to import and export data in a format that other software can use. In some cases, this function converts the data from one package's specialized format to another and in other cases it may have to be in some other format; for example, a comma delimited file or an ASCII (character) formatted file.

Statistical methodology continues to progress as new methods are implemented (e.g., for genomic analyses, see Chapter 26) and as computing speeds increase so that more complex models can be reasonably applied to actual datasets. Some of these models relax assumptions previously needed in order to make them computationally tractable. Another area of active statistical research is the development of methods for dealing with missing data—a problem frequently encountered in clinical research. Statistical software vendors frequently don't implement these newer methods until there has been general acceptance of the methods by the research community and the market for these methods is large enough to justify the investment. Thus, using these newer techniques is likely to require exporting data from the user's customary package.

The issue of the breadth of the software is more critical when the investigator is not collaborating with a statistician. The statistician is likely to have a broader spectrum of software available since almost all packages provide some capabilities for doing most analyses necessary for a "first pass" at looking at the data.

## STATISTICAL GRAPHICS

Many investigators are more comfortable with graphical representations of data than analyses that are restricted to summary numbers. Most statistical software packages have many graphical routines available to assist the data analyst.

One of the important uses of graphics in statistical analyses is for the user to become more familiar with the data and to be able to identify patterns in the data that may be scientifically meaningful. Almost all statistical packages contain modules to produce on-screen graphics with a wide variety of graph types. With contemporary high resolution color monitors, this feature is an invaluable component. Many will also allow three-dimensional graphics to be rotated in space in order to better view appropriate relationships.

Many users find that they want to produce data driven graphics for direct publication. Packages differ in their ability to produce graphics of an adequate quality for reproduction in a journal. Some packages have graphics editors available to allow manual editing of graphics in order to change fonts, add annotations, or make other similar enhancements. Some packages have the ability to export graphics images in formats to be edited with graphics programs or directly incorporated into word processing documents or electronic slide presentations.

## DOCUMENTATION AND SUPPORT

No matter how "easy to use" the software is described to be, it is still necessary to be able to refer to information about the specifics of the software. Most software systems today have at least the core manuals supplied in electronic format so they can either reside on the computer or a local server. Some manuals are even available in a searchable form on the vendor's websites. These electronic formats have the advantage of being able to be searched more easily, but some users have difficulties making the transition from paper-based documentation, so the availability of paper-based copies (or the documentation's being in a format suitable for printing locally) may be important.

Most software vendors provide some telephone or e-mail support for questions about the software and for reporting problems with using the software. Understanding the availability (and possible cost) for such support is an important ingredient in the choice of a particular set of software.

It is very desirable to have the ability to seek assistance locally. Many universities and institutions have help desks capable of providing assistance. Usually only a few statistical packages are supported in this fashion. Using the same software as one's colleagues may allow a researcher to seek assistance from one of them. If the user is collaborating with a statistician, that person may be able to help if they are familiar with the software.

With the easy, worldwide availability of e-mail, the definition of "local" has changed somewhat and there are e-mail lists for many of the more popular statistical software systems where users can submit problems that they are facing in using the software and receive answers from other helpful users.

Many users of statistical software find the manuals provided by the vendors inadequate and have written and published many books about specific aspects of the use of the software. Many of these books deal with the statistical theory and application of the software as well as how to actually specify the particular statistical model. Many vendors' websites list these books or searches at a good bookstore (or online equivalent) may help the user choose books that will aid in his or her productivity.

Training, whether in a classroom setting or on-line, is another important resource to consider. The user should inquire locally about opportunities. Most vendors provide training opportunities. Independent firms also provide training for the more popular software.

## COST

Comparing the costs of acquiring the software may actually take some effort because some software is only licensed with annual renewal charges for support and updates and other software may be sold with a perpetual license (shrink-wrapped). In addition, many vendors have special academic pricing or site licensing to institutions. Perhaps most importantly, however, is that the investigator needs to consider the "total costs of ownership," not just the price for the software per se, as detailed elsewhere in this chapter.

## SUMMARY

- When purchasing computer statistical software, the investigator should consider more than simply whether the program can perform routine statistical computations. These additional considerations are summarized in Table 28–2.

## TABLE 28-2

### Items to Consider When Purchasing Statistical Software

- Compatibility with software used by a statistical consultant
- Ease-of-use and comprehensiveness of the graphical user interface
- Ability to perform nonstatistical functions (e.g., interface with DBMS, generate reports)
- Data cleaning functionality
- Numerical accuracy of computations and diagnostics in the case of failures
- Breadth of the analytic models supported
- Graphical capabilities
- Documentation and support
- Cost

## REFERENCES

1. Longley JW. An appraisal of computer programs for the electronic computer from the point of view of the user. J Am Stat Assoc 1967;62(348):856–866.
2. McCullough BD. Assessing the reliability of statistical software: Part I. Amer Stat 1998;52(4):358–366.

# CHAPTER 29

# Presenting Data in Manuscripts

Karen L. Dodson, Dana R. Abendschein

*T he purpose of scientific publication is to communicate knowledge that has been gained through scientific research or observation. No study is complete until the results have been published and read by others. No series of observations of a patient or group of patients has achieved its fullest potential benefit until it has been not only published, but also read by others.*

—R. Michael Sly, MD, former Editor, Annals of Allergy (1)

One of the greatest contributions that researchers make to the field of science is to publish the results of their work. Equally important, a researcher's publication record is often the single most important criterion for advancement within academic medicine. In this chapter, we provide some guidance to new investigators on how to organize the effort to publish their work.

## CHOOSING THE RIGHT JOURNAL

It has been said that choosing the right journal is "arguably the most important aspect of publishing a manuscript, whatever the field of interest" (2). If a researcher chooses poorly, rejection and delay are inevitable. We suggest that authors browse through a few issues of candidate journals, checking the subject matter. They should scan the names on the editorial board. If some are familiar, it usually indicates that the journal represents the right reviewer pool and readership. Articles in the journal that cover topics similar to investigator's own research and are published by other experts in the field are also good signs. Finally, authors might try to find out which journals their colleagues read and respect.

Even though a biomedical manuscript can be submitted to only one journal at a time, it's smart to

select two or three candidate journals right from the beginning (2). Many experienced authors first consider submitting their work to a more selective journal (i.e., a journal with a relatively low ratio of accepted-to-submitted manuscripts) that has a relatively wide readership and greater prestige. But only an honest appraisal of the quality of the work itself can determine whether it is worth the risk of sending the paper to a more selective journal when the chances of its being rejected are relatively high and the time spent in the process—two or three months or more—can turn out to be wasted. Most journals publish annual statistics on acceptance rates, processing rates, and types of manuscripts received. Such information may help authors get a realistic picture of the chances that their manuscript will have at a particular journal. By selecting a second or third choice before submission to the first choice, time is saved if the manuscript is rejected because it can simply be reformatted and resubmitted quickly to the new journal. The advice of a respected colleague or mentor can be particularly helpful when choosing a journal for manuscript submission.

Biomedical journals accept case reports, invited review articles, editorials, and letters to the editor. However, published reports of original research are generally referred to as original articles, original contributions, or original reports.

## DEFINING THE RESEARCH QUESTION

Before beginning to write, it's important to identify the research question that the information in the manuscript answers. Most manuscripts represent the culmination of months, sometimes years, of work. The data to be presented usually represent the output of multiple individual experiments, each designed to answer its own individual research question or hypothesis. Yet when a researcher is finally ready to write a manuscript summarizing this work, these various experimental goals must be distilled into a single overall question or hypothesis that alerts the editors of the journal and the readers of the manuscript to the overall purpose of the research. Obviously, great care and considerable thought should be given to how this message is communicated.

Once the overall research question has been devised, it's useful to identify five or six main features of the study that readers of the manuscript should remember (3). As many as possible of these points should be noted in the title, and all of them must be covered in the abstract. Then, they should reappear logically throughout the manuscript so that the reader can easily follow what took place during the research study (3).

## DECIDING ON AUTHORSHIP

Generally, authors are members of the research team who have participated in one or more of the following "tasks" associated with the research project (3): making intellectual contributions to the project, participating in the actual writing of the manuscript, and reviewing and approving of the final version of the manuscript. All authors should be willing to take public responsibility for the contents of the manuscript (3). Disagreements over authorship are common and sometimes contentious given the importance that authorship—and place in authorship—can play in decisions concerning academic promotion. So, it's best to understand what the journal's requirements are and to decide on who qualifies to be an author, and their place in the listing of authors, before the manuscript is written. The most important criterion for authorship is the extent to which a team member makes an *intellectual contribution* to the research effort (3). A material contribution may be defined as at least one of the following:

1. *Formulating the research question or design of the study*. It is not necessary that all authors have participated in the project from the study's initiation. However, they should at least have been active participants at key points in the scientific development of the study. This participation might only involve a single important experiment or it may involve multiple experiments during the overall conduct of the study.
2. *Developing critical methodology*. The key word is *critical*. It should be apparent that without this methodology, an important component of the study would not have been possible.
3. *Planning the analysis or presentation of the data*. Specific ideas rather than vague generalizations should be the criterion here.

In general, the individual who provides the greatest intellectual contribution and writes the paper will be the first author, with the author who provides mentorship (not just money) to the research project serving as the last, or senior author. Department chairs and division chiefs do not automatically qualify as senior authors. Unless the manuscript reports the results of a multicenter trial, most journals become suspicious when more than seven authors are listed and may require justification for such authorship. Nurses, technicians, and students should not be included unless they meet the criteria for authorship. In general, their contributions are more appropriately recognized in the acknowledgments.

## STRUCTURE OF A SCIENTIFIC MANUSCRIPT

Most biomedical journals have a set structure in the way they wish information to be presented in their articles. In general, individual sections include the Title, Abstract, Introduction, Materials and Methods, Results, Discussion, Acknowledgments, and References—but authors should always consult the journal's Instructions for Authors (sometimes known as Guidelines for Authors) for specific information before writing their papers. These guidelines are now almost invariably available online at the journal's website. The journal's written guidelines will also include submission instructions, information about creating tables and figures, information about ethical policies, how to obtain permission to use copyrighted materials, cost of publication, and authorship changes. Some journals have manuscript checklists as a courtesy for their authors. Journals also require that authors use certain published style guides when creating the text, such as *The Chicago Manual of Style* or the *American Medical Association Manual of Style*. A list of the most-frequently used guides appears at the end of this chapter.

In planning the writing of the manuscript, it's useful to consider its expected overall length. Typically, the Methods, Results, and Discussion sections of an original article, which does not include the title and abstract pages, or pages devoted to references, tables and figures, are about 15 to 20 double-spaced pages of text (~3,000–3,500 words).

### Title

The title of the paper should clearly indicate the paper's content in as few words as possible. Some journals restrict the number of characters that can be included in the main title; some may not allow a subtitle. In general, the use of active verbs should be avoided and as many descriptive nouns as possible should be used (because many journals pull out the nouns for subject indexing). A tone of objectivity in the title is also desirable. Phrases such as "A study of..." should be avoided. Some authors use the title to indicate the overall purpose of the study (4) while others prefer to state what they consider to be the most important finding (5).

## Abstracts

An abstract should be viewed as a mini-version of the paper (6). The abstract must state concisely what was done and why, what was found (in terms of data), and what was concluded. Most journals require abstracts give at least the following key information:

- Introduction or Background: The abstract introduction should answer the question "Why is this study important?" It should be brief and concise and should include a one-sentence description of the research question or hypothesis that was tested.
- Methods: The methods section of the abstract should describe the study design, who was studied, what was measured, and how the data were analyzed. It should include information about where the volunteers came from and how they were selected. It is also important to specify the number of volunteers, by group if appropriate. All important measurement techniques should be described.
- Results: The results section of the abstract should describe the main findings of the study. When possible, quantitative data and not just qualitative descriptions should be included. The variability of the data (standard deviation or standard error of the mean) and statistics should be included, if available, to permit the reader to gauge the significance of the findings.
- Conclusions: This section of the abstract is meant to tell what the results mean. Its best to not repeat the results in slightly different words, but to instead use concise sentences to *interpret* how the results are important or insightful.

Some journals require so-called "structured abstracts" (7,8), especially for clinical articles and require authors to explicitly state the objective, basic research design, clinical setting, participants, interventions (if any), main outcome measurements, results, and conclusions. The intent of this structure is to facilitate peer review before publication, to assist the readership, and to allow more precise computerized literature searches (7).

Most journals strictly limit the number of words allowed in an abstract. The reason is that many published abstracts are available through computerized searches, but usually only for the first 250 words. The word limit is generally listed in the journal's author instructions and it is important to keep to that limit or the manuscript could be returned for correction before it even has a chance to be reviewed. In the abstract, it is not necessary to provide references to other work.

## Introduction

The introduction has two functions; one is to awaken the reader's interest and the other is to be informative enough to prepare readers, whether or not they are specialists in the field, to understand the paper (9). The ideal introduction is brief (approximately 1–2 double-spaced typewritten pages) and usually includes background material, a statement about the purpose of the study, and some references to previous work (by the authors or others) that support the study's importance or relevance. A critical error that junior investigators often make is to fail to include an explicit statement of the specific research hypothesis or research question in the introduction. This omission requires the readers or reviewers to figure out for themselves why the study was performed. If they are confused or wrong, they may reject the manuscript because, in their view, the results do not answer the hypothesis.

When writing the introduction (and indeed, all sections of the manuscript), it can be useful to keep in mind what a reviewer might ask when evaluating the manuscript. For example (10):

- Did the authors indicate why the study was undertaken?
- Was a specific hypothesis tested?
- Was the background information provided adequate to understand the aims of the study?

## Materials and Methods

In this section, the reader should be told what type of study was done (the design), who or what was studied (which research volunteers were recruited, what biologic materials were obtained), what was measured (which variables were chosen), and how the data were analyzed (3). The methods section (as well as other sections after the introduction) are usually written in the past tense (because after all, the study occurred at some time in the past) and consists of detailed descriptions of human subjects and other material (for example, blood or urine samples) that were used in the studies (with a statement that approval was obtained from the appropriate institutional review board); a description of the protocol (including the variables measured);

descriptions of the apparatus, chemicals, or other preparations employed; and any drugs used. The eligibility criteria for human research volunteers should be specified. Details of any randomization procedure should be given. The number of dropouts should be identified, if relevant, to give the reader a sense of the real conditions under which the data were collected and potential bias in the data set. Methods for blinding observers and eliminating bias during the analysis of results should be described.

A description of the statistical methods used (e.g., analysis of variance) should come at the end of this section. The computer programs used, as well as any nonstandard designs or applications, should be referenced.

Most journals strictly prohibit duplicate publication (i.e., the reporting of the same results in more than one journal) because research reports are characterized as "original" and not as "duplicates." However, it is not unusual for authors to include some material that overlaps with a previously published report. For instance, data from normal human volunteers may at times serve as control data for more than one study. When and if such overlap occurs, it is critically important that the editors of the journal be informed and that a statement describing the overlap, if allowed by the journal, be included in the methods section.

A journal's manuscript reviewers may be asked whether the methods section adequately answers the following questions (10):

- Were the methods described in sufficient detail for others to repeat or extend the study?
- If standard methods were used, were adequate references given?
- If methods were modified, were the modifications described carefully?
- Have the authors indicated the reasons why particular procedures were used?
- Have the authors clearly indicated the potential problems with the methods used?
- Have the authors indicated the limitations of the methods?
- Have the sources of the drugs or other specialized materials been given?
- Have the authors specified the statistical procedures used?
- Are the statistical procedures used appropriately?

## Results

This section embodies the major scientific contribution of the manuscript. More than any other section, it is likely to receive the most scrutiny by those the authors most want to read the paper. The narrative should proceed in a logical sequence (not necessarily representing the temporal sequence in which the data were actually acquired). In planning this section, it is useful to first create the figures and tables that will accompany the manuscript, and to place them in an order that will eventually allow the reader to understand (and hopefully, accept!) the final conclusions. Typically, the final figure or table is the most important, containing the key piece of information that supports the main conclusion of the study. Preceding figures, tables, and the narrative within the results section should be presented in a sequence that naturally and logically builds toward this goal.

Long lists of data in the narrative should be avoided (if necessary, these can be included in tables, an appendix, or in an online supplement); instead, representative examples should be discussed. In addition, data shown in tables or illustrated in figures (e.g., group means and standard deviations for a variable) should not be specified in the text. Rather, the main finding should be described (for example, "blood pressure fell significantly after group X received drug Y [Figure Z]").

If the study involves the use of an experimental intervention, it's important to note whether any complications occurred, and whether any data were obtained pertaining to protocol safety.

As with the other sections, the journal's reviewers will be asked whether the manuscript adequately answers questions such as the following about the study's results (10):

- Were the experiments done appropriately with respect to the objectives of the study?
- Do the results obtained make sense?
- Are the data in the figures clear?
- Do the legends to the figures clearly describe the data shown?
- Are the data presented in tabular form clear?
- Are the legends to the tables clear?
- Has appropriate statistical analysis been performed on the data?

## Discussion

The overall purpose of the discussion is to provide additional explication of the results and to provide a balanced context within which the results may be understood. Typically, this section begins with a statement or statements as to what are the main findings of the study. Next, technical or other methodologic issues are addressed, as necessary, especially if there is the possibility that these may have biased the results. In writing this portion of the discussion, the authors are expected to defend their choices and decisions about methodologic approach, but are also expected to honestly consider how the results may be limited by these same choices. In experimental studies, a discussion of the safety of the protocol, the nature of any complications, and the implication they may have for future use of the intervention should be included. The results themselves should be discussed relative to the already existing literature. Supportive studies may be mentioned, but more important are studies that appear to contradict the results of the authors' study. Though authors should resist the temptation to write the equivalent of a review article (i.e., an exhaustive analysis of the relevant literature), current and widely quoted articles should be included. The discussion section often ends with some speculation about the implications of the study's results. It is wise to keep such speculation under control and to limit inferences to those that are most likely to have an immediate impact. Finally, the researcher may wish to restate the key conclusions in the sentences that end the discussion section.

The following questions are usually considered by a journal's reviewers (10):

- Were the objectives of the study met?
- Did the authors discuss their results in relation to available information?
- Do the authors indulge in needless speculation?
- If the results obtained were statistically significant, were they also biologically significant?
- If the objectives were not met, do the authors have any explanation?
- Do the authors adequately interpret their data?
- Do the authors discuss the limitations of the methods used?
- Do the authors discuss only data presented or do they refer consistently to unpublished work?

## Acknowledgments

Contributions that need to be acknowledged, but do not justify authorship, such as general support by a department chairman, technical help, and financial or material support are described in this section of the manuscript. Financial relationships that may pose a conflict of interest such as consulting for industry-sponsored research should also be identified. People who have contributed intellectually to the paper (but who do not warrant authorship) can be named and their function described, but the authors are responsible for obtaining written permission to include their names in the manuscript because readers may infer their endorsement of the work.

## References

Accurate citations have always been important, but because most online journals now link references to the National Library of Medicine's PubMed, it's more important than ever to check author names, article titles, journal (or book) titles, and volume and page numbers. Journals provide formatting rules for their references, and these rules must be followed or the manuscript will be returned to the authors. Also, in most cases, journals do not verify reference information, so authors must do this before the manuscript is submitted, or the error will be published. Bibliography computer software, such as EndNote and Reference Manager, are helpful tools.

## Tables

Tables are used to list "hard" data that are not presented in the text. Again, it is not necessary to summarize data already given in the text. It's important that units of measure, abbreviations used, statistical tests applied to the data, or other information, be consistent with those in the narrative. Authors should strive to make each table self-explanatory so that it can be understood without having to read the text in the results section.

## Figures

Figures can be used to summarize and emphasize important findings. The type of figure that is chosen can help illustrate the points that are being made (bar graph or regression plot, for example). As with tables, each figure together with its figure legend should be fully self-explanatory. In general, it is unusual for a single manuscript to have more than 6–10 figures, and some journals actually require advance approval for figures above a set limit. Color is often desirable in a figure, and sometimes essential to its interpretation (for example, histologic slides), but journals may charge the authors hundreds of dollars (literally!) to reproduce each color figure.

## SUGGESTIONS FOR WRITING WELL

It should go without saying that writing clearly is an important goal, to ensure that the readers of the manuscript understand the intended message, but also to clarify one's own thinking (9). Many junior investigators are surprised to discover that during the writing process, as the direction of thought changes, there may be "an answer to a slightly different question from the one that [was] asked in the beginning of the research" (9). As the investigator is writing, this evolution of thought may expose lapses in logic and inconsistencies that will stimulate the writer to rethink what is meant.

Paragraphs should each begin with a topic sentence. Avoid "medspeak"—the use of complex words and phrases when simple ones will do. Examples include symptomatology instead of symptoms, prior to instead of before, and subsequent instead of after (11). Depersonalizing human research volunteers or participants by calling them cases or subjects should also be avoided.

Abbreviations are much loved by authors and often loathed by readers. Although some journals provide a list of abbreviations at the beginning of each article, most do not. Because many readers do not read an article from beginning to end but instead skip from one section to another (say, from abstract to results to methods to discussion), identifying the meaning of an abbreviation can be an exercise in frustration. Good advice is to limit abbreviations to a few at most, and to use standard abbreviations that are already widely understood by the readership whenever possible.

A similar issue is the naming of discrete experimental groups. Terms such as "Group 1" or "Group A" should be avoided; instead, more descriptive terms (such as, Controls or Drug A) should be used.

Finally, it's important of course to proofread for errors in spelling, grammar, and punctuation.

## SUBMITTING THE MANUSCRIPT

Before submitting the manuscript, the lead author should have all coauthors review the data for accuracy. Some journals also insist on signed documentation that all authors have read and approved of the manuscript's contents. It also helps to have other colleagues look at the paper critically so that problems can be caught before the review process. Most biomedical journals require that a cover letter accompany the manuscript. This letter provides an opportunity for the corresponding author to summarize the manuscript's key points. The letter should be brief and courteous and, most importantly, should contain the correct contact information for the corresponding author. Most journals also accept recommendations for possible reviewers and also consider requests to have certain reviewers excluded if there is a concern about possible bias. Many journals have a preset format for the letter that is available at their website.

## ONLINE SUBMISSION

Many journals now require that manuscripts be submitted electronically instead of by standard mail. This speeds the submission and review process, and makes it easier for authors to track the status of their papers. Online submission usually requires a confidential "User ID" and "Password" that is created by the author, and authors are usually notified by e-mail of the decision. Some journals supply templates for authors to follow when submitting their papers. Details can always be found in the Instructions for Authors at the journal's website.

## PEER REVIEW

Peer review is the process by which scientific articles are evaluated and selected for publication. Most manuscripts that are submitted to biomedical journals are evaluated by two or three "reviewers," also known as "referees," that are chosen within the author's field of study. At best, it takes two to three weeks for a decision to be made, but sometimes it can take longer depending on the number of referees, whether the referees are immediately available, and whether the editor decides that additional review is necessary. In general, the decision status ranges from "accepted" to "rejected," with "accepted with minor revisions," or "accepted with major revisions" as intermediate (but more common) levels of status. The journal can also decide whether to reject the manuscript outright without review if its content is more appropriate for another journal. It is rare indeed for a paper to be accepted without revision. The rejection rate may range from 50 to 90% of all manuscripts submitted to the journal.

## REVISING THE MANUSCRIPT

Reviewers and editors aren't always diplomatic in their critiques, but authors should resist the urge to be defensive or angry when responding to comments. Journals do not edit author responses, and revised manuscripts are usually returned to the original reviewers and editors for evaluation. The best strategy is to plan a response to each criticism. If it is appropriate to alter the manuscript according to the reviewer's suggestions, then the change should be made and acknowledged in the cover letter that will accompany the revision, even if the change is a simple correction of a typographical error. In the case where an author disagrees with the reviewer, a straightforward rebuttal should be included. Authors should avoid the temptation to engage in a prolonged argument over a single point. Authors invariably lose such arguments. Either the case is compelling or it is not.

## ACCEPTED MANUSCRIPTS

Once the manuscript is accepted, two things typically happen:

1. An approved PDF version is posted on the journal's website (often within 48 hours).
2. A copy of the accepted manuscript is sent to the journal's copy editors, who will then send

the copyedited version to a compositor for typesetting.

The compositor creates a page proof that will be sent to the authors, usually by e-mail. Authors are required to return proofs quickly, often within two to three days, or publication of the article may be delayed. After the proof is approved, the article is paginated into an issue of the journal, final corrections are made, and the files go to a printer that produces the bound journal for distribution.

## COPYRIGHT

Most biomedical journals require that authors sign a "copyright transfer" or "copyright release" form when submitting a manuscript, which turns ownership of the manuscript (and the information within) over to the journal. Copyright is a form of protection provided by the laws of the United States (title 17, U.S. Code) to the authors of "original works of authorship," including scientific, literary, dramatic, musical, artistic, and other certain intellectual works. This protection is available to both published and unpublished works and in the case of a biomedical article, gives the copyright owner exclusive rights to reproduce the work in copies and to prepare derivative works based on the original work. Any or all of the copyright owner's exclusive rights or any subdivision of those rights may be transferred, but the transfer of exclusive rights is not valid unless that transfer is in writing and is signed by the owner of the rights conveyed. Detailed information about copyright is contained at the website of the U.S. Copyright Office (http://www.copyright.gov/).

## EMBARGO POLICIES

Many journals have strict embargo policies that prohibit publication of a research report if the results of the study have already been disclosed to the media in any form. An exception is the presentation of material at a scientific meeting. Journals that have such policies will provide them in detail on their website.

## UNIFORM REQUIREMENTS FOR MANUSCRIPTS SUBMITTED TO BIOMEDICAL JOURNALS

In January 1978, a group of editors from several major biomedical journals met in Vancouver, British Columbia, and decided on uniform technical requirements for manuscripts to be submitted to their journals. These requirements, including formats for bibliographic references developed for what became known as the "Vancouver group" by the National Library of Medicine, were published in three

of the journals early in 1979. The Vancouver group later evolved into the International Committee of Medical Journal Editors (ICMJE) and the result was the Uniform Requirements for Manuscripts Submitted to Biomedical Journals. The Structured Abstract format referred to previously is one consequence of this group's deliberations.

## STANDARDS FOR REPORTING BIOMEDICAL RESEARCH

Many biomedical journals now require that their submitted papers conform to various standards by using checklists and flow diagrams that have been developed to improve the quality of reporting research results. The CONSORT (Consolidated Standards of Reporting Trials) statement (Table 29–1) and STARD (Standards for Reporting of Diagnostic Accuracy) (Table 29–2) are two such tools that have been adopted by many journals that report the results of clinical research. If a journal requires the use of either of these standards, it will be included in the journal's Instructions to Authors at their website.

### Consort

The CONSORT statement takes an evidence-based approach to improve the quality of reports of randomized trials (http://www.consort-statement.org/statement/revisedstatement.htm). Its critical value to researchers, health care providers, peer reviewers, journal editors, and health policy makers is the guarantee of integrity in the reported results of research. CONSORT comprises a checklist and flow diagram to provide a standard way for researchers to report trials. The checklist includes items, based on evidence, that need to be addressed in the report; the flow diagram provides readers with a clear picture of the progress of all participants in the trial, from the time they are randomized until the end of their involvement. The intent is to make the experimental process clearer, flawed or not, so that users of the data can more appropriately evaluate its validity for their purposes.

### Stard

STARD includes a 25-item checklist (http://www.consort-statement.org/stardstatement.htm). A prototypical flow diagram was developed, which provides information about the method of patient recruitment, the order of test execution and the numbers of patients undergoing the test under evaluation, the reference standard or both. The objective of STARD is to improve the quality of reporting of studies on diagnostic accuracy by using a checklist and flow

**TABLE 29-1**

**Consolidated Standards of Reporting Trials (CONSORT) checklist of items to include when reporting a randomized trial**

| PAPER SECTION AND TOPIC | Item | Description | Reported on Page # |
|---|---|---|---|
| *TITLE & ABSTRACT* | 1 | How participants were allocated to interventions (e.g., "random allocation," "randomized," or "randomly assigned"). | |
| *INTRODUCTION* Background | 2 | Scientific background and explanation of rationale. | |
| | | *METHODS* | |
| Participants | 3 | Eligibility criteria for participants and the settings and locations where the data were collected. | |
| Interventions | 4 | Precise details of the interventions intended for each group and how and when they were actually administered. | |
| Objectives | 5 | Specific objectives and hypotheses. | |
| Outcomes | 6 | Clearly defined primary and secondary outcome measures and, when applicable, any methods used to enhance the quality of measurements (e.g., multiple observations, training of assessors). | |
| Sample size | 7 | How sample size was determined and, when applicable, explanation of any interim analyses and stopping rules. | |
| Randomization— Sequence generation | 8 | Method used to generate the random allocation sequence, including details of any restrictions (e.g., blocking, stratification). | |
| Randomization— Allocation concealment | 9 | Method used to implement the random allocation sequence (e.g., numbered containers or central telephone), clarifying whether the sequence was concealed until interventions were assigned. | |
| Randomization— Implementation | 10 | Who generated the allocation sequence, who enrolled participants, and who assigned participants to their groups. | |
| Blinding (masking) | 11 | Whether or not participants, those administering the interventions, and those assessing the outcomes were blinded to group assignment. When relevant, how the success of blinding was evaluated. | |
| Statistical methods | 12 | Statistical methods used to compare groups for primary outcome(s); methods for additional analyses, such as subgroup analyses and adjusted analyses. | |
| | | RESULTS | |
| Participant flow | 13 | Flow of participants through each stage (a diagram is strongly recommended). Specifically, for each group report the numbers of participants randomly assigned, receiving intended treatment, completing the study protocol, and analyzed for the primary outcome. Describe protocol deviations from study as planned, together with reasons. | |
| Recruitment | 14 | Dates defining the periods of recruitment and follow-up. | |
| Baseline data | 15 | Baseline demographic and clinical characteristics of each group. | |
| Numbers analyzed | 16 | Number of participants (denominator) in each group included in each analysis and whether the analysis was by "intention-to-treat." State the results in absolute numbers when feasible (e.g., 10/20, not 50%). | |

*(Continued)*

## TABLE 29–1 (Continued)

**Consolidated Standards of Reporting Trials (CONSORT) checklist of items to include when reporting a randomized trial**

| PAPER SECTION AND TOPIC | Item | Description | Reported on Page # |
|---|---|---|---|
| Outcomes and estimation | 17 | For each primary and secondary outcome, a summary of results for each group, and the estimated effect size and its precision (e.g., 95% confidence interval). | |
| Ancillary analyses | 18 | Address multiplicity by reporting any other analyses performed, including subgroup analyses and adjusted analyses, indicating those prespecified and those exploratory. | |
| Adverse events | 19 | All important adverse events or side effects in each intervention group. | |

For the complete CONSORT table, visit http://www.consort-statement.org/statement/revisedstatement.htm

diagram. Complete and accurate reporting allows the reader to detect the potential for bias in the study and to evaluate the general application of the results. The STARD statement with the checklist and flow diagram has been published in several journals including: *Clinical Chemistry*, *Annals of Internal Medicine*, *Radiology*, *BMJ*, *Lancet*, *American Journal of Clinical Pathology*, *Clinical Biochemistry*, and *Clinical Chemistry and Laboratory Medicine*.

## ONLINE PUBLISHING VERSUS PAPER PUBLISHING

Most journals now present accepted manuscripts on their websites within 72 hours of acceptance, and journal offices do not copyedit the text before it goes online. Instead, a copy of the accepted manuscript is loaded onto the website in the standardized portable document format (PDF). In most cases, references are formatted so that they are directly linked to PubMed; therefore, it is important for authors to make sure that the bibliographic information is correct. Articles are usually citable through the use of a Digital Object Identifier (DOI) number. DOI is a system for identifying and exchanging intellectual property in the digital environment and it is managed and directed by the International DOI Foundation. More information on DOI can be found at their website (http://www.doi.org/).

Many journals, in an effort to publish more articles by limiting the overall length of each article, now allow authors to also submit additional information to the journal's online repository. In addition to additional details about methods, these repositories may also include movie clips or other material that won't reproduce well in a print format. Again, details are always available through the journal's website.

## OPEN ACCESS

There is a growing movement among some scientists to offer free access to published research. These individuals believe that open access to research is central to rapid and efficient progress in science. The following is the Bethesda Statement on Open Access Publishing (June 20, 2003):

*An Open Access Publication is one that meets the following two conditions: The author(s) and copyright holder(s) grant(s) to all users a free, irrevocable, worldwide, perpetual right of access to, and a license to copy, use, distribute, transmit and display the work publicly and to make and distribute derivative works, in any digital medium for any responsible purpose, subject to proper attribution of authorship, as well as the right to make small numbers of printed copies for their personal use. A complete version of the work and all supplemental materials, including a copy of the permission as stated above, in a suitable standard electronic format is deposited immediately upon initial publication in at least one online repository that is supported by an academic institution, scholarly society, government agency, or other well-established organization that seeks to enable open access, unrestricted distribution, interoperability, and long-term archiving (for the biomedical sciences, PubMed Central is such a repository).*

## TABLE 29–2

**Standards for Reporting of Diagnostic Accuracy (STARD) checklist of items to improve the reporting of studies on diagnostic accuracy**

| Section and Topic | Item | Describe | Reported on Page # |
|---|---|---|---|
| TITLE/ABSTRACT/ KEYWORDS | 1 | The article as a study on diagnostic accuracy (recommend MeSH heading "sensitivity and specificity"). | |
| INTRODUCTION | 2 | The research question(s), such as estimating diagnostic accuracy or comparing accuracy between tests or across participant groups. | |
| | | METHODS | |
| *Participants* | 3 | The study population: the inclusion and exclusion criteria, setting(s) and location(s) where the data were collected. | |
| | 4 | Participant recruitment: was this based on presenting symptoms, results from previous tests, or the fact that the participants had received the index test(s) or the reference standard? | |
| | 5 | Participant sampling: was this a consecutive series of patients defined by selection criteria in (3) and (4)? If not, specify how patients were further selected. | |
| | 6 | Data collection: were the participants identified and data collected before the index test(s) and reference standards were performed (prospective study) or after (retrospective study)? | |
| *Reference standard* | 7 | The reference standard and its rationale. | |
| *Test methods* | 8 | Technical specification of material and methods involved including how and when measurements were taken, and/or cite references for index test(s) and reference standard. | |
| | 9 | Definition and rationale for the units, cutoffs, and/or categories of the results of the index test(s) and the reference standard. | |
| | 10 | The number, training and expertise of the persons (a) executing and (b) reading the index test(s) and the reference standard. | |
| | 11 | Whether or not the reader(s) of the index test(s) and reference standard were blind (masked) to the results of the other test(s) and describe any information available to them. | |
| *Statistical methods* | 12 | Methods for calculating measures of diagnostic accuracy or making comparisons, and the statistical methods used to quantify uncertainty (e.g., 95% confidence intervals). | |
| | 13 | Methods for calculating test reproducibility, if done. | |
| | | RESULTS | |
| *Participants* | 14 | When study was done, including beginning and ending dates of recruitment. | |
| | 15 | Clinical and demographic characteristics (e.g., age, sex, spectrum of presenting symptom(s), comorbidity, current treatment(s), recruitment center). | |
| | 16 | How many participants satisfying the criteria for inclusion did or did not undergo the index test and/or the reference standard; describe why participants failed to receive either test (a flow diagram is strongly recommended). | |

## TABLE 29–2 (Continued)

**Standards for Reporting of Diagnostic Accuracy (STARD) checklist of items to improve the reporting of studies on diagnostic accuracy**

| Section and Topic | Item | Describe | Reported on Page # |
|---|---|---|---|
| *Reference standard* | 17 | Time interval and any treatment administered between index and reference standard. | |
| | 18 | Distribution of severity of disease (define criteria) in those with the target condition; describe other diagnoses in participants without the target condition. | |
| *Test results* | 19 | A cross-tabulation of the results of the index test(s) by the results of the reference standard; for continuous results, the distribution of the test results by the results of the reference standard. | |
| | 20 | Indeterminate results, missing responses and outliers of index test(s) stratified by reference standard result and how they were handled. | |
| | 21 | Adverse events of index test(s) and reference standard. | |
| *Estimation* | 22 | Estimates of diagnostic accuracy and measures of statistical uncertainty (e.g., 95% confidence intervals). | |
| | 23 | Estimates of variability of diagnostic accuracy between subgroups of participants, readers or centers, if done. | |
| | 24 | Measures of test reproducibility, if done. | |
| DISCUSSION | 25 | The clinical applicability of the study findings. | |

http://www.consort-statement.org/stardstatement.htm

A list of open access journals can be found at the Directory of Open Access Journals (DOAJ) website (http://www.doaj.org).

## SUMMARY

- Investigators about to publish their research should browse through a few issues of candidate journals to find out who is on the editorial board. It may also be useful to study journal statistics, such as acceptance rates, rates of processing, and types of manuscripts received. The advice of a mentor or respected colleague is almost always valuable.
- The research question that is to be answered by the information provided within the manuscript should be stated explicitly in the abstract and introduction sections of the manuscript.
- The article should be written according to the journal's Instructions for Authors. Specific standards such as CONSORT or STARD should be met. All data and references within the manuscript should be double-checked for accuracy.
- The text should be written clearly with correct use of paragraphing, grammar, spelling, and punctuation.
- If a revision is required, pay close attention to reviewer comments and respond with diplomatic clarity. Each concern raised by the reviewers should be addressed explicitly in a cover letter accompanying the revised manuscript.

## REFERENCES

1. Sly RM. How to present data for publication. Ann Allergy 1993;70:343–346.
2. Klein KP. The publication process at biomedical journals. Reston, VA: Council of Science Editors, Guidelines, 1999.
3. Browner WS. Publishing and Presenting Clinical Research. Baltimore: Lippincott, Williams & Wilkins, 1999.

4. Sandham JD, Hull RD, Brant RF et al. A randomized, controlled trial of the use of pulmonary-artery catheters in high-risk surgical patients. N Engl J Med 2003;348:5–14.

5. Gustavson SM, Chu CA, Nishizawa B et al. Glucagon's actions are modified by the combination of epinephrine and gluconeogenic precursor infusion. Am J Physiol Endocrinol Metab 2003;285:E534–44.

6. Day RA. How to Write & Publish a Scientific Paper. 5th Ed. Phoenix: Oryx,1998.

7. Haynes RB, Mulrow CD, Huth EJ et al. More informative abstracts revisited. Ann Intern Med 1990;113:69–76.

8. Bindman AB, Osmond D, Hecht FM et al. Multistate evaluation of anonymous HIV testing and access to medical care. JAMA 1998;280:1416–1420.

9. Zeiger M. Essentials of Writing Biomedical Research Papers 2nd Ed. San Francisco: McGraw-Hill, 2000.

10. Rangachari PK, Mierson S. A checklist to help students analyze published articles in basic medical sciences. Adv Physiol Educ 1995;268:S21–S25.

11. Christy NP. Sounding board: English is our second language. N Engl J Med 1979;300:979–981.

## SUGGESTED READINGS

American Medical Association Manual of Style. 9th Ed. Baltimore: Lippincott, Williams and Wilkins, 1998.

University of Chicago Press. The Chicago Manual of Style, 15th Ed. Chicago: Author, 2003.

Scientific Style and Format: The CBE Manual for Authors, Editors, and Publishers, 6th Ed. New York: Cambridge University Press, 1994.

Strunk Jr. W et al. The Elements of Style, 4th Ed. Needham Heights: Longman, 2000.

Browner, WS. Publishing and Presenting Clinical Research. Philadelphia: Lippincott Williams & Wilkins, 1999.

St. James, D. Writing and Speaking for Excellence: A Guide for Physicians. Boston: Jones & Bartlett, 1996.

Council of Biology Editors. Illustrating Science: Standards for Publication. Guidelines Series. Restin, VA: Author, 1998.

# CHAPTER 30

# Visual Presentation of Data

Vicki M. Friedman, Marcy H. Hartstein,
Andrea J. Myles, Lauren M. Rohde

Having spent an enormous amount of time planning, conducting, and analyzing a study, it only makes sense to invest additional time to plan a coherent scientific presentation of the study's results, be it a slide or poster presentation, at a departmental seminar or a national society meeting. Carefully gathered content, with an eye for aesthetics and clarity, maximizes understanding, increasing the likelihood that the material will be admired and remembered. Without such attention, it can just as easily be misunderstood and forgotten. No single presentation can satisfy all audiences and all levels of expertise—just as different methods have to be used to persuade peers or the reviewers for a grant, different techniques should be crafted for presentations as the audience varies. This chapter focuses on how to formulate the most visually effective and professional presentations.

## PRACTICAL FACTORS TO CONSIDER BEFORE CREATING A SLIDE PRESENTATION

Just like any statement or assertion, a presentation should have a goal. For example, presentations are used to inform, entertain, persuade, or some combination of these elements. Informative presentations tend to be heavy in monotonous data and statistics; they require an artistic layout and extra consideration to maintain audience interest when presenting quantitative data. Persuasive presentations often use quantitative data as a premise for changing attitudes or to elicit some action from the audience. Entertaining presentations have more levity and often use cartoons or similar presentation devices to elicit a more lighthearted response

(Table 30–1). Obviously, a single presentation might involve more than one category.

To develop these points more fully, we'll use a common example: a new faculty member presenting data at a large international conference. The goal is to inform the audience of new findings and to persuade them that the approach used is novel and scientifically sound. Because the aims are to inform and persuade, special attention needs to be paid to quantitative data.

As a first rule, graphs and figures should be consistent in color scheme, data formatting, and captioning (Figure 30–1). This uniformity allows the audience to focus on the data, not the style of each slide, which can otherwise easily distract the audience from the content and message of the presentation.

The next step is to identify the audience (Figure 30–2). Several audience factors to consider are the size, age or attention span, and knowledge base of the audience. A large audience often implies a large auditorium, which demands larger fonts and careful attention to (or removal of) paragraphs of plain text and small diagrams. Moreover, a large or dark auditorium demands greater color contrast between the foreground (fonts, diagrams) and the background. Audience age affects the presentation of data much the same way; an older audience will have trouble with small or poorly contrasted fonts as well as fast-moving text or pictures. Audience knowledge base affects the visual presentation of the content as much as it affects the content itself. Some diagrams or call-outs are common with certain expert audiences and appear regularly in textbooks or everyday lives. Using such diagrams can help expert audiences identify immediately with the data; in contrast, more amateur audiences can become alienated from such presentations.

## TABLE 30-1

### The Three Main Categories of Presentations

| | GOAL | |
|---|---|---|
| **Inform** | **Persuade** | **Entertain** |
| • Monotonous data/statistics | • Quantitative data | • More levity, e.g., cartoons |

In our example, the new faculty member is presenting to a large audience of experts. As a consequence, careful attention should be given to diagrams that represent state-of-the-art information in the given field of expertise. When possible, shapes, colors, and format of what might be considered classic visuals in the chosen field should be emulated. Moreover, the presenter probably should not focus too much time on the exposition or motivation for the research, as experts can be assumed to be already familiar with such information.

Another audience factor to consider is the time allotted for the presentation (often anywhere from 10 to 60 minutes); presentation length should be a powerful determinant of the number of slides used as well as the explanation allowed for each slide. Rushing or drudging through slides can cause the audience to become confused or bored. The visuals of a presentation should flow intuitively, like a speech. Each slide should be a new thought or sentence, and it should complement the vocals as such.

Ideally, before starting on the design or implementation of a presentation, technical and physical information about the presentation room and the equipment available should be known. The size and lighting of the room may be factors that should affect slide design. The presentation program software used (when slides are to be shown digitally, as with Power-Point®) can also have an impact on how the slides

should be designed. Various versions of PowerPoint display slides differently; that is, the animation, slide delay functions, and other aspects vary enough that the presenter should design (or at least preview) the slides on a workstation with the same PowerPoint version to be used during the presentation.

## ARTISTIC FACTORS TO CONSIDER WHEN DESIGNING A PRESENTATION

Artistic guidelines for creating an effective presentation aim to keep the audience connected with the presentation by appropriately accentuating key components of the gathered material. Effectively designed slides that appeal to the audience and complement the material should elicit favorable audience responses. By contrast, flashy presentation components that work against the material might make the audience admire the slides more for their look than their content.

A number of basic design principles should be considered for each and every slide. These guidelines affect which media (if any) will be used, how the slides will be laid out, and the typefaces and colors used (Table 30–2).

## TABLE 30-2

### Samples of Basic Design Principles

| Consistency | Balance and Composition | Color Choice |
|---|---|---|
| • Background color | • Amount of information | • Contrast |
| • Typeface formatting | • Simplicity | • Brightness |
| • Color scheme | | • Highlights |

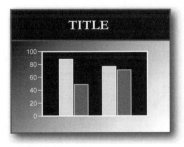 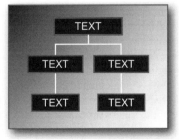

*FIGURE 30–1* ● Example of consistency within a presentation. The graph and the diagram share similar background, color scheme, and simplicity.

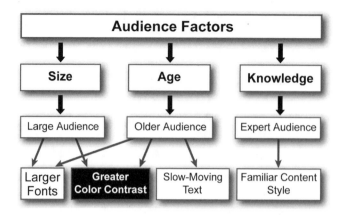

**FIGURE 30–2** ● Diagram of audience factors to consider in preparing a presentation. Size, age, and knowledge base demand sensitivity to each group.

*Consistency* in the visuals makes the slides flow more seamlessly from one to the next. Inconsistency, on the other hand, creates a disjointed and confusing presentation. Especially aspects such as background color, typeface formatting, and the way important concepts are emphasized should not vary without very good reason. When used consistently, the hierarchy and colors used in titles, subtitles, and bulleted points can create a mental map for the audience that helps guide them through the material.

*Balance* and *composition* in a slide is similar to composition in a sentence. If a sentence is too minimal, it fails to advance the argument; a convoluted sentence may be impossible to understand. Slides function in much the same way: the amount of information allowed on each slide will help keep the presentation assertive without being convoluted.

*Color choice* can affect both the professionalism and readability of the slides. Contrasting the background color with the foreground (diagrams, fonts) helps readability, as long as the colors vary in brightness and complement one another. Overlaying red on green or vice versa, regardless of brightness, can cause eye strain. Color is an excellent tool for highlighting important points and organizing contrasting information, but when used unnecessarily, especially within a single slide, can distract the audience and take away from the gravity or logic of the arguments.

Aside from choosing complementary colors for fonts, the *size* and *typeface* are also very important (Table 30–3). Often, presenters squeeze too much information onto a single slide and reduce the font size so everything fits neatly despite being difficult to read. If the material is difficult to read for the person designing the slides from a few steps back

from the monitor, the audience will have the same difficulty. In this situation, the only solution is to increase the font size and either adjust the remaining material accordingly or break it into multiple slides. Another helpful hint is to keep the presentation consistent with the way information is presented in people's everyday lives; namely, font size can be used as a tool to organize which headings embody others. This is a common tactic in media such as newspapers, websites, or posters, and people grow to expect information organized as such for better understanding.

The most important consideration when choosing the typefaces for slides is readability. An elaborate or unconventional font will distract the audience from the material, or in many cases, hinder their ability to read it at all. After considering readability, there are other decisions to make. Traditional fonts are either *serif* or *sans serif*. In general, serif fonts such as Times New Roman are used for text-heavy documents with complete paragraphs (i.e., any newspaper and almost every novel and textbook); they help the eye identify the important parts of a letter. Sans serif fonts

## TABLE 30–3

### Chart Exhibiting Font Usage

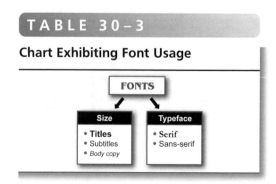

such as Arial are generally used for headings, large titles, tables, and call-outs in a diagram. If a paragraph of formatted block text is to be included (often a bad idea for a slide), a serif font is the best choice. Otherwise, sans serif is more pleasing to the eye.

## THE COMPOSITION OF THE PRESENTATION

How should slides be arranged for maximum effectiveness? A few rules of content and continuity that apply to any form of public speaking; digital presentations are no exception.

A common rule of thumb is to (1) tell the audience what is going to be discussed, (2) discuss it, and (3) then tell them what has just been discussed. For a digital slide show, this means including a title slide, an overview slide, and a conclusion slide (Figure 30–3). The title and overview slides do more than just tell the audience what content to expect—they set an expectation for a particular artistic style and slide format. It should be an accurate representation of the way information is to be presented and, as such, should affect the rest of the presentation's design.

The title slide should not expound on any of the points to be made in the rest of the presentation; similar to a report cover, it should contain simply the title, the presenter's name, the represented institution, and any appropriate institutional or other logos and colors. The main content slides that house the study's premises, data, and conclusions come after the overview slide.

A helpful strategy is to make a "master" slide that can act as a frame of reference for color, titles, subtitles, and body text. This slide is a home base of sorts from which to depart as needed; it should help the presenter develop a personalized look that can then be reused for other presentations.

The format and temporal presentation of slides presented in digital format (for example, with PowerPoint) can be different than with a normal transparency or traditional slide. For instance, the presenter can make bulleted points appear one at a time or use dynamically colored text labels to work hand in hand with the presentation. These so-called *transitions* between slides or *animations* within slides need careful thought and consideration, once again balancing judicious use that will enhance the presentation versus overuse that becomes distracting.

Optimally, this use of dynamic media can guide the audience during the verbal presentation. For instance, audiences tend to immediately read whatever is presented on a slide. Thus, an audience is likely to read an entire slide with multiple bulleted points that appear all at once although material only relevant to the first bullet is being discussed. Dynamic media can be used to highlight the current point or to hide future points, keeping the audience attuned to the verbal presentation. Likewise, if a topic or title needs an introduction, just the title of the slide can be shown before more complex content is shown.

In the case of image-heavy slides or detailed diagrams, the same rules apply. A tactic similar to showing bullets as they are discussed is to show a complex diagram by highlighting different regions of the diagram as they need to be explained. There are several effective strategies. For one, using arrows and text labels to highlight complex illustrations piece by piece is an effective technique for medical illustrations or photography. Showing a diagram in its entirety and zooming in on different regions one by one is also effective for photos and drawings, but only if each feature is easily separable and makes sense when viewed apart from context, such as an x-ray fragment. When discussing complex modular charts constructed with PowerPoint shapes, a good strategy is to overlay shapes and modules piecewise, and to discuss each feature as it is added to the view. In this way, the eyes of the audience are controlled using only artistic methods and not a laser pointer.

Reducing complexity with these strategies helps the audience stay attuned to the verbal presentation during explanatory slides, but even more of this attention should be used when data are presented. When using a pie chart or a timeline, adding pieces incrementally in tune with the narrative aids the audience in the walk-through of the process or the meaning of each component of data (Figure 30–4).

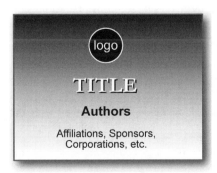

**FIGURE 30–3** ● Example of a title slide. Content incorporates the title, the presenter's name, the affiliations, corporations, and appropriate logos of the institution.

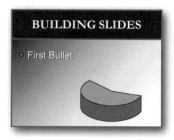
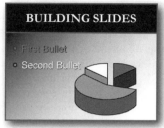
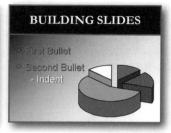

***FIGURE 30–4*** ●  Diagrams for building slides. A piece-by-piece effect in showing data will aid the audience in the meaning of each component as well as the use of highlighting type.

## SPECIAL CONSIDERATIONS FOR IMPORTING IMAGES

PowerPoint makes it easy to embed images into a presentation; it's important, however, to ensure compatibility and quality, especially with respect to file format, image complexity, image proportions, and image size, and resolution.

PowerPoint can import a variety of file formats, both with and without image compression. Both the format and compression level are factors of the exporting program, and can affect the sharpness, contrast, brightness, and saturation of the image. Most photo-editing and vector graphics suites have tools or sliders for modifying color attributes and sharpness, and it is usually a good idea to attend to these details before inserting images into Power-Point. Often, when exporting the image from a graphics application in a JPEG or GIF format, a prompt about compression will appear. Higher compression leads to a much smaller file size (and therefore faster loading), but can drastically reduce the quality of the color and sharpness. Unfortunately, there is no good rule of thumb for deciding compression level; it depends on the required complexity of the image. A good method, if possible, is to save images at different compression levels and examine each image to find the optimal compression to quality ratio.

Uncompressed or large images (e.g., TIFF files) can have an extremely large file size, which may take a noticeably long time to load during a presentation, especially on a slower computer. It can also cause flickering in slide animation or slide transition. Fortunately, PowerPoint allows image resizing within the slide design process. If after loading an image, resizing appears to be necessary, the image proportions (the ratio of height to width) and size (actual height and width) can be changed as needed. After resizing, it's a good idea to examine the image for quality; for instance, sometimes pixilation-blurring can occur, and in these cases, it pays to size the image in a more powerful graphics program.

## PRACTICAL FACTORS TO CONSIDER BEFORE CREATING A POSTER PRESENTATION

As with slide presentations, poster presentations also require careful planning and some specific information about the context and audience for the poster.

The sponsor or program coordinator for any specific poster session will usually publish specific preparation instructions (Figure 30–5). In almost all cases, these instructions include specifications for the size of board space allotted, as well as a method or materials for hanging or displaying the poster. They often also make typeface suggestions such as font size and font face. In some cases, they may include a layout plot of how the poster should be organized. In most cases, the typeface and layout suggestions are just that—suggestions. Often, its permissible to deviate from the prescribed layout as long as the basic poster components are implemented.

There are two general poster formats: traditional and one-piece. Both can be executed by an individual or by an outside company or department within most academic institutions. There are other nontraditional formats, such as computer-projections, but these will not be discussed here.

A *traditional poster* is a printout of all text, graphs, data, tables, or photos on either laser paper or photo quality paper. The print is then mounted on color boards (either with double-stick tape, glue stick, dry mount, or spray adhesive) (Figure 30–6). Some people merely print out $8 \frac{1}{2}$" $\times$ 11" pieces and mount them individually, leaving a thin $\frac{1}{2}$" aesthetic border of color around each piece. When using this method, it's useful to pick complementary colors that match or strengthen other visual elements in the poster

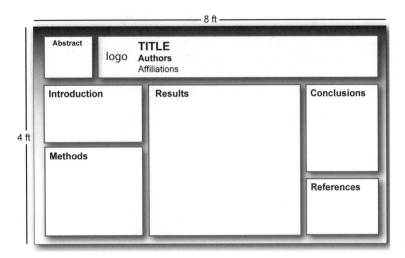

**FIGURE 30–5** ● Sample of preparation instructions for a poster session. Size is the most important factor, although the very general layout suggestions allow the opportunity to deviate from the layout.

pages. Some institutions mandate mounting board colors to emulate the colors of the institution's logo when considering borders and backgrounds.

The title of a traditional poster should be seen easily from a distance. Usually, this means that the title will stretch across a majority of the poster width. Because of the difficulty in seamlessly creating such a long "banner," some people choose to have only the title professionally executed, opposed to splicing it together with multiple smaller pages. Usually, the title is the most challenging aspect of a traditionally formatted poster.

The more professional- or current-looking method is the so-called *one-piece poster*, which is presently

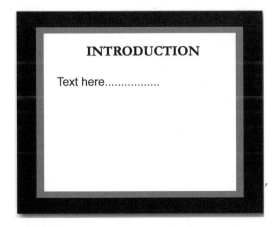

**FIGURE 30–6** ● Example of a traditional mounted poster piece. Colors can be used to reflect the institution's logo colors. Each piece of the poster is treated in a similar fashion.

the more popular method. One-piece posters are designed with a variety of computer software applications and printed out on a single large piece of paper (Figure 30–7). This allows for greater graphic options, integrated special effects, and a heightened sense of entirety. The one-piece method may even save time because fonts and images can be manipulated accurately and free of charge in digital media opposed to manipulating them after printing. Another advantage is that the poster can cover as much of the mounting surface as desired, dictated not only by the amount of information to be conveyed but also determined by the budget available for printing.

The components of a poster are dictated by the session organizer, the audience, the sponsoring organization, and, of course, the project itself. The same guidelines apply to both traditional and one-piece posters.

The *poster title* usually extends across the top length of the poster (Figure 30–8). It often includes the title of the abstract, the authors' names, and all of the necessary affiliations (universities, corporations, and sponsors). The authors' names are often presented exactly as they appear in the accepted abstract; the same applies to the affiliations. The amount of space allotted for the title should dictate how the author and organization information is formatted and what other content, if any, is included.

As seen in Figures 30–7 and 30–8, a *logo* is often included as a clean and professional design element. Logos are usually displayed in or near the title, though some posters benefit by displaying

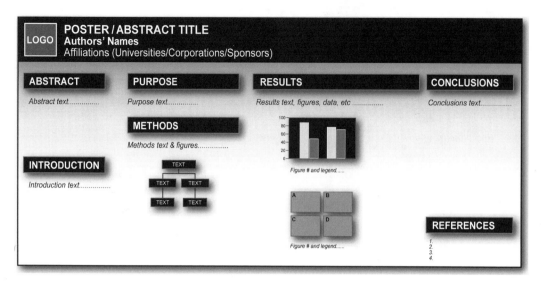

**FIGURE 30–7**  ●  Sample of a one-piece poster. As shown, this type of poster allows for greater graphic opportunities and special effects.

them in the acknowledgments or references. If more than one affiliation is listed, more than one logo may be displayed, but sometimes omitting logos altogether is the visually pleasing solution if consistency of color cannot be maintained. Institutions often have strict guidelines for logo usage, and reviewing these guidelines may not only improve the poster's consistency but avoid trouble with the institution's administration.

A conference poster almost always displays an *abstract*; some conferences are specific about its location on the poster. Some specify a given space (usually in the upper left part of the poster), and dictate how much blank room to leave for a provided printout. Some conferences simply require an abstract somewhere on the leftmost region of the poster; others will make no stringent requirements, including whether or not to include an abstract at all. Depending on space, the abstract may be printed in a smaller font size than the rest of the poster because the key information is usually presented in a more exciting manner somewhere else on the poster (as well as in a printing of the abstracts in a conference meeting booklet).

In addition to the title and abstract, several other distinct components of a poster should be considered individually: (1) Introduction, (2) Objectives, (3) Material and Methods, (4) Results, (5) Discussion, and (6) Conclusions.

Most or all of these segments will be included in any poster, but the format and method of presentation is up to the individual. Visual aids such as photos, graphs, and tables can be used to support the written text, along with headings to complement the body text and to guide the audience through the poster. Headings can be used as design elements to attract the eye to a specific section or simply to separate the section title from the text itself.

Some other poster components are usually optional, yet are included at times for completeness or legal reasons: (a) References, (b) Disclosure Statements, and (c) Acknowledgments. *References* are usually listed numerically in a common reference format. If many references are to be cited, some people print them in a smaller font size or on a separate 8.5 × 11" sheet. *Disclosure statements* and *acknowledgments* are necessary and appreciated in some instances; if used, they should be bold

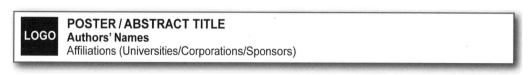

**FIGURE 30–8**  ●  Layout of title board. The length is determined by the size allocated in the specific preparation instructions. The final product can be scored and folded or rolled for transportation.

and noticeable enough to give adequate precaution and appreciation.

It's important to achieve some balance between text and figures in each section of the poster. A common rule of thumb is to minimize the text so it is still readable without compromising the effectiveness of the information or argument. An overly wordy poster will seem monotonous, while an overly sparse poster will not convey the intended message. Moreover, the font size should provide a comfortable read; that is, the text should be readable from a distance. Typically, this means 18 to 36 point type for body copy, larger for headings, and 100 point type or larger for titles. (Note that these font sizes are for the final print; smaller fonts should be used when composing the poster on a computer screen.) Images help to counter the monotony of text; they can add a splash of color and help guide the viewer's eye through the poster.

The actual typeface selection is an important consideration. Experience shows that most people use common fonts like Arial, Times New Roman, or variations therein. Occasionally, unique or uncommon fonts will be used for headings to add a fanciful design element—but the choice should be compatible with other font choices used elsewhere on the poster. In particular, all fonts should be available to the person or service printing the poster; checking with the printer regarding font choices may eliminate unpleasant surprises when the poster is delivered, especially if it's received just before leaving for the meeting.

When piecing these elements together, the overall layout of the traditional poster should be taken into consideration by grouping all the individual panel-by-panel elements together. When working with a one-piece poster, the whole poster "field" should be examined by having all the poster elements in a single working document for manipulation.

## CREATING THE ONE-PIECE POSTER

Because one-piece posters are now far more common and technologically challenging, we will use it as a vehicle to discuss steps in poster development.

Various computer *programs* can be used to create a one-piece poster; the decision about which one to use should depend on content and target output. Each program varies in tools, compatibility, user-friendliness, and output quality.

Microsoft PowerPoint is the preferred application of many investigators and illustration departments. First, PowerPoint offers excellent compatibility between client and department, and most are familiar and appreciative of its capabilities. Also, because many posters borrow figures and text from existing PowerPoint presentations, elements are easily swapped between projects. Finally, the graphic capabilities of PowerPoint are sufficient for small-scale image modification—the tools for alignment, cropping, graphing, and charting are easy to use and ample for poster formatting.

Adobe Illustrator® is a layout program with many design tools and interesting graphic functions. It is a more complex program to learn, but the graphic capabilities are much more sophisticated and rich than in PowerPoint.

Adobe Photoshop® is a graphics-rich raster application, used for image manipulation and photo editing. Photoshop is not intended to be used for the entire poster layout program but for putting together various visual elements contained in the poster, such as labeled photos, x-rays, gels, exported graphs, or scanned images. For text to be crisp when labeling a figure, the resolution should be at least 600 dpi. For this reason, we do not recommend Photoshop as a layout program because at this resolution, the file sizes become excessively large, taking a very long time to print, and the quality is generally not as "crisp" as a vector-based program like Illustrator or PowerPoint.

No matter which graphics suite is used, the generic step-by-step plan in Figure 30–9 can be used to execute the poster.

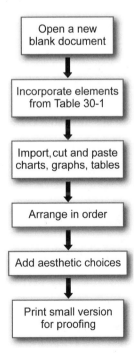

**FIGURE 30–9** ● Flow diagram of step-by-step plan for creating a one-piece poster. As indicated, aesthetic choices should be considered after all the components are factored into the layout.

In the program used for poster development, open a new, blank document or "slide." Specify the design scale at 50 percent of the final printed size (later, print at 200 percent magnification). This can be done in "page setup" or "document size," depending on the application.

Incorporate the components and specifications as described in the preceding sections.

Import images and figures from other applications. It is best to import images and artwork separately as TIFF or JPEG files, rather than by the rudimentary cut and paste method. If imagery is being exported from another application, it may be possible to simply do so by checking to see if that application has an *export* or *save as* function, in which case the figure or image should be exported in TIFF or JPEG format, preferably in 400–600 dpi resolution and below 5Mb in file size. (If the file size becomes prohibitive, one trick is to export to PDF format and then convert it later to a TIFF or JPEG format.)

Frustratingly, importing charts, graphs, and tables can be a headache or a breeze, depending on which programs are used for charting. Excel® and Word® data components are optimal when the poster is set up in PowerPoint; Microsoft makes data transfer between their programs clean and easy. By sticking with products from the Microsoft Office® family, data as well as font size, line width, alignment, and color—all of which determine readability and clarity during presentation—can all be edited easily.

A simple method of transferring a table into PowerPoint is selecting the table from Word or Excel and copying, then selecting "paste special" (as a picture) in PowerPoint. You will not be able to edit the table (unless you ungroup it), but it will be easy to resize.

Microsoft Word and PowerPoint are optimal for text formatting and layout. Some formatting (font size, color, bullets, boldness, or italics) will survive copying and pasting from other applications; the rest will require a reformatting of the text into the target application.

The most common tip from technical and artistic professionals is to first get all the elements into the poster document/slide before laying it out. Having all elements together will help assess the amount of text and figures that can be incorporated and will aid in determining space constraints. Content should not be packed too closely; some white space lends visual relief and cleanliness to data organization.

Poster elements should then be arranged in the order in which they should be read (top to bottom, left to right). When positioning text-heavy sections, keep in mind that audience members will not want to read a row of text the entire width of the poster (up to 8 feet). Columns of mixed width with images and charts will break up the monotony of text-heavy segments.

After loading and positioning all elements, aesthetic choices should be considered. For instance, the poster background can be a solid or gradient color, a photo image, or texture. Sometimes a solid white background will accentuate imagery and heighten headings, although a colorful photorealistic image can actually detract from the subject matter. Some posters use a solid background effectively with geometric entities, such as vertical or horizontal ruled or dotted lines. This technique is another method to help guide the eyes of the audience through the poster.

If the poster still looks unacceptably bland, adding borders or geometric figures to various sections may help. This also helps to separate and heighten text and data sections from an otherwise bland background.

Before final printing, print a small-scale poster proof—that is, print the poster in smaller dimensions. Printing a proof allows an opportunity to troubleshoot and to peruse the poster as a member of the audience. Many times, items from other applications cause problems by not printing as seen on the monitor or disappearing altogether (converting these to TIFF or JPEG format will usually solve this problem). Moreover, it's a useful way to catch typos and to inspect the print colors.

The final step after full-size printing is to roll the poster up (glossy side in) into a cardboard poster tote for transportation to the venue. Depending on the audience size and venue, some people opt to print a stack of tabloid-size posters as handouts.

## SUMMARY

- Whether presenting data in digital or physical media, format considerations (such as layout and chronology of elements), stylistic considerations (such as color, size, and typeface), and presentation considerations (such as the audience, time allotted, and presentation venue) should all be taken into account.
- When designing a slideshow, graphs and figures should be consistent in color scheme, data formatting and captioning.
- A useful rule of thumb is to arrange the slides to (1) tell the audience what is to be discussed,

(2) discuss it, and (3) then tell them what has just been discussed.

- Similar design considerations pertain to poster presentations; however, a poster requires extra layout attention. There are two main poster layouts—*traditional* and *one-piece*. Currently, the one-piece poster is the most commonly employed design and can be created with a step-by-step process.

- Poster elements (title, abstract, introduction, objectives, material and methods, results, discussion, conclusion, and references and other components) should be arranged in the order in which they should be read.

- Poster design is best accomplished within a computer-generated document or slide before the various elements are printed out for final presentation.

# Modern Techniques of Translational Clinical Research

# CHAPTER 31

# Fundamentals of Gene Expression

John Yang, Jeffrey Saffitz

With the advent of molecular medicine and the sequencing of the human genome, increased attention has been focused on the genetic basis of human disease and a more detailed understanding of how alterations in the DNA of human cells lead to clinical phenotypes. Some diseases, such as sickle cell anemia or familial hypercholesterolemia, have a direct genetic basis and can be attributed to specific mutations in a single gene. Other diseases, such as systemic hypertension, have a more complex familial pattern of inheritance that involves contributions of several or many genes that interact with other host and environmental factors. And finally, many diseases or responses to injury, such as cardiac hypertrophy, originate not primarily from changes in genetic material but from changes in the spectrum of proteins expressed by the diseased or injured organ.

Fundamental to all these scenarios is the concept of *gene expression*. Accordingly, the study of human disease in the modern era increasingly relies on methods to evaluate gene expression. Simply stated, gene expression can be ascertained at the level of RNA expression or protein expression. Measurements of the amount of messenger RNA (mRNA) of a specific gene reflect not only the level of gene *transcription* (synthesis of RNA from DNA), but also the rate of RNA turnover, both of which can be regulated to change the level of gene expression. Likewise, the amount of a given protein in cells or tissues reflects the balance between protein synthesis (*translation* of the mRNA template) and protein degradation.

The *rate* of mRNA transcription is probably the most direct measure of gene expression. However, a simple relationship between the *amount* of mRNA and the amount of protein for a given gene is not always present—and after all, it's the protein, not the DNA or RNA that is most directly linked to the clinical expression of the gene (phenotype). Differences may arise through posttranscriptional and posttranslational regulatory mechanisms. Thus, a complete understanding of a gene's expression often requires an analysis at multiple levels.

In characterizing the basic molecular features of a disease, it is almost always necessary to know whether the expression of one or more genes is affected and if so, how this contributes to disease pathogenesis. The methods to investigate gene expression discussed in this chapter are now so ubiquitous and fundamental that they are rarely used in isolation in research studies. Rather, they are usually combined with one or more of the most modern tools of biology (described in more detail in Chapters 33–37) to discover the basis for human disease.

## RNA EXPRESSION ASSAYS

Northern blotting was the first technique invented to measure RNA levels (1). It is a direct measurement of RNA content. To perform a Northern blot, total RNA is extracted from cells or tissues, usually by a phenol-based method, and loaded onto an agarose gel under denaturing conditions (which prevents the molecules from folding into complex secondary and tertiary structures that would interfere with the detection methods). Application of an electric field (electrophoresis) separates the various individual molecules of RNA within the gel based on their relative sizes.

It should be remembered that total cellular RNA consists of a mixture of ribosomal, transfer, and messenger RNAs. The mRNA is the RNA species that is of greatest interest because it specifically provides the template for translation of the gene into its protein gene product. The mRNA portion represents only a few percent of total cellular RNA and it is possible, although often not necessary, to purify the messenger RNA before loading it on the gel.

Once the RNA has been separated in the gel, it is transferred onto a solid matrix such as a nitrocellulose or nylon membrane. This membrane is then hybridized with a radiolabeled nucleic acid probe that has a sequence complementary to a sequence in the RNA of interest. Exposing the membrane to a radiosensitive film yields a signal in the shape of a band (Figure 31–1).

Northern blotting is often used as a quantitative assay, so it is important that equal amounts of RNA are loaded into each well in each lane of the agarose gel. This can be accomplished by stripping the membrane of the first radiolabeled probe and reprobing it with a new probe for a gene such as β-actin, which is not highly regulated at the transcriptional level. When the membrane is then exposed, separate bands should appear at the positions occupied by the different species of RNA

(one for the mRNA representing the gene transcript of interest and the other representing the transcript of the β-actin gene, or its equivalent). Bands of equal intensity for β-actin mRNA indicate comparable loading and strengthen the conclusion that mRNA levels for the gene of interest are present in different amounts in samples in which different band intensities are observed.

Primer extension is another method used to measure RNA levels in cells or tissues. A radiolabeled DNA oligonucleotide containing a sequence complementary to the RNA transcript of interest is incubated with total RNA isolated from the tissue sample. The oligonucleotide hybridizes to the RNA of interest and acts as a primer for extension along the RNA catalyzed by reverse transcriptase, an enzyme that synthesizes DNA from an RNA template. The resulting radiolabeled DNA/RNA hybrid is loaded onto a denaturing acrylamide gel and separated based on size. The gel is dried onto paper and exposed to film (Figure 31–2). Primer extension is a quantitative assay as long as there is primer excess. Equal loading can be checked with the use of a primer for an unregulated gene.

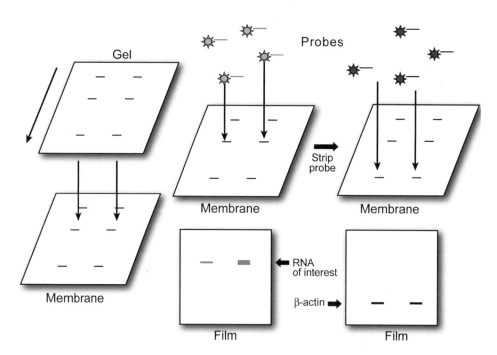

**FIGURE 31–1** ● Northern blotting. RNA samples are separated on a formaldehyde agarose gel and transferred to a membrane. The membrane is incubated with radioactive DNA probes (stars) that bind to the RNA transcript of interest. Two lanes are shown, each with three RNA transcripts of unknown identity. The blot is first probed with a cDNA to the RNA of interest (light gray); the blot is then stripped and reprobed with a cDNA to ß-actin (dark gray), a constitutively expressed housekeeping gene that is not expected to change its expression. The illustration shows an increase in expression of the gene of interest in the second lane.

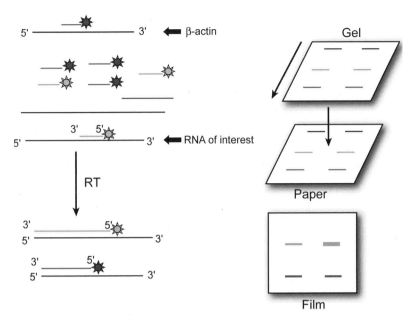

**FIGURE 31–2** ● Primer extension assay. Radioactive DNA primers (light and dark stars) bind to their target RNA transcript and are extended by reverse transcriptase (RT). The products are separated on an acrylamide gel and dried on filter paper. As in Figure 31–1, two lanes are shown, this time with three extended cDNAs, one of which includes the gene of interest (light gray) and another includes a cDNA to β-actin (lower row of dark gray). The illustration shows an increase in expression of the gene of interest in the second lane.

In a similar assay called the RNase protection assay, a radiolabeled RNA oligonucleotide is incubated with RNA that has been isolated from cells or tissues, and then treated with ribonuclease, which degrades all single-stranded RNA but not the double-stranded RNA in the hybrid. The radiolabeled double-stranded RNA is then loaded onto a denaturing acrylamide gel. The gel is dried onto paper and exposed to film (Figure 31–3). The RNase protection assay is especially good for purposes of quantitation but is technically more difficult than other assays because it involves manipulation of RNA throughout the procedure. RNA is more labile than DNA because it is vulnerable to degradation by RNase, which is widely present in the environment and is more difficult to neutralize than DNAase in test samples.

The methods just described for measuring RNA levels involve isolation of RNA from cells or tissues. Of course, normal human tissues are composed of multiple cell types including not only the parenchymal or primary differentiated cells of an organ (e.g., hepatocytes in the liver), but also the connective tissue cells of the organ stroma, cells of blood vessels, or nerves. Similarly, a sample of diseased tissue or tumor contains a heterogeneous population of cells.

Recognizing a particular mRNA species in a tissue does not necessarily identify the specific cell type in which the gene is expressed, nor does demonstrating a difference in mRNA expression between two tissues identify the cellular basis for the differences. For this reason, unless an investigator is using a purified sample (e.g., cells isolated from blood or bronchoalveolar lavage), simply demonstrating a change in mRNA levels in a tissue (say, from a patient with a particular disease) compared to some control sample is usually just the first step in a study of gene expression.

Another problem with these RNA assays is that they have limited sensitivity—they may not detect specific gene transcripts expressed at very low levels (with low concentrations in the target tissue). However, methods involving the polymerase chain reaction (PCR) have revolutionized molecular biology because they involve dramatic amplification of specific nucleic acid sequences of interest, making possible easy detection and measurement of rare sequences. A technique referred to as reverse transcriptase PCR (RT-PCR) is frequently used to detect low levels of gene expression at the RNA level. Before describing the RT-PCR method, it is worth reviewing the basic mechanism of PCR (Figure 31–4).

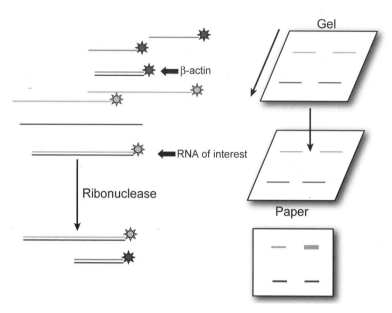

**FIGURE 31–3** ● RNase protection assay. Radioactive RNA probes (light and dark stars) bind to their target RNA transcript forming a double-stranded RNA. All RNA will be digested by ribonuclease except the double-stranded RNA. As in Figure 31–1, two lanes are shown, this time with two RNA probes left after digestion in each lane (light gray = gene of interest, dark gray = β-actin). The illustration shows an increase in expression of the gene of interest in the second lane.

With this technique, any segment of DNA that can be defined by hybridizing primers on either end of the sequence can be amplified exponentially with DNA polymerase. Primers are DNA oligonucleotides (usually 20 bases or longer) that hybridize to their complementary target DNA sequences and function as anchors for polymerases to begin synthesizing a copy of the original sequence of interest. Once the initial copy has been made, the complementary strands are separated by thermal denaturation and the process is repeated by again annealing primers to their complementary strands and making additional copies with the polymerase. This cycle is repeated approximately 30 times, resulting in massive amplification of the sequence of interest (Figure 31–5). Automation of PCR is made possible by the discovery of thermostable enzymes, such as those found in the bacteria *Thermus aquaticus*. These bacteria live in water temperatures that may exceed 72°C and their DNA polymerase is stable at temperatures as high as 94°C (2). This has made PCR practical for use in molecular genetics and cloning (e.g., see Chapter 33).

To detect and measure a specific mRNA sequence using RT-PCR, it is necessary first to make a DNA copy of the RNA of interest and then to use the DNA copy as the starting material for amplification by PCR. Thus, total RNA is isolated from cells or tissue of interest and a DNA copy of the RNA sequence of interest (cDNA) is prepared by incubating the isolated RNA with primers that flank the specific transcript. Then, reverse transcriptase is used to synthesize a DNA strand of the template provided by the mRNA of interest. Once the first DNA copy is synthesized, gene-specific primers are used in a conventional PCR assay to amplify the signal. The PCR products are run on an agarose gel, and the gel is stained with ethidium bromide, a fluorescent compound that binds in a specific molar ratio to DNA and allows ready identification of RT-PCR products when the gel is viewed under ultraviolet light (Figure 31–5).

The great power of RT-PCR is its sensitivity. Because of the vast amplification involved with this approach, even very rare transcripts can be readily identified and measured. This feature, in which DNA is amplified in an exponential manner, also makes it difficult to use RT-PCR to reliably quantify the amount of RNA in a tissue.

Recently, quantitative RT-PCR techniques have been developed using technology based on fluorescent chemical compounds such as SYBR®

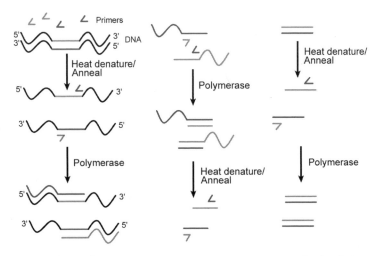

**FIGURE 31–4** ● Polymerase chain reaction (PCR). DNA primers bind to their complementary strands and extend along the template driven by DNA polymerase. This cycle is repeated multiple times resulting in an amplification of a DNA segment.

Green, a dye that becomes excited and fluoresces when bound to double-stranded DNA. With this modification, as the number of amplified sequences increases during PCR, the fluorescent signals increase correspondingly, allowing detection and sensitive measurement in real time. Because the dye binds to all double-stranded DNAs,

it is essential to show that nonspecific amplification is not occurring.

Another approach involves the design of a DNA probe that binds between the primer set and is linked to a fluorescent dye at its 5' end and a quencher at its 3' end (Figure 31–6). As PCR proceeds, the fluorescent dye is "released" from the

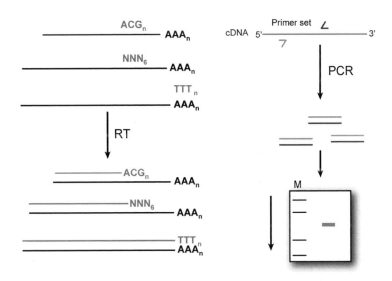

**FIGURE 31–5** ● Reverse transcriptase RT-PCR. First strand cDNA is synthesized from oligo-dT ($TTT_n$), random hexamer ($NNN_6$), or a gene-specific primer ($ACG_n$). Then, a segment of the cDNA is amplified by PCR. The illustration shows two lanes on an agarose gel, lane M = a molecular size marker lane, and lane 2 shows a band demonstrating the presence of the amplified product of the PCR reaction.

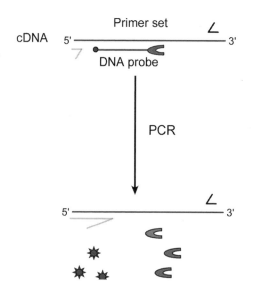

**FIGURE 31–6** ● TaqMan assay. A DNA probe is placed between two PCR primers. The probe has a fluorescent dye linked to its 5' end (small gray circle) and a quencher linked to its 3' end (gray semicircle). During PCR, the polymerase will release the dye from the quencher, producing fluorescence (dark stars) that can be detected and measured.

quencher (TaqMan®) by the nuclease activity of the polymerase. The presence of this third probe greatly enhances the specificity of the assay. With either "SYBR Green" or "TaqMan" PCR, increased amplification is reflected by changes in fluorescence that are measured in real time. The number of PCR cycles required to achieve an arbitrary threshold is, therefore, an indirect measure of the relative abundance of the RNA of interest.

As previously mentioned, RNA is highly labile because ribonucleases are abundant and particularly resistant to denaturation. Therefore, successful isolation of RNA from human tissues depends on processing samples as rapidly as possible. This limitation presents a significant challenge for clinical translational research studies because, in general, studies must be designed and conducted prospectively, not retrospectively on archived tissue. Autopsy tissues are usually suboptimal because of postmortem autolysis. Even tissues obtained from surgical specimens (e.g., diseased organs removed at the time of transplantation) require rapid processing and use of multiple RNase inhibitors. However, because of its great sensitivity, RT-PCR is well suited to the identification of RNA transcripts in human tissues, especially if they are present in low numbers.

Having demonstrated that the mRNA levels of a diseased tissue differ from the expression in a control tissue sample, a variety of other techniques have been developed to answer questions about where within an organ, and in which cells, a particular gene is being expressed, either at the RNA or protein level. In the case of RNA expression, identifying the spatial expression pattern of a certain gene can be accomplished by in situ hybridization of RNA (Chapter 36). In this technique, a sample of tissue is fixed to stabilize macromolecules and preserve tissue structure, and then embedded in paraffin for preparation of histologic sections. Alternatively, the tissue can be lightly fixed and then frozen in preparation for cryosectioning. A thin section of the specimen is mounted on a slide and hybridized with a radiolabeled RNA probe, referred to as a riboprobe, which has a sequence complementary to the unique sequence of the mRNA transcript of interest. By exposing the slide to radiosensitive film, a signal is created that corresponds to the precise location of the gene transcript of interest in the tissue. Such tissue-based techniques can be used to measure gene expression (explained in greater detail in Chapter 36).

## PROTEIN EXPRESSION ASSAYS

It is always important to compare gene expression at both the RNA and protein levels whenever possible because, as explained previously, a one-to-one correspondence between these two products of gene expression cannot be assumed. Whereas a measurement of mRNA transcript levels directly reflects the expression of a particular DNA sequence, the level of the protein directly reflects translation of that mRNA into the end product of gene expression. Because, in most cases, it is the protein that is responsible for the phenotype associated with expression of the gene, an analysis of gene expression at the RNA level alone is incomplete.

Techniques used to measure the expression of particular proteins are conceptually similar to those described above for RNA. In the case of the RNA methods, specificity depends on using specific *nucleic acid probes* to identify a unique mRNA sequence, thereby ensuring detection and measurement of a specific gene transcript. In the case of techniques designed to measure gene expression at the protein level, specificity generally depends on using a specific *antibody* that recognizes a unique protein. The use of antibodies as specific probes to detect and quantify protein levels in tissues is fundamental to many techniques, including those in which proteins are isolated from homogenates of biological samples and others in which tissue structure is preserved and the expression of a specific protein is detected (and, in some cases, quantified) using immunohistochemical techniques. This latter approach is described in Chapter 36, which also includes a detailed discussion of many important issues pertaining to the production and characterization of antibodies used for such assays. Here, only antibody-based techniques used to detect and quantify specific proteins in samples of total protein isolated from cells and tissues will be considered.

Like Northern blots, Western blots are designed to measure gene expression, first by separating a complex mixture of molecules according to size using gel electrophoresis, and then by using a probe, in this case an antibody, to detect the specific molecule of interest and create a signal that can be recognized and quantified (Figure 31–7). In Western blotting, cells or tissues are homogenized and the total proteins are isolated. An aliquot of isolated proteins is loaded onto an acrylamide gel under denaturing conditions, usually produced by including a detergent (such as sodium dodecyl sulfate, SDS) in the buffer, and then by separating the proteins via electrophoresis so that they are sorted on the basis of their relative size. The denaturing conditions ensure that the protein molecules do not fold, allowing them to migrate as a function of

their size. The separated proteins are then transferred or blotted onto a nylon or nitrocellulose membrane and incubated with a specific antibody that recognizes a single protein of interest. Typically, the primary antibody used to detect the protein of interest does not also contain or produce the signal used to detect and quantify the protein. Rather, a secondary antibody is used to recognize the primary antibody. The secondary antibody is typically linked to an enzyme such as horseradish peroxidase that can catalyze a reaction that emits light, which can in turn be detected and quantified when exposed to radiographic film (Figure 31–7).

In most Western blot studies, whole cells or tissues are homogenized and total proteins are analyzed. Obviously, as with Northern blotting, no conclusions can be reached about the specific cellular or subcellular site in which the protein resides. For this purpose, tissue-based techniques such as immunohistochemistry (Chapter 36) can be used to identify specific cells and, potentially, subcellular sites of protein distribution. Alternatively, it is possible to fractionate the cell or tissue sample before isolating the proteins for Western blotting, thereby, localizing expression of the protein to a specific site or sites. For example, if a

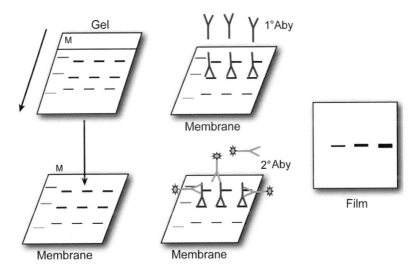

**FIGURE 31–7** ● Western blotting. Protein samples are separated on a denaturing acrylamide gel and transferred to a membrane. The membrane is incubated first with a primary antibody (1°Aby, dark gray) and then with a secondary antibody (2°Aby, light gray). The secondary antibody is typically linked to an enzyme such as horseradish peroxidase (gray stars) that can catalyze a reaction that emits light, which can in turn be detected and quantified when exposed to radiographic film. Shown in the illustration are four lanes. The left lane is a marker lane of molecular size. The other three lanes contain three peptides in each lane of different size, and the membrane is probed with an antibody to one of these peptides. The illustration shows increasing amounts of peptide detected in the right lanes.

researcher were investigating the expression of a transcription factor that was known to act within the nucleus to regulate gene expression, then it might be possible to isolate nuclei from a tissue sample and measure expression of the protein in the nuclear sample to better assess expression of the molecule of interest at its subcellular site of action.

One feature of the Western blotting technique is that the relative molecular weight of the signal can be determined by its migration pattern on the gel when compared to the migration pattern of a standard with proteins of known size. This provides an internal quality control if the molecular weight of the protein of interest is known.

As described in more detail in Chapter 36, there are many potential nonspecific interactions between antibodies and proteins. Controls for such nonspecific interactions are also important in performing Western blots. The best control is to use a tissue sample that either lacks the protein (a known negative control) or one in which the protein is known to be modified such that it no longer binds to the antibody or migrates at a different, known molecular weight.

A simpler version of the Western blot protein assay is called the enzyme-linked immunosorbent assay (ELISA). With this method, a multiwell plate is loaded with samples isolated from cells or tissues of interest. A primary antibody is added to the wells followed by an enzyme-linked secondary antibody. A substrate recognized by the enzyme is added to the wells, resulting in the formation of a colored product that reflects the amount of specific protein present. Although this assay is rather sensitive, it can be plagued by high background levels of signal.

A related approach is the radioimmunoassay (RIA) (Figure 31–8). In this technique, the amount of a specific protein of interest is measured by quantifying the amount of the same radioactively labeled protein that is displaced from a specific antibody. Thus, with this approach, it is necessary to have a radiolabeled sample of the protein of interest. RIA is used to measure proteins and peptides in clinical samples, such as peptide hormones in blood or other fluids. To perform RIA, a sample is added to a tube containing a specific antibody that is linked to a known amount of a radiolabled version of the protein of interest. The radiolabeled protein will be displaced from the specific antibody by the presence of the identical but unlabeled protein in the test sample. The extent to which the radiolabeled protein is displaced is directly proportional to the concentration of the protein in the test sample. To quantify the displacement, a secondary antibody that binds specifically to the primary antibody is added and the resultant complex is precipitated, leaving behind the supernatant and the displaced radioactive protein that can be measured with great sensitivity (Figure 31–8). This assay is particularly useful when a highly quantitative analysis is needed.

Proteins tend to be more stable than RNA, but this varies considerably among individual proteins. Although loss of enzyme activity may occur rapidly in isolated tissues, many protein

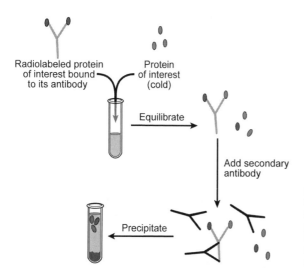

**FIGURE 31–8** ● Radioimmunoassay. Protein is added to a tube with radiolabeled protein linked to an antibody. With equilibration, some of the cold protein of interest displaces some of the radiolabel from the antibody. A secondary antibody is then added, and the complex is precipitated. The supernatant is measured for radioactivity.

molecules may still be identified by antibody-based techniques. Thus, autopsy tissues are often used to analyze protein expression in clinical investigations.

## PROTEIN AND RNA ASSAYS IN CLINICAL INVESTIGATION

Assays of both proteins and RNAs have become mainstays in clinical practice and research. Proteins have been used as biomarkers since the discovery of the Bence Jones' protein in multiple myeloma in 1873 (3). Most current biomarker analyses involve quantitative measurements in fluids such as blood, urine, or sputum (4). Perhaps, the most commonly used serum cancer biomarker is the prostate-specific antigen (PSA) (5,6). Most commercial assays are antibody based (RIA and ELISA), and the level of PSA in the serum reflects risk for prostate cancer. Many more cancer biomarkers are being discovered including products of tumor suppressor genes or oncogenes (4). Biomarkers are also being used increasingly in other clinical disciplines [e.g., brain natriuretic peptide (BNP) as a marker for heart failure] (7,8).

Assays of RNA have also been used recently as biomarkers. For example, RT-PCR has been used to identify mutations in tumor suppressor genes such as p53 and oncogenes such as K-ras (9). Quantitative RT-PCR has also been used to detect multiple biomarkers (10–12). A good example is the human telomerase reverse transcriptase (hTERT) assay. Elevated expression of hTERT, measured by quantitative RT-PCR, has been linked to lung, breast, and colon cancers (11,13). As previously mentioned, the great advantage of using RT-PCR to detect biomarkers is its sensitivity. This sensitivity facilitates use of limited amounts of tissues and bodily fluids in which the biomarkers are present in very low levels.

Even as assays for biomarkers become more sensitive and specific, it is likely that no one molecule will be specific for one and only one disease. Thus, a method for examining a *group* of gene expression changes; that is, a "profile," would be helpful. DNA microarray and proteomics technology (Chapter 34 and 35) provide ways to survey broad changes in RNA and protein expression patterns. Thus far, this technology has seen its greatest use in clinical investigations involving hematologic and solid malignancies (14–16), but examples from other organ systems are increasingly common. Although genomic and proteomic approaches are potentially very powerful, the results from such studies must be validated by the more established techniques described in this chapter.

## SUMMARY

- The study of modern disease in the modern era increasingly relies on methods to evaluate gene expression.
- Gene expression can be evaluated at different levels: transcription from DNA to messenger RNA, translation from RNA to a protein, and posttranslational modifications to the protein.
- Methods to measure RNA levels include Northern blotting, primer extension assays, RNase protection assays, the reverse transcriptase polymerase chain reaction (RT-PCR) assay (including so-called real-time PCR), and in situ hybridization.
- In situ hybridization is the only method that can be used to isolate RNA expression to a particular cell type in complex tissues. The assays that are based on PCR methods are the most sensitive.
- Methods to evaluate gene expression at the protein level include immunohistochemistry, Western blotting, enzyme-linked immunosorbent assays (ELISA), and radioimmunoassay.
- Immunohistochemistry is one of the best methods to identify the specific cell type associated with a change in protein levels, but is poorly quantitative. Radioimmunoassays are the most reliably quantitative method, but semiquantitative results can be obtained by either Western blotting or ELISA.
- Most recently, methods to evaluate the expression of groups of genes have been developed based on DNA microarrays and proteomic technology, as discussed in more detail in Chapters 34 and 35.

## REFERENCES

1. Alwine JC, Kemp DJ, Stark GR. Method for detection of specific RNAs in agarose gels by transfer to diazobenzyloxymethyl-paper and hybridization with DNA probes. Proc Natl Acad Sci 1977;74:5350–5354.
2. Eckert KA, Kunkel TA. High fidelity DNA synthesis by the *Thermus aquaticus* DNA polymerase. Nuc Acids Res 1990;18:3739–3744.
3. Roulston JE. Assessment of predictive values of tumor markers of cancer. Methods Mol Med 2004;97:13–27.
4. Wagner PD, Maruvada P, Srivastava S. Molecular diagnostics: a new frontier in cancer prevention. Expert Rev Mol Diagn 2004 Jul;4(4):503–511.
5. Hernandez J, Thompson IM. Prostate-specific antigen: a review of the validation of the most commonly used cancer biomarker. Cancer 2004;101(5):894–904.

6. Soderdahl DW, Hernandez J. Prostate cancer screening at an equal access tertiary care center: its impact 10 years after the introduction of PSA. Prostate Cancer Prostatic Dis 2002;5(1):32–35.

7. Yancy CW. Practical considerations for BNP use. Heart Fail Rev 2003;8(4):369–373.

8. Maewal P, de Lemos JA. Natriuretic peptide hormone measurement in acute coronary syndromes. Heart Fail Rev 2003;8(4):365–368.

9. Sidransky D. Nucleic acid-based methods for the detection of cancer. Science 1997;278(5340):1054–1059.

10. Chen XQ, Bonnefoi H, Pelte MF et al. Telomerase RNA as a detection marker in the serum of breast cancer patients. Clin Cancer Res 2000;6(10):3823–3826.

11. Kopreski MS, Benko FA, Gocke CD. Circulating RNA as a tumor marker: detection of 5T4 mRNA in breast and lung cancer patient serum. Ann N Y Acad Sci 2001; 945:172–178.

12. Ember I, Gyongyi Z, Kiss I et al. The possible relationship between onco/suppressor gene expression and carcinogen exposure in vivo: evaluation of a potential biomarker in preventive and predictive medicine. Anticancer Res 2002;22(4):2109–2116.

13. Hiyama E, Hiyama K. Telomerase as tumor marker. Cancer Lett 2003;194(2):221–233.

14. Staudt LM. Molecular diagnosis of the hematologic cancers. N Engl J Med 2003;348(18):1777–1785.

15. Wulfkuhle JD, Paweletz CP, Steeg PS et al. Proteomic approaches to the diagnosis, treatment, and monitoring of cancer. Adv Exp Med Biol 2003;532:59–68.

16. Hermeking H. Serial analysis of gene expression and cancer. Curr Opin Oncol 2003;15(1):44–49.

# CHAPTER 32

# Identifying Mutations and Polymorphisms

Sharon Cresci, Lisa de las Fuentes, Victor G. Davila-Roman

Increasingly in modern medicine, the identification of causative gene mutations forms the basis for diagnostic and prognostic tests. Identifying disease-related genes can lead to early diagnostic testing, thus enabling physicians to identify preclinical disease states; individuals from families with high disease prevalence may benefit from genetic testing to determine disease susceptibility risk. Interventions may then be instituted for individuals with disease-associated gene variants to mitigate or prevent the manifestation of the disease. For example, an infant identified as having phenylketonuria is at high risk of developing mental retardation, an outcome that can be all but eliminated if identified early and treated with dietary restrictions. An increased susceptibility for deep venous thrombosis is conferred by a genetic variant in which a single amino acid substitution in the factor V gene (factor V Leiden) increases the risk of venous thrombosis three- to eightfold for heterozygous and substantially more for homozygous individuals (1). In individuals found to harbor this genetic variant, extended anticoagulant therapy following a thrombotic event has been associated with decreased recurrent events (2).

## NOMENCLATURE

Family pedigree studies have traditionally focused predominantly on large families with multiple affected members. Therefore, rare diseases that follow Mendelian inheritance and have a high degree of penetrance are those most amenable to investigation. The genetic mutations found are thus strongly associated with a "disease phenotype." However, with the explosion of molecular techniques, and particularly DNA sequencing, it became evident that a distinct phenotype could not be ascribed to every alteration in DNA sequence and that a broader definition of mutation was needed. Single nucleotide base substitutions were defined as point mutations and further divided into *silent mutations* (single change in a nucleotide base resulting in no change in the amino acid sequence), *missense mutations* (change in a single nucleotide base resulting in the substitution of a similar amino acid [conservative missense mutation] or a dissimilar amino acid [nonconservative missense mutation]), *nonsense mutations* (change in a single nucleotide base resulting in a stop codon instead of an amino acid, thereby terminating the protein), and *frame shift mutations* (insertion or deletion of a single nucleotide base resulting in all subsequent codon reading frames being "shifted" by one, leading to amino acid sequence changes or termination). Using this broader definition, single base changes occurring in less than 1% of a given population were designated mutations, and those occurring in greater than 1% of the population were termed *single nucleotide polymorphisms (SNPs)*. Although this nomenclature system is often still used today, it should be emphasized that the classification of a particular base change as a mutation or SNP could change depending on its prevalence within a given population of interest, and therefore, the distinction between mutation and SNP is arbitrary.

For diseases that follow monogenic inheritance (i.e., inheritance according to Mendel's laws of inheritance), the altered DNA sequence is considered causative of the disease. For diseases that follow polygenic or complex inheritance patterns, single alterations in the DNA sequence are not sufficient to cause the disease. Instead, a complicated interaction between the DNA sequence change and the environment, or between the DNA sequence change and other sequence changes, is thought to occur. An example is the major histocompatibility gene complex. Individuals who inherit the B27 allele have a 121-fold increased risk of developing ankylosing spondylitis compared to individuals without the B27 allele (3). However, the B27 allele is not sufficient to cause ankylosing spondylitis because less than 15% of individuals who inherit the B27 allele develop ankylosing spondylitis. Thus, although individual nucleotide base changes may be identified that correlate with the disease, other individuals may have the same nucleotide base changes and yet not have the disease. Therefore, because these sequence changes may not cause the disease, the term *mutation* may not be accurate in this instance.

Given that the nomenclature systems listed above have some ambiguity, a more precise system has been proposed by The Nomenclature Working Group (4). The recommendation of this group is that the terms *mutation* and *SNP* be replaced with the term *sequence variation*. Sequence variations are given a prefix, such as g, c, m, r, or p, to specify the type of reference sequence (genomic, cDNA, mitochondrial, RNA, or protein, respectively). DNA nucleotides and amino acid one-letter codes are designated by capital letters and RNA nucleotides are designated by lowercase letters. DNA nucleotides are numbered with the ATG of the initiation codon corresponding to +1 and the nucleotide 5' to +1 being −1 (there is no 0). In this system, a single base change is designated by a greater than sign (>). For example, the single base substitution of a thymine for a cytosine at nucleotide 1019 in the connexin 37 gene (genomic sequence) recently associated with a significant risk of myocardial infarction in men (5) would be designated as g.1019 C>T. Deletions are designated by "del" after the nucleotides and insertions are designated by "ins" after the nucleotides. For example, the insertion of a single adenine nucleotide between nucleotides 1171 and 1172 5' of the ATG in the matrix metalloproteinase-3 (MMP3) gene, responsible for an improved response to statin therapy (5), would be designated as −1171_−1172insA. Although this system has largely been accepted in reporting sequence variations in publications, the term *SNP* has remained in common usage in written descriptions, publications, and in professional discourse.

## IDENTIFYING GENES OF INTEREST: GENOME-WIDE VERSUS CANDIDATE GENE APPROACH

Several approaches can be used to identify genes that are related to a particular disease. In a *genome-wide*

*approach*, the inheritance pattern of a disease trait is compared with the inheritance pattern of hundreds to thousands of markers interspersed throughout the genome. Chromosomal segments that do not influence disease segregate randomly according to Mendel's laws (i.e., 50:50 assortment of each copy to all offspring regardless of disease status). However, the closer two loci reside on the chromosome, the less likely they are to be separated by recombination during meiosis. Thus, the marker and the disease-causing gene are "linked," and the two loci are said to be in *linkage disequilibrium* (6). The strength of this linkage is identified by a significant LOD (logarithm of the odds) score, a statistical term that indicates whether two loci are linked; a score ≥ 3 is consistent with linkage and a score < −2 virtually excludes linkage. However, although fine-mapping with more narrowly interspersed markers may refine a region of interest, linkage analysis often suffers from relatively poor resolution, meaning that the regions identified are often quite large (approximately 20 million bases containing 200–500 genes), thus making it difficult to identify the specific disease-causing·gene by use of this method alone.

Nevertheless, family linkage studies are a powerful method for defining chromosomal regions associated with classic Mendelian disorders where the disease is attributed to a single gene mutation with a simple mode of inheritance. Mendelian disorders generally are characterized by (1) high *penetrance* (the proportion of individuals with the disease-causing allele that have the disease phenotype), (2) little *genetic heterogeneity* (different genetic variations resulting in similar phenotypes), and (3) very low disease prevalence in the general population.

Family linkage studies are statistically less powerful when investigating *complex traits*, where disease susceptibility is thought to result from multiple gene variants playing small and interactive roles with each other or the environment (7). Rather than tracking coinheritance of a chromosomal segment among affected family members (as in linkage analysis), case-control association studies consider the coincidence of genetic variants and disease traits within the population at large. Such genotype: phenotype association studies offer two main advantages: (1) greater statistical power in complex diseases, and (2) using samples and phenotype data from unrelated individuals, unlike linkage studies (8,9). Genotype:phenotype studies include an a priori selection of hypothesis-driven candidate genes and pathways. Thus, a *candidate gene approach* is often used when molecular biology studies implicate a specific enzyme, pathway, or molecule in the pathogenesis of the trait (see Chapters 33 and 34).

The existence of genetically modified animal models (such as those with knock-out or knock-in genes) having the phenotype of interest, may also be useful for candidate gene identification or selection (10). Candidate genes may also be selected on the basis of tissue-specific expression patterns (see Chapter 34), homology to other human genes, or the identification of similar genes in other species. Thus, the candidate gene approach represents a form of *translational clinical research* in which information from the bench is translated to clinical studies. An inherent limitation of the candidate gene strategy (both genotype:phenotype association and linkage:association approaches) is the assumption that the disease-related gene needs to have already been discovered and somehow implicated in the pathogenesis of disease. Thus, entirely new genes or pathways involved in disease susceptibility are not likely to be discovered by this method.

Combinations of genetic variants residing on a single chromosome, or *haplotypes*, may offer a substantial advantage in the search for susceptibility genes over the single variant-based approaches (9, 11–13). Within the sequence of the genome, sets of variants exist in more stable blocks that exhibit strong linkage disequilibrium, interrupted by apparent hot spots that appear to be remarkably more inclined to bear variants, partitioning each chromosome into blocks of linked variants (Figure 32–1) (6). Haplotype blocks contain far less diversity than would be predicted based on the number of variants within the block (Figure 32–2). Because the majority of variants within a haplotype block are often in tight linkage disequilibrium, a small number of haplotypes (typically three to five) capture approximately 90% of all chromosomes in the population (Figure 32–3) (14). Furthermore, new mutations arise on the background of specific chromosomal haplotypes. In subsequent generations, the association between the mutant allele and its ancestral haplotype is disrupted only by mutation and recombination. Thus, it should be possible to track each variant allele in the population by identifying the particular ancestral segment from which it arose. The International Haplotype Mapping Project (HapMap, http://www.hapmap.org), currently the largest single project in human population genetics, is a collaborative effort to chart variation within the human genome in an effort to

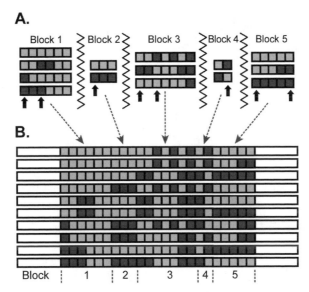

**FIGURE 32–1** ● Haplotype block structure. This diagram presents hypothetical data of 23 common SNPs in five individuals (10 chromosomes). Dark gray squares represent SNPs with the major allele; light gray squares represent the minor allele. **A.** The five haplotype "blocks" are represented by four, two, three, two, and three common haplotypes, respectively. When common variants are considered, the haplotype block paradigm portrays the genome as a series of short segments separated by recombination hotspots (zigzag lines in the figure). Within each block, there is little or no evidence for recombination, only a small number of distinct haplotypes is present in the population, and not all combinations of the various alleles are possible. **B.** Genome sequences can be portrayed as a series of common haplotype blocks representing the majority of genetic diversity. Within each block, tight linkage disequilibrium allows the selection of a reduced panel of representative SNPs, called "tag SNPs"—marked with small arrows in **A**. Most chromosomes in the population are a mosaic arrangement of the variants within each block. (Adapted from Cardon LR, Abecasis GR. Using haplotype blocks to map human complex trait loci. Trends Genet 2003;19:135–140.)

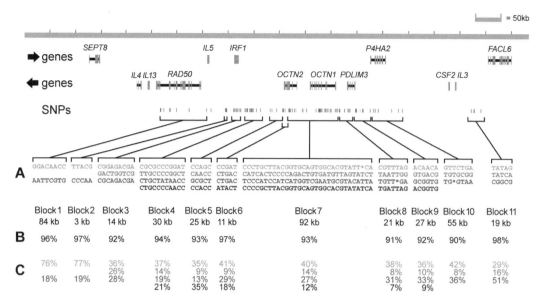

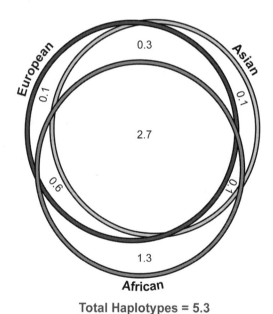

**FIGURE 32–2** ● Block-like haplotype diversity at 5q31, implicated in Crohn's disease. **A.** Each haplotype block is characterized by a number of common haplotype patterns. **B.** The percentage of all observed chromosomes that are exactly represented by one of these haplotypes. **C.** The percentage of chromosomes represented by each haplotype pattern. (Adapted from Daly MJ, Rioux JD, Schaffner SF et al. High-resolution haplotype structure in the human genome. Nature Genetics 2001;29:229–232.)

**Total Haplotypes = 5.3**

**FIGURE 32–3** ● Comparisons across populations reveals that although the majority of haplotypes are shared across populations, a small proportion appear to be unique to certain populations. The greater haplotype diversity among Africans is supportive of a single "out of Africa" origin. (Adapted from Gabriel SB, Schaffner SF, Nguyen H et al. The structure of haplotype blocks in the human genome. Science 2002;296:2225–2229.)

elucidate the genetic contributions to many common diseases. Algorithms applied to the HapMap data will identify the much smaller subsets of SNPs (*tag SNPs* or *htSNPs*) which can capture most of the genetic variation across sizable regions of DNA, theoretically enabling detection of the majority of haplotypes without significant loss of power (15,16).

It is possible to capitalize on the strengths of both linkage analysis and association studies. Once significant linkage is demonstrated on genome-wide and fine-marker mapping, a candidate gene is selected from within that chromosomal region. A recent description of the methods used for identifying genes related to the phenotype of premature atherosclerosis and myocardial infarction demonstrates how both of these methods can be combined (17). An unusual family characterized by premature coronary artery disease and early myocardial infarction was identified where the risk exhibited an autosomal dominant inheritance pattern (17). A genome-wide linkage scan using 382 markers spanning chromosomes 1–22 (with an average interval of 10 cM) was performed on DNA extracted from blood samples obtained from 13 members of this family. Linkage analysis identified the marker D15S120 and haplotype analysis with nearby markers confirmed the linkage. The putative genetic locus was given the designation adCAD1, for the first autosomal dominant coronary artery disease and myocardial infarction locus, and was localized to chromosome 15q26. The region of chromosome 15q26 contained approximately 93 genes, 43 of which were known. After assessment of the 43 known genes, myocyte enhancer factor-2α (MEF2α) was considered the strongest candidate gene (because MEF2α is an early marker for vasculogenesis and plays an important role in vascular morphogenesis). Systematic mutational screening of MEF2α gene in the 10 living affected members of the family demonstrated a 21 base-pair deletion (7aa) in exon 11 (using traditional sequencing methods) in all 10 members. Thus, a genome-wide approach established segregation of polymorphic DNA markers positioned throughout the genome with the severity of a phenotype and was followed by a candidate gene approach that identified the most likely gene responsible for the phenotype. Furthermore, these investigators demonstrated in functional studies that the Δ7aa MEF2α protein had decreased transcriptional activity compared to wild-type MEF2α protein in cotransfection studies. The Δ7aa MEF2α was also shown to have blocked entry into the nucleus, instead localizing to the endothelium of the coronary arteries where it may disrupt normal coronary endothelial function.

## CHOOSING CANDIDATE POLYMORPHISMS

Several strategies are available for selecting the specific genetic variants to be investigated. Although a review of published literature may be used to identify available data, much of the information regarding genetic sequence variants is found in a variety of online genomic databases. It is estimated that 10 million common sequence variations—approximately one sequence variation for every 200 base pairs—are present in the human genome (18,19). Greater than 90% of these are single base pair variations, generally referred to as SNPs in the literature (despite the recommendation for a more precise nomenclature system as described above). As of April 2005, nearly 10 million SNPs have been identified and deposited in public databases; however, many of these represent duplications and sequencing errors and only half have been "validated" (20). Unfortunately, at this time there is no standardization of validation or attempt made to enforce independent confirmation of the validity of SNPs deposited in most public databases. [One database, SNPper, http://snpper.chip.org does report

validation status, list of independent submissions, and reported minor allele frequencies for each SNP in its database (21).] In addition, very little overlap (between 1% and 2%) was found when SNPs from the most prolific sequencing laboratories were compared to each other for SNP content (20), and there is a lack of population diversity in many online databases, leading to inadequate representation of genetic variability. Therefore, a comprehensive search of several databases (see Table 32–1 for a partial list) should be completed to ensure that all potential putative SNPs are identified and given due consideration.

A search of such databases quickly reveals that there are more SNPs than can be realistically pursued at one time. It then becomes prudent to prioritize the SNPs of interest for further study. One straightforward approach is to first pursue genetic variants that lead to changes in the amino acid sequence of the protein (*coding* or *nonsynonymous* change); unfortunately these tend to be relatively more rare than variants in coding regions that do not create amino acid changes (*synonymous*) or than variants located in intron segments. Other high priority variants reside near the intron-exon splice sites and in the promoter regions, where nucleotide changes may lead to changes in protein structure or pattern of expression. It is increasingly evident that important variants are not restricted to coding and proximal promoter regulatory regions, which often presents a formidable challenge in selecting the most profitable variants to pursue.

For each SNP on the priority list, whether it has been identified from a database, by literature search, by direct sequencing, or by any other method, it is imperative to verify both the validity and frequency of the polymorphism in a control population. It has been shown by several authors that up to 17% of the sequences deposited in public databases failed to be confirmed by others (22,23). In addition, it has been repeatedly observed that there are often significant differences in the prevalence of SNPs across populations of different racial backgrounds and that the "minor" allele in one population may be the "major" allele in different population (24). Therefore, *the selection of the control population is as important as the selection of the study population.* The control population should be selected to match the study population as closely as possible—at the very least with respect to racial or ethnic background. In fact, the greater the penetrance the SNP has, the more important it is to select a control population that more closely matches the study population with respect to the

## TABLE 32–1

### Online Genome Resources

#### General Information

| | |
|---|---|
| NCBI | http://www.ncbi.nlm.nih.gov/ |
| GeneCards | http://bioinfo.weizmann.ac.il/cards/index.shtml |
| OMIM | http://www3.ncbi.nlm.nih.gov/entrez/query.fcgi?db=OMIM |
| HUGO | http://www.gene.ucl.ac.uk/cgi-bin/nomenclature/searchgenes.pl |

#### SNP Databases

http://www.ncbi.nlm.nih.gov/entrez/query.fcgi?db=snp
http://snpper.chip.org
http://gdb.jst.go.jp/HOWDY/
http://www.bioinformatics.ucla.edu/snp/
http://hgvbase.cgb.ki.se/
http://www.genome.utah.edu/genesnps/
http://pharmgkb.org

#### Sequence Alignment

| | |
|---|---|
| Genome-wide Blast | http://www.ncbi.nlm.nih.gov/blast/blast.cgi |
| Blast2 sequences | http://www.ncbi.nlm.nih.gov/blast/bl2seq/bl2.html |

disease being studied. As a general rule, the prevalence of an SNP should be greater than 5% in the control population to make it a reasonable candidate SNP for further investigation.

## VALUE OF HERITABILITY STUDIES

Investigators interested in the genetic underpinnings of disease should obtain reliable information suggesting that the disease in question is caused, at least in part, by heritable factors. In broad terms, *heritability* represents the proportion of phenotype variability that is attributed to genetic causes (25). In studies of monozygotic twins, heritability represents the upper limit of the genetic influence on disease susceptibility. For example, a twin study from the West of Scotland investigating the heritability of myocardial mass found that genetics may explain up to 53% of the variability in this population, after adjustment for covariates (26). More commonly, statistical calculations of heritability are performed from studies of nuclear families and siblings. Thus, heritability studies provide important proof of principle information regarding whether a phenotype is familial, and are therefore a useful adjunct to genetic studies. Although heritability studies are often available for

common diseases (such as hypertension, obesity, and a variety of neurologic and psychiatric disorders), that is often not the case for less common diseases.

## CHOOSING THE POPULATION TO BE STUDIED

Where practical, a common underlying pathology should be sought among study participants. For example, when studying the genetics of common forms of type 2 diabetes mellitus (T2DM), including individuals with corticosteroid-induced or hemochromatosis-associated diabetes would undermine the identification of important genes. It is imperative to stratify cases into well-defined phenotype categories that are homogeneous for the putative underlying biologic disease mechanism (e.g., separating ischemic from embolic strokes), especially when studying complex multifactorial diseases.

The validity of the candidate gene approach in association studies resides greatly on the selection of appropriate controls (also see Chapters 4 and 7). Misclassification of cases as controls significantly decreases the power of the study. For diseases with advanced age of onset or with variable penetrance, it is possible that an apparently unaffected individual may actually be either clinically asymptomatic (disease has not yet occurred) or the disease is present but the phenotypic abnormalities are not yet identified, either because of absent signs or symptoms, or due to insensitive diagnostic tests. Therefore, phenotypic characterization by use of highly sensitive techniques is as important for the controls as it is for the cases.

## CHOOSING DISEASE STATUS AND PHENOTYPE MARKERS

One of the greatest challenges of the candidate gene approach for association studies is the need to accurately characterize the *phenotype*, the observed characteristic or trait, especially when the overall magnitude of the genetic effect may be quite small. Many times, phenotype descriptors are poorly reproducible or are subject to significant inter- or intraobserver measurement variability (see Chapter 3). An investigator interested in studying the contribution of genetic variants to the risk of developing T2DM, for example, has several options for defining the phenotype. The most simplistic approach would be to just assign

phenotype on the basis of accepted clinical criteria, for example a fasting serum glucose > 125 mg/dL. Stronger genotype:phenotype associations, however, might be discovered if more sensitive or specific markers of disease were used, such as fasting serum glucose and insulin levels (as continuous variables), the response to physiologic challenges (such as an oral glucose tolerance test or hyperinsulinemic-euglycemic clamp), or calculated surrogates of insulin sensitivity such as the homeostasis model assessment of insulin resistance (HOMA-IR) (27).

Classifying populations according to intermediate or surrogate phenotypes (i.e., by quantitative measures of carotid plaque thickness rather than by history of stroke) increases the likelihood that a relationship between genotype and phenotype will be stronger because the path from genotype to intermediate phenotype (e.g., percent of carotid artery stenosis) is presumably more direct than the path to the composite phenotype (e.g., history of stroke). Quantitative measures of phenotype allow greater flexibility in statistical analyses over qualitative characterizations of disease severity. A list of variables that may be considered for analysis is shown in Table 32–2. Each

## TABLE 32–2

### Examples of Phenotype and Trait Characterization

| Demographics and Physical Exam Findings | Laboratory Findings | Imaging Studies |
|---|---|---|
| Age | Serum creatinine | Computed tomography (CT) |
| Gender | Fasting cholesterol panel | Magnetic resonance imaging (MRI) |
| Race/ethnicity | Complete blood count | Ultrasound |
| Heart rate | Hormones levels | Echocardiography |
| Blood pressure | Tumor markers (PSA) | Nuclear imaging |
| Height/weight | Inflammatory markers (CRP, TNFα) | Plain radiographs |
| Waist/hip circumference | | |

| Disease Traits | Physiologic Challenges | Surveys and Questionnaires |
|---|---|---|
| Age of diagnosis | Exercise testing | Mini-mental status exam |
| Severity | Oxygen consumption | Minnesota Living with Heart Failure |
| Tumor class | Six-minute walk | Functional Assessment of Cancer Therapy |
| Response to therapy | Oral glucose tolerance test | Addiction Severity Index |
| Family history of disease | | |
| NYHA class | | |

variable should be assessed for test and retest reliability, as well as for inter- and intraobserver variability where appropriate (see Chapter 3). Control subjects should also be tested to exclude asymptomatic disease. As with all observational studies (see Chapter 7), all possible confounders that may have effects equal to or greater than that of the candidate disease-associated gene being studied should be carefully considered.

## CHOOSING SOURCE OF DNA SAMPLING

Although DNA can be easily extracted from peripheral blood samples or buccal swabs, the challenge resides in collecting DNA from enough individuals with the disease or trait of interest. Genotyping should be performed on anonymized blood samples devoid of clinical data to assess the quality of the SNP detection assay and to gather initial information regarding the allelic frequency of the polymorphism. Proof-of-concept studies can often be accomplished with a relatively limited number of samples. Single-center studies can successfully recruit several hundred people for this purpose. The preliminary data gained though such efforts may generate enough plausible interest to justify larger DNA repositories to allow access to small aliquots of their DNA. Many industry or NIH-sponsored clinical trials and epidemiologic studies have collected DNA samples for several years, awaiting the inevitable opportunity to exploit that resource. A powerful design is the nested case-control study (see Chapter 7) built on an established cohort. DNA is only valuable, however, when coupled with quality clinical data. Many times, the requisite clinical data are not retrospectively available or retrievable.

## SAMPLES SIZE CALCULATIONS AND STATISTICAL ANALYSES

The central challenge of genetic association studies is to determine whether an observed difference in polymorphism frequency between cases and appropriately selected controls reflects true association rather than a chance event. Most association studies have focused on common polymorphisms (where the rare allele frequency is at least as great as the disease prevalence), where associations can be discovered in a modest-sized group of individuals (approximately 200); for more rare variants, a much larger group must be studied (13). For genotype:phenotype association studies, a detailed power calculation (Chapter 9) should be performed to determine how many cases and controls should be studied. These power calculations for genetic association studies are more difficult when the study is exploratory in nature. For example, reasonable power calculations require detailed information regarding the overall prevalence of disease in the population, the allelic frequency of the SNP, the penetrance of the disease trait with the SNP, and the relative risks afforded individuals heterozygous and homozygous for the SNP. Determining the genetic relative risks and disease trait penetrance is left to educated conjecture unless preliminary data are available.

Several types of risk estimates are used in genetic observational studies (28). The most common is relative risk, which provides an assessment of the association between the exposure (i.e., SNP) and disease that is independent of the prevalence of the exposure (i.e., allelic frequency) (29). The absolute risk is the overall risk in a particular population. The genetic attributable risk would indicate the proportion of a particular disease that may be attributed to a particular allele. The modest nature of the gene effects for complex disorders likely explains why case-control studies by different investigative groups of presumably similar populations frequently yield contradictory results. Reasons for this lack of reproducibility between studies include: (1) an insufficiently rigorous statistical threshold leading to false positives (Type I error); (2) small sample sizes limiting the statistical power to detect lower relative risks, thus increasing the chance for a false-negative result (Type II error); (3) true differences existing between the apparently similar populations; and (4) false positives due to population stratification. This latter phenomenon occurs when a trait that is present at a higher frequency in a particular racial group (or other subpopulation) shows a positive association with an allele that is also more common in that group (2,25,30). This problem can be averted in at least two ways: (1) analyze cases and controls in homogeneous groups (i.e., perform statistical analyses on racial groups separately), and (2) design an association study that uses family members as controls (called a *transmission disequilibrium test*) (30,31).

## PLACING DISEASE-ASSOCIATED ALLELES INTO AN APPROPRIATE CONTEXT

Finding a significant association between a tested polymorphism and a disease does not mean that a disease-causing polymorphism was found. Linkage disequilibrium between the two loci may increase the yield of association studies, but rarely determines the causative variant without further exploration. Once genetic dissection implicates a chromosomal region (by linkage analysis) or a gene or particular SNP (by association studies) as increasing disease susceptibility, there remains the formidable task of identifying the causative polymorphisms (Figure 32–4). Given the inevitable role played by linkage disequilibrium and the historic lack of reproducibility, associations detected in family linkage and genotype:phenotype studies should first be confirmed in large, population-based samples (25). If the initial results are duplicated, the SNPs residing on the same ancestral haplotype or those SNPs that exhibit strong linkage disequilibrium may help identify the causative variant. Resequencing the DNA segment of interest may be necessary to detect previously unreported SNPs. Once the suspected causative genetic locus has been identified, studies using genetically modified animals would be

desirable to demonstrate that introducing the relevant polymorphism alters gene expression or gene product function, resulting in the expected altered phenotype. In order to provide accurate risk estimates for the susceptibility allele, the next stage of research needs to move beyond affected individuals to the larger population.

## REGULATORY CONSIDERATIONS

Studies evaluating the genetic contributions to disease, by nature, constitute sensitive research (Chapter 14). Institutional Review Boards (IRBs) demand that stringent controls are taken to ensure that the results of genetic testing do not enter the public domain, or even into medical records, out of fear that the participant may encounter prejudice (either socially, or financially by termination of employment or refusal of insurance) if found to harbor a disease-associated genetic variant. With the advent of the Health Insurance Portability and Accountability Act (HIPAA), privacy concerns have become more heavily legislated. Although genetic testing itself is unlikely to cause physical harm to a research participant, other aspects of the study may pose physical risk, especially to a child or a pregnant woman. Particularly vulnerable are minors, women of childbearing potential or pregnant, institutionalized individuals, prisoners, non–native language speaking

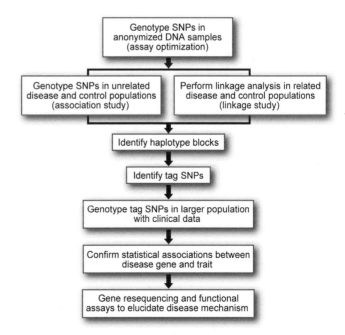

**FIGURE 32–4** ● Investigative strategy. Suggested steps to investigate a causal relationship between gene segments and complex disease traits. The strategy takes advantage of the linkage disassociation between tag SNPs and disease traits. Still unresolved are the best strategies for selecting the initial and tag SNPs.

individuals who lack proper access to translators, and in many cases, patients with life-threatening diseases for which treatment options are limited. In most genetic studies, separate written informed consent is required for study participation.

## METHODOLOGY OF SNP ANALYSIS

Almost all methods of SNP analysis have an *amplification step*, an *allele discrimination step*, and a *detection step* (32–34). The amplification step typically relies on the polymerase chain reaction (PCR) to amplify the DNA region of interest 10 billion–fold or greater (Chapter 31). The amplification step allows the use of minimal amounts of DNA (approximately 1–10 nanograms) for SNP analysis; however, the assay must be highly specific. PCR primers are designed to anneal to unique sites bordering the target DNA sequence. Before use, PCR primer sequences should be screened across the human genome using the NCBI Blast program (http://www.ncbi.nlm.nih.gov/blast/blast.cgi) to ensure their specificity for the gene of interest. This step is especially important when designing assays for highly homologous members of gene families. Hybridization conditions should be optimized and the assay tested prior to SNP analysis.

The allele discrimination step or genotyping step can be divided into those that give sequence (sequence-specific) and those that do not (sequence-nonspecific or sequence-free) (32). Sequence-nonspecific methods are often used in identifying polymorphisms in regions of low SNP density or in regions of DNA that have unknown sequence.

### Sequence-Nonspecific Methods of Allele Discrimination

The earliest method of sequence-nonspecific SNP analysis was *restriction fragment length polymorphism (RFLP) analysis*. RFLP relies on the gain or loss of a restriction enzyme recognition site at the site of the SNP. An example was identified in the glucose transporter-like protein 1 (Glut1) gene. A polymorphic Xba1 restriction enzyme site was found in intron 2 of this gene, and the presence of this restriction site was associated with increased risk of diabetic nephropathy in T2DM patients (35). The obvious limitation to this technique is that not all SNPs are within restriction enzyme recognition sites (although it is estimated that between one-fifth and one-half of all SNPs are) and restriction enzymes are expensive.

Another early method of sequence-nonspecific SNP analysis was *allele-specific PCR*. Allele-specific PCR is quick and gives direct visualization of the resulting product. An example of this method was used to identify the ACE insertion/deletion (I/D) polymorphism (36). This polymorphism has a 287 base pair insertion or deletion within intron 16 of the ACE gene. Allele-specific PCR relies on achieving specific primers for the variant alleles and resulting fragments must be run out on a gel. In addition, to avoid mistyping due to the preferential amplification of the deletion allele, it is often necessary to perform verification with an additional PCR reaction using insertion specific primers. The need for this verification step adds time and cost to this technique.

Two current-day examples of sequence-nonspecific SNP analysis method are *single-strand conformational polymorphism (SSCP) analysis* and *heteroduplex analysis*. SSCP analysis is the most common technique used for SNP analysis. This technique is based on the fact that single-stranded DNA has a secondary structure, or intramolecular conformation, that determines its mobility on a nondenaturing polyacrylamide gel. Under appropriate conditions, the conformation, and therefore mobility on a nondenaturing polyacrylamide gel, will be altered if even a single base differs between alleles. Benefits of this technique are that multiSNP alleles (alleles with more than one SNP in relatively close proximity to each other) can be differentiated from each other and the required laboratory materials are common and a large investment in specialized materials and equipment is not required. A disadvantage of this technique is that the gel conditions must be optimized and each reaction must be run out on a gel, resulting in more time requirement than some of the other methods.

Heteroduplex analysis takes advantage of the fact that, under appropriate conditions, heteroduplexes (a hybrid DNA complex, formed after heating the alleles and reannealing, consisting of wild type annealed to polymorphic DNA) will have different mobility on a gel or a different elution profile on a liquid matrix. Benefits of this technique are that multiSNP alleles can be differentiated from each other and that this technique has been mechanized, allowing for high-throughput SNP analysis.

### Sequence-Specific Methods of Allele Discrimination

Sequence specific methods are often divided into the following groups: (1) *allele-specific hybridization*, (2) *allele-specific nucleotide incorporation*,

(3) *allele-specific oligonucleotide ligation*, and (4) *allele-specific invasive cleavage* (32). The main advantage of these techniques is that they provide distinct sequence information.

The TaqMan assay is an example of allele-specific hybridization. This method makes use of the 5' nuclease activity of DNA polymerase. In this method, two oligonucleotide probes, one matching each allele, are each labeled twice. When the oligonucleotide probe that is specific for one allele anneals with the target DNA sequence (and matches it exactly), the probe is cleaved by DNA polymerase. Cleavage by DNA polymerase results in release of a fluorescent reporter. If, however, the other oligonucleotide probe anneals with the same target DNA sequence (and therefore, has a mismatch) it will not be cleaved but instead will be "pushed off" the target DNA sequence and the fluorescent reporter will not be released. If two distinct fluorescent dyes are used, the allele can be inferred by determining the fluorescence spectrum. An important key advantage of this method is that it is a *homogenous* assay method (i.e., amplification, genotyping, and detection steps are all carried out in a single solution). This saves both time and cost. The main disadvantage of this method is the need for optimization of probe design and of assay conditions. Also, because the genotype of the target DNA sequence is inferred, the assay may be affected by background if conditions are not optimal.

Two examples of the allele-specific nucleotide incorporation method are *Pyrosequencing*™ and the *template-directed dye-terminator incorporation (TDI) assay*. PCR with one of the primers containing a biotin tag is performed on genomic DNA to amplify and isolate the single-stranded DNA region containing the SNP. Genotyping using Pyrosequencing involves the addition of an internal primer and the separate addition of individual nucleotides to extend the primer using the PCR product as a template. Nucleotide incorporation liberates pyrophosphate, which acts as a substrate for ATP-sulfurylase, releasing ATP that is then used by luciferase, resulting in the emission of light. A cooled charge coupled device (CCD) camera records the light that is displayed as a peak on a Pyrogram™. The remaining nucleotides are removed from the assay by degradation with apyrase, and the reaction medium is regenerated for the next nucleotide addition. The main advantage of this technique is that alleles with more than one SNP in relatively close proximity to each other can be sequenced together. The primary disadvantage of this technique is that the Pyrosequencing reaction is costly and requires specialized equipment.

The TDI assay is an example of a homogenous allele-specific nucleotide incorporation assay detection method. The TDI assay uses 5'-fluorescein-labeled (donor-dye-labeled) primers designed to hybridize to the target DNA sequence adjacent to the SNP site. Acceptor-dye-labeled dideoxyribonucleoside triphosphate (ddNTP) and a modified Taq DNA polymerase are incubated with amplified DNA and the primer is extended one base with the specific acceptor-dye-labeled ddNTP. The method of detection is via fluorescence resonance energy transfer (FRET) (see below). The advantages of this assay include the lack of product separation, high sensitivity and specificity under optimized conditions, and high throughput. A disadvantage is that the genotype of the target DNA sequence is inferred and may be affected by background. In addition, there is the significant cost of two fluorescent labels per probe.

An example of the allele-specific oligonucleotide ligation SNP analysis method is homogenous ligation with FRET detection. This method uses allele-specific probes to discriminate between the two alleles, which takes advantage of the fact that, under optimized assay conditions, only the specific SNP will anneal with the correct probe. The advantage of this method is that it provides an amplification level of $10^9$-fold and therefore can be used directly on unamplified genomic DNA samples (although approximately 100 ng of genomic DNA is usually required). Other advantages are high specificity, and that it is a homogenous assay method.

An example of the allele-specific invasive cleavage method is the Invader® assay. The Invader assay is the only method of SNP assessment/identification that does not need amplification of the DNA region of interest prior to SNP identification. However, large amounts of genomic DNA must be used if this step is not performed (an obvious disadvantage if DNA quantities are limited). This homogenous assay method is very sensitive, also taking advantage of FRET detection. On the other hand, oligonucleotide probes used with this technique must be extremely pure to work well, and SNPs in highly repetitive target DNA sequences cannot be assayed by this method.

The biochemical reaction steps for allele identification are followed by a *detection step*. The detection step involves identification of the two alleles by *differences in light emission* (such as fluorescence or luminescence, as in Pyrosequencing), *mass*, or *electrical charge*. The most prevalent method of detection using fluorescence is fluorescence resonance energy transfer (FRET). This method uses two fluorescent dyes—a donor dye and an acceptor dye. It takes advantage of the fact that for FRET to occur the two dyes must be in close contact with each other. If the donor dye is near enough to the acceptor dye, the emission of the donor dye can excite the acceptor dye.

Mass spectrometry differentiates the two alleles by their differences in molecular weight. This method is so sensitive it can distinguish alleles that differ by only one base. In addition, the method is extremely fast, taking only milliseconds to analyze one sample. The main disadvantage of this method is that the product must be extremely pure for analysis and the equipment is costly.

## SUMMARY

- Several approaches can be used to identify disease-associated genes. Classic family linkage studies, while powerful at detecting highly penetrant Mendelian disorders, are yielding to genotype:phenotype association studies in unrelated populations to study complex disease traits.
- Genotype:phenotype studies rely on accurate and specific characterization of clinical traits in both the case and control populations, especially when the overall magnitude of the genetic effect may be small.
- *Haplotypes* may offer a substantial advantage in the search for susceptibility genes over the single variant-based approaches, significantly reducing the number of tested SNPs without reducing statistical power.
- Genes of interest may be identified by a genome-wide or a candidate gene approach.
- In a genome-wide approach, the inheritance pattern of a disease trait is compared with the inheritance pattern of hundreds to thousands of markers interspersed throughout the genome.
- A candidate gene approach is used if there is previous data implicating a specific enzyme, pathway, or molecule in the pathogenesis of the trait.
- Once a gene of interest has been identified, a comprehensive search of several databases should be employed to ensure that all putative SNPs are identified and given due consideration.
- For each SNP that will be pursued, whether it has been identified from a database, by literature search, by direct sequencing, or by any other method, it is imperative to verify both the validity and frequency of the polymorphism in a control population.
- In general, the prevalence of an SNP should be greater than 5% in the control population to qualify for further investigation.

- A variety of SNP analyses are available, most involving a DNA amplification step, allele discrimination, and a genotype-detection step. Sequence-nonspecific methods are gradually being replaced with sequence-specific methods as costs become more approachable.
- Identification of a disease-associated gene warrants confirmatory studies in another population. Gene sequencing and functional assays may be necessary to identify the exact disease-causing allele.
- Identification of causative gene mutations increasingly forms the basis for diagnostic and prognostic tests.

## REFERENCES

1. Bertina RM, Koeleman BPC, Koster T et al. Mutation in blood coagulation factor V associated with resistance to activated protein C. Nature 1994;369:64–67.
2. Marchetti M, Pistorio A, Barosi G. Extended anticoagulation for prevention of recurrent venous thromboembolism in carriers of factor V Leiden: cost-effectiveness analysis. Thromb Haemost 2000;84:752–757.
3. Reveille JD. The genetic basis of spondyloarthritis. Curr Rheumatol Rep 2004;6:117–125.
4. den Dunnen JT, Antonarakis SE. Nomenclature for the description of human sequence variations. Hum Genet 2001;109:121–124.
5. Yamada Y, Izawa H, Ichihara S et al. Prediction of the risk of myocardial infarction from polymorphisms in candidate genes. N Engl J Med 2002;347;1916–1923.
6. Cardon LR, Abecasis GR. Using haplotype blocks to map human complex trait loci. Trends Genet 2003; 19:135–140.
7. Risch N, Merikangas K. The future of genetic studies of complex human diseases. Science 1996;273:1516–1517.
8. Rosand J, Altshuler D. Human genome sequence variation and the search for genes influencing stroke. Stroke 2003;34:2512–2517.
9. Zhao H, Pfieffer R, Gail MH. Haplotype analysis in population genetics and association studies. Pharmacogenomics 2003;4:171–178.
10. Glazier AM, Nadeau JH, Aitman TJ. Finding genes that underlie complex traits. Science 2002;298:2345–2349.
11. Gabriel SB, Schaffner SF, Nguyen H et al. The structure of haplotype blocks in the human genome. Science 2002;296:2225–2229.
12. Patil N, Berno AJ, Hinds DA. Blocks of limited haplotype diversity revealed by high-resolution scanning of human chromosome 21. Science 2001;294:1719–1723.
13. Garner C, Slatkin M. On selecting markers for association studies: patterns of linkage disequilibrium between two and three diallelic loci. Genet Epidemiol 2003;24:57–67.
14. Wall JD, Pritchard JK. Haplotype blocks and linkage disequilibrium in the human genome. Nat Rev Genet 2003;4:587–597.
15. Zhang K, Calabrese P, Nordborg M et al. Haplotype block structure and its applications to association studies: power and study designs. Am J Hum Genet 2002;71: 1386–1394.
16. Schulze TG, Zhang K, Chen Y-S et al. Defining haplotype blocks and tag single-nucleotide polymorphisms in the human genome. Hum Mol Genet 2004;13: 335–342.

17. Wang L, Fan C, Topol SE et al. Mutation of MEF2α in an inherited disorder with features of coronary artery disease. Science 2003;302:1578–1581.

18. Venter JC, Adams MD, Myers EW et al. The sequence of the human genome. Science 2001;291:1304–1351.

19. Wang Z, Moult J. SNPs, protein structure, and disease. Hum Mutat 2001;17:263–270.

20. Marsh S, Kwok P, McLeod HL. SNP databases and pharmacogenetics: great start, but a long way to go. Hum Mutat 2002;20:174–179.

21. Riva A, Kohane IS. A SNP-centric database for the investigation of the human genome. BMC Bioinformatics 2004;5:33–40.

22. Reich DE, Gabriel SB, Altshuler D. Quality and completeness of SNP databases. Nat Genet 2003;33:457–458.

23. Mitchell AA, Zwick ME, Chakravarti A et al. Discrepancies in dbSNP confirmation rates and allele frequency distributions from varying genotyping error rates and patterns. Bioinformatics 2004;20:1022–1032.

24. Carlson CS, Eberle MA, Rieder MJ et al. Additional SNPs and linkage-disequilibrium analyses are necessary for whole-genome association studies in humans. Nat Genet 2003;33:518–521.

25. Merikangas KR, Risch N. Will the genomics revolution revolutionize psychiatry? Am J Psychiatry 2003;160:625–635.

26. Swan L, Birnie DH, Padmanabhan S et al. The genetic determination of left ventricular mass in healthy adults. Eur Heart J 2003;24:577–582.

27. Ferrannini E, Mari A. How to measure insulin sensitivity. J Hypertens 1998;16:895–906.

28. Lewis CM. Genetic association studies: design, analysis, and interpretation. Brief Bioinform 2002;3:146–153.

29. Falk CT, Rubinstein P. Haplotype relative risks: an easy reliable way to construct a proper control sample for risk calculations. Ann Hum Genet 1987;51:227–233.

30. Risch NJ. Searching for genetic determinants in the new millennium. Nature 2000;405:847–856.

31. Spielman RS, McGinnis RE, Ewens WJ. Transmission test for linkage disequilibrium: the insulin gene region and insulin-dependent diabetes mellitus (IDDM). Am J Hum Genet 1993;52:506–516.

32. Kwok PY. Methods for genotyping single nucleotide polymorphism. Annu Rev Genomics Hum Genet 2001;2:235–258.

33. Chen X, Sullivan PF. Single nucleotide polymorphism genotyping: biochemistry, protocol, cost and throughput. Pharmacogenomics J 2003;3:77–96.

34. Syvänen A-C. Accessing genetic variation: genotyping single nucleotide polymorphisms. Nat Rev Genet 2001;2:930–942.

35. Grzeszczak W, Moczulski DK, Zychma M et al. Role of GLUT1 gene in susceptibility to diabetic nephropathy in type 2 diabetes. Kidney Int 2001;59:631–636.

36. Rieder MJ, Taylor SL, Clark AG et al. Sequence variation in the human angiotensin converting enzyme. Nat Genet 1999;22:59–62.

# CHAPTER 33

# Cloning Methods

Janice Huss

O ften an important component of determining new mechanisms of disease involves identifying and characterizing genes and gene products that are essential for normal development and function, and similarly, genes and their products involved in pathologic processes. Commonly, to characterize a gene product, the gene of interest must first be cloned. Cloning refers to isolating recombinant DNA and transferring it to vectors (plasmid or viral), which allow the investigator to propagate, manipulate, and characterize the cloned DNA fragment. Genomic cloning and cDNA cloning are each distinctive tools for discovery. Cloning genomic DNA involves isolation of DNA segments directly from chromosomes, which includes all components of genes: introns, exons, and the regulatory regions surrounding genes. Cloning genomic DNA is often used to investigate gene structure, genetic variation (e.g., polymorphisms), and the regulation of gene expression. Cloning cDNA refers to isolating only the portion of DNA that encodes messenger RNA, which will then be translated into the final gene product; that is, a protein. Cloning cDNA is the focus of this chapter.

## GENERAL CLONING STRATEGIES

Cloning strategies vary, depending on what is known about the gene of interest (Figure 33–1). In a common scenario, an investigator wishes to isolate the human counterpart, or homolog, of a mouse gene (say, gene X) for which a cDNA clone already exists. In this case, a human cDNA library can be directly screened for human gene X by nucleic acid hybridization using a radiolabeled probe generated from the mouse gene. Novel genes or novel functions for known genes can be identified using functional cloning or cloning based on differential expression. With functional cloning, an assay is used to screen an expression library for a protein's activity. The yeast two-hybrid system, which is based on protein-protein interactions, is an example of functional cloning. Expression cloning identifies genes whose expression differs between cell or tissue types or is altered in a tissue during disease progression (i.e., tumor stages). The basis for differential expression cloning is selective isolation of only the differentially represented clones from the two populations being compared. The various techniques for cloning novel or known genes will be described in greater detail in the following sections and examples of relevant applications for each technique will be discussed.

## cDNA LIBRARIES

### Types of Libraries

A cDNA refers to a complementary DNA, the complement of RNA. A cDNA library represents the entire population of expressed mRNA transcripts in a certain cell, cell line, or tissue under a specific set of conditions (developmental stage, differentiation, or experimental condition). The vectors most commonly used in preparing cDNA libraries are plasmid or bacteriophage-based vectors ($\lambda$ vectors). Plasmid vectors are small vectors that episomally replicate in bacteria and can be directly purified from bacterial cultures. They are relatively easy to manipulate and many plasmid vectors can be used in both prokaryotic and eukaryotic hosts. These $\lambda$ vectors are viral vectors that are packaged into bacteriophage, which infect and propagate in bacteria. The most well known are the $\lambda$gt10 and $\lambda$gt11 vectors, which are used in the construction of nonexpression and expression libraries, respectively (discussed next). Library construction and subsequent isolation and manipulation of an identified clone of interest are

**Starting point:**

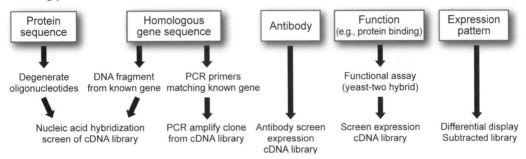

**FIGURE 33-1** ● Overview of general cloning strategies. The strategy employed for cloning genes is based on prior knowledge, if any, about the gene of interest and the reagents available for the screen.

more difficult with λ vectors than with plasmids. However, λ-based libraries are useful for cloning projects that require screening of a large number of recombinant clones (i.e., rare transcripts), due to the efficiency with which phage are taken up by bacteria and the ease of screening at high plaque densities by membrane hybridization. A major limitation of cloning from plasmid libraries is the relative inefficiency compared to λ-based libraries. The latest generation of cDNA library vectors is the combined excision vectors that are λ based, combining the desirable features of phage and plasmid vectors (1). Many molecular biotechnology companies offer variations of λ excision vectors (λZAP® series by Stratagene, λSCREEN™-1 by Novagen, λTriplEx™ by Clontech) that allow construction of high quality recombinant libraries that are easy to screen and facilitate subcloning of the cDNAs of interest into a plasmid vector.

One of the most important considerations when choosing an appropriate vector/host system for cloning is the means by which the clones of interest will be identified. Nonexpression libraries are screened by nucleic acid hybridization or by PCR amplification of the clone. Thus, prior sequence information from the gene itself or from homologous genes in other species is required. With the completion and public availability of sequence information from human, rodent, and microbial genomes and the continuous contribution of sequences from other species, having prior sequence information is no longer a limiting factor (2).

If the gene product (i.e., protein) can be detected using an antibody against the protein or a functional assay, then an expression library is appropriate. Expression libraries are the most versatile due to the variety of screening assays that can be used. Clone identification can be achieved by direct means, such as antibody recognition, or by more complex functional assays (e.g., membrane transport, ligand binding, or protein-protein interactions) to identify novel proteins. However, expression screening can be less efficient than nucleic acid screening. For example, if the expression vector used for the library expresses from a single reading frame, only $1/3$ of the library clones will synthesize a functional protein.

## Construction of cDNA Libraries

For a cDNA library to be complete, it must represent all the RNA species expressed in the tissue, including even rare transcripts present in only a few copies per cell. The number of distinct mRNA species represented in a mammalian cell varies but will range from 10 to 30,000 (3). By most estimates, a library should contain at least five times the expected number of distinct RNA species, knowing the relative abundance of the clone of interest in the original mRNA pool (4). For a transcript represented at 1/30,000 RNA species, at least 150,000 recombinants must be screened to detect that specific clone. Current cDNA cloning protocols starting with 5μg poly(A$^+$) RNA yield phage-based libraries of $10^6$–$10^8$ recombinants.

A cDNA library is constructed by "copying" poly(A$^+$) RNA isolated from the cells or tissue with reverse transcriptase that synthesizes DNA primed by oligo-dT annealed to the poly(A$^+$) tails of mRNA or by random short primers (random hexamers) distributed along the length of the RNA (Figure 33-2) (5). The copy DNA is made double-stranded using DNA polymerase followed by several enzymatic manipulations to prepare the cDNA for insertion (i.e., ligation) into λ or plasmid vectors. Once this population of reverse transcribed mRNA (i.e., the cDNA library) has been inserted into vectors, it is transferred into phage (packaging)

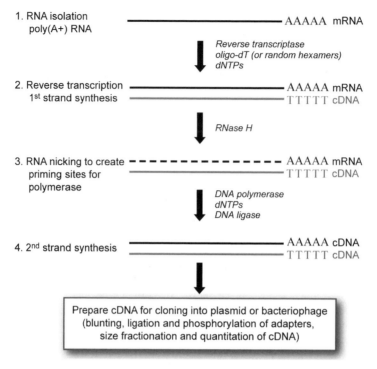

1. RNA isolation poly(A+) RNA ——————————————— AAAAA mRNA

*Reverse transcriptase*
*oligo-dT (or random hexamers)*
*dNTPs*

2. Reverse transcription 1st strand synthesis ——————————————— AAAAA mRNA
———————————————— TTTTT cDNA

*RNase H*

3. RNA nicking to create priming sites for polymerase – – – – – – – – – – – – → AAAAA mRNA
———————————————— TTTTT cDNA

*DNA polymerase*
*dNTPs*
*DNA ligase*

4. 2nd strand synthesis ——————————————— AAAAA cDNA
———————————————— TTTTT cDNA

Prepare cDNA for cloning into plasmid or bacteriophage
(blunting, ligation and phosphorylation of adapters,
size fractionation and quantitation of cDNA)

**FIGURE 33–2** ● Steps for the generation of double-stranded cDNA. Efficient synthesis of full-length double-stranded cDNA from poly(A⁺) RNA is the most important step in the production of a complete cDNA library.

or bacteria (transformation) to allow propagation and screening.

Construction of custom libraries is often necessary because a researcher is studying a specific disease model or experimental condition. However, a number of commercial sources provide libraries representing different species, tissue types, embryonic developmental stages, and cell lines that should be considered when deciding whether a custom library is necessary. In addition, clones can be directly purchased from a growing list of sources, such as the I.M.A.G.E. Consortium. A brief list of commercial and government-sponsored sources for libraries and clones is provided (Table 33–1).

## TABLE 33–1

### Sources for cDNA Libraries and Clones

| Company | Website |
| --- | --- |
| BD Biosciences (Clontech) | http://bdbiosciences.com/clontech.shtml/ |
| Invitrogen Life Technologies | http://invitrogen.com |
| EMD Biosciences (Novagen) | http://emdbiosciences.com |
| Stratagene | http://stratagene.com |
| NIH Mammalian Gene Collection Program | http://mgc.nci.nih.gov |
| I.M.A.G.E. Consortium | http://image.llnl.gov |
| NIA/NIH Mouse cDNA Project | http://lgsun.grc.nia.nih.gov |

## Screening of cDNA Libraries

This section briefly describes the basic technique for nucleic acid screening of nonexpression libraries or antibody screening of expression libraries. Understanding the traditional methods of library screening provides a theoretical foundation for currently applied techniques that will be discussed in subsequent sections. Nucleic acids or proteins expressed in bacteria or virus are immobilized on a membrane matrix that can be subsequently hybridized with a nucleic acid probe or antibody, respectively (Figure 33–3). For nucleic acid-based detection of clones, radiolabeled DNA or RNA probes are hybridized with the membrane-bound DNA and radioactive spots, corresponding to the cDNA clones of interest, are visualized by autoradiography (6). Selection of individual clones depends on a probe that specifically recognizes the cDNA of interest and is based on prior sequence information. Very often the gene of interest is the homolog of a cloned gene in another species, which can be used directly as a probe. Alternatively, structurally similar genes within a conserved gene family can be identified using a probe that corresponds to a highly conserved genetic region. A number of nuclear receptor transcription factors were cloned in this way, using the region of the gene encoding the DNA binding domain of known steroid receptors. The nucleotide sequence of this domain is highly conserved among members of this superfamily (7). If only the amino acid sequence of the protein of interest is known, nucleic acid–based methods can still be used but must take into account the inherent redundancy in the genetic code. In the case of membrane based screening, a small pool of degenerate oligonucleotides, representing all of the possible codon combinations for a short peptide stretch of the protein (6–8 amino acids), can be designed and serve as gene-specific probes (8,9).

### Screening Non-expression Libraries

With the complete sequence of the human genome now available, an experiment to identify a human homolog can often be done entirely *in silico*. In addition to numerous other databases, the National Center for Biotechnology Information (NCBI) curates the transcript and dbEST sequence data (10).

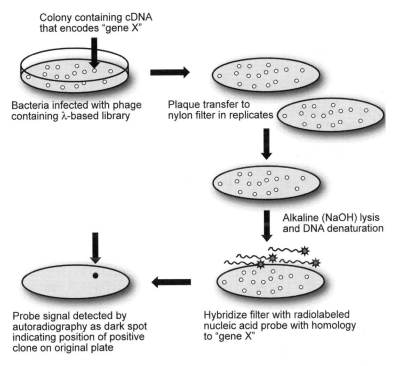

**FIGURE 33–3** ● Screening of a cDNA library by filter hybridization. Plaques or bacterial colonies carrying individual cDNAs from a library are transferred to nitrocellulose or nylon filters. Filters are treated with base to lyse bacteria and denature DNA for subsequent screening by hybridizing radiolabeled nucleic acids. The same process is used for antibody screening except that an expression library is hybridized with antibodies that specifically bind the protein of interest.

The International Protein Index (IPI) is a resource that collates protein sequences from numerous databases, providing a comprehensive set of human, mouse, and rat proteins (11).

Proteins involved in fundamental mechanisms, such as DNA replication, cell cycle control, and cell division, are frequently conserved between human and lower eukaryotes such as yeast. Yeast models provide an easily manipulated system in which to analyze such fundamental pathways. For example, Merkle et al. previously identified a complex of three proteins in yeast, CTF8, CTF18, and DCC1, involved in sister chromatid alignment during cell division, and predicted that homologs might exist in humans (12). The identity and function of proteins involved in genetic inheritance are relevant in human cancers, as chromosomal instability and aneuploidy, are observed in the earliest stages of tumor progression. Thus, the human proteins that mediate chromosomal stability are potential early mutational targets that predispose to the development of tumors.

The sequences of the yeast clones were used to search the NCBI human cDNA database and identify entries with significant sequence homology. These investigators performed their homology screen with the BLAST search tool, in which the database was queried using the sequence of each of the known yeast clones. The HomoloGene tool accessed through NCBI is a more recent system that performs automated homology searches among the completed eukaryotic genomes. Using this search tool, a homology search can be performed simply by entering a gene name or a Genbank accession number. Putative human homologs of the yeast genes were identified, and the cDNAs were acquired through the I.M.A.G.E. Consortium public collection of genes. Human cDNA clones acquired in this manner require subsequent validation to determine whether they are true functional homologs of the genes found in other species. In this study, the three human cDNAs were shown to express proteins of the appropriate size that formed a trimeric chromatin binding complex as predicted by behavior of the yeast homologs (12).

## Screening Expression Libraries

The process of antibody screening is analogous to that described above for nucleic acids (3,13). In an expression library (e.g., λgt11), protein is synthesized during phage growth and is transferred to nitrocellulose membranes by direct contact with plaques. The membranes are incubated with a protein solution to block nonspecific binding sites. Subsequent hybridization is performed with an antibody raised against the protein of interest. Detection can be performed using a radiolabeled or enzyme-linked secondary antibody for autoradiographic or chromogenic detection, respectively. It must be noted that positive clones identified by antibody screening may not represent the protein of interest but a protein containing the same epitope recognized by the antibody, an artifact of antibody cross-reactivity. For this reason, subsequent validation of potential clones must be performed using independent methods, such as expression analysis of the cloned protein using different antibody from that used in the initial screen.

This screening technique has proven to be particularly useful in the cloning of genes encoding serum antigens for which antibodies exist but for which the protein has not been identified. A serum assay based on antibody detection of the CA125 antigen has been used for over 20 years to monitor the clinical response of ovarian cancer patients (14). The CA125 antigen was thought to correspond to a high molecular weight glycoprotein that proved difficult to purify and clone. However, elucidating the molecular nature of the CA125 protein could lead to improvements in clinical detection of the antigen and more importantly may provide some insight into a mechanistic role for the protein in ovarian cancer development. A cDNA library constructed from mRNA isolated from an ovarian cancer cell line was screened using the antibody raised against a CA125 positive ovarian cell line. The cDNA sequence corresponded to a mucin family member (designated MUC16) and was verified by comparing the predicted amino acid sequence to that of a short peptide sequence of partially purified protein from the same ovarian cell line.

## PCR Cloning from cDNA Libraries

An entire chapter could be dedicated solely to describing the innovative use of PCR to screen libraries or other methods to clone genes of interest. The use of PCR in differential expression cloning will be discussed in a later section. The reader is referred to additional references for broader coverage of PCR cloning (15). The main advantages of screening cDNA libraries by PCR over hybridization-based techniques are efficiency, improved specificity (i.e. fewer false positives), and the ability to screen simultaneously for multiple genes (16). The screening method described here uses PCR to identify clones from pools of a cDNA library (17). As with nucleic acid hybridization, PCR screening requires sequence information about the gene of interest in order to design gene-specific PCR primers, preferably corresponding to a unique region of the gene.

Other optimization parameters to consider when designing PCR primers include annealing or melting temperature, GC content, primer length, and amplicon length (region amplified from cDNA). Amplification is most efficient if the amplicon is 200–500bp (18). The library is split into 10–20 aliquots, each of which is spread onto a single plate as performed for a hybridization library screen. When colonies (or plaques) have grown, they are scraped together and resuspended in growth media, giving 10–20 pools. Each pool is a subset of the library representing, for example, about 300,000 clones. PCR is performed on a small volume of each pool using the gene specific primers, and the pool containing the gene of interest is identified by agarose gel analysis of the PCR products. The positive pool is diluted $^{1}/_{10}$ and subdivided into aliquots containing approximately 3,000–5,000 clones using all the wells of a 96-well plate. Instead of performing PCR analysis on all 96 pools, the 96-well grid format can now be used to systematically screen additional pools (Figure 33–4). Small aliquots of each column and each row of wells are combined to give separate pools, respectively, giving 20 pools that represent all 96 wells. PCR is performed on these pools to identify the well containing the clone of interest. Using this strategy, a single positive pool, the intersection of a column and row (two positive pools in PCR screen), can be identified (Figure 33–4). The positive pool is then subdivided again, aliquoted into a 96-well plate (each well now contains 30–50 clones), and screened in 20 pools as before. The positive pool is spread onto bacterial plates so that the few remaining colonies or plaques can be individually screened by PCR.

## FUNCTIONAL CLONING

The completion of the human genome sequence has provided an estimate of the number of functional genes expressed in humans (approximately 25,000–30,000) (19). Sequence information from numerous important experimental model organisms, including mouse, arabidopsis, yeast, and recently rat, further contribute to researchers' knowledge about gene families. These sequence data serve as an important basis for the next step: to elucidate the function of uncharacterized expressed genes. Identification of genes based on function is fundamentally different from the cloning described earlier, which relies on some prior knowledge of related genes or proteins to the one being sought. Functional cloning is aimed at identifying novel genes involved in biological processes of interest without necessarily knowing anything about the protein. Virtually any protein that carries out or modulates a measurable process can be cloned this way. The two key requirements for a gene to be functionally cloned are (1) an efficient method to deliver and express the library or sublibraries (library pools or subtracted libraries) in the system, and (2) a robust assay system to accurately measure a functional endpoint. The two experimental applications discussed below highlight how this technique can be used very selectively to identify proteins involved in a specific cellular function or can be used to identify proteins that display a broader functional feature, such as an ability to associate with another protein, without assessment of functional relevance.

## Functional Cloning in a Cell Culture-Based Assay

Cells take up lipids for use in energy storage, signaling, membrane synthesis, and in oxidative ATP production. Recent studies have shown that, in addition to passive diffusion, transport mechanisms involving transmembrane proteins mediate uptake of lipids (20). Characterizing mechanisms of lipid uptake as an active, likely regulated, process has important implications for human disease. Diabetes,

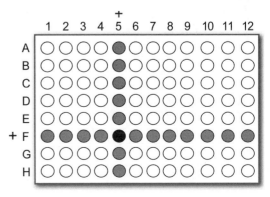

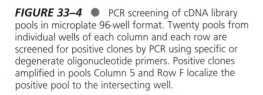

**FIGURE 33–4** ● PCR screening of cDNA library pools in microplate 96-well format. Twenty pools from individual wells of each column and each row are screened for positive clones by PCR using specific or degenerate oligonucleotide primers. Positive clones amplified in pools Column 5 and Row F localize the positive pool to the intersecting well.

atherosclerosis, and various forms of heart failure all involve an imbalance between lipid uptake and metabolism. Identification of the first member of a family of proteins involved in cellular long chain fatty acid transport included expression cloning (21). cDNAs from an adipocyte library were expressed in monkey kidney cells in culture to identify cDNAs that increased uptake of fatty acids. The primary screen involved delivering the entire cDNA expression library into cells using a chemical transfection technique. Uptake of a fluorescent fatty acid analog was measured by fluorescence-based cell sorting; the most fluorescent subpopulation of cells (0.03%) was collected. The cDNAs contained in these cells were isolated and the screen was repeated. The 0.03% most fluorescent cells from this second round of screening contained $10^3$ cDNA clones that were then divided into 50 pools of 20 clones each. The cDNA plasmids in these pools were then isolated and sequenced. The screen identified fatty acid transport protein (FATP1), that when expressed in cells, was localized to the plasma membrane and specifically increased uptake of long chain fatty acids. This relatively simple example highlights the specialized and potentially varied approaches to functional cloning. However, more generalized approaches have emerged based on assumptions about functionally related proteins, such as two-hybrid cloning, which is based on the notion that functionally related proteins often physically interact.

## Using the Two-Hybrid Assay to Identify Novel Interacting Proteins

The two-hybrid assay detects protein-protein interactions between a known protein and a protein from an expression cDNA library. This assay was originally described in yeast (22,23) but bacterial and eukaryotic cell-based systems have also been employed since the original method was described (24). The basic assay involves two fusion proteins (Figure 33–5). One fusion is created with the protein of interest, the "bait" protein, linked to a DNA binding domain (DBD) of a transcription factor (Gal4). The second set of fusion proteins (the "prey") are formed in the same way with cDNAs contained in a library fused to a transcriptional activation domain (AD). The DBD recognizes binding sites (UAS) located upstream of a selectable marker gene (or multiple marker genes) integrated into the host cell DNA. The selectable marker genes encode enzymes involved in purine or amino acid biosynthesis (*Ade* or *His*) or another easily measured enzyme (e.g., lacZ) not otherwise expressed in the host cells. Only when the *Ade* and *His* marker genes are expressed will the host cell grow on media lacking these nutrients. Expression of the selectable marker genes is activated when an AD fusion protein "prey", represented in the library, binds the Gal4-"bait" fusion protein. Unlike enzymes, the modular nature of transcription factors allows the DBD and AD to function independently of other domains usually present in the native

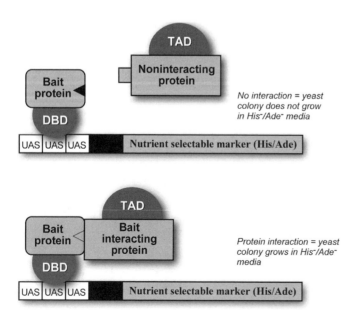

No interaction = yeast colony does not grow in His⁻/Ade⁻ media

Protein interaction = yeast colony grows in His⁻/Ade⁻ media

**FIGURE 33–5** ● Schematic of yeast two-hybrid screen for detecting protein-protein interactions. A known protein, the bait, is fused to a DNA binding domain (DBD) and coexpressed in yeast with a library that expresses prey proteins fused to a transcriptional activation domain (AD). Neither the bait-DBD nor the prey-AD individually can activate the reporter gene, which encodes biosynthetic genes (*Ade* or *His*). Only when the bait and prey interact, bringing the DBD and AD together, is there specific activation of *Ade* and *His* expression, permitting growth on media lacking adenine and histidine.

transcription factor, so recruitment of the AD to the promoter is sufficient to activate transcription of the *Ade* and *His* selectable marker genes. Cells expressing a protein from the cDNA library that interact with the "bait" protein are the only ones that will grow on selective media.

The two-hybrid assay is very sensitive because transient and weak interactions are often sufficient to produce small amounts of stable mRNA from the selectable marker genes. As high sensitivity can lead to false positives, all candidate interacting proteins identified in a two-hybrid assay must be verified by independent methods (e.g., coimmunoprecipitation, glutathione S-transferase (GST) pull down). Although the two-hybrid method has been widely applied, not all protein-protein interactions can be detected in this assay. Some proteins will not express or properly fold in yeast, and therefore will not adopt the proper conformation for interaction. Also, some protein-protein binding requires posttranslation modification, like phosphorylation; thus, these types of interactions will not be detected in this system unless modifying enzymes are coexpressed. The two-hybrid assay is based in the nucleus; thus, fused proteins that inhibit nuclear localization mediated by the nuclear localization signal contained in the DBD and AD domains cannot be assayed in this system.

### Translational Clinical Research Application

This technique has been a versatile tool in the transcription field, because enhancer elements bind high order protein complexes comprised of transcription factors, cofactors, and chromatin remodeling complexes. Additional interactions occur between enhancer proteins and the basal transcription factors (e.g., the RNA polymerase II complex) at the transcription initiation site. This system was used to clone a novel, cardiac-enriched transcription factor partner for the transcriptional coactivator peroxisome proliferator-activated receptor-$\gamma$ (PPAR$\gamma$) coactivator-1$\alpha$ (PGC-1$\alpha$), which is involved in regulating mitochondrial energy metabolism in heart and other highly oxidative tissues (25). A 182 amino acid region of the PGC-1$\alpha$ protein, encompassing domains shown to interact with other transcription factors, was fused to the Gal4 DBD and used as bait to screen an adult human heart cDNA AD fusion library in yeast. Of $4 \times 10^7$ transformants screened, approximately 150 colonies grew in selection media (*Ade-* or *His-*) media and were sequenced. The most frequent cDNA isolated (40% of clones representing two distinct cDNAs) encoded the nuclear receptor transcription factor, estrogen-related receptor $\alpha$ (ERR$\alpha$). Based on initial findings using two-hybrid cloning and subsequent functional studies, the

ERR family of receptors have emerged as important players in the developmental regulation of genes involved in mitochondrial metabolism.

## CLONING BASED ON DIFFERENTIAL EXPRESSION

The overall goal of cloning based on differential expression is to identify novel genes whose expression differs between distinct tissue or cell types, or is altered in response to an experimental treatment or a physiologic change. Several oncogenes and tumor suppressor genes have been discovered based on differential expression cloning strategies that include differential display, serial analysis of gene expression (SAGE), and various subtraction cloning methods (26–29). Expression profiling by DNA microarray analysis (Chapter 34), also allows nonbiased screening of thousands of expressed genes to detect changes between different mRNA populations. This technique requires specialized equipment and is costly to set up in an individual laboratory and the regulated genes identified by DNA array analysis must still be isolated either by cloning or by other means (collaboration, commercial, or public sources). Differential expression cloning and cDNA array analyses are often used in parallel to identify differentially expressed genes or in tandem to perform high throughput validation of candidates identified by differential expression library screening. The use of differential display and subtracted libraries to discover novel genes based on differential expression patterns will be discussed below. With any differential expression technique in which novel regulated genes are identified, the observed expression changes must be verified by independent methods, such as real-time PCR or Northern analysis (described in Chapter 31). Finally, it is essential to remember that in order to ascribe biological relevance to changes in transcript levels, it is necessary to link RNA expression with changes in protein expression.

### Differential Display Using PCR

Regardless of the specific method used, the general strategy of differential display involves reverse transcribing mRNA from two (or more) distinct biological samples, amplifying the cDNA with quantitative fidelity, and comparing the respective cDNA populations by high-resolution polyacrylamide gel electrophoresis (PAGE) (Figure 33–6). The differentially expressed clones can be subsequently recovered from the resolving gel, subcloned, and sequenced. There are many elegant variations of the differential display technique, but

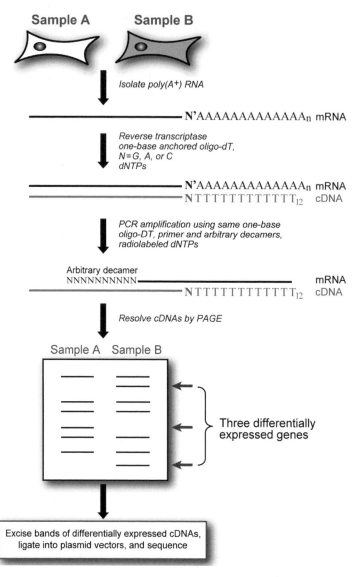

**Sample A      Sample B**

*Isolate poly(A$^+$) RNA*

————————————————— **N'**AAAAAAAAAAAAA$_n$ mRNA

*Reverse transcriptase*
*one-base anchored oligo-dT,*
*N=G, A, or C*
*dNTPs*

————————————————— **N'**AAAAAAAAAAAAA$_n$ mRNA
═══════════════════ **N** T T T T T T T T T T T$_{12}$ cDNA

*PCR amplification using same one-base*
*oligo-DT, primer and arbitrary decamers,*
*radiolabeled dNTPs*

Arbitrary decamer
NNNNNNNNNN ————————————————— mRNA
——————————— **N** T T T T T T T T T T T$_{12}$ cDNA

*Resolve cDNAs by PAGE*

Sample A    Sample B

Three differentially
expressed genes

Excise bands of differentially expressed cDNAs,
ligate into plasmid vectors, and sequence

**FIGURE 33–6** ● Steps involved in differential display by PCR. Poly(A$^+$) RNA
from two or more experimental samples are reverse transcribed with a one-base
anchored oligo-dT primer followed by PCR amplification in the presence of a radiolabeled dNTP using an arbitrary decamer and the same one-base oligo-dT primer.
The resulting cDNAs are resolved by high percentage, denaturing polyacrylamide
gel electrophoresis (PAGE). Bands are detected by autoradiography and can be
directly excised from the gel to isolate the differentially expressed cDNAs.

this relatively simple example is a modification of the original method (30,31). It serves to highlight the basic components of a differential display experiment. The poly(A$^+$) RNA isolated from each sample is reverse transcribed in three separate reactions using a single-nucleotide base anchored oligo-dT primer in which the 3′ nucleotide of the primer is C, G or A. Each of these primers selects different mRNA populations. PCR is then performed on the cDNA population in the presence of radiolabeled nucleotides using the same single-base oligo-dT primer in combination with an arbitrary sequence 10-base pair oligonucleotide (decamer) that theoretically can recognize any mRNA. Using this combination of primers for reverse transcription and PCR allows amplification from most of the mRNA species contained in the samples. The resulting amplified cDNAs from distinct samples are resolved side by side on a high percentage polyacrylamide gel to give fine resolution of differentially expressed transcripts (Figure 33–6). The radiolabeled cDNAs are visualized by autoradiography. A band that migrates the same distance but has different intensities between samples represents a differentially expressed gene. This band can be excised from the gel and the cDNA fragment isolated, cloned, and sequenced to determine its identity.

## Translational Clinical Research Application

In differential expression analyses, particularly relevant genes that are specifically activated or repressed in disease states are to be identified. Differentially expressed proteins may be involved in disease etiology and, therefore, present potential therapeutic targets. Alternatively, they may be coincidentally regulated genes that serve as valuable biomarkers for disease diagnosis and prognosis. A causal relationship between gene deregulation and disease development has been firmly established in human cancer. Altered expression of oncogenic and tumor suppressor genes is observed in many cancers and is linked to pathologic changes, such as cell cycle deregulation.

In a recent study, Kazemi-Noureini et al. sought to identify novel specific biomarkers for detecting esophageal cancer in order to improve early diagnosis and to identify potential molecular targets for therapeutic treatment. Differential display was used to screen altered expression of genes in RNA samples isolated from tumor tissue as well as normal tissue from an adjacent region in the esophagus of a single reference patient (32). Using PCR-based differential display (Figure 33–6) with three anchored oligo-dT and 24 arbitrary 13-mer primers, 6,000 genes were assayed for differential expression. Of 97 genes that showed altered expression in the tumors compared to normal esophageal tissue, seven were chosen for isolation, amplification, and cloning based on the high degree of expression change observed. Sequence data from the clones were compared to a transcript database to determine identity, and their predicted protein sequences were analyzed for putative structural domains. Importantly, because the screen was performed using tissue from a single individual, the expression of the cloned genes was assessed in normal and tumor tissue from nine additional patients. Of the seven cloned genes, four were regulated in 80% of the additional tumors samples similar to the pattern (upregulation or downregulation) observed in the differential display.

Validation to determine frequency of gene deregulation as well as to determine whether disease grade correlates with level of expression is critical to determine whether a gene will serve as a robust biomarker for diagnosis. The genes identified in this study are candidates for such validation, which could be performed on a larger scale using DNA microarrays spotted with candidate cDNAs to analyze the expression levels in samples collected from hundreds of patients.

## Subtractive Cloning

Differential expression cloning using subtraction methods selectively isolates cDNA clones that represent mRNAs present in one cell type or developmental stage but are absent in another. It involves two libraries: the (+) library, which expresses the transcript or transcript family of interest, and the (−) library, which contains transcripts present in both libraries. The (−) library of cDNAs is subtracted from the (+) library. Thus, transcripts common to both libraries will be selectively removed and the resulting subtracted library will only contain differentially expressed genes. A subtracted library is much smaller, generally containing 20 to 50% of the number of clones in the original (+) library, and therefore, is simpler to employ than full libraries when looking for tissue- or cell-specific mRNAs. A classic example using subtractive cloning allowed the isolation of cDNAs encoding T-cell-specific antigens by subtracting a B-cell library from a T-cell library, creating a library enriched for T-cell-specific cDNAs (33). The original technique will be described here to convey the conceptual basis for the subtractive cloning strategy.

In order to identify T-cell-specific proteins, a (+) cDNA library was constructed using mRNA from T cells, as described above, and modified to have sticky ends for cloning; while the (−) library was prepared from B-cell mRNA (Figure 33–7). The (−) library was cleaved with restriction enzymes that cut the DNA frequently and left blunt-ended fragments. The (+) and (−) libraries were mixed with the (−) library in excess, the cDNAs were heated to melt the double-strands, and the single-stranded cDNAs were allowed to rehybridize. The (−) cDNAs in excess reannealed with complementary sequences in the (+) library that represented transcripts common to both libraries. The remaining single-stranded (+) cDNAs that reannealed to create cDNAs with clonable sticky ends at both ends were those that were not represented in the (−) library. These clonable fragments were ligated into an appropriate λ or plasmid vector to generate the subtracted library. Typically, the library was plated, transferred to replicate filters, and differentially screened with radiolabeled

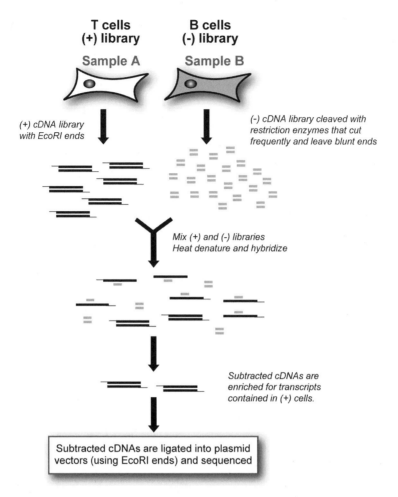

**FIGURE 33–7** ● Schematic of the subtractive cloning method. The (+) library (isolated from Sample A) expresses the cDNAs encoding protein(s) of interest, while the (–) library (isolated from Sample B) expresses cDNAs common to both libraries. The cDNAs from the (+) library are hybridized to cDNAs from the (–) library that have been blunt-ended and cleaved with frequent cutting restriction enzymes to create a molar excess of fragments. Only the (+) cDNAs represented in excess will reform double-stranded cDNAs with EcoRI overhangs that can be cloned to generate the subtracted library. The subtracted library is enriched cDNAs encoding transcripts specific to Sample A. Subtraction may be repeated to enrich for sample-specific cDNAs.

cDNAs from the original (+) and (–) libraries. The (–) cDNAs resulted in few clones, which corresponded to false positives, while the cDNAs from the (+) libraries hybridized with most of the clones in the subtracted library.

## Translational Clinical Research Application

The subtractive cloning method is particularly useful for profiling global differences in expression programs between distinct tissues or cell populations. The example below demonstrates how subtractive cloning can be used to distinguish transcript profiles within a cell type chronically exposed to different physiologic conditions.

Vascular endothelium is the site for development of atherosclerotic plaques, but all sites are not equally susceptible to plaque formation; lesions preferentially form at arterial branch points and curves. A contributing feature may be the differences in nonuniform shear stress experienced by endothelial cells at these sites. Yoshisue et al. predicted that gene expression changes in endothelial cell subpopulations exposed to greater nonuniform shear stress and that these microenvironments contribute to phenotypic changes involved in early lesion formation. They used subtractive cloning to generate a comprehensive list of genes upregulated in endothelial cells by shear stress (34). Human umbilical vein endothelial cells (HUVEC) were subjected to conditions simulating nonuniform shear stress using a model system in which cells were attached to beads and exposed to vortical flow. mRNA from the HUVEC exposed to shear stress were used to generate the (+) library and mRNA from the untreated cells were used for the (−) library. Thus, the experiment was designed to clone genes specifically present in the HUVEC exposed to nonuniform shear stress. Using a modified approach from that described in Figure 33–7, they identified 63 shear stress–upregulated genes. Demonstrating that the subtracted library contained genes previously shown to be upregulated by shear stress, such as laminin B1, validated their method. In addition, the regulation of 56 novel genes, identified in their screen, was verified in their own model by Northern analysis. More importantly, four of the novel genes were shown to be upregulated in human atherosclerotic tissue. Thus, this approach not only contributed to the basic understanding of relevant changes involved in early atherosclerosis but may have also identified potential therapeutic targets for preventing endothelial cell changes that allow plaque development.

### Comparison of Differential Expression Cloning Methods

The two differential expression methods for cloning described here have different advantages. Subtractive cloning allows cloning of cell- or tissue-specific cDNAs by comparing libraries from distinct cell types, while differential display is more appropriate for identifying regulated genes from a specific cell or tissue type subjected to experimental manipulation. The subtractive method allows only unidirectional comparisons between two libraries, but differential display detects induced and repressed genes from multiple samples. Finally, subtractive cloning is more sensitive than differential display and yields nearly a complete set of differentially expressed genes, while only a subset of cDNAs can be isolated by band excision from differentially displayed libraries resolved by PAGE.

### SUMMARY

- The appropriate method for cloning a gene of interest is largely determined by what is known about the protein of interest.
- A complete cDNA library is the most critical reagent in a cloning project. Often a custom library is needed; however, possible good libraries can be obtained commercially or from generous collaborators.

- Traditional library screening methods (i.e., nucleic acid screens) can often be performed using more efficient and specific PCR-based strategies.
- With the completed sequence of the human genome, the most important goal of cloning is to link predicted genes with their function.
- Functional cloning requires an experimental system in which cDNAs can be expressed and functional effects can be measured.
- Cloning based on differential expression is a powerful method for identifying genes involved in disease processes and genes that serve as diagnostic/prognostic biomarkers.
- Subtractive cloning results in a complete library of upregulated genes.
- Differential display identifies both upregulated and downregulated genes but only a subset of clones are typically isolated in a screen.

### REFERENCES

1. Short JM, Sorge JA. In vivo excision properties of bacteriophage λZAP expression vectors. In: Wu R, ed. Recombinant DNA Part G. Methods in Enzymology, vol 216. San Diego: Academic Press, 1992:495–509.
2. Williams, G. Nucleic acid and protein sequence databases. In: Bishop MJ, ed. Genetics Databases. London: Academic Press,1999:11–37.
3. Young RA, Davis RW. Efficient isolation of genes by using antibody probes. Proc Natl Acad Sci 1983;80:1194–1198.
4. Kimmel AR, Berger SL. Preparation of cDNA and the generation of cDNA libraries: overview. In: Berger SL, Kimmel AR, eds. Guide to Molecular Cloning Techniques: Methods in Enzymology, vol 152. London: Academic Press, 1987:307–316.
5. Bhattacharyya MK. Construction of a cDNA library. In: Brown TA, ed. Essential Molecular Biology: A Practical Approach, vol 2, 2nd Ed. Oxford: Oxford University Press, 2001:41–62.
6. Wahl GM, Berger SL. Screening colonies or plaques with radioactive nucleic acid probes In: Berger SL, Kimmel AR, eds. Guide to Molecular Cloning Techniques: Methods in Enzymology, vol 152. London: Academic Press, 1987:415–423.
7. Giguère V, Yang N, Segui P et al. Identification of a new class of steroid hormone receptors. Nature 1988;331: 91–94.
8. Lathe R. Synthetic oligonucleotide probes deduced from amino acid sequence data. J Mol Biol 1985;183: 1–12.
9. Lee CC, Wu XW, Giblos RA et al. Generation of cDNA probes directed by amino acid sequence: cloning of urate oxidase. Science 1988;239:1288–1291.
10. National Center for Biotechnology Information, National Library of Medicine. Bethesda, MD, 1996. http://www.ncbi.nlm.nih.gov. Accessed March 31, 2005.
11. Kersey PJ, Duarte J, Williams A et al. The International Protein Index: an integrated database for proteomics experiments. Proteomics 2004;4:1985–1988. http://www.ebi.ac.uk/IPI/. Accessed March 31, 2005.

12. Merkle CJ, Karnitz LM, Henry-Sanchez JT et al. Cloning and characterization of hCTF18, hCTF8, and hDCC1: human homologs of a Saccharomyces cerevisiae complex in sister chromatid cohesion establishment. J Biol Chem 2003;278:30051–30056.

13. St. John TP. In: Ausubel FM, Brent R, Kingston R et al., eds. Current protocols in molecular biology unit 6.7. New York: John Wiley and Sons, 1990.

14. Yin BWT, Lloyd KO. Molecular cloning of the CA125 ovarian cancer antigen. J Biol Chem 2001;276: 27371–27375.

15. Chen B-Y, Janes HW, eds. Methods in Molecular Biology: PCR Cloning Protocols: vol 192, 2nd Ed. Totowa, NJ: Humana 2002:353–358.

16. Zhu J. Use of PCR in library screening. In: Chen B-Y, Janes HW eds. Methods in Molecular Biology: PCR Cloning Protocols: vol 192, 2nd Ed. Totowa, NJ: Humana, 2002:353–358.

17. Takumi T, Lodish HF. Rapid cDNA cloning by PCR screening. Biotechniques 1994;17:443–444.

18. Hyndman DL, Mitsuhashi M. PCR primer design. In: Bartlett JMS, Stirling D, eds. Methods in Molecular Biology: PCR Protocols, vol 226, 2nd ed. Totowa, NJ: Humana,2003:81–88.

19. Southan C. Has the yo-yo stopped? An assessment of human protein-coding gene number. Proteomics 2004;4:1712–1726.

20. Schaffer JE. Fatty acid transport: the roads taken. Am J Physiol 2002;282:E239–E246.

21. Schaffer JE, Lodish HF. Expression cloning and characterization of a novel adipocyte long chain fatty acid transport protein. Cell 1994;79:427–436.

22. Fields S, Song O. A novel genetic system to detect protein-protein interactions. Nature 1989;340:245–246.

23. Chien CT, Bartel PL, Sternuglanz R et al. The two-hybrid system: a method to identify and clone genes for proteins that interact with a protein of interest. Proc Natl Acad Sci USA 1991;88:9578–9582.

24. Finkel T, Duc J, Fearon ER et al. Detection and modulation in vivo of helix-loop-helix protein-protein interactions. J Biol Chem 1993;268:5–8.

25. Huss JM, Kopp RP, Kelly DP. Peroxinsome proliferator-activated receptor coactivator-1α (PGC-1α) coactivates the cardiac-enriched nuclear receptors estrogen-related receptor-α and −γ. Identification of novel leucine-rich interaction motif within PGC-1α. J Biol Chem 2002;277:40265–40274.

26. Graveel CR, Jatkoe T, Madore SJ et al. Expression profiling and identification of novel genes in hepatocellular carcinomas. Oncogene 2001;20:2704–2712.

27. Lapointe J, Labrie C. Identification and cloning of a novel androgen-responsive gene, uridine diphosphoglucose dehydrogenase, in human breast cancer cells. Endocrinol 1999;140:4486–4493.

28. Zhang L, Zhou W, Velculescu VE et al. Gene expression profiles in normal and cancer cells. Science 1997;276: 1268–1272.

29. Lee SW, Tomasetto C, Sager R. Positive selection of candidate tumor-suppressor genes by subtractive hybridization. Proc Natl Acad Sci 1991;88:2825–2829.

30. Liang P, Pardee AB Differential display of eukaryotic messenger RNA by means of polymerase chain reaction. Science 1992;257:967–971.

31. Liang P, Zhu W, Zhang X et al. Differential display using one-base anchored oligo-dT primers. Nuc Acids Res 1994;22:5763–5764.

32. Kazemi-Noureini S, Colonna-Romano S, Ziaee A-A et al. Differential gene expression between squamous cell carcinoma of esophagus and its normal epithelium; altered pattern of mal, akr1c2 and rab11a expression. World J Gastroenterol 2004;10:1716–1721.

33. Hedrick SM, Cohen DI, Nielsen EA et al. Isolation of cDNA clones encoding T cell-specific membrane-associated proteins. Nature 1984;308:149–153.

34. Yoshisue H, Suzuki K, Kawabata A et al. Large scale isolation of non-uniform shear stress-responsive genes from cultured human endothelial cells through the preparation of a subtracted cDNA library. Atherosclerosis 2002;162:323–334.

# CHAPTER 34

# Transcriptional Profiling

Mark A. Watson

## MICROARRAY TECHNOLOGIES

In most general terms, a *microarray* refers to an ordered collection of objects, usually attached to a solid phase, two-dimensional surface of minimal area. Two basic configurations of microarrays are used for translational research studies (Figure 34–1). Reverse-phase (sample) microarrays represent collections of individual study samples arrayed onto a solid surface, to which a single biomarker probe is applied. In this application, many samples can be analyzed in a single experiment. Conversely, forward-phase (probe) microarrays represent collections of individual biomarker probes arrayed onto a solid surface, to which a single study sample is applied. These arrays allow hundreds or thousands of molecular biomarkers to be simultaneously assayed in a single sample.

*Tissue microarrays* are a commonly used form of a sample microarray designed to simultaneously measure protein expression in hundreds of study tissue samples (1). Individual 0.6-millimeter diameter tissue cores are harvested from either frozen or paraffin-embedded tissue blocks. Several hundred of these cylindrical tissue cores, each representative of an individual tissue specimen, are then arrayed into a grid and cast to form the tissue microarray block. When this block is sectioned, an array of individual tissue specimens is created that can be analyzed with antibody or nucleic acid probes for immunohistochemical protein expression studies (Chapter 36) or in situ hybridization analysis of gene dosage or expression (Chapter 36), respectively. The usefulness of this technique as applied to translational research is that many samples can be analyzed using only a small amount of reagent (e.g. antibody) and with a minimum amount of time and effort (a single slide may represent several hundred different study specimens). However, because only a single 0.6-millimeter diameter sample of the tissue specimen is analyzed (as compared to analysis of an entire section of tissue), staining or hybridization results from a tissue microarray may be confounded due to sampling error, particularly for tissue samples that are heterogeneous. Furthermore, although immunohistochemical or hybridization procedures can be performed rapidly on large numbers of tissue samples using this technology, each of the several hundred tissue spots present on the microarray must still be analyzed manually by an experienced histopathologist or in a semiautomated fashion using expensive image scanning hardware and quantification software.

*Protein microarrays* are a less commonly used form of reverse-phase microarrays that quantitatively measure protein expression in study samples (2). In this application, tissue protein homogenates from several hundred different study samples are spotted onto a solid surface using robotic, liquid handling equipment. The resulting slide of protein lysate spots is probed with an antibody corresponding to the biomarker of interest and quantification of the protein in each spot is performed using standard antibody-mediated detection techniques (Chapter 36). Unlike tissue microarrays, detection signals emanating from protein spots are homogeneous and easier to quantify, particularly when each protein sample is arrayed as a set of serial dilutions. Obviously, no histopathology expertise is required for data interpretation, but neither can any information be obtained with regard to protein expression relative to tissue histology.

Both tissue microarrays and protein microarrays are useful tools for *biomarker validation* studies. That is, one or a few biomarkers may be validated on a large number of study samples. In fact, tissue microarrays are frequently used to validate changes in gene expression discovered using nucleic acid

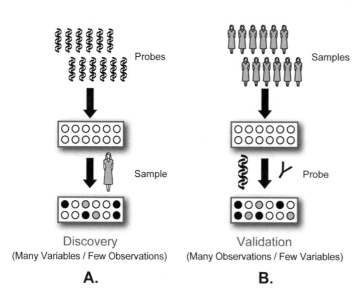

**FIGURE 34–1** ● Microarray applications. **A.** Probe, or forward-phase, microarrays contain a large number of biomarker probes such as antibodies or nucleic acid sequences to which one or two study samples are applied. They are generally used as biomarker discovery tools. **B.** Sample, or reverse-phase, microarrays contain a large number of study samples such as tissue cores to which one or two biomarker probes are applied. These arrays are excellent tools for biomarker validation.

microarrays (3). Because the data represent few variables (markers) and a large number of observations (samples), statistical analysis of reverse-phase array studies is fairly standard.

Forward-phase microarrays include both *antibody arrays* and *nucleic acid microarrays*. Nucleic acid arrays are discussed in the remainder of this chapter. Antibody arrays are the proteomic equivalent of nucleic acid arrays (4). In this application, spots of antibody solution are deposited onto a solid surface. An individual study sample of protein is then applied to the fabricated array. Specific proteins in the sample mixture bind to their cognate antibodies on the array and the amount of each protein bound to each antibody site can be measured. Thus, the concentration of a large number of individual proteins can be simultaneously measured within a single sample. Although many sources of commercial antibody arrays are now available, this technology is mainly limited by the number of high-performance, specific antibodies to proteins of interest. Antibody arrays represent a promising technology, but it is likely that they will be rapidly supplanted by other global proteomic methods (Chapter 35).

## NUCLEIC ACID MICROARRAYS

Nucleic acid (NA) microarrays are the most widely used form of forward-phase array. Routine and inexpensive chemical synthesis of nucleic acids and a fully sequenced and highly annotated human genome have made high-throughput, customized fabrication of NA microarrays possible for translational research. NA microarrays may be used to qualitatively or quantitatively assess the genome (genomic DNA)

or the transcriptome (mRNA). In all cases, a single nucleic acid study sample (or sometimes a pair of samples), commonly referred to as *target*, is applied to the solid array surface that contains thousands of sequence-specific, nucleic acid *probes*. These nucleic acid probes may be long stretches of chromosome-specific DNA (i.e., bacterial artificial chromosome -BAC- clones), cDNA clones representing expressed mRNAs, or sequence specific oligonucleotides ranging in length from 25 to 70 base pairs (5). In this last case, oligonucleotides may be chemically synthesized off-site and then physically spotted onto the array surface using robotic microfluidics instrumentation, or they may be synthesized in situ using light-directed combinatorial photochemistry (Figure 34–2).

NA microarrays are being used increasingly in translational research to perform highly multiplexed single nucleotide polymorphism (SNP) analysis (6) and DNA resequencing (7). SNP chips can simultaneously genotype patient samples at as many as 100,000 different loci, and are a powerful tool for gene association and linkage studies (Chapter 32). Genomic regions containing target polymorphic loci are amplified from the study sample using the polymerase chain reaction. Amplified, labeled DNA is then applied to the array where each amplified fragment containing one or more of the 100,000 polymorphic loci hybridizes specifically to one or both oligonucleotides representing the allelic variant sequence. This approach can be extended to determine the complete nucleotide sequence of a target gene or sets of genes, assuming that the reference sequence is known.

Using BAC clones to represent large regions of specific chromosomal loci, NA microarrays can be

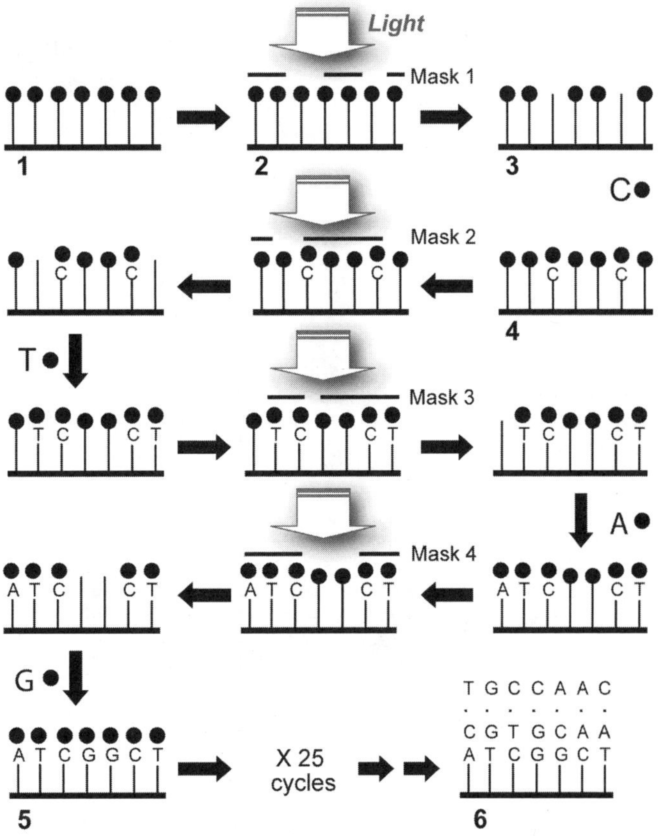

**FIGURE 34–2** ● Schema for in situ oligonucleotide microarray synthesis. Photochemical sites on a solid phase (1) are selectively activated by shining light through a patterned mask or grid (2). A reactive nucleotide is added to the surface (3), which is covalently bound to each activated site (4). This cycle is repeated four times with four independent masks for each possible nucleotide (C, T, A, G), until every site on the array is occupied (5). The entire cycle of four can then be repeated with four new sets of masks to build a unique oligonucleotide sequence at every position on the array (6). Depending on the technology used, each address on the array may be as small as 25 $\mu^2$. Using this scheme, 25 sets of masks could be used to build $1 \times 10^{15}$ unique sequences while $4 \times 10^6$ of these sequences could be arranged with a single 1 cm$^2$ microarray.

used to quantify specific changes in genome copy number (8). Also known as array comparative genome hybridization (array CGH), this method hybridizes labeled genomic DNA from a reference sample and an experimental sample to a single BAC clone array, representing the genome as a series of array elements. By comparing relative hybridization signal intensities of the reference and experimental samples at any given spot representing a specific chromosomal location, specific gains and losses of the genome can be assessed with very fine resolution (Figure 34–3).

The most popular use of NA microarrays in translational research to date has been for quantitative measurement of mRNA levels. For this reason, the remainder of this chapter will focus specifically on the use of NA microarrays for gene expression profiling.

## GENE EXPRESSION PROFILING USING MICROARRAYS

### Microarray Formats

As outlined above, there are many different methods for constructing NA microarrays, many of which are suitable for gene expression profiling studies. Many gene expression profiling studies use *cDNA microarrays*. Selected tissue mRNA is used to create a cDNA library (Chapter 33) and individual cDNA clones are physically spotted onto a chemically-treated glass slide using robotic microfluidics instrumentation (5). The use of cDNA arrays has two distinct experimental advantages. First, complete genomic sequence information is not a requisite for array preparation, although the sequence of each cDNA clone is eventually required for array annotation. For this reason, investigators frequently use cDNA arrays to study gene expression in organisms without extensive genome sequence data. Given the now completely sequenced and highly annotated human genome, this is not a particular advantage for translational research studies. Next, by representing only genes that are expressed in the tissue of interest (in the form of cDNAs), most probes on the array will provide useful information about differential gene expression in the study samples. For example, Alizadeh et al. used clones isolated from a variety of human lymphocyte-specific cDNA libraries to design a "lymphochip." This focused array was then used to classify molecular subtypes of diffuse large B-cell lymphoma (9).

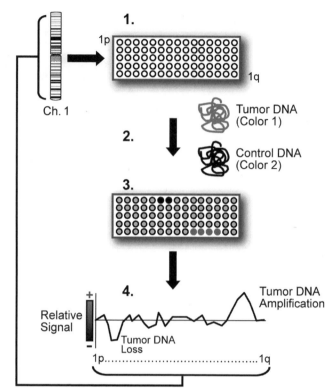

**FIGURE 34–3**  ●  Array comparative genomic hybridization (aCGH). Bacterial artificial chromosome (BAC) clones corresponding to known regions of chromosomal DNA are spotted onto a solid surface (1). Matched sample DNAs (e.g., tumor and nontumor genomic DNA from the same patient) are labeled with different fluorogenic dyes (2) and hybridized to the array (3). The relative fluorescent intensity at each spot is measured and mapped back to corresponding chromosomal location (4). Relatively increased fluorescent intensity of one dye versus the other indicates specific chromosomal regions of loss or amplification.

Although focused arrays may ultimately be useful as diagnostic instruments, high-density oligonucleotide array technology and a sequence-verified human genome have favored the use of "whole genome" expression arrays for translational research involving gene biomarker discovery.

In fact, most human gene expression microarrays used today are designed with either short or long oligonucleotide sequences. Because oligonucleotides are chemically synthesized based on known sequence, a fully sequenced genome and sophisticated bioinformatics tools to select optimal sequences for each transcript to be represented on the array are needed (5). Oligonucleotide sequences ranging from 50 to 70 nucleotides in length provide sufficient specificity to hybridize only to their intended target transcript. Many commercial vendors have developed catalogs of 35,000 to 45,000 oligonucleotide sequences, each representing a unique human gene transcript. These oligonucleotides, which are chemically synthesized off-site, may be purchased and physically spotted to a chemically treated glass slide using robotic microfluidics instruments that are available at many larger academic centers. More commonly, however, commercially prepared oligonucleotide microarrays are purchased directly. Added quality control, decreasing costs, and increasing flexibility

in generating customized arrays make commercial oligonucleotide microarrays an increasingly attractive alternative for translational research studies.

An alternate design of oligonucleotide microarray, the Affymetrix's GeneChip®, uses in situ synthesized oligonucleotides (Figure 34–2). Unlike spotted oligonucleotide arrays, GeneChip microarrays contain 25 nucleotide sequences, which in themselves do not provide sufficient sequence specificity to hybridize solely to their intended mRNA target. Therefore, multiple pairs of specific and mismatched sequences are used to detect a specific hybridization event. Although as many as 22 individual oligonucleotides may be required to assay a single transcript (compared to a single 50 base pair oligonucleotide on a spotted array), the ability to synthesize over one million discrete sequences on a single array more than compensates for this limitation (5).

### Sample Requirements

As the objective of a gene expression profile study is to quantify relative changes in gene expression between study samples, a finite amount of cellular RNA derived from each study sample is an obvious requirement. Using current methodology, total cellular RNA derived from cells or tissues is sufficient and does not need to be additionally enriched for the polyadenylated fraction of mRNA. For most microarray protocols, 1 to 5 micrograms of total cellular RNA is generally sufficient to perform a microarray experiment. However, it is also possible to perform experiments using as little as 1 ng of total RNA using molecular amplification techniques.

An even greater consideration than the quantity of RNA that can be retrieved from a biological specimen is the quality of the RNA. RNA itself is chemically labile and is also rapidly degraded by ubiquitous cellular RNAases. Use of substandard RNA preparations results in poor microarray performance. Furthermore, the use of varying qualities of RNA within an experiment can artificially create differential patterns of gene expression related to sample quality rather than biological or clinical correlates. Fortunately, many robust methods for isolating RNA from a variety of tissues and cell types exist, and new methods for quantitatively assessing RNA quality can provide stringent measures of quality control (Figure 34–4).

The highest quality RNA is derived from freshly isolated tissue or cell samples that are immediately snap frozen (using dry ice or liquid nitrogen) or properly homogenized in sample preparation buffer. Unfortunately, clinical specimens that are fixed in formalin and embedded in paraffin wax yield RNA that is highly fragmented and cross-linked due to the fixation and embedding process. RNA isolated from such specimens is generally (although not absolutely) unsuitable for gene expression microarray analysis. Furthermore, unlike genomic DNA, cellular RNA exists in a dynamic equilibrium. Small changes in cell state may dramatically change transcript abundance, particularly for genes associated with cell signaling in response to hypoxia and other environmental insults. Thus, in addition to protecting against general chemical or enzymatic degradation of the entire RNA pool, particular attention is required toward study sample collection and preparation (10). For example, collection of tissue specimens from surgical tumor resections may be associated with differing warm ischemia times, depending on the delay from resection to tissue freezing. Such delays can artificially produce differential patterns of gene expression related to differences in collection (11).

## Target Synthesis

In the nomenclature of NA microarrays, a *target* refers to the labeled material (i.e., study sample RNA) that is applied to the microarray containing nucleic acid *probes*. In its simplest form, target synthesis consists of converting sample RNA into cDNA in the presence of labeled nucleotides. This labeled cDNA is then hybridized to the array. Although this method is the most straightforward, it requires large amounts of mRNA-enriched, cellular RNA.

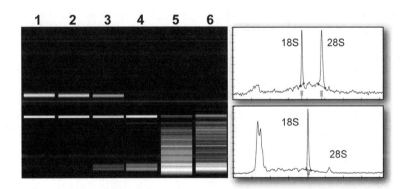

**FIGURE 34–4** ● Analysis of cellular RNA for microarray experiments. A number of methods are available to qualitatively assess RNA samples prior to their use in microarray experiments. On the left, a pseudo-electrophoretogram image generated using the Agilent Technologies, Lab-on-a-Chip RNA microelectrophoresis system. High quality RNA (lanes 1, 2) is indicated by sharp 28S and 18S ribosomal RNA bands in an intensity ratio of approximately 2:1, and the absence of low molecular weight nucleic acid. Slightly degraded RNA samples (lanes 3, 4) exhibit a relative decrease in 28S ribosomal RNA band intensity and the appearance of low molecular weight RNA fragments. Highly degraded RNA (lanes 5, 6) is characterized by a low molecular weight smear and the complete absence of detectable, full-length ribosomal RNA. On the right, chromatographic plots of samples in lanes 1 (top) and 4 (bottom). The intensity of nucleic acid signal is plotted as a function of migration time, from fastest (smallest) to slowest (largest) nucleic acid fragments. Note the decrease in 28S ribosomal RNA intensity and increase in fragmented RNA in the bottom plot (lane 4).

Most target synthesis methods use some form of molecular amplification technique. Although the polymerase chain reaction (PCR) is a frequently used method to amplify nucleic acids, this approach often distorts the relative abundance of original mRNAs represented in the amplified material. More recently, however, some PCR approaches have produced unbiased pools of amplification product suitable for quantitative gene expression microarray analysis. This represents a particularly attractive approach for performing gene expression profiling experiments from samples containing small cell numbers (12). Other approaches use isothermal polymerase reactions to achieve proportional amplification of gene transcripts for labeling and hybridization (13,14). In one popular method, polyadenylated mRNA is selectively converted into double-stranded cDNA using a chimeric poly-dT / T7 RNA polymerase promoter primer. The cDNA created from each initial mRNA contains a T7 RNA polymerase promoter site that, in the presence of T7 RNA polymerase, can be used to in vitro transcribe 300–1,000 copies of synthetic RNA from each individual cDNA. This amplified, antisense, or complementary RNA (aRNA or cRNA) can then be used as a substrate for labeling or an additional round of linear amplification. Because a theoretical amplification of 1,000-fold can be achieved with each round of synthesis, 1–5 μg of RNA can generate sufficient target for hybridization using a single round of amplification, whereas two successive rounds of amplification can generate labeled target from as little as 1–5 ng of RNA (15). Depending on cell type, this amount may represent RNA isolated from as few as 100 cells. Target amplification protocols have been tremendously helpful in applying microarray technology to translational studies. Using this approach, it is now routinely feasible to analyze gene expression profiles from limiting amounts of clinical biospecimens, such as fine needle aspirations or needle core biopsies, flow sorted and immunological selected cell populations, and cells isolated from solid tissues using laser microdissection (16–18).

Depending on the microarray technology platform that is used, several different target labeling strategies may be employed. These methods can be divided into one- or two-color labeling, and direct or indirect labeling. In one-color labeling methods, a single study sample is labeled and hybridized to one array. Differences in hybridization signal intensity between arrays are then compared to determine changes in gene expression between samples. In two-color labeling methods, two samples are labeled with two different fluorophores that have independent excitation and emission characteristics.

Nucleotide conjugates with the fluorophores Cy-3 and Cy-5 are commonly employed. Both samples are simultaneously hybridized to the same array and independent hybridization signal intensities from each sample are measured. One sample is usually a universal reference control, so that the relative hybridization signal intensity ratio (i.e., expression level) of the study sample to the reference sample is calculated. If dictated by experimental design, two study samples may also be directly compared to one another (e.g., before treatment sample and after treatment sample) on the same array using two-color labeling. In this experimental design, data are represented as ratiometric differences in gene expression between two time points or experimental conditions. One advantage of this approach is that half as many arrays are required for the study, as compared to hybridization of a single study sample to a single array. However, each fluorophore in the two-color labeling method does not incorporate into the target nucleic acid template with equal efficiency, thus leading to labeling bias. For this reason, well-controlled experimental studies often perform "dye swap" controls, where duplicate array hybridizations are performed with each study sample being labeled twice with each reciprocal dye. The relative necessity of performing duplicate array hybridizations essentially negates the cost benefit of hybridizing two study samples to a single array.

To eliminate biases associated with direct labeling, new methods employ indirect labeling. In these protocols, cDNA or cRNA targets are generated using a modified nucleotide containing a biotin or aminoallyl moiety. After synthesis, the target can be conjugated or chemically modified to accept the preferred fluorophore. For two-color microarray systems, both study sample targets are synthesized using the same modified nucleotide and then independently conjugated to two different fluorophores, thus eliminating dye incorporation bias. Although they involve additional steps and moderately increased cost, target synthesis protocols using amplification and indirect labeling are rapidly becoming the gold standard for gene expression microarray target synthesis.

## CONDUCTING A GENE EXPRESSION PROFILING EXPERIMENT

Figure 34–5 outlines the critical steps involved in performing a gene expression profiling experiment. Generally, translational studies using gene expression microarrays are designed to identify (i.e., discover) unique patterns of gene expression

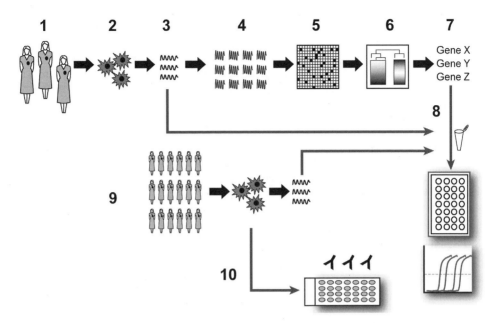

**FIGURE 34–5** ● Experimental steps for performing a gene expression profile study. A relatively small and select cohort of study participants is identified (1) and cell or tissue specimens are collected under optimized conditions (2). Cellular RNA is isolated from clinical specimens, quantified, and qualitatively assessed (3). Prepared RNA is used to generate amplified, fluorescently labeled target (4) that is then hybridized to the nucleic acid microarray (5). The entire microarray study dataset (often consisting of more than 4 million data points) is subjected to statistical data analysis and visualization using methods such as hierarchical clustering (6). Genomic annotation data (e.g., gene references to biological pathways and literature citations) is used to further facilitate the selection of gene sets with potential biological or clinical significance (7). Patterns of microarray gene expression for selected genes can be technically validated by using the same set of RNA samples with an alternate approach to quantify gene expression such as quantitative (real-time) reverse transcription or polymerase chain reaction, RT-PCR (8). Results can be biologically validated by selecting a larger number of independent specimens from a broader range of study participants (9). These specimens may be similarly used for RNA isolation and quantitative RT-PCR analysis of gene transcript expression. Alternatively, tissue specimens may be assembled into a tissue microarray and analyzed for corresponding protein expression using available antibody reagents (10).

that molecularly define a particular pathological or clinical phenotype within a set of study samples. Although the differential expression of one or two single genes may not adequately define a molecular classification scheme on their own, the expression pattern of a larger group of genes, considered as a whole, may provide diagnostic information. Accordingly, the successful application of gene expression microarray technology to translational research studies requires that three important principles be addressed: sample selection and experimental design, data analysis and informatics, and data validation. Each of these points is reviewed below.

## Sample Selection and Experimental Design

As discussed previously, expression profiling experiments require a high quality source of cellular RNA from samples that have been collected under

rigorous, quality controlled conditions (10). Although this may be easy to achieve with laboratory specimens, the challenges associated with collecting biospecimens from study participants are considerable. Cell and tissue specimens should be collected and processed (i.e., frozen or converted into RNA) as rapidly as possible, preferably within 30 minutes from the time of collection (11). It is important that biospecimen collection protocols are standardized and practiced uniformly, particularly for studies that involve collection of study material across multiple institutions. If study specimens are to be collected in remote areas, appropriate preservatives should be used to stabilize cellular mRNA populations until they can be processed. Several such RNA-stabilizing agents are commercially available (19).

If a study involves gene expression profile analysis of tissue biopsy specimens, careful histologic review of the actual study specimen is required.

Differences in the cellular composition of tissues can create artificial differences in gene expression between study samples. For example, identifying changes in gene expression between 30 lung adenocarcinoma samples collected from a clinical trial may be meaningless if 10 of the "tumor" biopsies contain less than 5 percent neoplastic cellularity and 10 other "tumor" biopsies contain a predominance of inflammatory cell infiltrate. When analyzing gene expression profiles from the cellular components of blood or body fluids, it may be desirable to enrich for uniform subpopulations of cells by immunological selection or other purification schemes (e.g., Ficoll density gradient centrifugation, flow cytometry, or immunomagnetic bead separation). Although these methods may enrich for the cell populations of interest, added manipulation of study samples may also artificially perturb patterns of gene expression.

For translational studies that will require several months or even years for sample accrual, it is important to consider when the actual target preparation and array hybridization will occur. For example, if expression microarray data are to be generated prospectively during the course of the study, differences in enzyme and microarray reagents used for samples prepared early in the study versus those that are used for sample preparation several months or years later can create large artificial differences in gene expression profiles. For this reason, whenever possible, it is preferable to complete study sample accrual prior to performing microarray experiments and to randomly batch target preparation and array hybridization of study samples, using as many uniform reagents as possible.

Finally, when simultaneously examining thousands of potential changes in gene expression, even the smallest differences in environmental conditions (e.g., time of sample collection, diet, gender, premedication) and much larger differences in genetic background between study participants can generate large random variability in gene expression patterns. Because most of this biological and environmental variability can not be controlled and because so many variables (i.e., gene expression values) are measured in a microarray experiment, it is important to include a sufficient number of replicates and independent observations (i.e., RNA study samples) to arrive at statistically significant conclusions.

*Replicates* are usually performed in one or more of three ways. *Array replicates* involve hybridization of the same labeled target to multiple arrays. This procedure is designed to quantify the experimental variability associated with the array itself. *Technical replicates* involve using the same RNA sample to generate duplicate targets that are then hybridized to independent arrays. This process estimates the total laboratory variability associated with the microarray experiment. Finally, *biological replicates* are samples taken from the same individual at the same time (such as two independent needle biopsy specimens) and then independently converted into RNA, labeled targets, and hybridized to microarrays. Such replicates are designed to measure total technical variability as well as intra-individual variability. The use of biological replicates is generally accepted practice for laboratory studies that involve genetically homogeneous cultured cell lines or inbred experimental organisms (20). However, in translational studies involving human research participants, inter-individual variability is so much greater than either technical or even intra-individual variability, that biological and technical replicates are rarely performed.

Instead, it is important that a sufficiently large sample size is analyzed to provide statistically reliable results. This principle is no different than in any other correlative science study design. However, because of the large number of variables (gene expression values) examined, Type I error, or the identification of false-positive results, is more problematic. Due to the relative expense of microarrays, a critical experimental design decision is whether to initially invest in a larger microarray sample set that will yield more true positives for subsequent validation studies or to minimize the initial investment in generating a microarray dataset, accepting that a large number of candidate biomarkers will be false positive. The number of samples needed in any given study to identify a statistically significant pattern of differential gene expression will depend in part on the anticipated biological magnitude of the difference between sample groups (21). For example, relatively few study samples may be necessary to identify fundamental differences in gene expression between acute myelogenous leukemia (AML) and acute lymphocytic leukemia (ALL), as these tumor cell types are biologically very distinct (22). On the other hand, a considerably larger study set may be required to identify differences in gene expression associated with clinical outcome within AML patients, if the intrinsic biological basis for patient outcome is more subtle (23). Although power calculations for sample size may be made based on assumptions about the magnitude of the biological effect on phenotype, a discussion of such calculations is outside the scope of this chapter (see Chapter 9).

## Data Analysis and Informatics

It can not be overemphasized that proper statistical and bioinformatics support must be identified *prior* to the initiation of any microarray experiment, particularly one associated with translational research questions. Statistical support involves expertise in study design and proper interpretation of numerical gene expression data. Bioinformatics support involves data warehousing, data mining, data visualization, and genomic data annotation. Both resources are complementary and essential to the successful conduct of a microarray experiment. In this chapter, a discussion of microarray analysis will focus on gene expression microarray data. However, many of the visualization tools and analytical approaches discussed below can be applied equally well to other types of microarray data.

Microarray data analysis can be viewed as four discrete tasks: image analysis, data visualization, statistical analysis, and functional annotation. Image analysis involves conversion of raw hybridization signal data, usually in the form of a large pixilated image file that is the output of the microarray scanner, into a set of gene-specific hybridization values. Because microarray formats can vary significantly (e.g., Affymetrix GeneChip®, one-color spotted microarray, two-color spotted microarray), software designed to perform image acquisition and analysis is usually proprietary or specifically designed for the array. Image analysis converts the pixilated microarray image into a set of intensity values, usually providing one or (in the case of two-color arrays) two values per probe or probe set represented on the array.

Subsequent to image analysis, signal values may be normalized, scaled, or otherwise transformed to allow direct comparison of data between arrays or across experiments. For example, inter-array normalization algorithms compensate for global differences in the signal intensity of arrays. If gene X has a signal intensity of 500 on array 1 with a total average intensity of 1,000, and gene X has a signal intensity of 1,000 on array 2 with a total average intensity of 2,000, inter-array normalization would correct signal intensities for gene X so that expression appeared equivalent between array 1 and array 2. Intergene normalization algorithms are useful for identifying common patterns of gene expression between study samples, even when absolute gene expression values are considerably different. One common transformation technique is the Z score calculation. For each probe or probe set on the array, the average signal for that probe across all arrays in an experiment is transformed to the value of zero with a standard deviation of 1.0. After such a transformation, gene X with signal values of 100, 500, 2,000, and 1,000 on arrays 1–4 is made comparable to gene Y with signal values of 1,000, 5,000, 20,000, and 10,000 on arrays 1–4. Other types of data transformation techniques, such as

log transformation of two-color signal ratios, may also be appropriate depending on the nature of the primary microarray dataset (24).

Visualization of microarray data also presents unique challenges. For a translational research microarray project involving 100 study samples applied to expression arrays representing 47,000 gene elements, it is obviously not practical to view all 4.7 million data points with common spreadsheet or scientific graphing software. Fortunately, biologists and statisticians alike have devised a number of visualization tools to allow a bird's-eye view of such immense datasets (25). Several of these visualization approaches are represented in Figure 34–6.

*Hierarchical clustering* (Chapter 26) is a data visualization approach that simultaneously organizes samples based on their similarity in gene expression across samples. Several different algorithms can be used to calculate similarity and no particular algorithm should be considered more "correct." In fact, although hierarchical clustering is a useful tool to provide a manageable view of immense datasets, it does not necessarily impart any underlying biological truth to microarray data. *Heat maps* (Figure 34–6) are a colorimetric representation of expression data, usually presented in combination with hierarchical clustering. This visualization scheme provides a convenient method to identify patterns or blocks of similarity between gene expression values and samples. *Principal components analysis* (Chapter 26) and *multidimensional scaling* are two methods used to perform data reduction. In principal components analysis, for example, samples may be plotted in a gene expression space where the distance between samples in this space is related to their similarity based on gene expression. However, for a 47,000-element microarray, gene expression space becomes 47,000 dimensions. Therefore, the goal of principal component analysis is to reduce 47,000 dimensions to two or three principal components. Then, relatedness between samples can be plotted (Figure 34–6).

Although these are all useful techniques for displaying data, other approaches are needed to define significant patterns of gene expression (26). The use of one or more methods for statistical analysis of gene expression microarray data depends on the experimental design and the hypothesis to be addressed. One of the most common applications of gene expression profiling in translational medicine involves *supervised clustering*, which may also be referred to as *class distinction* or *class prediction*. In this approach, samples belonging to study participants in two or more known clinical or pathological categories (e.g., good outcome versus bad outcome)

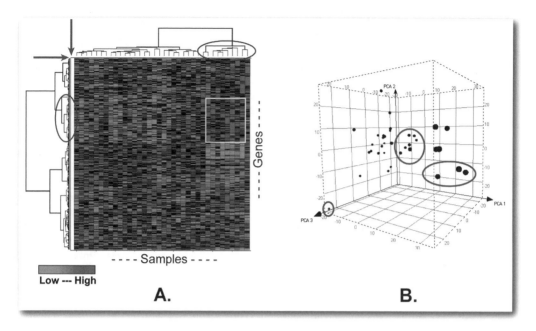

**FIGURE 34–6** ● Visualization of microarray data. **A.** In hierarchical clustering and heat-map visualization of microarray data, samples (represented here by 36 columns) are organized based on similarity of gene expression while genes (represented by approximately 9,000 rows) are simultaneously organized based on similarity of expression across all samples. In the heat map, green lines represent genes that are relatively less expressed in a sample while red lines represent genes that are relatively over expressed in a sample. The tree at the top quantifies the relative similarity between samples (vertical arrow). Samples with higher similarity to each other based on gene expression are depicted as lower branches on the tree (horizontal ellipse). Similarly, the tree on the left quantifies the relative similarity between gene expression patterns (horizontal arrow). Genes that show similar patterns of expression across all samples are depicted as smaller branches on the tree (vertical ellipse). Note subgroups of genes that demonstrate identical patterns of expression in subgroups of samples (yellow box). **B.** In principal components analysis, gene expression values may be condensed into two or three principal components that represent the majority of variation in gene expression across all samples. Each sample is plotted in two- or three-dimensional space (as shown here) based on the value of its principle expression components. Each point may be further color-coded based on other features of the sample (e.g., tumor grade, patient age). In this view, it is easy to demonstrate clusters of samples (green ellipses) that are very distinct in their gene expression profiles. Visualizations generated using DecisionSite for Functional Genomics software (Spotfire, Inc., Somerville, MA). **Note:** The color figure can be found following page 394.

are analyzed by gene expression microarrays, with the goal of identifying patterns of gene expression (or groups of genes) that can discriminate between the known classes. Intuitively, such an analysis could be performed by examining one gene at a time and calculating whether expression values for that gene are statistically significant between the defined sample classes using traditional statistics (e.g., ANOVA analysis). This approach, however, is flawed in two respects. First, by definition, using a traditional "significance threshold" of $p = 0.05$ allows for a 5% false-positive (false discovery) rate. Therefore, when analyzing 47,000 independent gene expression values, over 2,000 gene expression values will appear to be "significant" by chance alone. To contend with this problem of multiple testing, several methods have been applied to calculate a true significance threshold when analyzing thousands of variables in relatively few numbers of samples (27,28). At the

same time, applying standard statistical tests to microarray data results in over-reduction of the data. The true power of microarray data is that it allows the examination of multiple, independent gene expression values rather than examination of one gene at a time. However, traditional statistical analysis considers only a single gene at a time. Therefore, although three single sets of gene expression values may not discriminate between classes on their own, their combined expression pattern may be a statistically significant discriminator. One approach to this problem uses the concept of "metagenes" or groups of genes whose composite expression pattern provides discriminatory power (29).

Many translational studies also use *unsupervised clustering* or *class discovery* approaches to identify new subclassifications of study samples not previously recognized using traditional clinical or pathological data (22,26). However, this approach presents a conundrum; unless the group of identified genes suggests a previously unappreciated biological or clinical feature of the sample, it is difficult to determine whether the subclass discovered by gene expression profiling is simply fortuitous or whether it has some biological or clinical implication (9).

The final and undoubtedly the most difficult phase of microarray data analysis involves translating a list of statistically significant gene expression values into a biologically meaningful pattern of gene expression. In translational studies focused on identifying molecular biomarkers, it may be enough to simply identify a set of diagnostic gene expression patterns. However, to move beyond this requires defining how patterns of gene expression represent underlying cell signaling pathways. As annotation of the human genome continues to grow, the biological functions of specific gene products and gene-gene associations will become better characterized. Delineation of functional pathways based on gene expression in simple eukaryotes is now a reality (30) and is becoming increasingly more feasible in humans (31). Eventually, this knowledge will allow translational studies using gene expression microarrays to not only identify diagnostic biomarker patterns, but also to understand the biological basis of such patterns, making targeted therapeutics for many different disease processes a reality.

## Data Validation

As discussed above, the analysis of thousands of gene expression values in a relatively few number of study samples can frequently lead to a number of falsely significant results. Therefore, as in any good experimental design, data validation is absolutely necessary. There are several different methods for data validation. The simplest approach is to use the same microarray dataset for both discovery and validation of predictive markers. The "leave one out" cross validation algorithm is one such method. In an analysis of *N* study samples, *N–1* samples are used for supervised clustering analysis to identify groups of genes that effectively discriminate between defined classes. The ability of these genes to correctly classify the *N*th sample is then calculated and the gene list modified accordingly. This process is repeated, removing all *N* samples, one at a time, until a list of genes with the best class prediction score is created (26). The advantage of this method is that no additional data or experimentation are needed for validation. However, because the cross-validation is still applied to a single set of experimental samples, the ability to generalize conclusions to independent or larger sample sets

may still be limited. If an initial microarray data set is large enough, it is also possible to divide the experiment into independent sets of test data and validation data. In this scheme, patterns of "significant" gene expression are identified using the first set of microarrays and patterns are validated in a second set of arrays. Although this approach uses two truly independent datasets, it necessarily limits the number of datasets used for the discovery phase and validation phase. Microarray data results may also be validated electronically. As an increasing number of microarray expression studies are published and corresponding datasets are made publicly available in gene expression microarray repositories, it has become increasingly possible to validate patterns of gene expression identified in one experiment using other microarray experiments in the published literature. In fact, meta-analyses of microarray data are becoming more frequent, and although some studies demonstrate that significant patterns of gene expression can be validated in experiments conducted by independent investigators (32), other such analyses have demonstrated clear differences between studies (9,33).

Perhaps the most convincing method for validating microarray data is through the use of an alternative technology for assessing gene expression. *Quantitative RT-PCR* (qRT-PCR) and tissue microarrays are popular approaches for data confirmation. Much like conventional RT-PCR (Chapter 31), qRT-PCR is performed by converting RNA into first strand cDNA. The first strand cDNA is then used as a template for PCR, where accumulation of gene-specific amplification product is monitored by direct or indirect fluorescent detection in real time. Any number of fluorescent chemistries may be employed in qRT-PCR assays. SYBR Green is a dye that fluoresces when bound to double-stranded DNA. When added to a PCR reaction, increasing SYBR Green fluorescence is proportional to accumulation of double-stranded amplification product, presumably that of the specific gene transcript to which amplification primers have been designed. The advantage of the SYBR Green approach is that it is relatively inexpensive, requiring only one pair of standard amplification primers. The disadvantage of this method is that SYBR Green lacks sequence-binding specificity such that fluorescence from nonspecific amplification products is indistinguishable from that generated by the sequence specific amplicon. This translates into a generally lower signal to noise ratio and a need to carefully validate primers before using them.

An alternative to using SYBR Green dye is the use of sequence-specific fluorescent probes. In this approach, transcript amplification occurs through the use of a pair of standard PCR primers, but a third fluorescent probe is required to bind to the amplified product to generate a fluorescent signal. This signal may be generated by polymerase cleavage of a fluorescent quencher (e.g., TaqMan assay) or through a conformational change of the probe on binding to the amplified product (e.g., molecular beacons). In either case, the use of a third gene-specific sequence greatly increases the specificity of the assay. Furthermore, prevalidated primer and probe sets for many human transcripts are commercially available, making assay set-up quick and convenient. The main disadvantage of this method is the expense associated with fluorescent probes, particularly when attempting to initially validate a large number of genes identified in a microarray experiment.

Regardless of the fluorescent chemistry employed, with each subsequent PCR cycle, the amount of amplification product increases and so does the fluorescence. At some cycle number, fluorescent intensity exceeds an arbitrarily defined threshold. This is referred to as the cycle threshold ($C_T$). The number of PCR cycles required to reach this threshold is inversely proportional to the starting amount of gene-specific cDNA (and hence RNA) template present in the reaction. By comparing normalized $C_T$ values between samples, the relative (or absolute) abundance of original RNA present in the sample can be calculated (34).

As discussed at the beginning of this chapter, tissue microarrays are also a powerful approach for performing gene expression validation studies (1,3). The use of prefabricated tissue microarrays (either commercially available or prepared by an academic core facility) can be used to rapidly validate differential patterns of gene expression at the level of protein expression. Tissue microarrays allow independent validation in a large number of tissue samples potentially available from diagnostic pathology blocks, and provide additional information about the cellular location of gene expression in the tissue of interest. However, use of tissue microarrays for immunohistochemical (IHC) validation of gene expression requires a robust antibody for the gene of interest, which can often be a significant limiting factor (Chapter 36). Furthermore, data from IHC analysis of tissue microarrays is less quantitative, and it may be difficult to validate small changes in gene expression identified by microarray data analysis using IHC analysis of tissue. Finally, because gene expression microarrays evaluate changes in gene expression at the RNA level and IHC evaluates gene expression at the protein level, it is possible that posttranscriptional regulation of protein expression will lead to disparate results between methods, without any one set of data being 'invalid.'

## Limitations of Gene Expression Profiling Experiments

Although microarray technology is certainly a useful discovery tool to identify gene expression profiles that may serve as clinically useful biomarkers, several points discussed earlier clearly demonstrate the limitations of this technology. First, the power of microarray technology lies in its ability to perform assays on thousands of genes simultaneously, but not in the performance of any one assay on a single gene with optimal sensitivity and specificity. As a result, subtle changes in gene expression that may be biologically important or diagnostically useful will be missed using gene expression microarray technology. Second, because of the current expense associated with microarray technology, the exacting requirements for samples that are to be analyzed, and the complexity of the resulting data sets, studies are necessarily limited to relatively few numbers of samples. Although it may be easy to analyze 1,000 study samples for the expression of a single biomarker, a study of this proportion is currently not practical using gene expression microarrays. As technology becomes less expensive, as increasing standardization of microarray platforms and data formats allow more robust meta-analyses, and as new sample collection and preparation methods allow access to larger numbers of study samples, the ability to examine expression microarray data in very large sample sets may become a reality. Finally, most functional units of the cell are proteins, and, therefore, direct measurements of protein abundance, protein modification, and protein-protein interaction are more likely to provide direct information about the molecular pathology of disease in translational studies. Although nucleic acid microarray technology is now widely available, it is likely that global proteomic techniques (Chapter 35) will eventually become a more favored approach for biomarker discovery.

## APPLICATION OF GENE EXPRESSION PROFILING TO TRANSLATIONAL RESEARCH

Gene expression profiling using nucleic acid microarrays is being used with increasing frequency in translational medicine research studies. Most of these studies have focused on clinical and biological issues related to solid and hematological malignancies (35). In one approach, gene expression profiling can be used simply as a high-throughput screen to identify previously unappreciated, individual gene transcripts that are associated with specific disease processes. The expression of these single gene transcripts and their potential as disease biomarkers may then be independently validated using traditional approaches (3,36,37). However, the real power of gene expression microarray analysis is that the composite expression pattern of a larger group of genes may serve as a useful biomarker, when individual gene expression patterns fail to provide satisfactory diagnostic power on their own. Using supervised statistical analysis, as outlined above, many studies have identified patterns of tumor gene expression that correlate with organ site (38,39), tumor grade, metastatic potential (40), and clinical outcome (41,42). Of even greater clinical interest, patterns of gene expression may also predict tumor response to specific therapies (43), suggesting that diagnostic gene expression profiles may soon be an important tool for personalized molecular medicine (44). Several studies employing unsupervised statistical analyses of microarray data have identified novel molecular subclasses of tumors that may have clinical significance, independent of other pathological or clinical biomarkers (9,45).

Although each of these and other similar studies provide exciting data on their own to suggest the utility of gene expression profiling in patient management, a number of caveats still exist. Most studies that have defined patterns of gene expression associated with clinical correlates have not comprehensively validated their results in independent trials. For those studies that have done so, data suggest that diagnostic genes expression profiles are not completely concordant between studies (32,33). Nonconcordant results may be related to nonstandardized methods used between studies or simply the relatively few number of specimens that have been evaluated in each study. There are also few data to suggest that gene expression profiles will have truly independent predictive power over traditional histopathological analysis. What is clearly needed in the field are new, prospective studies that use gene expression profile data to make treatment management decisions and to determine whether such an approach can favorably affect patient outcome. Although such studies are now actively under development or in progress, it may still be several years before robust gene expression profiles can be used for routine clinical management of diseases like cancer.

Beyond the field of medical oncology, the use of gene expression profiling in translational research has been less pronounced. Several studies have identified patterns of gene expression associated with human neurological disease (Alzheimer's, Parkinson's, epilepsy, schizophrenia), autoimmunity (systemic lupus, multiple sclerosis), transplant rejection, reproductive biology, tissue regeneration and wound healing, cardiovascular disease, and pathogen/host interactions in infectious disease (46–52). However, a number of restrictions exist when applying gene expression profiling approaches to translational research in these other disease systems. First, identifying the appropriate target cell population for study can be difficult. In cancer research, the tumor itself is usually the target of molecular analysis. In more systemic diseases such as diabetes or multiple sclerosis, the target cell population is less well defined. Unlike cancer studies where large collections of surgically resected, fresh tumor tissue specimens may be readily available, acquisition of large numbers of specimens may be difficult for diseases such as Parkinson's, diabetic nephropathy, and idiopathic cardiac hypertrophy. Because of the cost of current microarray technology and limited access to adequate clinical specimens, most translational microarray studies focusing on noncancer disease processes have been limited to very small sample sizes. Together with the fact that studies have been performed using a wide variety of microarray platforms and technologies, it has been difficult to collect a sufficiently large number of study samples to make statistically valid conclusions regarding associations between gene expression patterns and disease phenotype. Known and unknown variability within disease processes and between patient participants makes establishing definitive patterns of gene expression associated with disease phenotype difficult as well. In the future, therefore, it will be important for microarray-based translational research studies to address specific diagnostic questions, to carefully consider what and how biospecimens are collected for analysis, and to use a sufficient number of clinical samples on a standardized microarray platform to ensure that statistically meaningful gene expression data can be generated that relate to specific clinical issues in treatment or diagnosis of human disease.

## FUTURE APPLICATIONS

Microarray technology continues to improve. Nucleic acid arrays are being designed at increasingly higher probe density and decreasing cost, similar to the evolution of the semiconductor industry (Moore's law). These advances will allow comprehensive human transcriptome analysis on a single array. More importantly, it will allow microarrays to perform even more complex analyses such as quantitation of alternate mRNA splicing events, simultaneous detection of SNPs at over 100,000 independent loci, and direct sequencing of over 500 kb of DNA sequence using a single array.

Methods are now available for amplifying and labeling nanogram quantities of nucleic acids samples derived from microscopic biopsy specimens that are either fresh or archived in paraffin (12–15). These advances will be tremendously important for translational research studies. The ability to use small numbers of cells obtained from minimally invasive procedures such as fine needle aspiration, swabs, and lavages will allow the design of sophisticated prospective studies that can use serial samples collected from a single study participant to analyze changes in gene expression over time (53). Use of archival tissue specimens, fixed and embedded in paraffin, will increase the number of specimens available for translational studies by several orders of magnitude. These advances will open access to diagnostic clinical specimens associated with a wealth of clinical information, which are ideal for retrospective, clinical correlative studies.

Continuing annotation of the human genome will provide new information about relevant disease-related SNPs and haplotypes (Chapter 33). Data from these studies will be useful for designing new array formats that eliminate redundancy and provide more comprehensive coverage of the genome. Similarly, knowledge of gene exon structure and alternative mRNA splicing patterns will allow independent quantitation of multiple mRNA transcripts originating from a single genomic locus. The advances in microarray fabrication discussed above will be necessary to harness this explosion of genomic information.

Finally, although most translation studies that use microarray technology today may still be considered biomarker discovery experiments, it is foreseeable that an eventual critical mass of such data will lead to robust genomic signatures in the form of gene mutations, polymorphisms, methylation patterns, or transcriptional patterns that can effectively predict disease outcome or therapeutic response. Once such patterns are indeed validated, it is probable that a new era of microarray application will begin, one that will use this powerful technology for the routine clinical management of human disease (54).

## SUMMARY

- Microarray technology can be used to screen a large number of arrayed biomarkers in a single sample (probe arrays) or to screen a large number of arrayed samples using a single biomarker (samples arrays). Nucleic acid microarrays and antibody microarrays are examples of probe arrays while tissue microarrays are the most commonly used type of sample array.
- Nucleic acid microarrays are arrayed collections of nucleic acid probes to which a biological

sample is applied for analysis. Nucleic acid probes may be long stretches of genomic DNA, cDNA clones, or short oligonucleotide sequences that are either physically spotted to the array surface or synthesized in situ. Nucleic acid microarrays may be used to analyze gene copy number, DNA sequence, and gene transcript (RNA) abundance.

- Gene expression profiling uses nucleic acid microarrays to characterize patterns of RNA abundance in biological samples. A number of different microarray formats are available and investigators use a number of different molecular biology protocols to prepare labeled samples for microarray analysis. Technologies exist for performing gene expression profiling on limited amounts of clinical material, but the dynamic nature of gene transcription and the chemical and enzymatic instability of RNA necessitates careful attention to sample quality.
- The implementation of microarray technology in translational research requires consideration of experimental design, data analysis, and data validation. Proper experimental design is the most critical requisite for a successful microarray experiment. Many software tools (both commercial and academic) exist to process, visualize, and statistically analyze microarray data. Ultimately, however, expression profiling using nucleic acid microarrays is a biomarker discovery experiment, the data from which must be independently validated. Gene expression profiles may be confirmed electronically, by comparison with other published expression profile data sets. Alternatively, other high-throughput laboratory methods such as quantitative RT-PCR or *tissue* microarrays may be used to validate patterns of gene expression in larger, independent sets of biological specimens.
- Gene expression profiling has now been used in numerous translational studies to identify biomarkers associated with tumor phenotype, disease progression, and clinical outcome. Although the majority of microarray studies in translational research have been focused on the field of oncology, this technology is also being applied to identify biomarkers and to better understand biology in other areas of medicine such as cardiovascular and neurological disease.
- Microarray technology continues to evolve. Lower cost, higher density nucleic acid microarrays and novel sample labeling protocols will allow for a more comprehensive analysis of the transcriptome in larger numbers and diversity of clinical biospecimens. Further annotation of the human genome and advanced array technology will also allow other microarray-based

approaches such as quantification of alternative RNA splicing, DNA methylation profiling, genotyping, and DNA sequencing to become more efficient and cost effective. At the same time, accumulating data from translational studies should crystallize definitive sets of genetic biomarkers that will be useful in disease-specific diagnostic microarrays.

# REFERENCES

1. Packeisen J, Korsching E, Herbst H et al. Demystified...tissue microarray technology. Mol Pathol 2003; 56(4):198–204.
2. Nishizuka S, Charboneau L, Young L et al. Proteomic profiling of the NCI-60 cancer cell lines using new high-density reverse-phase lysate microarrays. Proc Natl Acad Sci USA 2003;100(24):14229–14234.
3. Hao X, Sun B, Hu L et al. Differential gene and protein expression in primary breast malignancies and their lymph node metastases as revealed by combined cDNA microarray and tissue microarray analysis. Cancer 2004;100(6):1110–1122.
4. Liotta LA, Espina V, Mehta AI et al. Protein microarrays: meeting analytical challenges for clinical applications. Cancer Cell 2003;3(4):317–325.
5. Schulze A, Downward J. Navigating gene expression using microarrays—a technology review. Nat Cell Biol 2001;3(8):E190–195.
6. Matsuzaki H, Loi H, Dong S et al. Parallel genotyping of over 10,000 SNPs using a one-primer assay on a high-density oligonucleotide array. Genome Res 2004;14(3):414–425.
7. Wong CW, Albert TJ, Vega VB et al. Tracking the evolution of the SARS coronavirus using high-throughput, high-density resequencing arrays. Genome Res 2004; 14(3):398–405.
8. Albertson DG, Pinkel D. Genomic microarrays in human genetic disease and cancer. Hum Mol Genet 2003;12 Spec No 2:R145–152.
9. Alizadeh AA, Eisen MB, Davis RE et al. Distinct types of diffuse large B-cell lymphoma identified by gene expression profiling. Nature 2000;403(6769):503–511.
10. Emmert-Buck MR, Strausberg RL, Krizman DB et al. Molecular profiling of clinical tissue specimens: feasibility and applications. J Mol Diagn 2000;2(2):60–66.
11. Dash A, Maine IP, Varambally S et al. Changes in differential gene expression because of warm ischemia time of radical prostatectomy specimens. Am J Pathol 2002;161(5):1743–1748.
12. Iscove NN, Barbara M, Gu M et al. Representation is faithfully preserved in global cDNA amplified exponentially from sub-picogram quantities of mRNA. Nat Biotechnol 2002;20(9):940–943.
13. Xiang CC, Chen M, Ma L et al. A new strategy to amplify degraded RNA from small tissue samples for microarray studies. Nucleic Acids Res 2003;31(9):e53.
14. Glanzer JG, Eberwine JH. Expression profiling of small cellular samples in cancer: less is more. Br J Cancer 2004;90(6):1111–1114.
15. Luzzi V, Mahadevappa M, Raja R et al. Accurate and reproducible gene expression profiles from laser capture microdissection, transcript amplification, and high density oligonucleotide microarray analysis. J Mol Diagn 2003;5(1):9–14.
16. Pusztai L, Ayers M, Stec J et al. Gene expression profiles obtained from fine-needle aspirations of breast cancer reliably identify routine prognostic markers and reveal large-scale molecular differences between estrogen-negative and estrogen-positive tumors. Clin Cancer Res 2003;9(7):2406–2415.
17. Barrett MT, Glogovac J, Prevo LJ et al. High-quality RNA and DNA from flow cytometrically sorted human epithelial cells and tissues. Biotechniques 2002;32(4):888–890, 892, 894, 896.
18. Luzzi V, Holtschlag V, Watson MA. Expression profiling of ductal carcinoma in situ by laser capture microdissection and high-density oligonucleotide arrays. Am J Pathol 2001;158(6):2005–2010.
19. Florell SR, Coffin CM, Holden JA et al. Preservation of RNA for functional genomic studies: a multidisciplinary tumor bank protocol. Mod Pathol 2001; 14(2):116–128.
20. Churchill GA. Fundamentals of experimental design for cDNA microarrays. Nat Genet 2002;32 Suppl:490–495.
21. Yang YH, Speed T. Design issues for cDNA microarray experiments. Nat Rev Genet 2002;3(8):579–588.
22. Golub TR, Slonim DK, Tamayo P et al. Molecular classification of cancer: class discovery and class prediction by gene expression monitoring. Science 1999; 286(5439):531–537.
23. Bullinger L, Dohner K, Bair E et al. Use of gene-expression profiling to identify prognostic subclasses in adult acute myeloid leukemia. N Engl J Med 2004; 350(16):1605–1616.
24. Quackenbush J. Microarray data normalization and transformation. Nat Genet 2002;32 Suppl:496–501.
25. Gilbert DR, Schroeder M, van Helden J. Interactive visualization and exploration of relationships between biological objects. Trends Biotechnol 2000;18(12):487–494.
26. Cui X, Churchill GA. Statistical tests for differential expression in cDNA microarray experiments. Genome Biol 2003;4(4):210.
27. Reiner A, Yekutieli D, Benjamini Y. Identifying differentially expressed genes using false discovery rate controlling procedures. Bioinformatics 2003;19(3):368–375.
28. Tusher VG, Tibshirani R, Chu G. Significance analysis of microarrays applied to the ionizing radiation response. Proc Natl Acad Sci USA 2001;98(9):5116–5121.
29. Pittman J, Huang E, Dressman H et al. Integrated modeling of clinical and gene expression information for personalized prediction of disease outcomes. Proc Natl Acad Sci USA 2004;101(22):8431–8436.
30. Lee TI, Rinaldi NJ, Robert F et al. Transcriptional regulatory networks in Saccharomyces cerevisiae. Science 2002;298(5594):799–804.
31. Stuart JM, Segal E, Koller D et al. A gene-coexpression network for global discovery of conserved genetic modules. Science 2003;302(5643):249–255.
32. Sorlie T, Tibshirani R, Parker J et al. Repeated observation of breast tumor subtypes in independent gene expression data sets. Proc Natl Acad Sci USA 2003; 100(14):8418–8423.
33. Shipp MA, Ross KN, Tamayo P et al. Diffuse large B-cell lymphoma outcome prediction by gene-expression profiling and supervised machine learning. Nat Med 2002;8(1):68–74.
34. Bustin SA. Quantification of mRNA using real-time reverse transcription PCR (RT-PCR): trends and problems. J Mol Endocrinol 2002;29(1):23–39.
35. Chung CH, Bernard PS, Perou CM. Molecular portraits and the family tree of cancer. Nat Genet 2002;32 Suppl:533–540.
36. Shen-Ong GL, Feng Y, Troyer DA. Expression profiling identifies a novel alpha-methylacyl-CoA racemase exon

with fumarate hydratase homology. Cancer Res 2003; 63(12):3296–3301.

37. Dhanasekaran SM, Barrette TR, Ghosh D et al. Delineation of prognostic biomarkers in prostate cancer. Nature 2001;412(6849):822–826.

38. Shedden KA, Taylor JM, Giordano TJ et al. Accurate molecular classification of human cancers based on gene expression using a simple classifier with a pathological tree-based framework. Am J Pathol 2003;163(5):1985–1995.

39. Khan J, Wei JS, Ringner M et al. Classification and diagnostic prediction of cancers using gene expression profiling and artificial neural networks. Nat Med 2001;7(6):673–679.

40. Ramaswamy S, Ross KN, Lander ES et al. A molecular signature of metastasis in primary solid tumors. Nat Genet 2003;33(1):49–54.

41. van de Vijver MJ, He YD, van't Veer LJ et al. A gene-expression signature as a predictor of survival in breast cancer. N Engl J Med 2002;347(25):1999–2009.

42. Beer DG, Kardia SL, Huang CC et al. Gene-expression profiles predict survival of patients with lung adenocarcinoma. Nat Med 2002;8(8):816–824.

43. Chang JC, Wooten EC, Tsimelzon A et al. Gene expression profiling for the prediction of therapeutic response to docetaxel in patients with breast cancer. Lancet 2003;362(9381):362–369.

44. Langheier JM, Snyderman R. Prospective medicine: the role for genomics in personalized health planning. Pharmacogenomics 2004;5(1):1–8.

45. Sorlie T, Perou CM, Tibshirani R et al. Gene expression patterns of breast carcinomas distinguish tumor subclasses with clinical implications. Proc Natl Acad Sci USA 2001;98(19):10869–10874.

46. Blalock EM, Geddes JW, Chen KC et al. Incipient Alzheimer's disease: microarray correlation analyses reveal major transcriptional and tumor suppressor responses. Proc Natl Acad Sci USA 2004;101(7):2173–2178.

47. Lock C, Hermans G, Pedotti R et al. Gene-microarray analysis of multiple sclerosis lesions yields new targets validated in autoimmune encephalomyelitis. Nat Med 2002;8(5):500–508.

48. Sarwal M, Chua MS, Kambham N et al. Molecular heterogeneity in acute renal allograft rejection identified by DNA microarray profiling. N Engl J Med 2003; 349(2):125–138.

49. Kao LC, Tulac S, Lobo S et al. Global gene profiling in human endometrium during the window of implantation. Endocrinology 2002;143(6):2119–2138.

50. Theilgaard-Monch K, Knudsen S, Follin P et al. The transcriptional activation program of human neutrophils in skin lesions supports their important role in wound healing. J Immunol 2004;172(12):7684–7693.

51. Chen Y, Park S, Li Y et al. Alterations of gene expression in failing myocardium following left ventricular assist device support. Physiol Genomics 2003;14(3):251–260.

52. Bryant PA, Venter D, Robins-Browne R et al. Chips with everything: DNA microarrays in infectious diseases. Lancet Infect Dis 2004;4(2):100–111.

53. Sotiriou C, Powles TJ, Dowsett M et al. Gene expression profiles derived from fine needle aspiration correlate with response to systemic chemotherapy in breast cancer. Breast Cancer Res 2002;4(3):R3.

54. Petricoin EF III, Hackett JL, Lesko LJ et al. Medical applications of microarray technologies: a regulatory science perspective. Nat Genet 2002;32 Suppl:474–479.

# CHAPTER 35

# Proteomics

R. Reid Townsend

$\mathbf{A}$s seen in Chapter 34, the focus of biological and medical research in many instances is changing. Now, instead of studying one gene and its products, the scientific community is increasingly aspiring to understand biological systems that consist of many genes, many mRNA transcripts, many proteins, many protein modifications, and many metabolites (1). The realization that many diseases are likely to involve multiple genes interacting with environmental factors has given added impetus to this paradigm shift.

The ultimate goal of proteomics is to be able to analyze the full complement of proteins produced by an individual's genome (2). However, proteomics currently lacks the necessary tools to measure all the proteins produced by a genome. Current platforms limit analysis to "only" several hundred proteins at one time, although the ability to analyze the expression of many proteins continues to improve with increasing levels of sensitivity, specificity, and speed. However, as with gene expression array analysis (Chapter 34), even this level of productivity produces reams of information that provide a tremendous challenge for conversion into clinically useful knowledge.

Proteomics is likely to impact clinical care initially by facilitating the discovery of protein biomarkers for diagnosis, disease classification, customization of therapy, prognosis, and as predictors of treatment response (3). In a manner analogous to the Human Genome Project, a Human Proteome Project is currently underway, with an initial focus on characterizing all the proteins in serum (4). A primary goal of this chapter is to provide a description of the analytical workflow that is required for the proteomic analysis of clinical samples. The focus will be on an established gel-based method that is linked to high-performance mass spectrometry. As will be emphasized, the performance of proteomic experiments requires multiple analytical methods and a bioinformatics infrastructure.

## WHY PROTEOMICS?

A simple answer to this question is that proteins and their products are the effectors of a genome. A corollary is that protein dysfunction, or the lack of one or more proteins, is often a primary etiologic factor for disease. Unfortunately, even complete knowledge of the sequence of a genome cannot predict the protein forms that are expressed, the co- and posttranslational modifications, the protein subunit interactions, subcellular locations and intracellular trafficking, or the roles played in cellular function. Knowledge of the portion of the genome that is expressed as mRNA is certainly useful, but does not necessarily predict translation of the transcript, and cannot address the previously mentioned aspects of protein form and function.

The discovery that humans have only 30,000 to 35,000 genes is an unexpected finding from the sequencing of the human genome (5). Understanding how so few genes can produce a complex organism will undoubtedly be a major focus in the postgenomic era. Detailed studies of a few proteins suggest how so few genes may give rise to the considerable complexity associated with multicellular organisms. Figure 35–1 depicts a single gene producing multiple splice variants at the transcription level and then each transcript undergoing posttranslational modifications (e.g., phosphorylation, proteolytic trimming) and multimerization to produce many protein forms from a single gene. The

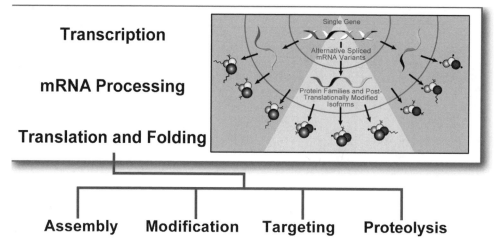

**FIGURE 35–1** ● Protein expression—one gene, many forms.

reader is directed to a review on acetylcholinesterase for a detailed discussion of these processing events (6). In addition a complex bidirectional flow of information from proteins to nucleic acids regulate gene expression. The potential for enormous structural complexity via posttranslational modifications is well known. A major challenge for proteomics is the development of high-throughput analyses that not only identify proteins, but also characterize the plethora of protein forms.

Why can't complete proteomes be easily defined? Although it is now possible to measure mRNA transcripts from every gene in the human genome on a microarray of nucleic acid sequences (Chapter 34), protein array technology is not as advanced, although it is progressing rapidly (for review, see reference (7)). Moreover, the large concentration range of proteins in cells and biological fluids (over 11–12 orders of magnitude), the absence of general amplification methods for proteins, and the greater chemical diversity (20 naturally occurring amino acids and modifications) require fundamentally different analytical approaches that are currently limited and involve multiple analytical steps.

Figure 35–2 shows a generic workflow for proteomic analysis. In step 1, a complex mixture of thousands of proteins or peptides must be separated for biochemical characterization of each component. Electrophoresis, liquid chromatography (LC), and affinity purification are examples of key technologies that are used to separate proteins and peptides, and these methods have been implemented in tandem to perform multidimensional separations (8). Quantification can be accomplished using either two-gel electrophoresis or mass spectrometry. A recent review summarizes the strengths and weaknesses of several quantitative methods in proteomics (9).

Identifying proteins by Edman degradation has largely been supplanted by mass spectrometric methods. Orders of magnitude increases in speed, sensitivity, and tolerance for the analysis of peptide mixtures have been achieved using electrospray ionization (ESI) mass spectrometry and matrix-assisted laser desorption/ionization (MALDI) mass spectrometry, deployed for protein identification either individually or in combination (10). Another important advantage of mass spectrometry is the ability to characterize protein and peptide modifications, either those that occur naturally or those introduced by targeted chemical modifications. Another approach that can be incorporated into this workflow is to perform affinity enrichment, with identification and quantification at the peptide level using multidimensional LC coupled to mass spectrometry (MS) after labeling with stable isotopes (11). This approach is especially useful for analyzing proteins not amenable to 2-D gel electrophoresis (e.g., hydrophobic and very basic proteins) and is not limited by protein molecular weight; however, this method does not provide information on protein isoforms. Additional development will still be required to extend this technique to analyzing modified peptides.

In Figure 35–2, step 3, bioinformatics methods are used to assemble and analyze all the data from the previous steps and to search databases for information on the identified proteins. These data are best organized and stored in a relational database that is part of a laboratory information management system (LIMS) and linked to bar-coded samples. Commonly employed queries include (1) identification of related proteins and genes; (2) identification of candidate interacting proteins; (3) prediction of secondary and tertiary structures;

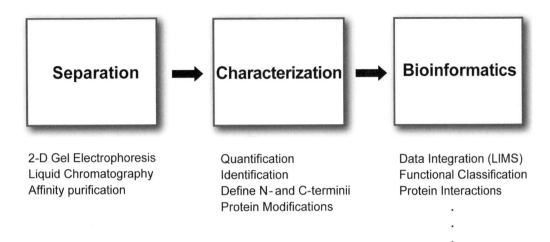

**Separation**  →  **Characterization**  →  **Bioinformatics**

2-D Gel Electrophoresis
Liquid Chromatography
Affinity purification

Quantification
Identification
Define N- and C-terminii
Protein Modifications

Data Integration (LIMS)
Functional Classification
Protein Interactions
.
.
.

*FIGURE 35–2* ● Overview of proteomic analysis.

and (4) consensus sequences that suggest post-translational modifications and functional domains. It is hoped that the coherent assembly of these data will produce candidate protein biomarkers and lead to new hypotheses about disease pathogenesis.

## A PROTEOMICS WORKFLOW

Of the protein separation methods, two-dimensional gel electrophoresis makes visualization and quantification of thousands of protein forms possible in a single digital image (9). The sensitivity and robustness of this established method has continued to improve significantly since it was first introduced (13). An important technical problem is experimental variation in image patterns that occurs among gels and the associated tedious effort that is required to minimize gel artifacts (14). Image artifacts from poor resolution, vertical and horizontal streaking, and particularly local geometric distortions impair accurate software matching and, thus, quantitation. Instead, time-consuming software-assisted manual inspection is required to identify incorrect alignment of features among individual gels. Furthermore, for each pair-wise image analysis, a significant percentage of features cannot be aligned, resulting in a significant loss of these 'orphan' features as images are matched to the master (15).

Recently, the adaptation of multiplex fluorescent labeling methods to proteins (16) has been shown to be an improved method for distinguishing between experimental and biological variation in 2-D gel analyses (17–19). Figure 35–3 shows a two-dimensional difference gel analysis of three samples in a single physical gel. In the first step, each of the samples is labeled with one of three fluorometrically

distinct cyanine dyes (Cy2, Cy3, or Cy5). The samples are then combined and equilibrated to a strip containing immobilized ampholytes. After applying current, the proteins move until they reach a pH region that equals their isoelectric point. The strip containing the focused proteins is then overlayered onto a slab gel that has been immobilized to a low fluorescent glass plate. Electrophoresis is carried out in the presence of SDS and proteins are separated on the basis of molecular weight. The gel is scanned at the appropriate excitation and emission wavelengths for the cyanine dyes and three images are produced. Because the samples are analyzed in the same gel, quantitative, sample dependent artifacts associated with, for example, equilibration of proteins with the immobilized pH gradient strip or the efficiency of transfer of proteins from the strip to the second dimension slab gel are practically eliminated. These images can be readily matched and the gel features quantified using software without manual intervention. The pixel counts are summed, and the relative quantization of each feature is determined. In the superimposed image, the red and green spots indicate proteins that are increased in the sample labeled with Cy5 and Cy3, respectively. The close similarities among the images translates to user independent, nearly perfect matching of features across images and the use of improved algorithms for distinguishing between experimental and biological variation (19).

An example of using this method to compare protein differences in the serum from different individuals is shown in Figure 35–4. Serum samples were collected from two patients and depleted of albumin, IgG, IgA, transferrin, haptoglogin, and $\alpha_1$-antitrypsin using a multi-affinity method. Depleted serum samples from individuals A and B

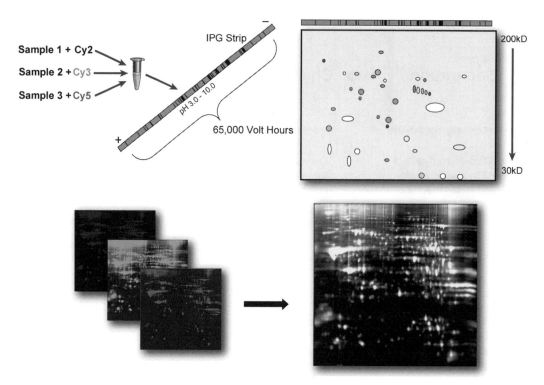

**FIGURE 35–3** ● Two-dimensional difference gel electrophoresis. **Note:** The color figure can be found following page 394.

were labeled with Cy3 and Cy5, respectively. The superimposition of the images shows that most of the protein abundances in the two individuals are similar as indicated by the yellow-colored features. However, prominent green and red spots are apparent indicating differences in the relative amounts of these proteins. Three-dimensional views of normalized features further illustrate increases and decreases between these two samples.

The ability to produce multiple images in a single gel also has advantages for inter-gel comparisons. Gel image analysis is based on the premise that features are accurately matched across the experimental set, a difficult task as discussed above. Using difference gel electropheresis (DIGE), a pooled sample can be included as an internal standard into each gel to serve as both an intra-gel master image and as an internal standard for quantitative purposes (17). Figure 35–5 shows an experimental design in which a pooled sample from longitudinal samplings from the same patient are included in all gels within an experiment. The feature volumes (total pixel counts) from the pooled standard are used to calculate ratios for each of the matched features from the other two images. The same operation is carried out on all physical gels, and it is the ratios that are used to quantify across gels instead of raw feature volumes that are sensitive

to inter-gel variability (15). Applying the above basic design to longitudinal samplings from the same patient in clinical studies could minimize the false positives and false negatives that result from the technical drawbacks still present in proteomic analyses.

After image analysis, the molecular identity of the gel features is determined. The ability to identify the proteins in a gel feature, using mass spectrometric methods and sequence databases, represents a major advance in proteomics. Currently, the sensitivity of fluorometric detection exceeds that of mass spectrometry (approximately 50 ng compared to approximately 200 pg). However, the recent development of sensitive linear trap mass spectrometers may result in similar limits of detection for the two methods.

Analysis then proceeds by excising those portions of the gel that are of interest using a robotic cutter. As part of image analysis, the coordinates of each feature are produced relative to alignment markers that are fixed within the gel onto a low fluorescent glass plate. A gel cylinder (approximately 2 mm in diameter) is excised and transferred to a 96-well plate as shown in Figure 35–6. The plate is then loaded into an auto-pipetting robot where a series of washes occurs to remove MS interfering substances (Figure 35–6, step 2). The gel plug is dehydrated with organic solvents prior

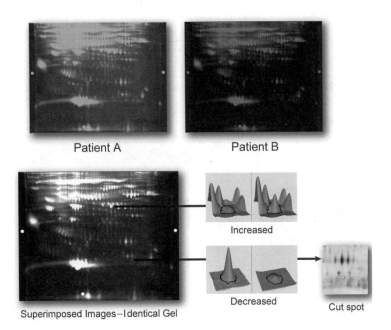

Patient A          Patient B

Superimposed Images—Identical Gel

Increased

Decreased          Cut spot

***FIGURE 35–4*** ● Two-dimensional difference gel electrophoresis of depleted serum from two individuals. **Note:** The color figure can be found following page 394.

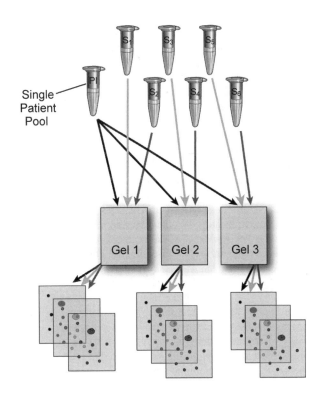

Single Patient Pool

***FIGURE 35–5*** ● A design for proteomic analysis in longitudinal clinical studies.

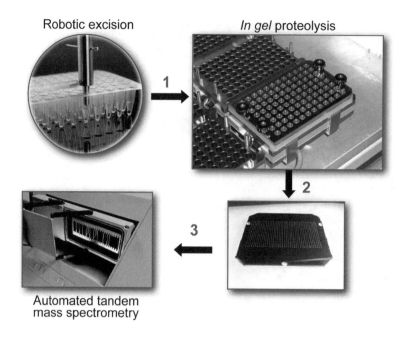

Robotic excision

*In gel* proteolysis

Automated tandem
mass spectrometry

**FIGURE 35–6** ● Automated protein identification using tandem mass spectrometry.

to introduction of a high concentration of trypsin solution. After incubation, an aliquot containing the released peptides is combined with a UV absorbing matrix for MALDI analysis and spotted as an array onto a target plate (Figure 35–6, step 2). The plate is loaded into a MALDI-TOF/TOF mass spectrometer (20) that produces mass spectra of the peptides in each spot, corresponding to the proteins in individual gel features.

Figure 35–7A shows a MALDI mass spectrum of the peptides prepared from an excised gel feature using in situ gel digestion. Using the MALDI-TOF/TOF instrument the masses of the peptides are determined to six significant figures or to a mass accuracy of approximately 10 ppm. The set of masses can be used to identify the parent protein in a database using "mass matching" algorithms. As databases have dramatically increased in size, however, the specificity of the "mass matching" database searching method has decreased and tandem mass spectrometry is becoming the method of choice to identify proteins (21). With this approach, software directs the instrument to select masses for tandem mass spectrometry. Ions at designated *m/z* values are isolated in a collision cell and subjected to fragmentation. In this example, gas-phase fragmentation of the ion at *m/z* 1195.49 produces the spectrum shown in Figure 35–7B. The spectrum can be interpreted manually by calculating the differences between signals. For example, the signal at *m/z* 1082.59 minus the one at 995.57 equals 87.08 that is

the mass of a Ser residue. The difference between the next two most intense signals gives a value of 2120.08, which does not correspond to the residue mass of any one of the 20 naturally occurring amino acid residues. The *m/z* between the signal at 783.43 and 597.33 equals the residue mass of a Trp residue and a partial sequence of S[XY]W. These gaps often occur in tandem spectra and prevent deduction of an unambiguous amino acid sequence. For a more detailed discussion of other issues in the interpretation of peptide fragmentation spectra, the reader is referred to reference 21.

With the introduction of sequence databases, manual interpretation has largely been supplanted with software that can match the information in the spectrum to theoretical spectra or sequences. A database search of the spectrum shown in Figure 35–7 gave the sequence ASPDWGYDDK with acetylation of the amino terminal. As a quality check, the sequence is used to assign ions in the spectrum. The gap of 212.08 is the sum of the masses of Pro and Asp. The sequence is consistent with the series of *y* ions (Figure 35–7, Panel B).

Once a protein has been identified, the masses in the parent MS spectrum can be assigned to tryptic peptides as shown in Table 35–1. The high mass accuracy is useful in reducing the false-positive assignments based on peptide mass. In this case, an investigator can conclude that at least residues 1–228 of carbonic anhydrase are present in the excised gel feature.

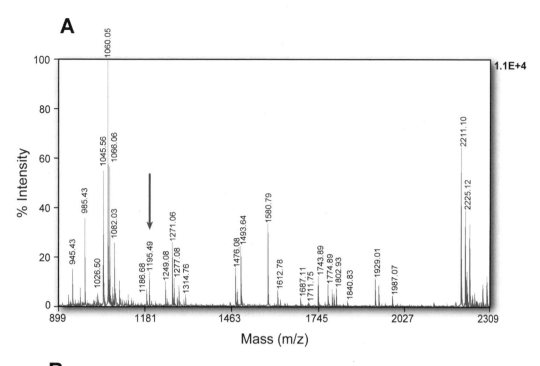

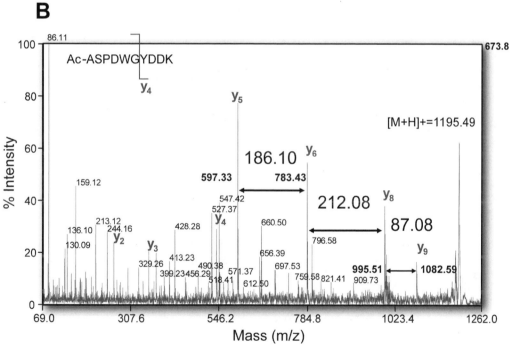

**FIGURE 35–7** ● Mass spectral analysis of a two-dimensional gel feature.

What if the peptide sequence is not in a sequence database? A sequence may not be present in a database because (1) the available genome sequence is incomplete; (2) a mutation has occurred that changes the amino acid sequence; or (3) the peptide has been modified either naturally or through degradation processes. Despite the impressive number of completed genomes (approaching 100), there remain organisms for which their nucleic acid sequences are not available or there is limited

## Comparison of Observed and Theoretical Masses of Tryptic Peptides from a Gel Feature Identified as Human Carbonic Anhydrase

| Tryptic peptide sequence | $[M+H]^+$ observed | $[M+H]^+$ theoretical |
|---|---|---|
| NGPEQWSK | 945.43 | 945.44 |
| GGPFSDSYR | 985.43 | 985.44 |
| ADGLAVIGVLMK | 1,186.68 | 1,186.69 |
| AcASPDWGYDDK | 1,195.49 | 1,195.50 |
| ESISVSSEQLAQFR | 1,580.79 | 1,580.79 |
| YSAELHVAHENSAK | 1,612.78 | 1,612.79 |
| HDTSLKPISVSYNPATAK | 1,929.01 | 1,929.01 |

sequence information. Databases have scant information on posttranslational modifications and search algorithms have not been designed for the comprehensive coverage of described posttranslational modifications (23). In cases where high quality spectra do not return a hit from a database, *de novo* sequencing can be performed and the resulting sequences used in BLAST type searches in order to identify related sequences or sequelogs (24). Figure 35–8 summarizes a data flow from a relational database that contains the mass spectra for protein identification using search algorithms and de novo sequences. The files of raw spectra that contain the acquired MS data as digitally defined peaks are converted to spectra in which the signals are represented as single, centroided masses (preprocessing). The fragmentation spectra are then used to search databases (protein or conceptually translated nucleic acid sequences). The protein identifications, coverage maps, and sequelogs are used to annotate gel features and are entered into a proteomics database for cross-queries with other "omics" databases.

The emerging field of proteomic bioinformatics endeavors to (1) manage and organize the multiplicity of data types from proteomic experiments; (2) standardize data formats for data sharing across databases; (3) build databases containing information on differential protein expression, protein-protein interactions, and posttranslational modifications; and (4) develop new algorithms for improved specificity, quantitation, and statistical analyses of large datasets. The reader is referred to the January 2004 issue of *Nucleic Acids Research* for a compendium of web-accessible proteomics databases.

Figure 35–9 shows a workflow with the instrumentation and data types that are needed to perform a proteomics experiment. Diverse data types are produced and stored as (1) text files that describe the experiment, sample preparation; (2) files that contain quantitative information; (3) mass spectra of peptides and proteins; and (4) lists of peptide sequences from database searches. The scale and diversity of data requires a bioinformatics infrastructure for even proteomic operations performing a few complete proteomics experiments annually. The overarching goal is the integration of functional genomic and clinical data into data warehouses that are accessible to clinical investigators (25–27).

## APPLICATION OF PROTEOMICS TO TRANSLATIONAL MEDICINE

The capability of analyzing the expression of large numbers of proteins and the potential to characterize posttranslational modifications at the molecular level has generated considerable enthusiasm within the biomedical community. Proteomics holds promise for the discovery of new disease markers, better and more rapid understanding of disease mechanisms, and enhanced drug development with customization of therapeutic protocols (for reviews, see references 28,29). Initial large-scale studies to find protein biomarkers have used mass spectral patterns to distinguish between normal and diseased individuals without requiring molecular characterization of the altered proteins. Although the pattern recognition approach has adequate through-put for clinical studies, there are many unaddressed issues, some of which apply to clinical proteomics studies in general (30). There is currently intense debate regarding the use of mass spectrometric patterns alone as a diagnostic and biomarker discovery tool (3,31).

Alternative proteomics methods that incorporate molecular characterization of disease-associated proteins continue to undergo significant advances. For example, recent improvements in two-dimensional gel electrophoresis, as discussed above, and multidimensional high-performance liquid chromatographic separations with high-resolution mass spectrometry have demonstrated that large sets of proteins can be detected in serum over concentration ranges of approximately 8 orders of magnitude with limits of detection of approximately 10 ng/mL of serum. Adkins et al. (32) performed reversed phase LC-MS/MS of strong cation exchange fractions of tryptic peptides from immunoglobulin-depleted serum, reporting 490 proteins. Pieper et al. (33) combined multi-affinity removal of high abundance proteins with ion exchange, 2-DE and LC-MS/MS to find 325 serum proteins in 3,700 gel

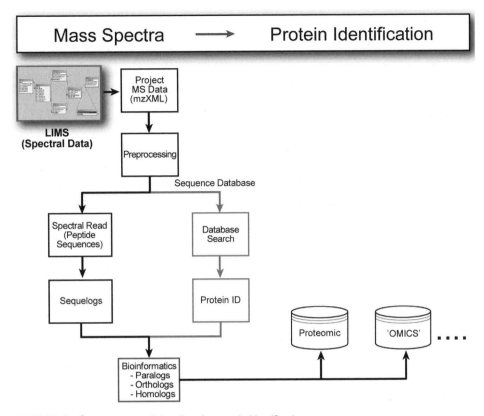

**FIGURE 35–8** ● Mass spectral data flow for protein identification.

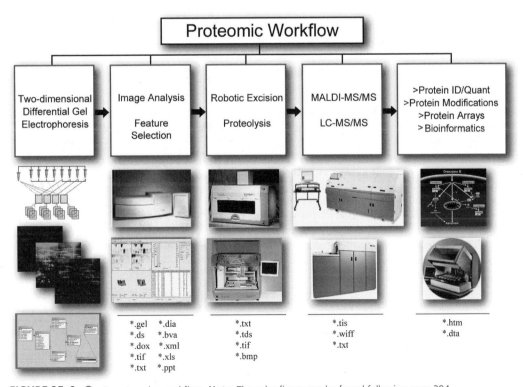

**FIGURE 35–9** ● A proteomics workflow. **Note:** The color figure can be found following page 394.

features. Most recently, Shen et al. (34) used capillary multidimensional LC (strong cation exchange-reversed-phase LC) interfaced to an ion trap mass spectrometer to identify > 800 human plasma proteins from approximately 5 uL of sample. With the introduction of linear ion-trap-Fourier transform ion cyclotron tandem mass spectrometry (FTICR-MS/MS) in the past year, the limits of detection have decreased by two to three orders of magnitude to the "routine" attomole level. The coupling of multidimensional capillary liquid chromatography and high field Fourier transform ion cyclotron mass spectrometry combines continuous orthogonal separations of peptides to mass accuracies sufficient to determine elemental composition from mass alone (35). High mass accuracy (approximately 1 ppm) reduces the required number of tandem experiments in a chromatographic analysis and produces more accurate mass tags for improved (reduction in search time and false-positives) identification of database proteins (36).

These newer methods, however, do not have the through-put to enable biomarker development beyond the stage of discovering candidate biomarkers. Proteomics discovery by its very nature yields a large number of potential biomarkers that must undergo grading, iterative clinical application, and quality control (37,38). Protein and antibody arrays are promising approaches to develop a panel of markers (39); however, there are no proteomic-scale libraries of specific reagents such as antibodies to manufacture arrays that can be tailored to a discovery arm of a clinical proteomics study.

Fundamental issues regarding standardization of collection and sample handling procedures for clinical proteomic studies have not been developed. For example, a recent study showed dramatic changes in the low molecular weight ($m/z$ approximately 100–7,000) spectral pattern of sera treated with serine protease inhibitors prior to analysis, and the changes were disease dependent (39). Additional studies need to be performed to identify the steps in routine blood collection that significantly alter proteomic data. Guidelines for the creation of appropriate normal controls for comparative proteomic analyses have not yet been systematically addressed.

## SUMMARY

- The convergence of separation technologies, mass spectrometry, large-scale genomic sequencing, and bioinformatics has spawned the emerging field of proteomics.
- Current proteomics technologies enable the analysis (identification and relative quantification) of approximately 1,000 protein forms in a single analysis. Thus, in contrast to microarray technologies, proteomics technologies measure a smaller percentage of gene products at a significantly lower through-put.
- Proteomics methods are capable of identifying established and discovering new post-translational modifications.
- Fundamental issues of sample procurement, sample preparation, analysis reproducibility, appropriate statistical models have yet to be addressed and will likely be guided by previous experience in microarray analysis (see Chapter 34).
- The first translational medicine applications will likely be the discovery of biomarkers with validation using immunometric methods.
- Significant advances in proteomics technology are needed for more rapid discovery of protein biomarkers, to understand disease mechanisms in the context of systems biology, and to enhance drug development and customization of therapeutic protocols.

## REFERENCES

1. Ge H, Walhout AJM, Vidal M. Integrating "omic" information: a bridge between genomics and systems biology. TIG 2003;19:551–560.
2. Kenyon GL, DeMarini DM, Fuchs E et al. Defining the mandate of proteomics in the post-genomic era: workshop report. Mol Cell Proteomics 2002;1:763–780.
3. Petricoin III E, Liotta L. The vision for a new diagnostic paradigm. Clin Chem 2003;49:1276–1278.
4. Hanash S. HUPO Initiatives relevant to clinical proteomics. Mol Cell Proteomics 2004;3:298–301.
5. Guttmacher AE, Collins FS. Genomic medicine: a primer. N Eng J Med 2002;347:1512–1520.
6. Nalivaeva NN, Turner AJ. Post-translational modifications of proteins: acetylcholinesterase as a model system. Proteomics 2001;1:735–747.
7. Phelan ML, Nock S. Generation of bioreagents for protein chips. Proteomics 2003;3:2123–2134.
8. Link AJ. Multidimensional peptide separations in proteomics. Trends Biotechnol 2002;20:S8–S13.
9. Hamdan M, Righetti PG. Modern strategies for protein quantification in proteome analysis: advantages and limitations. Mass Spectrom Rev 2002;21:287–302.
10. Aebersold R, Mann M. Mass spectrometry-based proteomics. Nature 2003;422:198–207.
11. Tao WA, Aebersold R. Advances in quantitative proteomics via stable isotope tagging and mass spectrometry. Curr Opin Biotechnol 2003;14:110–118.
12. O'Farrell PH. High resolution two-dimensional electrophoresis of proteins. J Biol Chem 1975;250:4007–4021.
13. Görg A, Obermaier C, Boguth G et al. Recent developments in two-dimensional electrophoresis with immobilized pH gradients: wide pH gradients up to pH 12, longer separation distances and simplified procedures. Electrophoresis 1999;20:712–717.
14. Asirvatham VS, Watson BS, Sumner LW. Analytical and biological variances associated with proteomic studies of *Medicago truncatula* by two-dimensional polyacrylamide gel electrophoresis. Proteomics 2002;2:960–968.

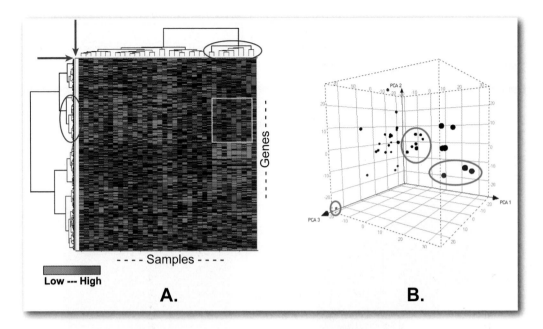

**FIGURE 34–6** ● Visualization of microarray data. **A.** In hierarchical clustering and heat-map visualization of microarray data, samples (represented here by 36 columns) are organized based on similarity of gene expression while genes (represented by approximately 9,000 rows) are simultaneously organized based on similarity of expression across all samples. In the heat map, green lines represent genes that are relatively less expressed in a sample while red lines represent genes that are relatively over expressed in a sample. The tree at the top quantifies the relative similarity between samples (vertical arrow). Samples with higher similarity to each other based on gene expression are depicted as lower branches on the tree (horizontal ellipse). Similarly, the tree on the left quantifies the relative similarity between gene expression patterns (horizontal arrow). Genes that show similar patterns of expression across all samples are depicted as smaller branches on the tree (vertical ellipse). Note subgroups of genes that demonstrate identical patterns of expression in subgroups of samples (yellow box). **B.** In principal components analysis, gene expression values may be condensed into two or three principal components that represent the majority of variation in gene expression across all samples. Each sample is plotted in two- or three-dimensional space (as shown here) based on the value of its principle expression components. Each point may be further color-coded based on other features of the sample (e.g., tumor grade, patient age). In this view, it is easy to demonstrate clusters of samples (green ellipses) that are very distinct in their gene expression profiles. Visualizations generated using DecisionSite for Functional Genomics software (Spotfire, Inc., Somerville, MA).

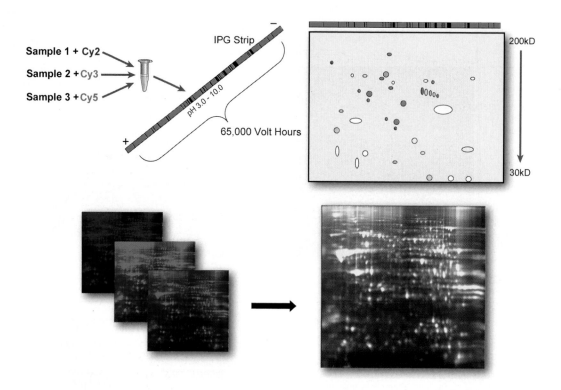

**FIGURE 35–3** ● Two-dimensional difference gel electrophoresis.

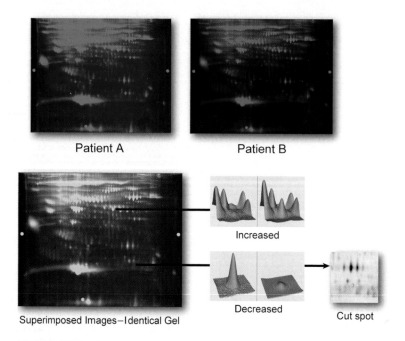

**FIGURE 35–4** ● Two-dimensional difference gel electrophoresis of depleted serum from two individuals.

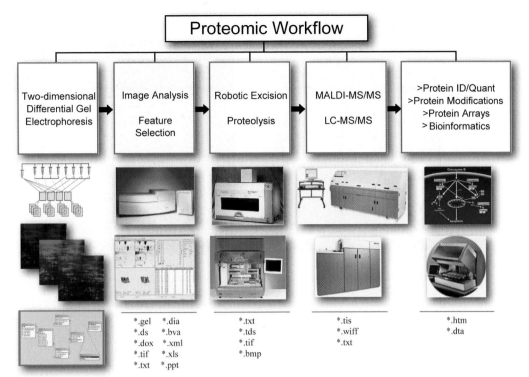

# Proteomic Workflow

| Two-dimensional Differential Gel Electrophoresis | Image Analysis<br><br>Feature Selection | Robotic Excision<br><br>Proteolysis | MALDI-MS/MS<br><br>LC-MS/MS | >Protein ID/Quant<br>>Protein Modifications<br>>Protein Arrays<br>> Bioinformatics |

```
*.gel   *.dia       *.txt       *.tis       *.htm
*.ds    *.bva       *.tds       *.wiff      *.dta
*.dox   *.xml       *.tif       *.txt
*.tif   *.xls       *.bmp
*.txt   *.ppt
```

**FIGURE 35–9** ● A proteomics workflow.

**FIGURE 36–6** ● Representative FISH hybridizations performed on paraffin sections from various tumors. **A.** This glioma assayed with DNA probes against PTEN (green) and DMBT1 (red) displayed the normal disomic (two copies) state for chromosome 10q. **B.** Polysomy 7 or chromosome 7 gain (three to four signals in some cells) is seen in this glioblastoma tested with probes against the centromere 7 (green) and EGFR gene (red). This is thought to represent a progression-associated alteration and the signals appear paired because the two probes are in close proximity within the same chromosome. **C.** Chromosome 1p deletion (one green 1p32 and two red 1q42 signals in most nuclei) identifies this oligodendroglioma as "genetically favorable," associated with both improved prognosis and increased therapeutic responsiveness. **D.** In contrast, this high-grade oligodendroglioma had evidence of homozygous p16 deletion, a progression-associated alteration linked with aggressive behavior. The two non-neoplastic endothelial cells on the left have the normal two copies of the centromere 9 (green) and p16 (red), whereas the tumor cells on the right have no p16 signals. **E.** This medulloblastoma had evidence of c-myc gene amplification (innumerable red c-myc signals; centromere 8 in green), consistent with a more aggressive subtype. **F.** The diagnosis of synovial sarcoma was confirmed in this case using SYT break-apart probes in order to detect its signature X;18 translocation. The red and green probes are localized just proximal and distal to the breakpoint involving the SYT gene on chromosome 18. Therefore, the yellow fusion (overlapping green and red) signals represent the normal, whereas the split red and green confirm an SYT-containing translocation. In some cells represented in these figures, there are fewer than expected signals due to either nuclear truncation artifact or their presence in a plane of focus beyond that captured in the photographs.

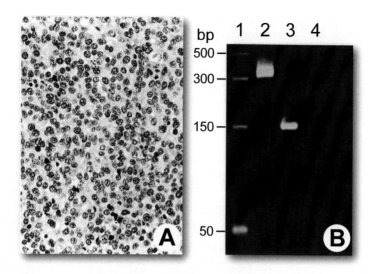

**FIGURE 37–3** ● Example of molecular genetic analysis of Ewing's sarcoma/peripheral neuroectodermal tumor (ES/PNET) arising in the kidney of a 60-year-old woman. **A.** H&E stained section of the tumor. **B.** RT-PCR of formalin-fixed, paraffin-embedded tissue demonstrates the presence of an *EWS-FLI1* gene fusion transcript that is characteristic of ES/PNET. Lane 1, molecular size markers; lane 2, positive control RT-PCR product from an ES/PNET cell line (*EWS* exon 7 to *FLI1* exon 5 fusion); lane 3, renal tumor (*EWS* exon 7 to *FLI1* exon 8 fusion); lane 4, negative control. This type of analysis has been used in translational research studies of ES/PNET to demonstrate that fusion transcript type correlates with prognosis (118,119).

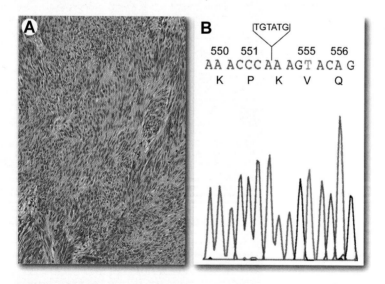

**FIGURE 37–4** ● Example of the use of cycle sequencing to characterize the genotype of a gastrointestinal stromal tumor (GIST). **A.** H&E stained section of the tumor. **B.** DNA was extracted from formalin-fixed paraffin embedded sections of the tumor, and direct DNA sequence analysis of the KIT gene was performed. The computer-generated base sequence (top) inferred from the automated sequencing electropherogram (bottom) is shown; comparison with the wild-type KIT sequence demonstrates a six base deletion that changes codons 552 through 554 but maintains the gene's open reading frame, a mutation characteristic of GIST.

15. Voss T, Habert P. Observations on the reproducibility and matching efficiency of two-dimensional electrophoresis gels: consequences for comprehensive data analysis. Electrophoresis 2000;21:3345–3350.

16. Ünlü M, Morgan ME, Minden JS. Difference gel electrophoresis: a single gel method for detecting changes in protein extracts. Electrophoresis 1997;18;2071–2077.

17. Alban A, David SO, Bjorkesten L et al. A novel experimental design for comparative two-dimensional gel analysis: two-dimensional difference gel electrophoresis incorporating a pooled internal standard. Proteomics 2003;3:36–44.

18. Karp NA, Kreil DP, Lilley KS. Determining a significant change in protein expression with DeCyder™ during a pair-wise comparison using two dimensional difference gel electrophoresis. Proteomics 2004;4:1421–1432.

19. Tonge R, Shaw J, Middleton B. et al. Validation and development of fluorescence two-dimensional differential gel electrophoresis proteomics technology. Proteomics 2001;1:377–396.

20. Medzihradszky KF, Campbell JM, Baldwin MA et al. The characteristics of peptide collision-induced dissociation using a high-performance MALDI-TOF/TOF tandem mass spectrometer. Anal Chem 2000;72:552–558.

21. Baldwin MA. Protein identification by mass spectrometry: issues to be considered. Mol Cell Proteomics 2004;3:1–9.

22. Medzihradszky F, Burlingame AL. The advantages and versatility of a high-energy collision-induced dissociation-based strategy for the sequence and structural determination of proteins. Methods Comp Methods Enzymol 1994;6:284–303.

23. Garavelli JS. The RESID database of protein modifications as a resource and annotation tool. Proteomics 2004;4:1527–1533.

24. Habermann B, Oegema J, Sunyaev S et al. The power and the limitations of cross-species protein identification by mass spectrometry-driven sequence similarity searches. Mol Cell Proteomics 2004;3:238–249.

25. Celis JE, Gromov P, Gromova I et al. Integrating proteomic and functional genomic technologies in discovery-driven translational breast cancer research. Mol Cell Proteomics 2003;2:369–377.

26. Mouridsen HT, Brünner N. Clinical infrastructure to support proteomic studies of tissue and fluids in breast cancer. Mol Cell Proteomics 2004;3:302–310.

27. Celis J, Gromov P. Proteomics in translational cancer research: toward an integrated approach. Cancer Cell 2003;3:9–15.

28. Hanash S. Disease proteomics. Nature 2003;422:226–232.

29. Petricoin E, Wulfkuhle J, Espina V et al. Clinical proteomics: revolutionizing disease detection and patient tailoring therapy. J Proteome Res 2004;3:209–217.

30. Diamandis EP. Mass spectrometry as a diagnostic and a cancer biomarker discovery tool. Mol Cell Proteomics 2004;3:367–378.

31. Diamandis EP. Proteomic patterns in biological fluids: do they represent the future of cancer diagnostics? Clin Chem 2003;49:1272–1275.

32. Adkins JN, Varnum SM, Auberry KJ, et al. Toward a human blood serum proteome: analysis by multidimensional separation coupled with mass spectrometry. Mol Cell Proteomics 2002;1:947–955.

33. Pieper R, Su Q, Gatlin CL, et al. Multi-component immunoaffinity subtraction chromatography: an innovative step towards a comprehensive survey of the human plasma proteome. Proteomics 2003;3:422–432.

34. Shen Y, Jacobs JM, Camp II DG, et al Ultra-high-efficiency strong cation exchange LC/RPLC/MS/MS for high dynamic range characterization of the human plasma proteome. Anal Chem 2004;76:1134–1144.

35. Bogdanov B, Smith RD. Proteomics by FTICR mass spectrometry: Top down and bottom up. Mass Spectrom Rev 2005;24:168–200.

36. Rodland KD. Proteomics and cancer diagnosis: the potential of mass spectrometry. Clin Biochem 2004; 37:579–583.

37. Hayes DF, Bast RC, Desch CE et al. Tumor marker utility grading system: a framework to evaluate clinical utility of tumor markers. J Nat Cancer Inst 1996;88:1456–1466.

38. Sweep FC, Fritsche HA, Gion M, et al. Considerations on development, validation, application, and quality control of immuno(metric) biomarker assays in clinical cancer research: an EORTC-NCI working group report. Int J Oncol 2003;23:1715–1726.

39. Marshall J, Kupchak P, Zhu W et al. Processing of serum proteins underlies the mass spectral fingerprinting of myocardial infarction. J Proteome Res 2003;2:361–372.

# CHAPTER 36

# Cell and Tissue Imaging Techniques

Kevin A. Roth, Arie Perry

Immunohistochemistry (IHC) and in situ hybridization (ISH) techniques are powerful tools for detecting expression of specific proteins and nucleic acid sequences in cells and tissues of interest. Successful application of these methods in translational and experimental medicine requires at least a basic understanding of the theory that forms the foundation for their use and practical concerns that may limit their interpretation. The first part of this chapter will focus on IHC detection and localization of proteins in human tissue sections followed by a brief discussion of mRNA ISH. The second part of the chapter will describe and illustrate fluorescence ISH (FISH) detection of genomic DNA dosages.

## IMMUNOHISTOCHEMISTRY

### Introduction

Immunohistochemistry (IHC) can be defined as a technique in which antibodies are used in conjunction with other reagents to localize the expression of specific antigens in tissues. In most cases, the antigen is a protein but it can be any molecule recognized by an antibody (e.g., a carbohydrate, lipid, nucleic acid, biological amine). The term *immunocytochemistry* refers to the use of antibodies to localize antigens within cells either in cell culture, cytological specimens, or tissue sections. For the purpose of this chapter, we will define IHC as a technique using antibodies to localize specific antigens in cells or tissue sections (Figure 36–1).

IHC is widely used in diagnostic pathology to define the lineage of tumors, assess cell proliferation and death rates, and detect expression of prognostically significant antigens (Figure 36–2). Many of these routinely used diagnostic tests arose from translational studies identifying and validating an association between antigen expression and specific disease conditions. IHC applications and the design of studies employing IHC techniques vary widely but the two major factors determining the success of virtually all IHC studies are antibody specificity and a critical approach to IHC data interpretation.

### Antibodies

Antibodies are produced by terminally differentiated B-cells known as plasma cells (for a review of antigens and antibodies in IHC see reference (1), pp. 31–51). Each plasma cell makes a single antibody species that recognizes a single antigenic epitope and, thus, all antibodies derived from a plasma cell clone are identical and are referred to as monoclonal antibodies. Antibodies can be of five different immunoglobulin subtypes: IgG, IgA, IgM, IgD, and IgE. The vast majority of monoclonal antibodies used in IHC are of the IgG subtype. Most monoclonal antibodies are generated from mouse plasma cell clones but plasma cells from rat, hamster, and other species may also be used for monoclonal antibody production. Typically, monoclonal antibodies are generated from in vivo immunized B cells that are subsequently fused to myeloma cells in culture to generate hybridoma cells that can be propagated in vitro or alternatively, be expanded in vivo in the peritoneal cavity of mice. The hybridoma supernatant or ascitic fluid containing the monoclonal antibody species can then be used directly or be further purified or concentrated prior to use in IHC.

Alternatively, antibodies derived from the response of multiple plasma cells to antigen exposure (i.e., polyclonal antibodies) can be used for IHC.

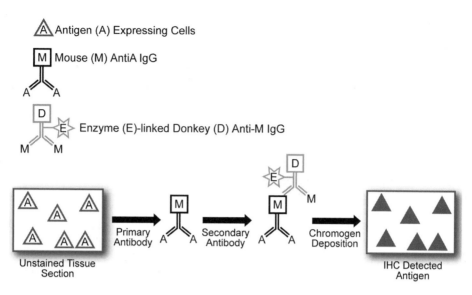

**FIGURE 36–1** ● Schematic illustration of immunohistochemical detection. In this illustration, tissue sections are incubated with a primary mouse antibody, then with a secondary donkey antibody conjugated to an enzyme that permits enzymatic conversion of soluble substrates into insoluble colored reaction products, which can be detected when examined microscopically. Horseradish peroxidase (HRP) is the most frequently used enzyme in IHC.

Most often, polyclonal antibodies are generated in rabbits, although sheep, donkeys, goats, and other species are also used. Unlike monoclonal antibodies, which by definition recognize a single epitope on an antigen, polyclonal antibodies contain multiple antibody populations that recognize various epitopes on the antigen. Antiserum containing polyclonal antibodies can be used directly in IHC studies, or the antibodies can be further concentrated using antigen affinity columns or immunoglobulin purification procedures.

There is no set preference for monoclonal or polyclonal antibodies in IHC because each has advantages and disadvantages. It is a common misconception that monoclonal antibodies are more "specific" than polyclonal antibodies because they recognize only a single epitope. As explained in greater detail later, IHC specificity depends on many factors and must be experimentally determined. Monoclonal antibodies do have the advantage of being clonally produced in vitro, which eliminates any immunoglobulin contribution from

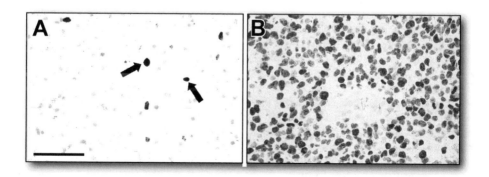

**FIGURE 36–2** ● **A.** IHC detection of Ki-67 antigen, a nuclear protein associated with cell proliferation, shows only scattered immunoreactive cells in a well-differentiated astrocytoma (examples indicated by arrows). **B.** In contrast, Ki-67 immunolabeling of a glioblastoma multiforme demonstrates extensive tumor cell labeling. Elevated Ki-67 labeling has been associated with increased tumor grade in human brain tumors.

antigen irrelevant plasma cells and serum constituents that can cause nonspecific staining. Monoclonal antibodies also have potentially increased reproducibility of IHC staining results because, unlike polyclonal antisera that may be collected from an animal at various times postimmunization or be derived from multiple animals, monoclonal antibodies are always generated by the same plasma cell clone. In contrast, polyclonal antibodies may prove more useful than monoclonals in IHC because multiple antigen epitopes can be detected that potentially increase the number of antibodies bound to the antigen of interest and the probability that tissue fixation will not eliminate all potential antibody recognition sites. Thus, when planning an IHC experiment for which both monoclonal and polyclonal antibodies are available, it is wise to experimentally determine which works best.

## Fixation

Numerous factors affect IHC results and the design of IHC experiments. Many IHC investigations involve the use of human archival tissue samples, and this material will most likely have been fixed in formalin and paraffin-embedded. If tissue processed in this fashion is all that is available for IHC, determining the fixation conditions for optimal antibody staining in frozen tissue sections will be of little value and researchers' efforts should be focused on obtaining interpretable results with formalin-fixed paraffin-embedded tissue sections. Greater experimental flexibility is possible if the tissue to be stained will be prospectively obtained from patients at surgery or autopsy.

The first step in successful IHC is rapid and appropriate fixation of tissue to preserve antigenicity of the target antigen (reference (1), pp. 53–69). The most widely used fixative in pathology is formalin, which preserves tissue by forming cross-links between proteins. The extent of cross-linking depends on the concentration of formaldehyde in the formalin fixative, the length and temperature of fixation, and the presence of a sufficient volume of fixative to adequately penetrate and react with the tissue specimen. Although suitable for many antigens, formalin fixation is suboptimal or useless for preserving others. If antibodies recognizing the antigen of interest have been reported to effectively label formalin-fixed paraffin-embedded tissue, extensive testing of other fixatives may not be necessary. Other useful IHC fixatives include aldehyde-based solutions such as Bouin's fixative or nonaldehyde-based solutions such as Methacarn, acetone, or methanol. These latter solutions preserve tissue by precipitating rather than

cross-linking proteins. The downside to such precipitating fixatives is poor tissue penetration, which limits their use to small samples, and inferior histologic preservation compared to aldehyde-based fixatives. Paraffin embedding of fixed tissue specimens may also diminish the IHC detection of some antigens. This is particularly true for membrane-associated antigens because many cellular lipids and lipoproteins are extracted during the paraffin processing procedure. Many cell surface associated receptors and molecules are most readily detected in acetone or methanol fixed cryostat sections.

The IHC detection of most antigens in formalin-fixed paraffin-embedded tissue sections is dramatically improved by antigen retrieval methods (2). These methods involve either partial enzymatic digestion of the tissue section or more commonly, heat-induced epitope retrieval. Antigen retrieval works in part by reversing excess formalin-induced protein cross-linking. By breaking these cross-links, antigen retrieval facilitates antibody penetration of the tissue section and unmasks previously inaccessible epitopes. Antigen retrieval techniques have made possible the localization of some antigens in formalin-fixed paraffin-embedded tissue sections that had previously been undetectable in such samples. One cautionary note, however, is that antigen retrieval of tissue sections can significantly increase nonspecific background staining if the IHC detection procedure is not appropriately optimized.

## Detection

IHC localization of antigen expression requires visualization of antibody-specific binding in the tissue section of interest (Figure 36–1, Table 36–1). This can be accomplished using either fluorescence or chromogenic detection (3). Although directly labeled primary antibodies can be used if available, in most IHC applications a secondary antibody recognizing the species-specific Fc portion of the primary antibody is used. Thus, following incubation with antigen-specific primary antibodies, a secondary antibody conjugated to a fluorophore or to an enzyme is applied to the tissue section. Fluorescently labeled secondary antibodies bound to the tissue can then be visualized with a fluorescence microscope equipped with filters of the appropriate excitation and emission characteristics. Chromogenic detection is accomplished via the enzymatic conversion of soluble substrates into insoluble colored reaction products. Horseradish peroxidase (HRP) is the most frequently used enzyme in IHC. HRP substrates producing various colored reaction products have been described, and diaminobenzidine (DAB) is the one that is most commonly used.

**TABLE 36–1**

## Outline of a Standard IHC Detection Procedure

- Four micron thick sections are cut from formalin-fixed, paraffin-embedded tissue samples and adhered to glass slides
- Sections are deparaffinized in xylene and rehydrated in graded alcohol solutions and water
- Antigen retrieval in hot 0.01M citrate buffer, pH 6
- Primary antibody incubation
- Incubation with HRP-linked secondary antibody
- Chromogen deposition
- Hematoxylin counterstain
- Coverslip
- Examine under the microscope

The choice of fluorescence or chromogenic detection method is dependent on several variables including the availability of equipment (i.e., a fluorescence microscope), tissue-specific background considerations (e.g., the presence of autofluorescent signals), and the need for archival capability (fluorescent staining typically requires aqueous mounting medium and fades over time). Regardless whether fluorescence or chromogenic detection is preferred, the sensitivity of IHC localization can be improved by a variety of techniques. In standard fluorescence detection, sensitivity is dramatically affected by the choice of fluorophore. The recent commercial development of photostable and sensitive nanocrystal reagents (e.g., Qdots: Quantum Dot Corporation) increases the utility of fluorescence-based IHC (4). Traditionally, "layering" techniques such as peroxidase-anti-peroxidase (PAP) or avidin-biotin complexes (ABC) have been used in combination with enzyme amplification to increase the sensitivity of chromogenic detection. The development of tyramide signal amplification (TSA; Perkin-Elmer Life Sciences) reagents and procedures over the last 10 years has dramatically improved the sensitivity of both chromogenic and fluorescence IHC detection (5,6).

TSA is based on the enzymatic conversion of a labeled tyramine-containing HRP substrate into an oxidized, short-lived free radical that can covalently bind to tyrosine residues in cellular proteins at or near the site of HRP conjugated antibody (7). For fluorescence detection, fluorophore-labeled tyramide is used and provides dramatically improved IHC sensitivity over standard fluorescence techniques due to the enzyme catalyzed deposition of large numbers of fluorescent molecules at the site of antibody binding. For TSA chromogenic detection, hapten labeled tyramide, typically biotinylated tyramide, is used and the deposited reaction product is localized using enzyme conjugated hapten binding reagent, typically HRP labeled streptavidin, and subsequent chromogen deposition. Dramatic increases in IHC sensitivity have been reported with TSA methods and the combined application of antigen retrieval, TSA, and quantum dots can produce remarkable IHC results (8). These improvements in IHC sensitivity, however, necessitate greater vigilance in interpretation of IHC results because the possibility for false-positive results is also dramatically increased.

### Controls

A variety of controls must be performed if IHC findings are to be interpreted accurately. Before even considering the specificity of the IHC signal generated by the primary antibody, it is essential to determine the extent of primary antibody-independent signal produced by the chosen IHC detection method. When performing IHC immunofluorescence, autofluorescent materials such as lipofuscin are present in many cells and tissues; these fluorescent signals should not be confused for "real" signals. Similarly, endogenous biotin and peroxidases will generate primary antibody-independent signals in chromogenic IHC procedures using streptavidin or HRP conjugated reagents. Techniques to reduce the contribution of these factors are available and include the use of avidin-biotin blocking reagents to mask endogenous biotin, $H_2O_2$ pretreatment of tissue sections to diminish endogenous peroxidase activity, and the use of fluorophores that have excitation-emission spectra different from that of autofluorescent materials.

To monitor these nonspecific signals, in every IHC staining experiment and for every independent sample, negative control sections should be included. Minimally, primary antibody should be omitted from these negative control sections or preferably, immunoglobulin of the same isotype and concentration as the monoclonal antibody or non-immune serum from the same species and at the same dilution as the polyclonal antiserum should be substituted for primary antibody. Such negative controls should be thoroughly examined and compared with primary antibody stained sections to avoid false-positive results.

Equally important for accurate IHC interpretation is the use of positive controls. Such controls are run to answer two questions: first, did the primary antibody and detection system perform appropriately? And second, is the tissue section of interest adequately fixed and processed to permit IHC detection? If a primary antibody has previously been well characterized and reported to stain a particular cell type or tissue, positive control sections from such tissue should be included in every IHC run. To verify that the individual samples possess at least some antigenicity, each sample should be stained with a well-characterized cell or tissue-specific antibody. Virtually all cells contain cytoskeletal elements, and antibodies against cytokeratin, vimentin, actin, or other proteins can be useful positive controls. However, it is critical to realize that fixation sensitivity varies widely between proteins and even for different epitopes on the same protein. Therefore, "positive" staining in the control section does not necessarily mean that the antigen of interest to the study has been adequately preserved. A negative result, however, indicates that tissue preservation is inadequate (i.e., the tissue could be underfixed, overfixed, or inappropriately fixed) and the sample should not be used for an IHC study.

## Antibody Specificity

Assuming that appropriate positive and negative controls were performed and stained as expected, the major question to address in all IHC experiments is the specificity of staining produced by the primary antibody (9,10). Due to remarkable advances in antigen retrieval techniques, signal amplification methods, and detection procedures (e.g., high resolution cameras and image processing software), an IHC signal can be generated from virtually any antibody, monoclonal or polyclonal.

In many cases however, the signal will be of unclear or dubious specificity. Several common misunderstandings about IHC specificity can seriously jeopardize an experiment in translational and experimental medicine, particularly when new or previously unvalidated antibodies are being used. It is important to realize that just because an antibody against a particular protein of interest is commercially available does not mean the purchased antibody will be useful for IHC detection or that it even recognizes the endogenous antigen of interest. Reasons are numerous and include fixation sensitive epitopes, cross-reactive proteins, nonspecific antibody binding, inaccessible epitopes, and low antibody binding affinity. Some antibodies have been well characterized and are extensively used in diagnostic pathology, including antibodies recognizing HER-2-*neu*, Ki-67, progesterone receptors, and many other antigens (11); (Figures 36–2 and 36–3). Such antibodies can be used without undue concern about specificity as long as appropriate positive and negative controls are included in the study design.

When new or poorly characterized antibodies are used for IHC investigations, substantial effort must be devoted to addressing staining specificity. It is critical to appreciate that the conditions used for IHC localization of antigen expression in tissue sections is dramatically different from those used to show antigen specificity in a Western blot. The fact that an antibody recognizes a band of an appropriate molecular weight on a Western blot of protein extracted from cells overexpressing the protein in culture has little relevance to IHC detection of the same protein in the complex environment of a fixed tissue section. Similarly, demonstrating that an antibody generates an IHC signal in cultured cells transfected with the gene encoding the protein of

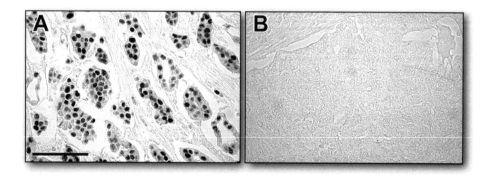

**FIGURE 36–3** ● **A.** and **B.** Progesterone receptor IHC detection was performed on tissue sections from two human breast cancer specimens biochemically determined to have either high levels **(A)** or absent **(B)** progesterone receptor expression. Numerous progesterone receptor immunoreactive tumor nuclei are seen in sample A but no immunoreactivity is observed in the identically processed and stained sample B.

interest but not in nontransfected cells simply indicates that under some experimental conditions the antibody is capable of recognizing its specific target, not that it actually does so under other experimental conditions. Finally, many investigators mistakenly feel that IHC specificity can be proven by demonstrating that primary antibody-dependent signal is abolished by pre-absorption of the antibody with the antigen against which it was raised. Although it is a useful control, pre-absorption can not rule out that the IHC signal generated in the tissue section is from a protein that shares a common epitope with the antigen of interest. Shared IHC epitopes can be independent of shared primary amino acid sequences because antigen epitopes are three-dimensional structures and can not be predicted solely on the linear amino acid sequence.

Under some exceptional experimental conditions, IHC specificity can be proven directly (12). Using mice with targeted disruptions of genes encoding specific proteins of interest, it has been possible to demonstrate a complete abolition of IHC staining in tissues from "protein negative" knockout mice compared to tissues derived from identically-processed control tissues from wild-type mice (Figure 36–4). Even these results can be misleading however, because expression of cross-reacting proteins may be cell-, developmental stage-, or species-specific.

Despite the complexities of proving absolute IHC specificity, investigators can take several steps to gain confidence in their IHC results. First, if multiple independently generated antibodies against the protein of interest demonstrate an identical IHC expression pattern, particularly when the antibodies were raised in different species and recognize different epitopes, it is likely that the IHC detection is specific. Second, the cell- or tissue-specific pattern of IHC staining should correlate with protein expression as determined by Western

blots, although this correlation is suspect if the same antibody is used for both determinations. Third, the pattern of IHC staining should correlate, at least grossly, with expression of mRNA for the protein. Fourth, IHC results should be reproducible.

Although IHC has sometimes been referred to as an "art," it is not. IHC is a science that requires careful attention to experimental detail. Unfortunately, in translational medicine, some of the critical steps may be difficult to control if the samples are processed "routinely" in the diagnostic pathology laboratory (e.g., the length of fixation, the ratio of sample size to fixative volume, variations in tissue processing parameters, or postmortem intervals). However, when done appropriately, IHC remains one of the most powerful tools in translational and experimental medicine.

## IHC Studies in Translational and Experimental Medicine

IHC can be used in many ways to address specific hypotheses in translational and experimental medicine. One of the most common is to test the relationship between a specific disease condition or histopathologic feature and expression of a particular molecule. For example, the IHC localization of alpha-synuclein immunoreactivity in substantia nigra neurons of patients with Parkinson's disease helped define the relationship between this molecule, Lewy bodies, and disease pathogenesis (13). Similarly, the identification of activated caspase-3-like immunoreactivity in hippocampal neurons undergoing granulovacuolar degeneration in autopsy brain sections from patients with Alzheimer's disease suggested a relationship between apoptosis-associated molecules and neurodegeneration (14). Such correlative studies do not require extensive quantitation of the amount of immunoreactivity present because it is the association

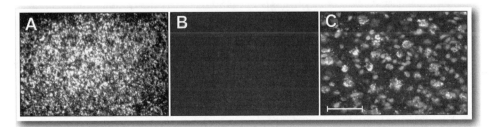

**FIGURE 36–4** ● **A.** IHC detection of Bcl-X$_L$, an anti-apoptotic member of the Bcl-2 family, shows strong diffuse reactivity in the wild-type embryonic mouse spinal cord. **B.** In contrast, identical staining performed on a spinal cord section from an embryonic mouse homozygous for a *Bcl-X* targeted gene disruption (i.e., a Bcl-X$_L$ knockout mouse) shows no immunoreactivity demonstrating the specificity of the Bcl-X$_L$ antibody. **C.** IHC staining of a section from a human glioblastoma multiforme shows numerous Bcl-X$_L$ immunoreactive tumor cells.

of immunoreactivity with particular pathological structures that is important.

A second and more common type of IHC investigation involves a comparison of relative labeling intensity or frequency between experimental groups. Such studies may involve IHC detection of cell proliferation markers, for example, Ki-67 (Figure 36–2), specific receptors, progesterone receptors (Figure 36–3), or molecules associated with defined cellular functions, such as the anti-apoptotic molecule, Bcl-X$_L$ (Figure 36–4). Each of these applications may require a different type of quantitation for accurate data assessment. For a marker like Ki-67, which is largely binary (i.e., a cell is either positive or negative), determination of the frequency of positive cells in each sample yields quantitative data with which to perform statistical comparisons between groups. In contrast, if IHC staining intensity varies widely between cells or exhibits significant regional heterogeneity within a given sample, a simple determination of "percent positive cells" may be inaccurate or misleading.

Under certain experimental conditions, truly quantitative IHC results are possible but these conditions are rarely met in translational medicine. The relationship between the concentration of an antigen present in a tissue section and the amount of chromogen deposited or fluorescence intensity measured in an IHC procedure is complex and affected by many parameters. Variation in tissue sample handling, fixation, processing, and IHC labeling make absolute antigen quantitation difficult if not impossible to perform. A realistic compromise to this problem is to perform semiquantitative analyses in which an arbitrary but defined IHC grading scheme is used to score the amount of immunoreactivity in each sample. The scoring system used will depend on the study design and characteristics of the IHC signal but might include an assessment of relative staining intensity, frequency of immunoreactive cells, or subcellular distribution of immunoreactivity. The critical factor in such semiquantitative scoring systems is minimization of experimenter bias. Samples should be coded and IHC scores determined by an observer blinded to the study design. If possible, all IHC staining for a particular antigen should be performed on all samples at the same time, positive and negative controls performed, replicate samples included, and the scoring system be validated by independent observers. Appropriate tests can then be performed on the data to determine their statistical significance.

## mRNA ISH

Compared with IHC detection of proteins, ISH detection of mRNA is much less frequently performed in translational medicine due to the paucity of commercially available probes and the increased complexity of the mRNA detection procedure. mRNAs are fairly labile and in relatively low abundance in comparison with their protein products. In the past, most mRNA ISH required using radiolabeled probes, typically riboprobes, to produce sufficient signal to permit mRNA localization in tissue sections. Recently, several nonradioactive mRNA ISH protocols have been developed using TSA alone or in combination with other enzyme amplification strategies to improve nonradioactive mRNA ISH detection (15–17). To date, most of these applications have focused on experimental animal tissues because rapid fixation and careful attention to processing conditions can be accomplished. However, as nonradioactive mRNA ISH detection techniques improve and specific probes become more widely available, mRNA localization in human tissue sections will become of significant experimental and diagnostic interest. Given the explosion in genomics and identification of disease-associated genes and mRNAs, it will be particularly important to develop still more sensitive mRNA ISH techniques and more user-friendly probes (18). As in the IHC detection of proteins, ISH detection of mRNA requires careful attention to probe specificity, positive and negative control samples, and standardized experimental conditions.

## FLUORESCENCE IN SITU HYBRIDIZATION (FISH)

### Introduction

Although in situ hybridization (ISH) has been around for more than 30 years, its application to the study of DNA alterations in solid tissue has only become popular over the last decade. It is somewhat unique among molecular techniques due to its basis in morphology, using direct microscopic visualization of probe-specific, intranuclear signals with either chromogenic (CISH) or fluorescence (FISH) detection (19) (Figure 36–5). The latter is used more frequently due to its superior sensitivity and spatial resolution. Given that nonmitotic nuclei are analyzed and metaphase chromosomes are not required for interpretation, this technique has also been referred to as interphase cytogenetics. In clinical cytogenetics laboratories, it is most often used for either prenatal detection of germline alterations (e.g., aneusomy or microdeletion syndromes) or the detection of somatic cancer-associated alterations that have known diagnostic, prognostic, or therapeutic implications (Table 36–2). In anatomic pathology laboratories, the oncology-associated

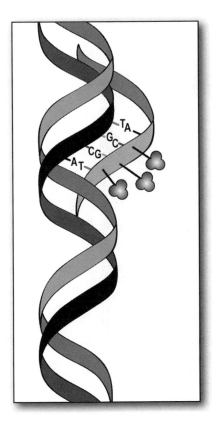

**FIGURE 36–5** ● Schematic illustration of end result of fluorescence in situ hybridization (FISH). The method begins with a mixture of native double helix DNA in the target tissue and intact but separate fragments of fluorochrome-labeled probe (also double-stranded, but linear DNA). In the denaturation step, the strands of the double helix separate and the two strands of the labeled probe similarly come apart. Lastly, in the hybridization step, linear fragments of single stranded labeled probe hybridize to the target DNA (forming a new double helix with the fluorochrome attached to the probe strand) as illustrated.

| **TABLE 36–2** |
|---|

**Examples of Specimen Types and Tests Applicable to FISH**

- Fresh/frozen tissue
- Cytology specimens
  - Body fluids (urine)
  - Intraoperative smears
  - Cell culture preparations
- FFPE tissue
  - Thin sections
  - Disaggregated nuclei
- Prenatal testing
  - Trisomy 13, 18, 21
  - XY aneusomies
- Microdeletion syndromes
  - Cri-du-chat (5p)
  - Prader-Wili/Angelman (15q)
  - Di George syndrome (22q)
- Transplant pathology
  - Male versus female bone marrow cells after cross-gender transplant
- Oncology (diagnostic, prognostic, or therapeutic markers)
  - Chromosomal aneusomies
  - Gene/locus deletions
  - Gene amplifications
  - Translocations

applications are typically of greatest interest. FISH provides data on intranuclear target DNA localization and copy number. Therefore, with the exception of some sex-chromosome determinations, two signals per nucleus are normally expected and four common alterations are detectable: aneusomy (gain or loss of a chromosome or chromosomal region), gene deletion, amplification, and translocation (Figure 36–6).

## Advantages and Limitations of FISH

FISH is applicable to a variety of specimen types, including fresh or frozen tissue, cytologic preparations, and formalin-fixed paraffin-embedded (FFPE) tissue. The latter provides a particularly rich source of archival material and may be performed using either thin (4–6μ) sections, such as those cut for immunohistochemistry or intact nuclei extracted from thick sections (e.g., 50μ), such as those normally prepared for flow cytometry. Although adjustments must be made for nuclear truncation (discussed next), thin sections preserve architecture, are simpler to prepare, and waste less tissue.

For translational research, morphologic preservation is probably the greatest advantage, and is particularly attractive for studies on heterogeneous tissue samples without the need for microdissection. For example, a morphologically mixed tumor recently studied by FISH is the gliosarcoma (20,21). The finding of identical genetic alterations in both components refuted the notion of a collision tumor and supported the hypothesis that both elements originate from a single clone, with the mesenchymal component presumably representing metaplasia. An extension of this morphologic advantage

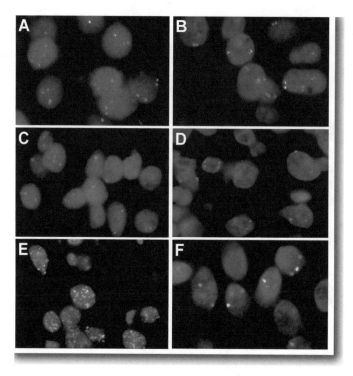

**FIGURE 36–6** ● Representative FISH hybridizations performed on paraffin sections from various tumors. **A.** This glioma assayed with DNA probes against PTEN (green) and DMBT1 (red) displayed the normal disomic (two copies) state for chromosome 10q. **B.** Polysomy 7 or chromosome 7 gain (three to four signals in some cells) is seen in this glioblastoma tested with probes against the centromere 7 (green) and EGFR gene (red). This is thought to represent a progression-associated alteration and the signals appear paired because the two probes are in close proximity within the same chromosome. **C.** Chromosome 1p deletion (one green 1p32 and two red 1q42 signals in most nuclei) identifies this oligodendroglioma as "genetically favorable," associated with both improved prognosis and increased therapeutic responsiveness. **D.** In contrast, this high-grade oligodendroglioma had evidence of homozygous p16 deletion, a progression-associated alteration linked with aggressive behavior. The two non-neoplastic endothelial cells on the left have the normal two copies of the centromere 9 (green) and p16 (red), whereas the tumor cells on the right have no p16 signals. **E.** This medulloblastoma had evidence of c-myc gene amplification (innumerable red c-myc signals; centromere 8 in green), consistent with a more aggressive subtype. **F.** The diagnosis of synovial sarcoma was confirmed in this case using SYT break-apart probes in order to detect its signature X;18 translocation. The red and green probes are localized just proximal and distal to the breakpoint involving the SYT gene on chromosome 18. Therefore, the yellow fusion (overlapping green and red) signals represent the normal, whereas the split red and green confirm an SYT-containing translocation. In some cells represented in these figures, there are fewer than expected signals due to either nuclear truncation artifact or their presence in a plane of focus beyond that captured in the photographs. **Note:** The color figure can be found following page 394.

comes from the possibility of combining FISH with immunohistochemistry, wherein separate counts are rendered in immunopositive and negative cells. For example, this approach, coined FICTION (fluorescence immunophenotyping and interphase cytogenetics as a tool for investigation of neoplasms), was required to demonstrate numerical chromosomal alterations in the CD30-positive Reed-Sternberg cells of Hodgkin's lymphoma (22,23). Because these neoplastic cells typically constitute only a minor fraction of the lymphoid population, clonal alterations are not amenable to detection by "averaging" techniques such as flow cytometry and PCR. Using this dual FISH-immunohistochemistry approach, *NF1* deletions have been shown to be restricted to the S-100 protein positive, Schwann cell elements in another cellularly and immunophenotypically heterogeneous neoplasm, the plexiform neurofibroma (24). Lastly, Tubbs et al. used this technique to simultaneously visualize HER-2/*neu* gene amplification and protein overexpression in breast carcinomas (25). They coined the acronym CODFISH (concomitant oncoprotein detection with FISH) for this particular application.

Another distinct advantage is the similarity of FISH to immunohistochemistry, which is already familiar and widely applied in many laboratories. The two techniques are analogous, except that FISH uses DNA probes, rather than antibodies. Unlike the typical qualitative or semiquantitative immunohistochemical interpretation schemes (e.g., ± or 0–3+), FISH provides quantitative results that are therefore, more objective (i.e., actual copy numbers of target DNA per cell, see examples in Figure 36–6). Nevertheless, FISH on paraffin tissue has at least as many artifacts as immunohistochemistry and researchers must similarly be aware of these in order to avoid false positives and false negatives.

Compared to classic metaphase cytogenetics (i.e., karyotyping), FISH has several advantages, most importantly, the lack of requirements for mitotically active cells and culturing. Because only cells capable of proliferating in vitro are assessable on karyotype, significant growth selection biases can occur during such studies, including overgrowth of nonneoplastic elements (particularly when analyzing benign or low-grade neoplasms). On the other hand, FISH is not a genomic screening tool; it simply provides a more targeted approach for alterations that have been initially identified by more global assessments, such as conventional cytogenetics, loss of heterozygosity (LOH) screening, comparative genomic hybridization (CGH), CGH array (aCGH) and gene expression profiling.

In terms of sensitivity and resolution, FISH is better than karyotyping and CGH, but worse than PCR-based assays for detecting small alterations. The former is limited to alterations of several Mb in size, whereas the latter can be designed to detect even single base pair mutations. Because FISH probes are typically at least 20 Kb in size, alterations need to be equally large for reliable detection. For this reason, FISH cannot detect small intragenic mutations and is best reserved for alterations that occur at the "cytogenetic" level. PCR is also more sensitive than FISH for detecting abnormal fusion transcripts resulting from chromosomal translocations, picking up as few as one per million cells. This is particularly useful when attempting to detect "minimal residual disease" or early recurrence, though the biologic relevance of such small tumoral fractions is not always clear. In contrast, FISH is more sensitive than PCR at identifying gene deletions or amplifications from samples of mixed cellularity, such as neoplasms with clonal heterogeneity or contaminating nonneoplastic elements (26). It is estimated that sample purity must reach at least 70% tumor for quantitative PCR, which is sometimes difficult to achieve in highly infiltrative neoplasms or tumors with abundant stroma or inflammation. FISH, on the other hand, can typically identify gains, translocations, or amplifications in as few as 5% and deletions in 15 to 30% of the cells within a sample.

In comparison to LOH studies, FISH results are similar or complementary, but not identical and each has its advantages and disadvantages. A common misconception is to equate the two techniques, stating that "FISH demonstrates LOH" for a region of interest. Because FISH measures absolute copy number rather than allele status, such a statement is inaccurate. Whereas LOH often results from a simple deletion, this is not always the case. For example, mitotic recombination of chromosome 17p may lead to loss of the wild-type p53 allele and duplication of the mutated allele. Although one "allele" (maternal or paternal) would be lost in this scenario (i.e., LOH), there would still be two copies of the p53 gene, simulating the normal disomic situation by FISH analysis. This was in fact, found to be the most common mechanism for p53 inactivation in gliomas (27) and therefore, FISH is not a suitable assay for detecting this type of loss in these tumors (28). Another advantage of the LOH studies is the ease of evaluating large numbers of markers spanning the entire length of a chromosome or chromosomal arm. As emphasized above however, morphologic correlation is not possible unless regions of interest are microdissected first. Additionally, LOH requires matching germline DNA from the patient's leukocytes or microdissected normal tissue and this is not always available.

A recent and particularly advantageous application of FISH uses high-throughput analysis via tissue microarray (TMA). This technology takes advantage of multispecimen paraffin blocks constructed from up to 1,000 0.6-mm neoplastic, nonneoplastic, and control tissue cores of interest. Therefore, hundreds of specimens can be simultaneously evaluated on a single slide using TMA-FISH, markedly increasing efficiency and reducing data acquisition time, probe, reagent, and storage space requirements. A recently popularized approach is to initially screen a small number of tumors with gene expression profiling and then verify the resulting candidate genes in a large number of tumors, using TMA-immunohisto-chemistry and TMA-FISH (29,30). Recent TMA studies have shown excellent morphologic, anti-genic, and genomic preservation with high levels of concordance compared to the traditional whole slide approach (30–34). Tumor heterogeneity can still be a problem, but adequate sampling can be optimized by using multiple cores from each specimen. For gene amplifications, TMA-FISH is particularly appealing, because interpretations are rapid, typically requiring only seconds per tissue core. For aneusomies and deletions, manual signal counts still remain tedious and time consuming. However, software programs for automated spot counting are currently being de-veloped and promise to increase the efficiency of this technique considerably.

As discussed earlier, recent technical advances have greatly enhanced the applicability of FISH, though a number of limitations remain. One of the main disadvantages of FISH as a clinical tool is sig-nal fading. By storing hybridized slides in a freezer and avoiding prolonged exposure to light, hybridiza-tion signals remain visible for up to two to three years or longer. However, a permanent record is gen-erally not achieved, unless chromogenic detection is used. Therefore, clinical labs routinely capture digi-tal images as a permanent record of case results. Un-fortunately, multicolor CISH is not as simple as multicolor FISH and currently available chromogens lack the spectral versatility, sensitivity and spatial resolution attainable with fluorochromes. However, the recently developed photostable quantum dots offer another potential alternative for permanent sig-nals in future FISH applications (8).

Other limitations include a variety of artifacts, particularly common in paraffin sections. It is for this reason that while the FISH protocol itself is often mastered quickly, interpretation requires sig-nificantly more experience. Most troublesome are truncation artifacts, aneuploidy, autofluorescence, and partial hybridization failure. Truncation arti-fact refers to the underestimation of target copy numbers due to incomplete DNA complements in transected nuclei. Therefore, it is important to in-clude controls cut at the same thickness. Cutoffs for hemizygous deletion are often based on mean percentages of control nuclei with less than two signals plus three standard deviations (requirement of >50% nuclei with one signal is typical). How-ever, a number of other approaches have also been applied and currently, there are no consensus crite-ria published. Homozygous deletions are defined by the complete lack of test probe signals in tumor cells. Partial hybridization failure is ruled out by the presence of reference probe signals in the tumor cells, as well as test probe signals in adjacent

non-neoplastic elements, such as vascular en-dothelial cells (Figure 36–6D).

Aneuploidy and polyploidy are particularly com-mon in malignant neoplasms and can result in con-fusing signal counts. The inclusion of reference probes is extremely helpful in such situations. Al-though the simplest approach is to interpret absolute losses (<2 copies) and gains (>2 copies), researchers may opt to delineate "relative" losses and gains com-pared with a reference ploidy, obtained either by flow cytometry or the assessment of multiple chro-mosomes by FISH. For example, the finding of three copies would be considered a relative gain in a diploid tumor, normal in a triploid tumor, and a rela-tive loss in a tetraploid tumor. Lastly, investigators may combine a centromere and locus-specific probe from a single chromosome and determine their ratios. For example, cells with four chromosome 9 centromeres and two copies of the p16 region on 9p21 would be interpreted as having polysomy 9 and a hemizygous p16 deletion. A similar tumor with 4 centromere and no p16 signals would be inter-preted as polysomy 9 with homozygous p16 dele-tion. Similarly, cells with six copies of HER-2/*neu* might be interpreted as low-level amplification if there were only two chromosome 17 centromeres, but would represent polysomy 17 without gene am-plification if there were six centromeres.

Autofluorescence is a common problem in paraf-fin sections. Because autofluorescent tissue frag-ments are typically larger and more irregular than true signals, they can often be disregarded. However, some fragments present at just the right size to simu-late signals. In this case, the use of multiple filters is helpful, because autofluorescence will typically ap-pear on both green and red filters, whereas true sig-nals only fluoresce under one or the other. The problem of partial hybridization failure can be mini-mized by counting only in regions where the major-ity of cells have detectable signals.

## FISH Assay: Technical Considerations

A number of FISH protocols have been published and vary depending on individual preferences and specimen type. In general, the simpler protocols are preferable, because they require less "hands-on" time, have fewer steps in which errors may be intro-duced, and are easier to troubleshoot. Additionally, automated instruments are now available to further minimize hands-on time. Generally, the basic steps are similar to those of immunohistochemistry and include deparaffinization, pretreatment or target re-trieval, denaturation of probe and target DNA, hy-bridization (usually overnight), posthybridization washes, detection, and microscopy/imaging. This is typically a two-day assay, which requires roughly 3–4 hours the first day and 30 minutes the second day. Alternatively, same day protocols are possible with particularly robust probes.

A few technical caveats should be kept in mind. Similar to immunohistochemistry, microwave or heat-induced target retrieval often works better than chemical forms of pretreatment and significantly improves hybridization efficiency (26,35,36). When this step is included, protein digestion may often be reduced or eliminated altogether. Nevertheless, optimal pretreatment and digestion varies from one specimen to another, depending on methods of fixation or processing. Some hybridization buffers are significantly more efficient than others and therefore work with lower probe concentration requirements (e.g., DenHyb™ from Insitus, http://www.insitus.com). This is particularly useful when using expensive commercial probes, because they may last 5 to 20 times as long as they would when using the manufacturers recommended dilutions. This same company now offers a product called SkipDewax™, which allows investigators to deparaffinize and pretreat all in one step. Lastly, a variety of amplification steps are available for cases with weak signals. However, such steps are rarely necessary and the simpler protocol and cleaner background associated with directly labeled fluorochrome probes (e.g., FITC, rhodamine) is preferred, in contrast to indirectly labeled probes (e.g., digoxigenin, biotin) that require an additional step (e.g., fluorochrome-labeled secondary antibody) with or without further amplification. Nevertheless, just as discussed in the prior section on immunohistochemistry, dramatic levels of FISH signal amplification are now achievable with tyramide signal amplification (TSA) or catalyzed reporter deposition (CARD) (5,15,37,38). This technique takes advantage of peroxidase-mediated deposition of haptenized tyramine molecules, not only in the precise site of hybridization, but also in the nearby vicinity. This results in increases of signal size, up to 1,000-fold or greater amplification. Although one possible application is marked reductions of probe concentration requirements, the more exciting potential is the use of smaller probes, perhaps down to the level of 1 Kb or less (39). Therefore, TSA could potentially increase the sensitivity for small alterations, such as those detectable by PCR, while maintaining the morphologic advantage of FISH.

## FISH Probes and Probe Development

A number of different probe types are currently available for FISH. Centromere enumerating probes (CEPs) were among the first to be developed and are ideal for detecting whole chromosome gains and losses, such as monosomy, trisomy, and other polysomies. Because they target highly repetitive 171 bp sequences of α-satellite DNA, they are associated with excellent hybridization efficiencies and typically yield large, bright signals. However, sequence similarities in some pericentromeric regions result in cross-hybridization artifacts. Because of the inevitable cross-hybridization between centromeres 13 and 21 or between centromeres 14 and 22, these CEPs have been previously used as probes with four expected signals rather than two. A better solution is to use locus-specific or painting probes to enumerate these individual chromosomes. Anecdotally, researchers also occasionally encounter cross-hybridization problems with other centromere probes, though the nonspecific signals are usually dimmer and using either more stringent washes or lower probe concentrations often resolves this problem. Also, an interesting phenomenon in nonneoplastic brain is that certain chromosomes are packaged into interphase nuclei with paired centromeres in close proximity, a concept known as somatic pairing (40,41). This is most dramatic with CEP17, but may be encountered to a lesser extent with other centromeres as well, including CEP1 and CEP8. Because of this close proximity, FISH yields an unexpected fraction of cells harboring a single large signal rather than two smaller ones, an artifact that could potentially lead to overinterpretation of monosomy. For unknown reasons, somatic pairing is not typically seen in neoplasms. Nonetheless, interpretations with these CEPs are problematic if using normal brain controls to establish cutoffs for monosomy. Despite these technical limitations, CEPs remain extremely useful for detecting aneusomies and are still among the best FISH probes available. The presence of similarly repetitive DNA sequences in subtelomeric regions has led to the development of commercially available probes for each chromosomal arm as well.

Another chromosome-specific probe is the whole chromosome paint (WCP), in which a cocktail of DNA fragments is created to target all the nonrepetitive DNA sequences in an entire chromosome. Because they cover such a large region of DNA, they yield more diffuse signals in interphase nuclei and are primarily used on metaphase spreads for resolving complex structural alterations. However, some of the smaller, acrocentric chromosomes yield sufficiently discrete signals for enumeration in interphase nuclei. The WCPs also form the basis for advanced applications such as spectral karyotyping (SKY) and multiplex FISH (M-FISH), where each chromosome is painted with its own unique mixture of fluorescent colors. This is a particularly useful technique for identifying complex structural alterations, such as translocations involving multiple chromosomes, "marker chromosomes" that are unidentifiable on routine karyotype banding. In contrast, another advanced application, comparative genomic hybridization (CGH), uses entire genomes as the "probe." Genomic tumor DNA is labeled in one color, normal DNA is labeled in another color, and equal quantities of both are competitively hybridized to a normal human metaphase in order to screen for regions of relative tumoral losses and gains. This is a very useful methodology for cytogenetic screening of rare tumors where nothing is known about the genetics. However, the resolution is fairly limited, and therefore only large alterations are typically identified. Techniques such as FISH, CGH, M-FISH, and SKY are sometimes referred to collectively as molecular cytogenetics.

Today, some of the most versatile and commonly used FISH probes are the locus-specific (LSI) or gene-specific probes. These probes target specific regions of interest and use single copy rather than repetitive DNA sequences. Therefore, in order to yield signals large enough to be detected in tissue sections, the probe typically needs to be at least 20 Kb in size. The largest FISH probes are often >1 Mb and most fall into the 100–300 Kb range. Until recently, commercially available LSI probes have been limited in scope. Therefore, cloning vectors have been exploited for developing homemade FISH probes, including cosmids, bacterial artificial chromosomes (BACs), P1 artificial chromosomes (PACs), and yeast artificial chromosomes (YACs). Whereas in the past, this required a rather lengthy and tedious process of screening vector libraries with PCR primers, the recent human genome project and sequencing of entire BAC libraries has enabled rapid internet screening, using DNA sequences of interest, gene names, or physical maps of chromosomes (e.g., http://genome.ucsc.edu, http://gdbwww.gdb.org). Similarly, mapped BAC clones spread throughout the human genome at 1-Mb intervals have also become available (http://www.ncbi.nlm.nih.gov/ncicgap; http://mp.invitrogen.com/). Therefore, it is now relatively simple to obtain a BAC clone localizing to virtually any region of interest, label the DNA with commercially available kits, and use it as a FISH probe. These developments will no doubt enhance the rate of future discoveries significantly and greatly facilitate the ability to perform translational research.

## Application of FISH to Translational Research

Over the past decade, FISH has been applied to many translational studies. Typical hypotheses tested include (1) a cytogenetic alteration (deletion, gain, amplification, translocation) is highly sensitive and specific for a single tumor type (i.e., has diagnostic value); (2) within a single diagnostic category (e.g., ductal breast carcinoma), a specific cytogenetic alteration can predict which tumors will be clinically aggressive versus indolent (i.e., has prognostic value); and (3) within a single diagnostic category, a cytogenetic alteration will predict which tumors will respond to either general, nontargeted forms of chemotherapy (e.g., alkylating agent) or targeted therapy (e.g., antibody against a unique surface protein expressed by the patient's tumor) (i.e., genetic biomarker serves as a guide to patient therapy). The most common applications today include HER-2/*neu* amplification testing in breast cancer, 1p/19q deletion testing in gliomas (a form of brain cancer), and testing for signature translocations associated with specific hematologic, soft tissue, or pediatric malignancies. The first two applications are discussed below as examples of translational FISH studies in the literature.

Of all the current applications of FISH analysis in diagnostic tumor pathology, the assessment of HER-2/*neu* status in breast cancer has attracted the greatest attention and application (42). Although there is now agreement that HER-2/*neu* assessment provides clinically useful information, the optimal diagnostic approach is still widely debated. The HER-2/*neu* gene ("HER-2" for human EGF receptor 2, "neu" for rat neuroblastoma/glioblastoma-associated oncogene, a.k.a. *c-erb-B2*) on chromosome 17q21 is a member of the EGFR family of tyrosine kinases and encodes a 185 kD transmembrane protein implicated in the regulation of cell growth. It has no known ligand and normally requires heterodimerization with other ErbB coreceptors, such as EGFR (ErbB1) or ErbB3 for activation. HER-2/*neu* protein overexpression, primarily due to gene amplification is thought to be involved in the malignant progression of several tumor types and has been identified in 20 to 35% of breast carcinomas, primarily of high-grade ductal type (42–44). HER-2/*neu* gene amplification and protein expression status is thought to provide both prognostic and therapeutic information and the current rationale for HER-2/*neu* testing is based on the following observations: (1) overexpression/amplification is an independent prognostic variable, associated with reduced patient survival, especially in lymph node positive, but also in node negative cases; (2) overexpression/amplification is associated with increased responsiveness to adriamycin-based therapeutic regimens; (3) overexpression/amplification is associated with increased responsiveness to Herceptin®

(trastuzumab), which specifically targets the overexpressed surface protein; (4) overexpression/amplification is associated with decreased responsiveness to radiation therapy, cyclophosphamide, methotrexate, 5-FU, hormonal therapy, and taxol (unless administered with Herceptin); and (5) there is significant risk of cardiotoxicity with adriamycin and Herceptin therapy and this combination should therefore, be avoided in patients with low probability of response.

Presently, the two primary modalities for assessing HER-2/*neu* status in routinely processed breast cancer biopsies are immunohistochemistry and FISH. Each technique has its advantages and disadvantages, and both FDA-approved antibodies and DNA probes are now commercially available. Although immunohistochemistry is simpler, cheaper, and more widely available than FISH, concerns have been raised regarding the variable antibody specificities and sensitivities, as well as the subjectivity involved in semiquantitative interpretations, such as the 0–3+ scale recommended with the FDA-approved Dako HercepTest™ antibody. Due to the increased objectivity, reproducibility, accuracy, and associations with clinical behavior, FISH is now playing an increasing role in these assessments.

FISH has also proved clinically valuable for primary brain tumors in the genetic profiling of one specific type of glioma, known as oligodendroglioma. It is named as such due to the resemblance of the tumor cells to nonneoplastic oligodendrocytes. Comprising approximately 20 to 25% of adult gliomas, oligodendrogliomas tend to progress more slowly than astrocytomas, and are associated with longer patient survival (45). The diagnosis of these tumors is particularly critical given that many anaplastic oligodendrogliomas respond favorably to chemotherapy, especially the PCV regimen [procarbazine, lomustine (CCNU), and vincristine] and more recently, temozolamide, a newer alkylating agent with a lower side effect profile. Translational LOH, CGH, and FISH studies have shown that 50 to 85% of oligodendrogliomas are characterized by a distinctive genetic pattern, consisting of combined deletions of the entire 1p and 19q chromosomal arms (45). These molecular alterations have potential diagnostic, prognostic, and even therapeutic relevance, because they are associated with histologically classic oligodendroglioma morphology, prolonged patient survival irrespective of grade, and a higher degree of therapeutic responsiveness.

The basic steps in designing a translational FISH study are highlighted in Table 36–3. The first critical piece of information is the identification of molecular cytogenetic alterations associated with a particular tumor type or a genetic syndrome. This typically comes from initial basic science or

---

> ## TABLE 36–3
>
> ### Experimental Design for Translational FISH Studies
>
> - Identification of a cytogenetic biomarker
>   - Chromosomal gain/loss
>   - Gene/locus deletion
>   - Gene amplification
>   - Translocation
> - Selection/design of test and reference DNA probes
>   - Commercial
>   - Homemade (e.g., BAC clones)
> - Assess potential clinical relevance
>   - Diagnostic aid
>   - Prognostic aid
>   - Guide to patient therapy
> - Determine appropriate specimen cohort to test and clinical endpoints needed
>   - Archival paraffin-embedded tissue versus fresh/frozen versus cytology
>   - Retrospective versus prospective
>   - Morphologically similar tumors to assess specificity
>   - Times to progression, metastasis, or death
>   - Patient age or other demographically relevant prognosticators
>   - Extent of resection
>   - Types of therapy administered
>   - Biostatistics needed to answer study questions

---

translational studies using genomic screening techniques such as karyotyping, CGH, LOH, or expression profiling.

The next question that must be answered is appropriate DNA probe availability. If it is commercially available, then there is no problem, but if not, then homemade probes can still be fashioned using human BAC clones of known sequence and cytogenetic localization. For deletions, chromosomal arm losses and gains, or gene amplifications, the CEP from the same chromosome is often used as a reference probe, such that the copy number for the locus of interest can be compared with the copy number of the chromosome from which it originates. Alternatively, a marker on the opposite chromosomal arm may serve as a copy number reference. For chromosomal translocations, significant knowledge of breakpoints is needed for probe design, though many of the common translocation probes are already commercially available. One common strategy is to look for fusion signals, where two markers or genes from two different chromosomes (e.g., BCR on 22q and ABL on 9q) that normally yield separate green and red signals form fusion yellow or red-green signals in the presence of a translocation. However, investigators must be careful not to overinterpret occasional cells where the signals are overlapping purely by chance.

The opposite (break apart) strategy uses two probes localizing just proximal and distal to one of the two breakpoints of interest. Because the two probes are spatially so close to each other, this results in two fusion signals normally, but split green and red signals if there is a translocation. The advantages of this approach are that split signals shouldn't occur by chance alone and it will still be positive in variant translocations where multiple different partner genes may be fused to the same primary gene of interest (e.g., EWS can fuse with several other genes). The disadvantage is that one does not know the exact partner gene.

In any case, once the appropriate DNA probes are obtained, a clinically relevant question should be tested. If the diagnostic value is being evaluated, then a large number of other tumor types of similar morphology should also be assessed in order to determine the sensitivity and specificity of the biomarker in question. If the prognostic value is tested, then only one tumor type needs to be tested, but there must be sufficient clinical follow-up to determine variable patient outcomes, such as time to tumor recurrence, presence/absence of metastases, and patient death. Lastly, if therapeutic responsiveness is being tested, then it is critical that patients are treated in a uniform manner in addition to knowing times to recurrence, radiographic parameters of response versus progression, and survival times. The latter type of study is often the most rewarding, but is also the most difficult to design, often requiring large clinical trials with multidisciplinary expertise and biostatistics support.

The usual confounding variables that affect prognosis should also be considered ahead of time (e.g., patient age, relevant demographics, extent of surgery, or forms of adjuvant therapy). In fact, depending on the complexity of the clinical question addressed, it is often helpful to consult a biostatistician ahead of time to determine the sample numbers that will be required to provide sufficiently robust statistical power.

## SUMMARY

- Immunohistochemistry (IHC) and in situ hybridization (ISH) techniques are particularly

useful for detecting the expression of a particular protein or nucleic acid sequence in a specific cell or tissue type.

- With IHC, antibodies are used to localize the expression of specific antigens (usually, but not always, a protein) in tissues.
- The antibodies can be mono- or polyclonal; the best choice for a specific application must often be determined empirically.
- In most IHC applications, a secondary antibody that recognizes the Fc portion of the primary antibody is used to visualize and detect binding of the primary antibody to the antigen of interest.
- Proper interpretation of any IHC study will usually depend on carefully chosen negative and positive controls, and on the steps taken to document staining specificity of the primary antibody.
- A common application of IHC in translational medicine includes a test of the relationship between a disease or a histopathologic feature and the expression of a particular molecule. Another application involves a comparison of the relative labeling intensity in a tissue of interest among different patient groups.
- Fluorescence in situ hybridization (FISH) is a tissue-based method for imaging DNA localization and copy number (i.e., to detect chromosomal gain or loss, gene deletion, amplification, or translocation). Thus, it is a quantitative alternative to classic chromosomal karyotyping.
- The method of FISH is analogous to IHC, except FISH uses DNA probes instead of antibodies.
- FISH methods are commonly used in clinical cancer studies. Common applications include determining whether a specific cytogenetic alteration is sensitive or specific for a particular tumor type, whether a specific cytogenetic alteration can predict which tumors will be particularly aggressive clinically, and determining whether a particular cytogenetic abnormality can predict treatment efficacy.

## REFERENCES

1. Hayat MA. Microscopy, Immunohistochemistry, and Antigen Retrieval Methods: for Light and Electron Microscopy. New York: Kluwer Academic/Plenum, 2002.
2. Shi SR, Cote RJ, Taylor CR. Antigen retrieval techniques: current perspectives. J Histochem Cytochem 2001;49(8):931–937.
3. Roth KA. In situ detection of apoptotic neurons. In: LeBlanc AC Ed. Neuromethods: Apoptosis Techniques and Protocols, vol 37. Totowa, NJ: Humana, 2002:205–224.
4. Wu X, Liu H, Liu J et al. Immunofluorescent labeling of cancer marker Her2 and other cellular targets with semiconductor quantum dots. Nat Biotechnol 2003;21:41–46.

5. van Gijlswijk RPM, Zijlmans HJ, Weigant J et al. Fluorochrome-labeled tyramides: use in immunocytochemistry and fluorescence in situ hybridization. J Histochem Cytochem 1997;45:375–382.

6. Shindler KS, Roth KA., Double immunofluorescent staining using two unconjugated primary antisera raised in the same species. J Histochem Cytochem 1996;44:1331–1335.

7. Bobrow MN, Litt GJ, Shaughnessy KJ et al. The use of catalyzed reporter deposition as a means of signal amplification in a variety of formats. J Immunol Meth 1992;150:145–149.

8. Ness JM, Akhtar RS, Latham CB et al. Combined tyramide signal amplification and quantum dots for sensitive and photostable immunofluorescence detection. J Histochem Cytochem 2003;51:981–987.

9. Willingham MC. Conditional epitopes: is your antibody always specific? J Histochem Cytochem 1999; 47:1233–1235.

10. Burry RW, Specificity controls for immunocytochemical methods. J Histochem Cytochem 2000;48:163–165.

11. Roth KA, Brenner JW, Selznick LA et al. Enzyme-based antigen localization and quantitation in cell and tissue samples (midwestern assay). J Histochem Cytochem 1997;45:1629–1641.

12. Srinivasan A, Roth KA, Sayers RO et al. *In situ* immunodetection of activated caspase-3 in apoptotic neurons in the developing nervous system. Cell Death Differ 1998;5:1004–1016.

13. Spillantini MG, Schmidt ML, Lee VM-Y et al. A-synuclein in Lewy bodies. Nature 1997;388:839–840.

14. Selznick LA, Holtzman DM, Han BH et al. *In situ* immunodetection of neuronal caspase-3 activation in Alzheimer's disease. J Neuropathol Exp Neurol 1999; 58:1020–1026.

15. Speel EJM, Hopman AHN, Komminoth P. Amplification methods to increase the sensitivity of in situ hybridization: play CARD(S). J Histochem Cytochem 1999;47:281–288.

16. Zaidi AU, Enomoto H, Milbrandt J et al. Dual fluorescent in situ hybridization and immunohistochemical detection with tyramide signal amplification J Histochem Cytochem 2000;48:1369–1376.

17. Breininger JF, Baskin DG. Fluorescence in situ hybridization of scarce leptin receptor mRNA using the enzyme-labeled fluorescent substrate method and tyramide signal amplification. J Histochem Cytochem 2000;48:1593–1599.

18. Mills JC, Roth KA, Cagan RL et al. DNA microarrays and more: completing the journey from tissue to cell. Nature Cell Biol 2001;3:E175–E178.

19. Fuller CE, Perry A. Fluorescence in situ hybridization (FISH) in diagnostic and investigative neuropathology. Brain Pathol 2002;12:67–86.

20. Paulus W, Bayas A, Ott G et al. Interphase cytogenetics of glioblastoma and gliosarcoma. Acta Neuropathol 1994;88:420–425.

21. Boerman RH, Anderl K, Herath J et al. The glial and mesenchymal elements of gliosarcomas share similar genetic alteration. J Neuropathol Exp Neurol 1996: 55:973–981.

22. Weber-Matthiesen K, Deerberg J, Poetsch M et al. Numerical chromosome aberrations are present within the CD30+ Hodgkin and Reed-Sternberg cells in 100% of analyzed cases of Hodgkin's disease. Blood 1995; 86:1464–1468.

23. Nolte M, Werner M, Vonwasielewski R et al. Detection of numerical karyotype changes in the giant cells of Hodgkin's lymphomas by a combination of FISH and immunohistochemistry applied to paraffin sections. Histochem Cell Biol 1996;105:401–404.

24. Perry A, Roth KA, Banerjee R et al. NF1 deletions in S-100 protein-positive and negative cells of sporadic and neurofibromatosis 1 (NF1)-associated plexiform neurofibromas and Malignant Peripheral Nerve Sheath Tumors. Am J Pathol 2001;159:57–61.

25. Tubbs RR, Pettay J, Roche P et al. Concomitant oncoprotein detection with fluorescence *in situ* hybridization (CODFISH): a fluorescence-based assay enabling simultaneous visualization of gene amplification and encoded protein expression. J Mol Diagn 2000;2:78–83.

26. Perry A, Nobori T, Ru N et al. Detection of p16 gene deletions in gliomas: a comparison of fluorescence *in situ* hybridization (FISH) versus quantitative PCR. J Neuropathol Exp Neurol 1997;56:999–1008.

27. James CD, Carlbom E, Nordenskjold M, et al. Mitotic recombination of chromosome 17 in astrocytomas. Proc Natl Acad Sci USA 1989;86:2858–2862.

28. Perry A, Anderl KA, Borell TJ et al. Detection of p16, RB, CDK4, and p53 gene deletion and amplification by fluorescence in situ hybridization in 96 gliomas. Am J Clin Pathol 1999;112:801–809.

29. Sallinen S-L, Sallinen PK, Haapasalo HK et al. Identification of differentially expressed genes in human gliomas by DNA microarray and tissue chip techniques. Cancer Res 2000;60:6617–6622.

30. Moch H, Kallioniemi O-P, Sauter G et al. Tissue microarrays: what will they bring to molecular and anatomic pathology? Adv Anat Pathol 2001;8:14–20.

31. Kononen J, Bubendorf L, Kallioniemi A et al. Tissue microarrays for high-throughput molecular profiling of tumor specimens. Nat Med 1998;4:844–847.

32. Schraml P, Kononen J, Bubendorf L et al. Tissue microarrays for gene amplification surveys in many different tumor types. Clin Cancer Res 1999;5:1966–1975.

33. Camp RL, Charette LA, Rimm DL. Validation of tissue microarray technology in breast carcinoma. Lab Invest 2000;80:1943–1949.

34. Hoos A, Urist MJ, Stojadinovic A et al. Validation of tissue microarrays for immunohistochemical profiling of cancer specimens using the example of human fibroblastic tumors. Am J Pathol 2001;158:1245–1251.

35. Henke RP, Ayhan N. Enhancement of hybridization efficiency in interphase cytogenetics on paraffin-embedded tissue sections by microwave treatment. Anal Cell Pathol 1994;6:319–325.

36. Shi S-R, Cote RJ, and Taylor CR. Antigen retrieval techniques: current perspectives. J Histochem Cytochem 2001;49:931–937.

37. Macechko PT, Krueger L, Hirsch B et al. Comparison of immunologic amplification vs enzymatic deposition of fluorochrome-conjugated tyramide as detection systems for FISH. J Histochem Cytochem 1997;45:359–364.

38. Schmidt BF, Chao J, Zhu Z et al. Signal amplification in the detection of single-copy DNA and RNA by enzyme-catalyzed deposition (CARD) of the novel fluorescent reporter substrate Cy3.29-Tyramide. J Histochem Cytochem 1997;45:365–374.

39. Schriml LM, Padilla-Nash HM, Coleman A et al. Tyramide signal amplification (TSA)-FISH applied to mapping PCR-labeled probes less than 1 Kb in size. BioTechniques 1999;27:608–613.

40. Arnoldus EPJ, Peters ACB, Bots GTAM et al. Somatic pairing of chromosome 1 centromeres in interphase nuclei of human cerebellum. Hum Genet 1989;83:231–234.

41. Arnoldus EPJ, Noordermeer IA, Peters ACB et al. Interphase cytogenetics reveals somatic pairing of chromosome 17 centromeres in normal human brain tissue, but

no trisomy 7 or sex-chromosome loss. Cytogenet Cell Genet 1991;56:214–216.

42. Schnitt SJ. Breast cancer in the 21st century: neu opportunities and neu challenges. Mod Pathol. 2001;14;213–218.

43. Pauletti G, Dandekar S, Rong HM et al. Assessment of methods for tissue-based detection of the HER-2/*neu* alteration in human breast cancer: a direct comparison of fluorescence in situ hybridization and immunohistochemistry. J Clin Oncol 2000;18:3651–3664.

44. Yu D, Hung M-C. Overexpression of ErbB2 in cancer and ErbB2-targeting strategies. Oncogene 2000;19: 6115–6121.

45. Perry A, Fuller CE, Banerjee R, Brat DJ, Scheithauer BW. Ancillary FISH analysis for 1p and 19q status: preliminary observations in 287 gliomas and oligodendroglioma mimics. Front. BioSci 2003;8:a1–9.

# CHAPTER 37

# Non-Imaging Cell and Tissue Techniques and Tissue Banking

W. Richard Burack, John D. Pfeifer

T raditionally, translational research that required the evaluation of cells and tissues was based on morphologic features alone. However, a number of other techniques are now widely used to supplement analysis of patient specimens, including flow cytometry, electron microscopy, and molecular genetic testing. The methodologies are versatile and can be used to address a wide variety of questions in many different tissue types including tumors, peripheral blood, cytology specimens, and cultured cells (Table 37–1). However, as with all techniques, the methods have limitations which can decrease their usefulness, especially in some clinical research settings.

## MORPHOLOGY-BASED TECHNIQUES

### Routine Pathologic Processing

Processing of tissue specimens for routine microscopic evaluation of hematoxylin and eosin (H&E) stained sections requires a minimum period of fixation in formalin, or any of a number of more specialized alternative mordants. These alternative fixatives achieve superior preservation of cellular or nuclear detail that is required to address specific questions. Following fixation, slices of the tissue are dehydrated and saturated with hot paraffin wax, an automated process that takes several hours to complete. Finally, the processed tissue is embedded in a small block of paraffin wax, cut on a microtome into sections that are about five microns thick, and stained.

Routine processing offers several advantages. It provides optimum preservation of the architectural and cytologic features of tissues, enabling very detailed histomorphologic examination. In addition, a broad range of histochemical stains can be performed on routinely processed tissue. Routinely processed tissue can also be used as a substrate for testing by other methodologies, including electron microscopic examination or even molecular genetic analysis.

Morphologic evaluation of H&E stained sections of formalin-fixed, paraffin-embedded tissue has been, and remains, the fundamental technique to characterize the features of a disease at the tissue and cellular level. When routine histopathologic examination fails to identify specific changes, special stains or electron microscopy can be used to rule out alterations that are below the resolution of light microscopy.

### Histochemical Stains

While the standard stain used to prepare tissue sections from formalin-fixed, paraffin-embedded tissue is the H&E stain, a huge number of specialized histochemical stains have been developed that can be used to detect specific tissue components (Table 37–2). Although many histochemical stains can be performed on routinely processed samples, some require special tissue processing (1).

### Immunohistochemical Stains

As discussed in more detail in Chapter 36, immunohistochemistry is a powerful method that can be used to detect specific gene products or antigens within tissue sections that cannot be detected by routine or specialized histochemical stains. A wide range of antibodies are available that can be used for immunohistochemical analysis of structural components of the cell and interstitial matrix,

## TABLE 37–1

### Examples of Clinical Research Questions Addressed by Cell and Tissue-Based Techniques

| Technique | Sample Clinical Research Questions |
|---|---|
| *Morphology-Based Techniques* | |
| Routine H&E stained sections, frozen sections | Which organs or tissues are abnormal as a result of a specific mutation, drug toxicity, or infectious disease? What morphologic features of a disease or tumor correlate with prognosis or response to therapy? |
| Histochemical stains | What biochemical changes occur in the tissue as a result of altered gene expression? As a result of therapy? As a result of infection? |
| Immunohistochemical stains | Which molecules, and at what level of abundance, correlate with the presence of disease, prognosis, or response to therapy? |
| Electron microscopy | Which cellular organelles are abnormal as a result of a specific mutation, drug toxicity, or infectious disease? |
| Immuno-electron microscopy | Do changes in cellular localization or trafficking of a specific protein correlate with disease? With infection? |
| *Flow Cytometric and Cell Sorting Techniques* | |
| Flow cytometry using antibodies against specific molecules | What cell activation, proliferation, hormone receptor, oncoprotein, or tumor suppressor genes are expressed by the abnormal cells? How does the level of expression change with specific mutations? Does the level of expression correlate with prognosis or response to therapy? |
| Flow cytometry with intercalating dyes | How does a mutation or disease affect the cell cycle? Are the abnormal cells aneuploid? |
| Bead-based cell separation; FACS | Which population of cells harbors the mutation? Do different cell populations respond differently to different drugs? |
| *Molecular Genetic Techniques* | |
| Routine cytogenetic analysis | What abnormalities in chromosomal structure or number are characteristic of the disease or neoplasm? |
| Southern blot hybridization; PCR | Is a specific gene abnormal due to a rearrangement, amplification, or mutation? Does the mutation correlate with disease susceptibility or severity, prognosis, or response to therapy? Does the mutation correlate with a specific tumor type? |
| Northern blot hybridization; RT-PCR; quantitative RT-PCR | Do changes in mRNA structure or abundance correlate with disease? |
| Interphase FISH; PCR; RT-PCR | Which individual cells harbor a specific abnormality in chromosomal structure or chromosomal number? |
| Comparative genomic hybridization | Do changes in copy number at specific chromosomal regions correlate with disease, prognosis, or response to therapy? |
| PCR; RT-PCR | Does the presence of submicroscopic disease correlate with prognosis or predict relapse? Does the pattern of gene methylation predict response to therapy? |
| Clonality assays | Is a neoplasm clonal? Is a disease due to mosaicism? |
| Microsatellite instability assays | Are defects in DNA mismatch repair involved in the development of the tumor? |
| DNA sequence analysis | Which specific mutations correlate with tumor type, disease severity, age of onset, prognosis, or response to treatment? |

### Selected Specialized Histochemical Stains That Can Be Used to Identify Tissue Components

| Stain | Specificity | Use |
|---|---|---|
| Alcian blue | Acid mucosubstances | Demonstration of stromal mucin production by mesotheliomas |
| Period acid-Schiff | Glycogen (with appropriate control); neutral mucosubstances | Demonstration of mucus or glycogen production |
| Oil red-O | Neutral lipids | Demonstration of lipids (useful for distinguishing, for example, between ovarian fibroma and thecoma); cannot be used on paraffin-embedded tissue |
| Fontana-Masson (argentaffin) | Catecholamines or indolamines | Demonstration of neurosecretory differentiation and of melanin; some modifications require special fixatives |
| Grimelius (argyrophilic) | A subset of neurosecretory granules | Demonstration of neurosecretory differentiation |
| Trichrome | Nuclei, cytoplasm, and collagen | Nonspecific; often can demonstrate immature skeletal muscle cells in poorly differentiated mesenchymal tumors |
| Leder | Requires the presence of enzyme choloacetate esterase | Demonstration of cells of myeloid lineage and mast cells (is actually an enzymatic histochemical technique) |
| Congo red | Amyloid | Demonstration of amyloid deposition in neuroendocrine tumors or associated with plasma cell tumors, immunocyte dyscrasias, chronic inflammatory conditions, chronic renal failure, etc. |

cell proliferation markers, hormone receptors, oncoproteins, and tumor suppressor genes, either alone or in combination. Although most immunohistochemical stains can be performed on routinely processed tissue, some antibodies can only be used on frozen sections (discussed next). In addition, because no antibody employed in immunohistochemical staining is 100% sensitive or 100% specific, a detailed survey of the immunoreactivity of an antibody is required in order to ensure that the immunohistochemical result is correctly interpreted.

### Electron Microscopy

Although light microscopy is best suited to study groups of cells, electron microscopy is best suited to study individual cells. To achieve ideal fixation for electron microscopy, tissue is fixed in glutaraldehyde (which better preserves proteins) followed by osmium tetroxide (to better preserve lipids), but tissue initially fixed in formalin can also be reprocessed for electron microscopy (2). Following fixation, the tissue is dehydrated and embedded in an epoxy resin so that much thinner sections can be cut than is possible with the soft paraffin wax used in routine tissue processing. Sections less than 0.1 microns thick are cut on an ultra-microtome using a blade made of diamond or glass rather than steel, and then incubated in heavy metal solutions (usually uranium and lead) which selectively add contrast to the various subcellular components (3–5).

Electron microscopy (EM) makes it possible to produce an image of the extracellular space, cell membrane, and intracellular contents magnified 200,000 times or more. Thus, EM is useful in many types of translational research. For example, studies of the type and abundance of various cellular organelles and structural components (Table 37–3) make it possible to characterize tumors in the absence of definitive findings by routine light microscopy, histochemistry, or immunohistochemistry (5). In nonneoplastic tissue, EM can be used to demonstrate morphologic changes in cellular components that correlate with disease but that are not evident by light microscopy, as in the study of the

## TABLE 37–3

### Selected Features for Cell and Disease Identification by Electron Microscopy

| Subcellular Feature | Cell of Tissue Type | Use |
|---|---|---|
| *Characterization of Neoplasms* | | |
| Intercellular junctions | Epithelial cells; selected mesenchymal nonlymphoid tumors | Distinction between lymphoma and carcinoma |
| External pericellular basal lamina | Epithelial cells; selected mesenchymal nonlymphoid tumors | Distinction between lymphoma and carcinoma; identification of some soft-tissue sarcomas |
| Intracellular or intercellular lumina | Glandular epithelium | Identification of adenocarcinomas |
| Microvillous care rootlets | Glandular epithelium of alimentary tract | Identification of gastrointestinal origin of metastatic carcinomas |
| Cytoplasmic tonofibrils | Squamous epithelium | Identification of squamous differentiation in epithelial tumors |
| Premelanosomes | Melanocytic cells | Identification of melanomas |
| Neurosecretory granules | Neuroendocrine cells | Identification of euroendocrine neoplasms |
| *Characterization of Medical Diseases* | | |
| Siderosomes | Mitochondria | Sideroblastic anemia |
| Peroxisomes | Liver | Increased number in alcoholic liver disease, chronic passive congestion, use of oral contraceptives, various hepatitides |
| *Characterization of Genetic Diseases* | | |
| Cilia | Epithelial cells | Identification of ciliary dysfunction |
| Lysosomes | Neurons | Identification of lipoidosis and several types of mucopolysaccharidoses |
| Lysosomes | Hepatocytes | Identification of several types of mucopolysaccharidoses |
| Glycogenosomes | Striated muscle | Identification of glycogenosis type II |
| Peroxisomes | Liver and kidney | Identification of adrenoleucodystrophy and lipodystrophy |
| *Other* | | |
| Viruses and parasites | Solid tissues, fecal specimens, body fluids | Identification of infectious agent |
| Electron dense deposits | Glomeruli | Identification and classification of glomerular diseases |

mechanisms of drug toxicity. EM can be coupled with immunohistochemistry through the use of antibodies coupled with very small gold particles; this technique, known as immuno-electron microscopy, can be used to localize defined molecules with extremely high resolution. In translational research, immuno-electron microscopy can be used, for example, to investigate altered trafficking of specific molecules as a result of drug toxicity or DNA mutations.

### Frozen Sections

Tissue sections made from fresh unfixed specimens are known as frozen sections, and are quickly and easily produced. The tissue sample is simply cooled to a temperature of about –20°C, a temperature at which the tissue is solid enough that histologic sections can be cut using a refrigerated microtome known as a cryostat. The tissue components in the frozen sections can be visualized by a variety of stains, including the routine H&E stain, many histochemical stains, and numerous immunohistochemical stains. In fact, some special stains (for example, stains for lipids) and certain immunohistochemical stains (especially in the evaluation of hematolymphoid malignancies) can only be performed on frozen sections because routine processing destroys the targeted tissue components.

In the setting of translational research, frozen sections have several advantages over sections of routinely processed tissue. Because they are performed on fresh tissue without fixation, the tissue remains amenable to testing by virtually any other laboratory technique, minimizing the need to collect multiple samples from the same patient. In addition, because the frozen section itself is a permanent record of the morphologic features of the tissue, it can be used as a control for comparison with the results of subsequent laboratory tests that necessarily consume the tissue, such as molecular genetic analysis.

Limitations to the use of frozen sections in clinical research, beyond those of all light microscopy-based methods, are mainly logistical (Table 37–4). Patient specimens must be frozen within several minutes after collection, and they must be not subjected to subsequent freeze-thaw cycles. For multi-institutional studies, an organized plan for specimen collection and handling, including shipping, is therefore an absolute necessity.

## FLOW CYTOMETRY-BASED TECHNIQUES

Flow cytometry makes it possible to rapidly, quantitatively, and simultaneously measure a variety of cellular characteristics (such as size, granularity, and surface molecule expression) and intracellular components (such as protein, DNA, and RNA). Briefly, the principle of flow cytometry is as follows (6,7,8): After staining with the appropriate fluorochromes, a suspension of single cells in an aqueous buffer is passed through a flow chamber designed to align the stream of cells so that each cell is struck individually by a focused laser beam. Simultaneous multiparametric analysis is possible by using two or more fluorophores that emit light of different wavelengths, in combination with multiple lasers of different wavelengths. The scattered light and fluorescent emissions from each cell are separated according to appropriate filters and mirrors, and directed to detectors that convert the emissions into electronic signals that are displayed on a video screen, and analyzed and stored by a computer. Through the process of gating (the placement of an electronic boundary around a specific cell population that is of interest), data can be acquired on only a subset of cells, a technique that can be used to take full advantage of multiparametric analysis (Figure 37–1). After the data are collected, they can be displayed as a frequency histogram (the number of cells versus intensity of fluorescence) for single-parameter analysis, or as a scatter graph (one cell parameter versus another) for multiparametric analysis.

In vivo single-cell suspensions such as peripheral blood or bone marrow are easily analyzed by flow cytometry. Solid tissues, such as lymph nodes and even solid tumors, require enzymatic, detergent, or mechanical treatment prior to analysis in order to produce a disaggregated sample of individual cells that is suitable for analysis. Methods have even been developed that make it possible to analyze single-cell suspensions derived from archival formalin-fixed, paraffin-embedded tissue (9).

Fluorophores used in flow cytometric analysis include two broad classes of compounds. Those that bind stoichiometrically to nucleic acids, but that fluoresce at different wavelengths when bound to DNA versus RNA, are used to evaluate cell cycle stage and ploidy status. Those that can be conjugated to antibodies against specific cell antigens are used to evaluate structural components of the cell, cell activation or proliferation markers, hormone receptors, oncoproteins, and tumor suppressor genes. Simultaneous multiparametric analysis is possible by using two or more fluorophores that emit light of different wavelengths (8,10–12), as noted above.

### Flow Cytometry Versus Fluorescence Activated Cell Sorting (FACS)

Flow cytometry and FACS are often confused. As discussed above, flow cytometry is used to analyze

## TABLE 37-4

### Key Issues for Planning Clinical Research Using Cell- and Tissue-Based Techniques

| Technique | Special Requirements and Limitations |
|---|---|
| *Morphology-Based Techniques* | |
| Routine H&E stained sections | Optimal evaluation requires a pathologist |
| Frozen sections | Fresh tissue is required, so specimen collection must be coordinated in advance, especially for multi-institutional trials; requires a crytostat; optimal evaluation requires a pathologist |
| Histochemical stains | May entail nonstandard processing; optimal evaluation requires a pathologist |
| Immunohistochemical stains | An antiserum must be produced if it is not commercially available; some antibodies only work on frozen sections |
| Electron microscopy | Nonstandard sample processing is necessary, as is access to an electron microscopy lab |
| *Flow Cytometric and Cell Sorting Techniques* | |
| Flow cytometry | Fresh, viable cell or tissue specimen is required |
| Adhesion- or bead-based separation | Fresh, viable cell or tissue specimen is required; is not ideal for investigation of signal transduction events because the separation may activate signaling pathways |
| FACS | Fresh, viable cell or tissue specimen is required; is slow and harsh, so recovery of a sufficient number of cells requires an abundant cell source |
| *Molecular Genetic Techniques* | |
| Routine cytogenetic analysis | Fresh, viable tissue sample that will grow in vitro is required; genetic aberration must be larger than about 3 Mb to be detected |
| Southern blot hybridization | Relatively large sample of fresh tissue is required for analysis; a probe that is specific for the target DNA locus is also required |
| Northern blot hybridization | Relatively large sample of fresh tissue is required for analysis; a probe that is specific for the target DNA locus is also required |
| FISH | Metaphase chromosome spreads are needed for chromosome FISH; recuts of fresh tissue or frozen sections are needed for interphase FISH; a probe that is specific for the target DNA locus is also required; a specialized microscope is necessary to analyze the results |
| Comparative genomic hybridization | Fresh or fixed diseased tissue and normal control tissue are both required; metaphase chromosome spreads or BAC arrays are needed for the hybridization, and a specialized microscope and computer software are necessary to analyze the results |
| PCR, RT-PCR, and quantitative variations | Sequence of target region must be known; strict attention to laboratory technique is required to avoid contamination |
| Clonality assays | X-linked assays are only informative for female patients |

the characteristics of a cell population. FACS is used when a highly specific population of cells must be purified from the whole sample based on a subtle feature or combination of features. Because many cell purifications performed in translational research are not based on subtle differences between cells, but rather on very obvious distinctions, FACS is often not required and can be supplanted by other methods that are simpler, more robust, and less expensive.

The FACS instrument is built around a flow cytometer (8) and makes it possible to physically separate cell populations that have different

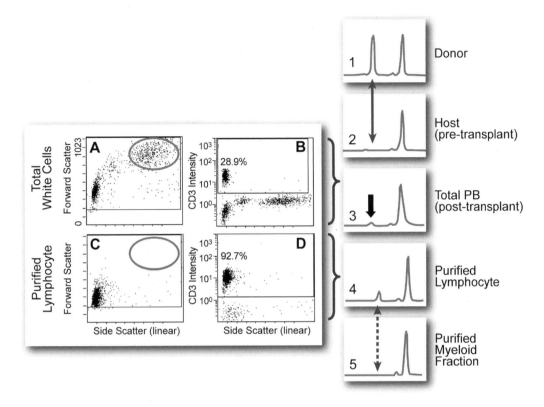

**FIGURE 37–1** ● Example of cell purification in clinical research, in which a study designed to address factors that affect lineage-specific bone marrow engraftment requires a method to assess the engraftment. Hurler's syndrome is a lysosomal storage disease caused by the deficiency of an enzyme required for glycosaminoglycan catabolism in macrophages. Storage diseases of this type can be treated by "nonmyeloablative" bone marrow transplants: the patient is given an infusion of donor marrow (or stem cells) to create a host/donor chimeric marrow. This procedure avoids the complications of marrow ablation and can supply the patient with sufficient donor-derived macrophages to slow or halt disease progression. The figure shows analysis of the donor and host composition of lymphoid and myeloid cells after a nonmyeloablative transplant for Hurler's syndrome. Analysis of engraftment uses PCR amplification of polymorphic regions called "short tandem repeats" (STR). The donor (tracing 1) and host pre-transplant (tracing 2) show a single informative STR peak in the donor that is not present in the host (double-headed solid arrow). Analysis of total peripheral blood from the host post-transplant (tracing 3) shows that very few cells are derived from the donor (short arrow). However, the critical question is whether this minor donor-derived population is myeloid. If yes, it would imply that the chimeric marrow can make other myeloid-derived cells including the macrophages that the patient needs; if instead the cells are donor-derived T-lymphocytes in excess over host T-lymphocytes, the minor donor-derived population may herald graft versus host disease. To assess the contribution of donor and host stem cells to the lymphocyte and myeloid fractions, lymphocytes and myeloid cells were purified from total peripheral blood by a simple affinity based method. The oval in panel **A** of the flow dot plots identifies the region of granulocytes, a myeloid-derived population. Panel **C** shows that these myeloid-derived cells have been almost entirely removed by the purification. Panel **B** shows that T-lymphocytes initially comprised about 29% of the total cells in the peripheral blood, and panel **D** shows that T-lymphocytes comprise about 93% of the purified lymphocyte fraction. STR analysis of the cell population in panels **C** and **D** (tracing 4) shows that the lymphocyte fraction is relatively enriched for donor cells (double-headed dotted arrow). STR analysis of the myeloid fraction (the cells from the oval region in panel **A**) shows that none are derived from the donor (double-headed dotted arrow, tracing 5), an unfortunate result for this patient with Hurler's syndrome.

characteristics based on flow cytometric analysis. For example, if distinct populations of tumor infiltrating CD8[+] T cells are needed that differ in the level of surface expression of CD3, FACS would be required to separate "bright" from "dim" from "negative" cells. In actual practice, FACS is slow and harsh on the cell populations under study. And, because only small numbers of viable cells are often recovered from a FACS separation, the method is not ideal for analysis of small or unique tumor specimens.

Although FACS is ideal for purification of cells based on the *relative* expression of a specific antigen, when the distinction between the cells of interest and the rest of the cells in the population is quite coarse (e.g., metastatic carcinoma cells versus lymphocytes; or T cells versus B cells; or CD4[+] versus CD8[+] T cells), a number of other approaches are of greater utility, including differential adherence to tissue culture plates or bead-based purification based on surface marker expression (13–15). Commercially available reagents greatly simplify the separation of numerous subtypes of hematopoietic cells, endothelial cells, epithelial cells, and fibroblasts by plate- or bead-based approaches. In terms of experimental design, separations can be either positive (select the cells with the phenotype of interest), negative (select cells without the phenotype of interest), or a combination of the two.

Although the purified cells from plate- or bead-based separations are excellent sources of DNA or RNA, they are not ideal for studies of signal transduction because the cross-linking of surface receptors that occurs during the purification processes may result in activation of specific signaling pathways.

## CYTOGENETIC TECHNIQUES

The fundamental tool of cytogenetics is the karyotype, which is the chromosomal complement of a somatic cell displayed in standard sequence on the basis of size, centromere location, and banding pattern (Figure 37–2). Although the individual banding techniques vary, all require in vitro culture of a cell suspension prepared from the tissue sample, arrest of cell division in metaphase, lysis of the cells to provide enhanced spreading of the chromosomes, fixation, and finally staining to produce bands that can be visualized by light microscopy. The most

widely used staining techniques, termed G-, Q-, and R-banding, produce 350 to 550 bands per haploid set of chromosomes, permitting a detailed description of both normal and abnormal chromosomal structures (16,17). More refined description of karyotypic abnormalities can be achieved by spectral karyotyping (also know as SKY), a hybridization-based approach in which probes specific for individual chromosomes are hybridized to the metaphase chromosome spreads (18).

As long as the cells in a specimen are capable of growth and division in vitro, cytogenetic analysis can be performed on the sample. Consequently, a wide variety of tissues can be analyzed, including products of conception, fetal cells from amniotic fluid, chorionic villi, fetal blood, peripheral blood (one of the easiest and most accessible specimens for cytogenetic analysis), skin fibroblasts, bone marrow, lymph nodes, and solid tissues including solid tissue tumors. Often, only a subset of the cell clones that are generated during in vitro growth are required to produce the karyotype; the extra clones are a valuable resource for additional study and can frequently be used to produce an immortalized cell line.

The power of conventional cytogenetic analysis lies in its ability to provide a simultaneous low-resolution analysis of multiple chromosomes without prior knowledge of the regions of the genome that are mutated. Consequently, cytogenetics is a genome-wide screening technique that can be used to identify sites of recurrent numerical or structural abnormalities in a number of different translational

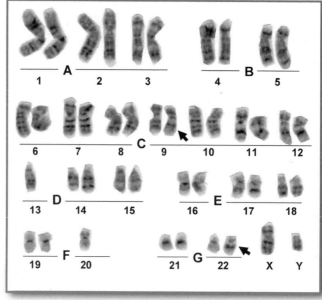

**FIGURE 37–2** ● Example of conventional cytogenetic analysis of a soft tissue mass involving the foot of a 54-year-old man. The karyotype shows a t(9;22)(q22;q12) translocation that is characteristic of extraskeletal myxoid chondrosarcoma (EMC), a result that is obviously helpful from a diagnostic point of view. However, cytogenetic analysis is also a useful technique for identifying groups of tumors with the same or similar genetic aberrations for research questions that focus on oncogenic mechanisms.

**46,XY,t(9;22)(q22;q12),-13,-20**

research settings. For example, cytogenetics can be used to correlate the presence or absence of recurrent chromosomal aberrations with drug, toxin, or mutagen exposure; with specific tumors; or with prognosis or response to a particular treatment regimen. In many cases, the type and location of the chromosomal abnormality can be used to direct additional testing, and can provide clues to direct further research into the gene-specific mechanisms involved.

However, the sensitivity of cytogenetic analysis constrains its utility. For example, it may be difficult to obtain viable tissue for the short-term in vitro growth of cells necessary to produce a karyotype (19). In addition, because routine cytogenetic analysis can only demonstrate large structural or numerical chromosomal aberrations, the technique lacks the sensitivity to detect chromosomal abnormalities smaller than about 3 Mb in size. Because cytogenetics can not detect smaller mutations, such as point mutations or microsatellite instability, many diseases and tumors are not amenable to study by this technique.

## MOLECULAR GENETIC TECHNIQUES

### Southern and Northern Blot Hybridization

Southern blot hybridization and Northern blot hybridization are similar in principle. Purified nucleic acids (DNA for Southern blots, RNA for Northern blots) are size fractionated by gel electrophoresis, transferred and immobilized on a synthetic membrane made of nitrocellulose or nylon, and then hybridized to a specific nucleic acid probe. The probe can be visualized by either radioactive or nonradioactive methods, and the location of the probe indicates not only the presence of the target DNA sequence, but the size of the fragment in which it is contained.

Southern blot hybridization is a reliable and versatile method for sequence specific DNA analysis, and can be used to provide information about the presence of deletions, insertions, and rearrangements, and, because the method is quantitative, can even provide information on gene copy number. Northern blotting, though technically demanding, simultaneously provides information on both mRNA transcript abundance (a measure of a gene's level of expression) and structure, including the utilization of alternative transcript initiation or termination sites, alternative splicing patterns, and mutations. Because Northern blots are quantitative, they also indicate the relative abundance of the different transcript types. The technique of Northern blotting has been described in more detail in Chapter 31.

Southern and Northern blots are limited to those translational research questions in which a target genetic locus has already been identified. The use of blotting in clinical studies is further limited by the fact that both Southern and Northern blots require a relatively large tissue sample, usually in the range of about 0.5-1 cubic centimeter of tissue from a solid tumor, or about 20 mL of peripheral blood for hematolymphoid malignancies. In addition, Southern and Northern blotting can only be performed on fresh tissue specimens. PCR-based methods have replaced Southern and Northern blot hybridization in many settings because PCR-based methods are as sensitive and reliable, but faster, less cumbersome, and require less tissue.

### In Situ Hybridization

In situ hybridization (ISH) makes it possible to detect mRNA and DNA in histologic sections of tissue that has been formalin-fixed and routinely processed (20,21). The advantage of ISH methods is that they make it possible to directly correlate the morphology of individual cells with the presence or absence of the target sequence.

ISH methods for detecting mRNA can be used, for example, to correlate the expression level of a specific gene (22,23) with the tissue changes characteristic of a disease, with a tumor's phenotype, or to monitor transgene expression in gene therapy regimens (24,25). There is no doubt that ISH for mRNA is a versatile technique; however, the method is technically demanding. Commercial kits have simplified mRNA ISH assays, but the technique remains cumbersome and, even when optimized, has a sensitivity below that of PCR-based methods. Both of these practical issues limit the utility of ISH for measurement of gene expression in tissue sections. More information about the technique of ISH can be found in Chapter 36.

ISH can also be used to detect DNA and is especially useful for demonstrating abnormalities in chromosomal structure. FISH is often used to demonstrate genetic aberrations in metaphase chromosome spreads. However, as discussed more fully in Chapter 36, it is the application of fluorescent ISH (FISH) to interphase cells that has revolutionized the detection of abnormalities in chromosome number and chromosome structure. Because FISH analysis eliminates the need for in vitro cell culture, the technique can be used to study a broader range of cell and tissue types (and therefore a broader range of diseases and tumors) than can be evaluated by conventional cytogenetic analysis. In addition, FISH can be used on standard tissue sections to detect the nucleic acids of a wide variety of infectious diseases such as hepatitis virus, Epstein-Barr virus, and human papilloma virus.

Although probes can easily be generated to any region of interest in either RNA or DNA, and several probes can be used in the same hybridization to simultaneously evaluate multiple genetic loci, ISH is limited to analysis of specific genetic loci that have already been well characterized. Even using optimized probes, ISH usually lacks the resolution to detect structural or numerical chromosomal aberrations that are less than about 50–100 Kb in size; consequently, the technique cannot be used to evaluate smaller mutations such as single base pair changes.

## Comparative Genomic Hybridization

Comparative genomic hybridization (CGH) is a modification of ISH that makes it possible to survey the genome of even fixed tissue for chromosomal deletions and amplifications (26). For a typical CGH test, genomic DNA from the tumor sample is labeled with a green fluorophore, and genomic DNA from a paired normal tissue sample is labeled with a red fluorophore. The green and red DNA (referred to as the probe) are mixed, and then used in a single hybridization reaction to either metaphase chromosome spreads (standard CGH) or an array of defined DNA sequences (array CGH).

Standard CGH is essentially a variation of chromosomal FISH. The mixture of green and red probes is hybridized to metaphase chromosome spreads prepared from normal peripheral blood lymphocytes, and the ratio of the green to red fluorescent signals is measured along the length of each chromosome. Regions where the ratio deviates significantly from the expected one-to-one relationship are areas where there has been a change in DNA copy number in the tumor versus the paired normal tissue; regions where the green to red ratio is significantly greater than one are areas of chromosomal gain (amplifications); and regions where the green to red ratio is significantly lower than one are areas of chromosomal loss (deletions). In practice, the smallest chromosomal alterations that can be detected by standard CGH are about 3 Mb.

For array CGH, known DNA sequences are arrayed on a support. The mixture of green and red probes is hybridized to the array, and because each DNA sequence on the array has been mapped to a specific region of the genome, the ratio of the green to red fluorescent signals for each of the DNA sequences provides information on the gain or loss of the corresponding chromosomal region. Array CGH offers much higher resolution than standard CGH, and is in theory limited only by the number and length of the DNA sequences in the array. Arrays that contain about 30,000 nonoverlapping sequences, each roughly 150–250 Kb long, give approximately 100 Kb resolution (27). More information about array technology can be found in Chapter 34.

Although a number of studies have shown that CGH often has a higher sensitivity than conventional cytogenetic analysis (26,28,29), the real advantage of CGH in translational research is that the technique can be performed using DNA extracted from fixed as well as fresh tumor samples. Consequently, CGH makes it possible to perform a genome-wide scan for structural alterations on even those cases for which conventional cytogenetic analysis is not feasible or is unsuccessful. CGH essentially opens the entire formalin-fixed tissue archive to at least limited cytogenetic analysis.

The limited resolution of CGH makes the technique unsuitable for translational studies focused on identifying small genetic changes such as point mutations. In addition, it is important to keep in mind that, unlike conventional cytogenetic analysis, CGH can only detect changes in copy number. Structural aberrations that do not result in gains or losses of chromosomal regions, such as inversions or balanced translocations, are not detected.

## Polymerase Chain Reaction (PCR)

PCR can be performed on a variety of tissue types, including solid tissue, biopsies, peripheral blood, cytology specimens, and cell lines. Although the optimal substrate for PCR-based testing is fresh tissue (ultra-low temperature frozen storage at –70°C permits indefinite preservation of samples with virtually no effect on the quality of the extracted RNA or DNA), nucleic acids can also be extracted from fixed tissue, although the type of fixative and length of fixation have a profound effect on their recovery. Non-cross-linking fixatives such as ethanol provide the most consistent preservation of amplifiable DNA, with more variability from tissues fixed with formalin, Zamboni's and Clark's fixatives, paraformaldehyde, and formalin-alcohol-acetic acid. Tissues processed in Carnoy's, Zenker's, Bouin's and B-5 fixatives are poor substrates for PCR testing because little amplifiable DNA can be recovered from them (30–32). In general, tissue fixed in neutral buffered formalin for less than 8 hours contains DNA and RNA from which PCR products up to about 600 bp in length can be reliably amplified, but fixation extended for greater than 8–12 hours decreases the length of the PCR product that can consistently be amplified. A number of protocols have been developed to optimize the recovery of nucleic acids from fixed tissue, but the degradation and cross-linking of nucleic acids that is a consequence of fixation, especially formalin-fixation, still require modifications in PCR design, including reoptimization of primer sequences, shorter amplicon lengths, a greater number of cycles in the amplification, and often a nested approach. The basic technique of PCR is described in Chapter 31.

## Advantages of PCR

With appropriate primers and reaction conditions, the application of PCR to tissue specimens in translational research brings all the advantages of PCR performed in a basic science laboratory setting. The technique is simple, quick, inexpensive, and provides a method for detecting a broad range of genetic abnormalities ranging from gross structural alterations such as translocations and deletions, to mutations due to individual base pair changes. Because of the inherent sensitivity and specificity in optimized PCR amplifications, the technique can be used to detect abnormal cells that may comprise only a minority population within a background of normal cells; when optimized, PCR can detect one abnormal cell in a background of $10^5$ normal cells (33). PCR can even be used to analyze single copy genes from individual cells (34–36).

PCR is obviously ideally suited for clinical studies that require detection of specific genetic changes that correlate with disease, and the utility of the technique has been enhanced by a number of variations of the basic methodology. For example, multiplex PCR (the simultaneous amplification of multiple target sequences in a single PCR through the use of multiple primer pairs) can be used to evaluate a number of different sites for the presence of a mutation in a single reaction, and is therefore a practical screening method in many translational studies. The multiplex PCR approach also conserves sample DNA, which can be helpful when the patient specimen is very small. Methylation-specific PCR (which makes it possible to evaluate the methylation status of individual CpG sites) can be used to evaluate how imprinting or gene regulation correlates with disease, and the telomeric repeat amplification protocol assay can be used to determine the relationships between structural alterations in telomeres and tumor development.

A number of techniques for PCR-based analysis of tissue samples make it possible to correlate the morphology of individual cells with the presence or absence of a specific mutation. Microdissection, in which the region of interest is simply carved out of the formalin-fixed paraffin-embedded tissue block, scraped from a tissue section, or collected with a micromanipulator apparatus, provides

some enrichment for morphologic-genetic correlations (37–40). Even more precise phenotypic-genotypic analysis is achieved by collecting individual cells by laser capture microdissection (36,41), by flow cytometry (42), or even immunomagnetic techniques (43). Although these methods make it possible to analyze single cells, the correlations are still, strictly speaking, indirect because the tissue is destroyed when the nucleic acids are extracted. In contrast, in situ PCR is performed directly on histologic tissue sections themselves, and is perhaps the ultimate method for correlating specific mutations with individual cells (44). Although technically demanding (45,46), in situ PCR has a sensitivity that makes it possible to detect low-level gene expression in individual cells at a copy number below that which can be detected by conventional ISH.

## Limitations of PCR

Because PCR only amplifies the target region bounded by the specific primer set employed, PCR will fail to identify genetic changes that lie outside the target region (known as the amplicon).

PCR analysis can also be limited by amplification bias. Amplification bias refers to the fact that, within the same reaction, some DNA templates are preferentially amplified versus other templates. PCR bias can be caused by differences in template length (in general, shorter amplicons are preferentially amplified), random variations in template number (especially with very low target abundance, producing an artifact known as allele dropout), and random variations in PCR efficiency with each cycle (40,47). Amplification bias can even result from differences in the target sequence itself that are as small as a single base change (48–50). The magnitude of PCR bias, which can cause 10- to 30-fold differences in amplification efficiency in some settings, is easily large enough to influence quantitative PCR test results and loss of heterozygosity analysis, and can be a particularly troublesome problem in multiplex PCR (51,52).

Technical factors intrinsic to analysis of patient specimens can decrease the sensitivity of PCR in translational research. Nonspecific, uncharacterized inhibitors of PCR are often present in CSF, urine, and sputum. However, the most important technical limitation on analysis of tissue specimens is degradation of target nucleic acids, especially when extracted from necrotic tissue, or from fixed tissue (as discussed above).

Although the sensitivity of PCR underlies its utility, the high sensitivity also greatly increases the risk of erroneous results due to contamination of samples, especially cross-contamination due to

PCR product carryover (53–56). The risk of contamination is another important technical limitation of PCR, the significance of which cannot be overstated in terms of analysis of clinical samples. Problems due to contamination can be largely avoided by strict attention to laboratory technique, physical separation of the various stages of testing, use of aerosol barrier pipette tips, regular ultraviolet radiation of laboratory workspaces and instruments to degrade any transient uncontained DNA, and rigorous use of appropriate positive and negative controls (56–59).

## Reverse Transcriptase PCR (RT-PCR)

RT-PCR makes it possible to amplify mRNA from fresh tissue, fixed tissue, and cytology specimens (60,61). Consequently, RT-PCR has many uses in translational research. RT-PCR makes is possible to directly amplify multi-exon sequences by eliminating the intervening introns, and thus greatly simplifies mutation scanning methods that would require multiple reactions to evaluate exons individually from genomic DNA. Similarly, RT-PCR makes it much simpler to demonstrate the presence of translocations that create fusion genes by making it possible to directly detect the fusion transcripts encoded by the translocations (Figure 37–3); because

the precise breakpoint often ranges over dozens of Kb, detection of the translocations by standard PCR based on genomic DNA would be unwieldy. RT-PCR can also be used to detect changes in mRNA structure that may be correlated with disease, including changes due to alternative splicing or aberrant splicing. It can also be used to evaluate the level of gene expression through the quantitative methods discussed below. And finally, because the methods used to collect specific cells for PCR analysis can also be used to collect specific cells for RT-PCR, changes in RNA structure or abundance can be correlated with defined cell populations in tissue sections (62,63) or even cytology smears (64,65).

## Quantitative PCR

RNA and DNA extracted from a wide variety of patient specimens, including solid tissue, tissue sections, cytology specimens, and single cell suspensions, can be used for analysis by the many different quantitative PCR chemistries discussed in Chapter 31, including TaqMan (also known as 5' exonuclease or hydrolysis real-time PCR), molecular beacons (66,67), scorpions (68,69), hybridization probes (70), and intercalating dyes such as SYBR Green. Quantitative PCR (Q-PCR), therefore, has a broad range of applications in translational

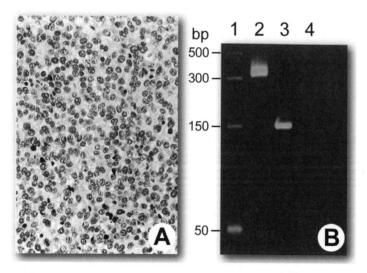

**FIGURE 37–3** ● Example of molecular genetic analysis of Ewing's sarcoma/peripheral neuroectodermal tumor (ES/PNET) arising in the kidney of a 60-year-old woman. **A.** H&E stained section of the tumor. **B.** RT-PCR of formalin-fixed, paraffin-embedded tissue demonstrates the presence of an *EWS-FLI1* gene fusion transcript that is characteristic of ES/PNET. Lane 1, molecular size markers; lane 2, positive control RT-PCR product from an ES/PNET cell line (*EWS* exon 7 to *FLI1* exon 5 fusion); lane 3, renal tumor (*EWS* exon 7 to *FLI1* exon 8 fusion); lane 4, negative control. This type of analysis has been used in translational research studies of ES/PNET to demonstrate that fusion transcript type correlates with prognosis (118,119). **Note:** The color figure can be found following page 394.

research. For example, when DNA is the substrate, the technique can be used to demonstrate gene amplifications that may have prognostic or therapeutic implications for a particular tumor type. When mRNA is the substrate, quantitative RT-PCR can be used to correlate changes in gene expression with the clinical features of a disease or a specific tumor type (71). Quantitative methods can be used to address these issues in specific cell types through the use of laser capture microdissection, flow cytometry, or immunomagnetic techniques to collect defined cell populations for analysis, from either fresh or fixed tissue.

However, the reliability of Q-PCR is very dependent on the purity of the input nucleic acid preparation, primer and probe design [greatly facilitated by a number of internet websites (72)], choice of thermostable polymerase, cycle parameters, and buffer conditions. Consequently, real-time PCR assays must be optimized to ensure their reproducibility in routine use. One parameter of quantitative RT-PCR that is often overlooked is the reverse transcription step itself; a lack of attention to detail in the reverse transcription reaction can introduce variables into quantitative RT-PCR that prevent accurate measurement of the level of gene expression in even well designed assays (72–76).

## Clonality Assays

According to the clonal model of carcinogenesis, all tumors arise from a single founder cell that acquires an initial mutation that provides its progeny with a selective growth advantage, and from within this expanded population, another single cell acquires a second mutation that provides an additional growth advantage, and so on, until a fully developed malignant tumor emerges (77,78). Demonstration that the cells in a lesion share a common genetic alteration can therefore be used to support classification of a lesion as a neoplasm rather than as a polyclonal reactive process, although clonal neoplasms are not necessarily malignant. Because of its sensitivity and specificity, PCR-based testing has found wide application in clonality assays using two different approaches.

### Loss of Heterozygosity Assays

PCR-based approaches to loss of heterozygosity (LOH) analysis can be used to identify a clonal pattern of gene inactivation at a target locus (X-linked assays), or to detect the clonal loss of one allele at a target locus (microsatellite-based assays).

X-linked clonality assays have their basis in Lyon's hypothesis (79) which states that one of the two X chromosomes in every normal human female

cell is inactivated on a random basis during early embryogenesis, and that the pattern of inactivation is stable and perpetuated through subsequent cycles. Different patterns of X inactivation can be distinguished by gene expression analysis because mRNA is only transcribed from genes on the active X chromosome (80). However, in practice it is much easier to distinguish the active and inactive X chromosomes through use of methylation-sensitive restriction endonucleases to cleave the genomic DNA, followed by PCR amplification of the region of the gene that includes the restriction sites to determine the pattern of X chromosome inactivation (81). X-linked clonality assays are obviously limited by the fact that they are only informative for female patients.

Microsatellites (also known as short tandem repeats or STRs) are hypervariable regions of DNA composed of repetitive short sequences that belong to the family of highly polymorphic and repetitive noncoding DNA sequences. Microsatellites are particularly well suited for use in PCR-based clonality assays because of their ubiquity in the genome, easy amplification by PCR-based techniques, Mendelian codominant inheritance, and extreme polymorphism (82,83). Although any microsatellites can function as a target, those linked to tumor suppressor genes involved in malignant transformation are often the most informative. Nonetheless, analyses of tissue samples are often complicated by a background level of LOH, present in from 4 to 20% of some normal tissue (84,85), and by variability in the frequency of LOH at individual test loci (86–88). Consequently, reliable assessment of clonality using microsatellite-based assays usually requires evaluation of more than one STR locus.

## Microsatellite Instability Assays

The characteristic feature of microsatellite instability (MSI) is the presence of short increases or decreases in the length of microsatellite sequences. MSI is caused by defects in the DNA mismatch repair system, but direct analysis of the genes responsible for mismatch repair is an inefficient approach for detecting mutations in the repair system because several genes are involved in the repair pathway, inactivating mutations do not cluster at specific sites in the repair genes, and the genes may be inactive as a result of epigenetic silencing rather than mutations (89–92). PCR-based identification of alterations in the length of microsatellite sequences can be used as a more efficient method to identify defects in the mismatch repair system.

MSI assays are usually performed to investigate the relationship between defects in DNA mismatch repair and the development of sporadic or familial cases of a specific tumor type, and to correlate prognosis or response to therapy with the level of MSI. Only a few technical issues limit analysis of patient specimens in translational research, including the presence of contaminating nonneoplastic tissue (93), biased amplification of different alleles of the same microsatellite (94), and different frequencies of MSI of the same microsatellite within different regions of individual tumors (95). The affect of these limitations can usually be minimized by careful experimental design.

## DNA SEQUENCE ANALYSIS

### Direct DNA Sequence Analysis

Virtually all routine direct DNA sequence analysis in translational research is automated, and is performed on templates generated by the enzymatic chain termination method using the methodology known as cycle sequencing (96). Even though cycle sequencing reactions require a very low quantity of template DNA to generate enough product for subsequent automated DNA sequence analysis, the amount of DNA present in most patient specimens is usually still insufficient for analysis without a preliminary amplification step, usually via PCR. Direct DNA sequence analysis remains the gold standard for characterizing point mutations, small insertions and deletions, and the boundaries of larger structural changes that are characteristic of many diseases and tumor types. DNA sequence analysis is also used to correlate specific mutations with prognosis or response to therapy.

DNA sequence analysis is occasionally complicated by errors that are introduced during production of the DNA template. These introduced errors are almost exclusively the result of template amplification by PCR and are due to the intrinsic error rate of thermostable DNA polymerases. Even polymerases with a proofreading function have an intrinsic error rate that is highly dependent on the precise reaction conditions, including the buffer composition, salt concentration, dNTP concentration, reaction pH, and even the template sequence itself (97–100). The computerized algorithms used to produce the DNA sequence via automated analysis can also introduce errors. Regardless of the algorithm, all currently available methods have an error rate [that includes both base substitution errors as well as insertion/deletion errors) in the range of less than 0.3% to over 4% (101,102)]. Consequently, putative sequence changes must always be confirmed in order to exclude technical artifacts.

### Indirect Methods of DNA Sequence Analysis

Once normal and mutant alleles at a specific locus have been characterized by direct DNA sequence analysis, indirect methods can often provide enough DNA sequence information to be of clinical utility. These indirect techniques include allelic discrimination by size, restriction fragment length polymorphism analysis, allele-specific PCR, single-strand conformational polymorphism analysis, heteroduplex analysis, denaturing gradient gel electrophoresis, cleavage of mismatched nucleotides, ligase chain reaction, the protein truncation test, and numerous variants, used either alone or in combination. Because these indirect methods are based on PCR, they can be applied to a broad range of clinical specimens and so are especially useful in translational research. In addition, because many of the indirect methods are quicker and less expensive than direct sequence analysis, they are ideally suited for screening large numbers of patient samples. The specific advantages and disadvantages of the different methods are summarized in Table 37–5.

### Sequence Analysis by Microarray Technology

High-density DNA micoarrays have found their greatest use in hybridization-based evaluation of gene expression as discussed in Chapter 34, but chip-based hybridization analysis is also a promising technology for sequence analysis. Hybridization-based and minisequencing-based approaches to microarray sequence analysis are the two methods that have been most widely employed (103,104). Both employ custom-designed arrays to evaluate specific sequences, and both have a variety of applications for the evaluation of clinical specimens, including de novo sequencing, mutation and single nucleotide polymorphism discovery, and genotyping (103,105,106). Both methods have been shown to have a high concordance with DNA sequence obtained by the traditional chain termination methods (107,108), but the time and expense involved in the design and production of the sequencing microarrays severely limits their use.

### Internet Resources for DNA Sequence Analysis

Numerous internet resources are available that greatly simplify the process of DNA sequence interpretation and mutation identification. The utility of these sites is enhanced by the fact that DNA sequence from automated analysis can be submitted

## TABLE 37–5

### Advantages and Disadvantages of the Different Methods for DNA Sequence Analysis in Clinical Research

| Method | Advantages | Disadvantages |
|---|---|---|
| *Direct Methods* | | |
| Dideoxy enzymatic sequencing | Detects and fully characterizes changes; inexpensive and quick; is automated | Computer generated inferred base sequence can contain errors |
| Oligonucleotide arrays | Quick, high through-put analysis | Requires expensive equipment; individual arrays are expensive and available for only a limited number of genes; arrays do not characterize all changes |
| Southern blotting | Only method that can detect large structural rearrangements | Cumbersome; requires large quantities of DNA from fresh tissue |
| *Indirect Methods* | | |
| Allelic discrimination based on size | Quick; simple; high through-put | Only detects insertions or deletions, does not reveal position of change |
| Allelic discrimination based on RFLP analysis | Quick; simple; high through-put | Only detects targeted change |
| Allele-specific PCR | Quick; simple, useful for screening | Only detects targeted change |
| Single-strand conformational polymorphism (SSCP) analysis | Simple; useful for screening | Limited sensitivity; limited to sequences <200 bp long; does not reveal position or type of change |
| Heteroduplex analysis | Simple; inexpensive | Limited sensitivity; limited to sequences <200 bp long; does not reveal position or type of change |
| Denaturing gradient gel electrophoresis (DGGE) | High sensitivity; useful for screening | Requires optimization for each individual DNA region; does not reveal position or type of change |
| Ligase chain reaction (LCR) | Quick; simple; useful for screening | Only detects targeted change |
| Protein truncation test (PTT) | High sensitivity for truncating mutations; indicates general position of change; useful for screening | Only detects terminating mutations; technically difficult |
| Cleavage of mismatched nucleotides by chemical or enzymatic methods | High sensitivity; useful for screening | Cumbersome methodology |

electronically, eliminating the need for time consuming (and error prone) manual entry. The http://www.ncbi.nlm.nih.gov/BLAST website is particularly useful for identifying sequence changes (109), and other useful websites are listed in Table 37–6.

There are several caveats regarding the use of Internet resources for sequence analysis. First, the accuracy of many accessioned sequences in the databases is unknown, and some accessioned sequences contain outright errors. Sequences produced as part of the human genome project were subjected to rigorous quality control standards, and so are some of the most reliable. Second, the accessioning information that accompanies each sequence may not provide detailed information on the experimental or tissue source, which can complicate interpretation of the importance of putative sequence differences. Third, the significance of even genuine sequence differences is uncertain without detailed knowledge of the biology of the gene product and associated

## TABLE 37–6

### Internet Resources for Evaluating DNA Sequence Changes

| | |
|---|---|
| http://www.ncbi.nlm.nih.gov/ | National Center for Biotechnology Information homepage; links to PubMed, Entrez, BLAST, OMIM, and other sites |
| http://www.ncbi.nlm.nih.gov/Entrez | A versatile cross-database search engine |
| http://www.ncbi.nlm.nih.gov/entrez/query.fcgi | PubMed homepage; provides links to other NCBI sites |
| http://www.ncbi.nlm.nih.gov/BLAST/ | BLAST nucleotide similarity search homepage |
| http://www.ncbi.nlm.nih.gov/projects/geo/ | The Gene Expression Omnibus, a gene expression and hybridization array data repository |
| http://www.ncbi.nlm.nih.gov/LocusLink/ | Interface to curated sequence and descriptive information about genetic loci |
| http://www.ncbi.nlm.nih.gov/omim | Online Mendelian Inheritance in Man (OMIM), a catalog of human genes and genetic disorders |
| http://www.ncbi.nlm.nih.gov/genome/guide/human/ | Views of chromosomes, maps, and loci with links to other NCBI resources |
| http://www.ncbi.nlm.nih.gov/ projects/SNP/ | A database of single nucleotide polymorphisms (SNPs) and other nucleotide variations |
| http://snp.cshl.org/ | Provides a variety of methods to query for SNPs in the human genome |
| http://genome.ucsc.edu/ | University of California Santa Cruz Genome Bioinformatics homepage; links to Human BLAT homology search and genome browser |
| http://genome.wustl.edu/ | Washington University School of Medicine Genome Sequencing Center homepage; links to multiple human genome sites |
| http://www.ensembl.org | Ensembl Genome Browser at the Wellcome Trust Sanger Institute |
| http://www.gdb.org | A genome database useful for identifying microsatellite loci |
| http://gai.nci.nih.gov/CHLC/ | Useful for identifying microsatellites linked to loci of interest |

disease process. For example, single base pair substitutions may merely represent different alleles rather than disease causing mutations, insertions or deletions in cDNA may simply reflect alternative mRNA processing that is a normal component of developmental or tissue-specific gene regulation, and so on.

## TISSUE BANKING

Tissue banks are organized to facilitate the collection, storage, and distribution of human tissues for use in basic science and translational research. Most well-developed tissue banks focus on oncologic applications (tumor banks), and these are described in more detail next. However, the general principles involved are applicable to any formal tissue bank, be it comprised of biopsy material or blood samples.

Most tumor banks are organized around fresh/frozen tissue (for the simple fact that fresh or frozen tissue is the most versatile substrate for a wide variety of experimental techniques), but formalin-fixed paraffin-embedded tissue blocks are also a very valuable part of the archive of many tumor banks. A tumor bank's usefulness also depends on the accuracy, extent, and availability of information that is stored with the tissues, including patient history and clinical data, tumor type and stage, response to treatment, and follow-up (110–113). Tumor banks are an especially valuable resource for translational research involving the analysis of mutations that correlate with tumor type, prognosis, or response to therapy; for research seeking to identify tumor markers that can be used for screening, diagnosis, or identification of early relapse; and for research focused on patient subgroups that may respond to novel drug therapies (111).

Most tumor banks provide additional services related to the collection and storage of diseased tissue, including the collection and distribution of normal tissues for control studies; histology services for fresh, frozen, and formalin-fixed, paraffin-embedded tissues; and preparation of DNA, RNA, and protein from tissue specimens. Most tumor banks also have associated equipment resources such as microscopes for laser capture microdissection, quantitative PCR machines, and platforms for microarray analysis. A good tumor bank is also an invaluable source of information on the applicability of various methodologies to a wide variety of translational research.

Collection and storage of tissue samples, along with the related clinical data, has raised a number of ethical and legal issues. Some issues relate to informed consent and whether the same procedures for clinical research participants should also be applied to samples collected for tumor banks (110, 111). Other ethical concerns revolve around the balance of the interests of science and society versus an individual donor's right to autonomy and privacy. Privacy rights are especially important; patient confidentiality is necessary to avoid potential discrimination that could result if insurance carriers or employers gained access to experimental results that have an impact on the risk of disease in the patient or the patient's family. The ethical aspects of commercial use of patient specimens, and whether donors should share in the profits that may result from commercial use of their tissues, are additional issues that have recently been raised. These ethical and legal questions must be considered in the design of the experimental approach to a translational research question. Additional information on this issue is available in Chapter 14.

## EXAMPLES OF THE USE OF CELL AND TISSUE TECHNIQUES IN TRANSLATIONAL RESEARCH

### Use of Flow Cytometry or FACS

**Example 1:** Determine the level of MAP kinase activation in tumor infiltrating CD4$^+$ T cells versus tumor infiltrating CD8$^+$ cells. This example only requires quantification of the level of various cellular proteins, which is easily performed without any physical purification of the tumor sample into different cellular populations. All that is needed are antibodies that are specific for CD4, CD8, and the phosphorylated (active) form of the kinase. This is an excellent example of an experimental question that requires flow cytometry without a need for FACS.

**Example 2:** Prepare a population of circulating breast cancer cells for mRNA expression analysis or proteomic analysis. Although this example clearly requires purification of a specific cell population, FACS is still not the technique of choice. FACS is needed only when the distinction between cells required for the purification is very subtle. When enriching tumor cells from peripheral blood, the tumor cells are easily distinguished from blood cells by the expression of a host of epithelial markers, and by the lack of expression of hematopoietic markers. The technique of choice is therefore an adhesion- or bead-based method, such as differential adherence to tissue culture plates (a method to separate sticky epithelial cells from nonadherent lymphocytes) or a bead-based separation (based on the expression of specific surface markers) would be better approaches.

**Example 3:** Assess whether, in a single tumor specimen, the gene expression profile varies with the amount of MHC class I expressed on the surface of the malignant cells. This study obviously requires purification of the populations of cells that express the lowest and highest amounts of MHC-I. In addition, those cells that express near mean values of MHC-I need to be eliminated from the analysis. And, because all cells express MHC-I, contaminating nontumor cells such as tumor infiltrating lymphocytes also need to be eliminated from the analysis. This is the type of application for which FACS is ideal. Multiple parameters are used to select the cells of interest, namely those that are positive for epithelial membrane antigen expression (EMA$^+$) but negative for the leukocyte common antigen expression (CD45$^-$), and from within this group, the 10% that stain most intensely for MHC-I (MHC-I high), and the 10% that stain least intensely (MHC-I low, but greater than background).

Compared to bead or affinity-mediated purification methods, FACS is often slow and harsh on the cells. Even using well-defined cultured cell lines, only a small fraction of cells survive FACS separation. Consequently, FACS is risky, especially if the initial tissue sample is a small or unique clinical specimen.

### Use of Molecular Genetic Analysis

**Example:** Assess whether specific mutations correlate with the clinical behavior of GIST, or with tumor response to imatinib mesylate. By way of background, gastrointestinal stromal tumor (GIST) is a neoplasm of mesenchymal origin that is the most common nonepithelial tumor of the gastrointestinal tract. GISTs have a characteristic morphology and immunohistochemical profile, and so the diagnosis is straightforward by pathologic evaluation of routinely processed tissue sections. However, morphologic features have a very low accuracy for predicting whether an individual GIST will behave in a benign or malignant fashion. Because many GIST harbor mutations in the KIT receptor kinase (114), it is of interest to know if specific mutations correlate with the tumor's clinical behavior or with the therapeutic response to imatinib mesylate (Gleevec®), a drug that is a potent inhibitor of the KIT receptor tyrosine kinase (115).

Direct DNA sequence analysis is the most efficient way to address this question. The coding regions of the KIT gene can be PCR amplified from fixed or fresh tissue, which eliminates any need for special tissue procurement procedures, and also permits retrospective as well as prospective case analysis. Automated sequence analysis followed by a computerized homology search can then be used to identify the site and type of the mutation in each tumor (Figure 37–4). Note that although indirect methods of DNA sequence analysis could be used to screen the samples for mutations, the high percentage of GIST that harbor mutations makes the screening step unnecessary. In addition, because indirect methods only demonstrate the presence of a mutation without defining the site and type, follow-up direct sequence analysis of positive cases would still be required.

Analysis of this type has shown that the presence of KIT mutations is not a highly sensitive or specific predictor of malignant behavior (116), but that imatinib mesylate has a better therapeutic effect on GISTs with juxtamembrane KIT mutations compared with GISTs without KIT mutations (117).

## SUMMARY

- A variety of tissue-based techniques can be applied to translational clinical research studies, including those based on morphology, flow cytometry, electron microscopy, and molecular genetic testing.
- Immunohistochemical methods are used to detect specific gene products or antigens within tissue sections that cannot be detected by routine histochemical stains.
- Light microsopy is best suited for studies of cell groups, while electron microscopy is best suited for studies of individual cells.
- Flow cytometry is used to analyze the characteristics of a cell population. Fluorescence activated cell sorting is used when a highly specific population of cells must be purified from a larger sample based on a subtle feature or combination of features.
- Southern and Northern blotting are molecular genetic techniques used in a broad range of

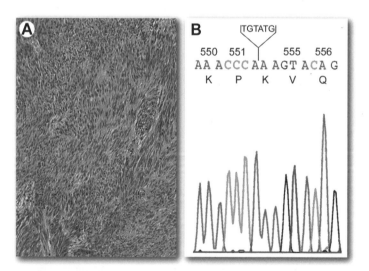

**FIGURE 37–4**  ●  Example of the use of cycle sequencing to characterize the genotype of a gastrointestinal stromal tumor (GIST). **A.** H&E stained section of the tumor. **B.** DNA was extracted from formalin-fixed paraffin embedded sections of the tumor, and direct DNA sequence analysis of the KIT gene was performed. The computer-generated base sequence (top) inferred from the automated sequencing electropherogram (bottom) is shown; comparison with the wild-type KIT sequence demonstrates a six base deletion that changes codons 552 through 554 but maintains the gene's open reading frame, a mutation characteristic of GIST. **Note:** The color figure can be found following page 394.

translational studies. Southern hybridization can be used to provide information about the presence of gene deletions, insertions, and re-arrangements. Northern blotting can be used to provide information on a gene's level of expression and structure. With in situ methods, it is possible to directly correlate the morphology of individual cells with gene expression.

● The polymerase chain reaction (PCR) is a revolutionary technique that is ideally suited to detect specific genetic changes that correlate with disease. A number of PCR-based techniques make it possible to correlate the morphology of individual cells with the presence or absence of a specific mutation.

● Tissue banks are organized to facilitate the collection, storage, and distribution of human tissues for research. A tissue bank's usefulness depends on the accuracy, extent and availability of information that is stored with the tissues, including patient history and clinical data, tumor type and stage, response to treatment, and follow-up. Ethical issues include questions about ownership of and privacy rights to the information derived from analyses of banked tissues.

## REFERENCES

1. Sheehan DC, Hrapchak BB. Theory and Practice of Histotechnology, 2nd Ed. Columbus, OH: Battelle, 1987.
2. Johannessen JV. Use of paraffin material for electron microscopy. Pathol Annu 1977;12:189–224.
3. Dardick I, Herrera GA. Diagnostic electron microscopy of neoplasms. Hum Pathol 1998;29:1335–1338.
4. Kandel R, Bedard YC, Fan QH. Value of electron microscopy and immunohistochemistry in the diagnosis of soft tissue tumors. Ultrastruct Pathol 1998;22:141–146.
5. Bozzola JJ, Russell LD. Electron Microscopy. Principles and techniques for biologists. Sudbury, MA: Jones and Bartlett, 1992.
6. McCoy JP. Basic principles in clinical flow cytometry. In: Keren DF, Hanson CA, Hurtubise PE, eds. Flow Cytometry and Clinical Diagnosis. Chicago: ASCP, 1994:26–55.
7. Shapiro HM. Practical Flow Cytometry. 3rd Ed. New York: Wiley-Liss, 1995:179–216.
8. Herzenberg LA, Parks D, Sahaf B et al. The history and future of the fluorescence activated cell sorter and flow cytometry: a view from Stanford. Clin Chem 2002;48:1819–1827.
9. Koss LG, Czerniak B, Herz F et al. Flow cytometric measurements of DNA and other cell components in human tumors: a critical appraisal. Hum Pathol 1989;20:528–548.
10. Krutzik PO, Nolan GP. Intracellular phospho-protein staining techniques for flow cytometry: monitoring single cell signaling events. Cytometry 2003;55A:61–70.
11. Nap M, Brockhoff G, Brandt B et al. Flow cytometric DNA and phenotype analysis in pathology. A meeting report of a symposium at the annual conference of the German Society of Pathology, Kiel, Germany, 6–9 June 2000. Virchows Arch 2001;438:425–432.
12. Perez OD, Nolan GP. Simultaneous measurement of multiple active kinase states using polychromatic flow cytometry. Nat Biotechnol 2002;20:155–162.
13. Bilkenroth U, Taubert H, Riemann D et al. Detection and enrichment of disseminated renal carcinoma cells from peripheral blood by immunomagnetic cell separation. Int J Cancer 2001;92:577–582.
14. Engle H, Kleespies C, Friedrich J et al. Detection of circulating tumor cells in patients with breast or ovarian cancer by molecular cytogenetics. Br J Cancer 1999;81:1165–1173.
15. Wang ZP, Eisenberger MA, Carducci MA et al. Identification and characterization of circulating prostate carcinoma cells. Cancer 2000;88:2787–2795.
16. Harnden DG, Klinger HP. An International System for Human Cytogenetic Nomenclature (1985): ISCN (1985): Report of the Standing Committee on Human Cytogenetic Nomenclature. Basel: Karger, 1995:1–117.
17. Mitelman F, ed. ISCN(1991): Guidelines for cancer cytogenetics: supplement to an international system for human cytogenetic nomenclature. Basel: Karger, 1991.
18. Khoury H, Lestou VS, Gascoyne RD et al. Multicolor karyotyping and clinicopathological analysis of three intravascular lymphoma cases. Mod Pathol 2003; 16:716–724.
19. Mandahl M. Methods in solid tumor cytogenetics. In: Rooney DE, Czepulkowski BH, eds. Human cytogenetics: a practical approach. Oxford: IRL, 1992:155–188.
20. Wilkinson D. In Situ Hybridization: A Practical Approach. Oxford: IRL, 1998.
21. Szakacs JG, Livingston SK. mRNA in-situ hybridization using biotinylated oligonucleotide probes: implications for the diagnostic laboratory. Ann Clin Lab Sci 1994;24:324–338.
22. Gowans EJ, Arthur J, Blight K et al. Application of in situ hybridization for the detection of virus nucleic acids. Methods Mol Biol 1994;33:395–408.
23. DeLellis RA. In situ hybridization techniques for the analysis of gene expression: applications in tumor pathology. Hum Pathol 1994;25:580–585.
24. Gazit G, Kane SE, Nichols P et al. Use of the stress-inducible grp78/BiP promoter in targeting high level gene expression in fibrosarcoma in vivo. Cancer Res 1995;55:1660–1663.
25. Lisziewicz J, Sun D, Smythe J et al. Inhibition of human immunodeficiency virus type 1 replication by regulated expression of a polymeric Tat activation response RNA decoy as a strategy for gene therapy in AIDS. Proc Natl Acad Sci USA 1993;90:8000–8004.
26. Kallioniemi A, Kallioniemi O, Sudar D et al. Comparative genomic hybridization for molecular cytogenetic analysis of solid tumors. Science 1992;258:818–821.
27. Ishkanian AS, Malloff CA, Watson SK et al. A tiling resolution DNA microarray with complete coverage of the human genome. Nat Genet 2004;36:299–303.
28. Knuutila S, Bjorkqvist AM, Autio K et al. DNA copy number amplifications in human neoplasms: review of comparative genomic hybridization studies. Am J Pathol 1998;152:1107–1123.
29. Knuutila S, Aalto Y, Autio K et al. DNA copy number losses in human neoplasms. Am J Pathol 1999; 155: 683–694.
30. Jackson DP, Lewis FA, Taylor GR et al. Tissue extraction of DNA and RNA and analysis by the polymerase chain reaction. J Clin Pathol 1990;43:499–504.
31. Greer CE, Peterson SL, Kiviat NB et al. PCR amplification from paraffin-embedded tissues. Effects of fixative and fixation time. Am J Clin Pathol 1991;95:117–124.

32. Ben-Ezra J, Johnson DA, Rossi J, et al. Effect of fixation on the amplification of nucleic acids from paraffin-embedded material by the polymerase chain reaction. J Histochem Cytochem 1991;39:351–354.

33. Kohler S, Galili N, Sklar JL et al. Expression of bcr-abl fusion transcripts following bone marrow transplantation for Philadelphia chromosome-positive leukemia. Leukemia 1990;4:541–547.

34. Li H, Gyllensten UB, Cui X et al. Amplification and analysis of DNA sequences in single human sperm and diploid cells. Nature 1988;335:414–417.

35. Chong SS, Gore-Langton RE, Hughes MR. Single-cell DNA analysis for application to preimplantation genetic diagnosis. In: Dracopoli NC, Haines JL, Korf BR et al., eds. Current Protocols in Human Genetics. New York: John Wiley and Sons, 1996:9.10.1–9.10.26.

36. Hahn S, Zhong XY, Holzgreve W. Single cell PCR in laser capture microscopy. Methods Enzymol 2002; 356:295–301.

37. Mutter GL, Chaponot ML, Fletcher JA. A polymerase chain reaction assay for nonrandom X chromosome inactivation identifies monoclonal endometrial cancers and precancers. Am J Pathol 1995;146:501–508.

38. Maitra A, Wistuba II, Virmani AK et al. Enrichment of epithelial cells for molecular studies. Nat Med 1999; 5:459–463.

39. Serth J, Kuczyk MA, Paeslack U et al. Quantitation of DNA extracted after micropreparation of cells from frozen and formalin-fixed tissue sections. Am J Pathol 2000;156:1189–1196.

40. Heinmoller E, Liu Q, Sun Y et al. Toward efficient analysis of mutations in single cells from ethanol-fixed, paraffin-embedded, and immunohistochemically stained tissues. Lab Invest 2002;82:443–453.

41. Simone NL, Bonner RF, Gillespie JW et al. Laser-capture microdissection: opening the microscopic frontier to molecular analysis. Trends Genet 1998;14:272–276.

42. Thompson L, Chang B, Barsky SH. Monoclonal origins of malignant mixed tumors (carcinosarcomas). Evidence for a divergent histogenesis. Am J Surg Pathol 1996; 20:277–285.

43. Yaremko ML, Kelemen PR, Kutza C et al. Immunomagnetic separation can enrich fixed solid tumors for epithelial cells. Am J Pathol 1996;148:95–104.

44. Retzel E, Staskus KA, Embretson JE et al. The in situ PCR: amplification and detection of DNA in a cellular context. In: Innis MA, Gelfand DH, eds. PCR Strategies. San Diego: Academic Press, 1995:199–212.

45. Nuovo GJ, MacConnell P, Gallery F. Analysis of nonspecific DNA synthesis during in situ PCR and solution-phase PCR. PCR Methods Appl 1994;4:89–96.

46. Zehbe I, Sallstrom JF, Hacker GW et al. Indirect and direct in-situ PCR for the detection of human papillomavirus. An evaluation of two methods and a double staining technique. Cell Vision 1994;1:163–167.

47. Walsh PS, Erlich HA, Higuchi R. Preferential PCR amplification of alleles: mechanisms and solutions. PCR Methods Appl 1992;1:241–250.

48. Barnard R, Futo V, Pecheniuk N et al. PCR bias toward the wild-type k-ras and p53 sequences: implications for PCR detection of mutations and cancer diagnosis. Biotechniques 1998;25:684–691.

49. Ogino S, Wilson RB. Quantification of PCR bias caused by a single nucleotide polymorphism in SMN gene dosage analysis. J Mol Diagn 2002;4:185–190.

50. Liu Q, Thorland EC, Sommer SS. Inhibition of PCR amplification by a point mutation downstream of a primer. Biotechniques 1997;22:292–294, 296, 298.

51. Polz MF, Cavanaugh CM. Bias in template-to-product ratios in multitemplate PCR. Appl Environ Microbiol 1998;64:3724–3730.

52. Warnecke PM, Stirzaker C, Melki JR et al. Detection and measurement of PCR bias in quantitative methylation analysis of bisulphite-treated DNA. Nucleic Acids Res 1997;25:4422–4426.

53. Niederhauser C, Hofelein C, Wegmuller B et al. Reliability of PCR decontamination systems. PCR Methods Appl 1994;4:117–123.

54. Lehman U, Kreipe H. Real-time PCR analysis of DNA and RNA extracted from formalin-fixed and paraffin-embedded biopsies. Methods 2001;25:409–418.

55. Rys PN, Persing DH. Preventing false positives: quantitative evaluation of three protocols for inactivation of polymerase chain reaction amplification products. J Clin Microbiol 1993;31:2356–2360.

56. Kwok S, Higuchi R. Avoiding false positives with PCR. Nature 1989;339:237–238.

57. Hill DA, O'Sullivan MJ, Zhu X et al. Practical application of molecular genetic testing as an aid to the surgical pathologic diagnosis of sarcomas: a prospective study. Am J Surg Pathol 2002;26:965–977.

58. Burkardt H. Standardization and quality control of PCR analyses. Clin Chem Lab Med 2000;38:87–91.

59. Sarkar G, Sommer SS. Shedding light on PCR contamination. Nature 1990;343:27.

60. Klebe RJ, Grant GM, Grant AM et al. RT-PCR without RNA isolation. Biotechniques 1996;21:1094–1100.

61. Chuaqui R, Cole K, Cuello M et al. Analysis of mRNA quality in freshly prepared and archival Papanicolaou samples. Acta Cytol 1999;43:831–836.

62. Fend F, Emmert-Buck MR, Chuaqui R et al. Immuno-LCM: laser capture microdissection of immunostained frozen sections for mRNA analysis. Am J Pathol 1999; 154:61–66.

63. Kohda Y, Murakami H, Moe OW. Analysis of segmental renal gene expression by laser capture microdissection. Kidney Int 2000;57:321–331.

64. Schlott T, Nagel H, Ruschenburg I et al. Reverse transcriptase polymerase chain reaction for detecting Ewing's sarcoma in archival fine needle aspiration biopsies. Acta Cytol 1997;41:795–801.

65. Inagaki H, Murase T, Otsuka T et al. Detection of SYT-SSX fusion transcript in synovial sarcoma using archival cytologic specimens. Am J Clin Pathol 1999;111:528–533.

66. Lewis F, Maughan NJ, Smith V et al. Unlocking the archive—gene expression in paraffin-embedded tissue. J Pathol 2001;195:66–71.

67. Mhlanga MM, Malmberg L. Using molecular beacons to detect single-nucleotide polymorphisms with real-time PCR. Methods 2001;25:463–471.

68. Thelwell N, Millington S, Solinas A et al. Mode of action and application of Scorpion primers to mutation detection. Nucleic Acids Res 2000;28:3752–3761.

69. Whitcombe D, Theaker J, Guy SP. Detection of PCR products using self-probing amplicons and fluorescence. Nat Biotechnol 1999;17:804–807.

70. Wittwer CT, Herrmann MG, Gundry CN et al. Real-time multiplex PCR assays. Methods 2001;25:430–442.

71. Luthra R, Sanchez-Vega B, Medeiros LJ. TaqMan RT-PCR assay coupled with capillary electrophoresis for quantification and identification of bcr-abl transcript type. Mod Pathol 2004;17:96–103.

72. Ginzinger DG. Gene quantification using real-time quantitative PCR: an emerging technology hits the mainstream. Exp Hematol 2002;30:503–512.

73. Specht K, Richter T, Muller U et al. Quantitative gene expression analysis in microdissected archival formalin-fixed and paraffin-embedded tumor tissue. Am J Pathol 2001;158:419–429.

74. Godfrey TE, Kim SH, Chavira M et al. Quantitative mRNA expression analysis from formalin-fixed, paraffin-embedded tissues using 5' nuclease quantitative reverse transcription-polymerase chain reaction. J Mol Diagn 2000;2:84–91.

75. Lehmann U, Bock O, Glockner S. Quantitative molecular analysis of laser-microdissected paraffin-embedded human tissues. Pathobiology 2000;68:202–208.

76. Freeman WM, Walker SJ, Vrana KE. Quantitative RT-PCR: pitfalls and potential. Biotechniques 1999; 26:112–122, 124–125.

77. Nowell PC. The clonal evolution of tumor cell populations. Science 1976;194:23–28.

78. Fialkow PJ. Clonal origin of human tumors. Biochim Biophys Acta 1976;458:283–321.

79. Lyon MF. Sex chromatin and gene action in the mammalian X-chromosome. Am J Hum Genet 1962; 14:135–148.

80. Gale RE, Wheadon H, Linch DC. X-chromosome inactivation patterns using HPRT and PGK polymorphisms in haematologically normal and post-chemotherapy females. Br J Haematol 1991;79:193–197.

81. Allen RC, Zoghbi HY, Moseley AB et al. Methylation of HpaII and HhaI sites near the polymorphic CAG repeat in the human androgen-receptor gene correlates with X chromosome inactivation. Am J Hum Genet 1992;51:1229–1239.

82. Boland CR. Setting microsatellites free. Nat Med 1996;2:972–974.

83. Koreth J, O'Leary JJ, O'D McGee J. Microsatellites and PCR genomic analysis. J Pathol 1996;178:239–248.

84. Chen LC, Kurisu W, Ljung BM et al. Heterogeneity for allelic loss in human breast cancer. J Natl Cancer Inst 1992;84:506–510.

85. Deng G, Lu Y, Zlotnikov G et al. Loss of heterozygosity in normal tissue adjacent to breast carcinomas. Science 1996;274:2057–2059.

86. Califano J, van der Riet P, Westra W et al. Genetic progression model for head and neck cancer: implications for field cancerization. Cancer Res 1996;56:2488–2492.

87. Jones PA, Droller MJ. Pathways of development and progression in bladder cancer: new correlations between clinical observations and molecular mechanisms. Semin Urol 1993;11:177–192.

88. Liloglou T, Maloney P, Xinarianos G et al. Sensitivity and limitations of high throughput fluorescent microsatellite analysis for the detection of allelic imbalance: application in lung tumors. Int J Oncol 2000;16:5–14.

89. Liu B, Parsons R, Papadopoulos N et al. Analysis of mismatch repair genes in hereditary non-polyposis colorectal cancer patients. Nat Med 1996;2:169–174.

90. Weber TK, Conlon W, Petrelli NJ et al. Genomic DNA-based hMSH2 and hMLH1 mutation screening in 32 Eastern United States hereditary nonpolyposis colorectal cancer pedigrees. Cancer Res 1997;57:3798–3803.

91. Ahuja N, Mohan A, Li Q et al. Association between CpG island methylation and microsatellite instability in colorectal cancer. Cancer Res 1997; 57:3370–3374.

92. Kane MF, Loda M, Gaida GM et al. Methylation of the hMLH1 promoter correlates with lack of expression of hMLH1 in sporadic colon tumors and mismatch repair-defective human tumor cell lines. Cancer Res 1997;57:808–811.

93. Sieben NL, ter Haar NT, Cornelisse CJ et al. PCR artifacts in LOH and MSI analysis of microdissected tumor cells. Hum Pathol 2000;31:1414–1419.

94. Liu J, Zabarovska VI, Braga E et al. Loss of heterozygosity in tumor cells requires re-evaluation: the data are biased by the size-dependent differential sensitivity of allele detection. FEBS Lett 1999; 462:121–128.

95. Wild P, Knuechel R, Dietmaier W et al. Laser microdissection and microsatellite analyses of breast cancer reveal a high degree of tumor heterogeneity. Pathobiology 2000;68:180–190.

96. Innis MA, Myambo KB, Gelfand DH et al. DNA sequencing with *Thermus aquaticus* DNA polymerase and direct sequencing of polymerase chain reaction-amplified DNA. Proc Natl Acad Sci USA 1988; 85:9436–9440.

97. Jacobs G, Tscholl E, Sek A et al. Enrichment polymerase chain reaction for the detection of Ki-ras mutations: relevance of Taq polymerase error rate, initial DNA copy number, and reaction conditions on the emergence of false-positive mutant bands. J Cancer Res Clin Oncol 1999;125:395–401.

98. Eckert KA, Kunkel TA. DNA polymerase fidelity and the polymerase chain reaction. PCR Methods Appl 1991;1:17–24.

99. Clarke LA, Rebelo CS, Goncalves J et al. PCR amplification introduces errors into mononucleotide and dinucleotide repeat sequences. Mol Pathol 2001;54:351–353.

100. Krawczak M, Reiss J, Schmidtke J et al. Polymerase chain reaction: replication errors and reliability of gene diagnosis. Nucleic Acids Res 1989;17:2197–2201.

101. Richterich P. Estimation of errors in "raw" DNA sequences: a validation study. Genome Res 1998; 8: 251–259.

102. Durbin R, Dear S. Base qualities help sequencing software. Genome Res 1998;8:161–162.

103. McGall GH, Christians FC. High-density genechip oligonucleotide probe arrays. Adv Biochem Eng Biotechnol 2002;77:21–42.

104. Goto S, Takahashi A, Kamisango K et al. Single-nucleotide polymorphism analysis by hybridization protection assay on solid support. Anal Biochem 2002; 307:25–32.

105. Hacia JG. Resequencing and mutational analysis using oligonucleotide microarrays. Nat Genet 1999;21:42–47.

106. Warrington JA, Shah NA, Chein X et al. New developments in high-throughput resequencing and variation detection using high density microarrays. Hum Mutat 2002;19:402–409.

107. Gunthard HF, Wong JK, Ignacio CC et al. Comparative performance of high-density oligonucleotide sequencing and dideoxynucleotide sequencing of HIV type 1 pol from clinical samples. AIDS Res Hum Retroviruses 1998;14:869–876.

108. Ahrendt SA, Halachmi S, Chow JT et al. Rapid p53 sequence analysis in primary lung cancer using an oligonucleotide probe array. Proc Natl Acad Sci USA 1999;96:7382–7387.

109. Altschul SF, Madden TL, Schaffer AA et al. Gapped BLAST and PSI-BLAST: a new generation of protein database search programs. Nucleic Acids Res 1997;25: 3389–3402.

110. Oosterhuis JW, Coebergh JW, van Veen, EB. Tumour banks: well-guarded treasures in the interest of patients. Nat Rev Cancer 2003;3:73–77.

111. Teodorovic I, Therasse P, Spatz A et al. Human tissue research: EORTC recommendations on its practical consequences. Eur J Cancer 2003;39:2256–2263.

112. Florell SR, Coffin CM, Holden JA et al. Preservation of RNA for functional genomic studies: a multidisciplinary tumor bank protocol. Mod Pathol 2001;14:116–128.

113. Adams D. Online tumour bank aims to offer ready route to tissues. Nature 2002;416:464.

114. Rubin BP, Singer S, Tsao C et al. KIT activation is a ubiquitous feature of gastrointestinal stromal tumors. Cancer Res 2001;61:8118–8121.

115. Buchdunger E, Cioffi CL, Law N et al. Abl protein-tyrosine kinase inhibitor STI571 inhibits in vitro signal transduction mediated by c-kit and platelet-derived growth factor receptors. J Pharmacol Exp Ther 2000; 295:139–145.

116. Corless CL, McGreevey L, Haley A et al. KIT mutations are common in incidental gastrointestinal stromal tumors one centimeter or less in size. Am J Pathol 2002;160:1567–1572.

117. Dematteo RP, Heinrich MC, El-Rifai WM et al. Clinical management of gastrointestinal stromal tumors: before and after STI-571. Hum Pathol 2002;33:466–477.

118. Zoubek A, Dockhorn-Dworniczak B, Delattre O et al. Does expression of different EWS chimeric transcripts define clinically distinct risk groups of Ewing tumor patients? J Clin Oncol 1996;14:1245–1251.

119. de Alava E, Kawai A, Healey JH et al. EWS-FLI1 fusion transcript structure is an independent determinant of prognosis in Ewing's sarcoma. J Clin Oncol 1998; 16:1248–1255.

# CHAPTER 38

# Evaluating Substrate Metabolism

## Andrew R. Coggan, Bettina Mittendorfer, Samuel Klein

$\mathbf{R}$elatively noninvasive but powerful new tools now enable researchers to obtain insights into the regulation of intermediate substrate metabolism, and how it is altered by physiological (e.g., exercise) and pathophysiological (e.g., critical illness) challenges, in humans. In this chapter, we discuss the basic principles of methods that allow investigators to obtain information on metabolism in its most genuine sense (i.e., assessment of dynamic changes and rates). Considerable insights into the regulation of substrate metabolism can be obtained by using appropriate and often many different approaches simultaneously. A summary of the methods discussed in this chapter, outlining their advantages and disadvantages, is presented in Table 38–1, and Figure 38–1 depicts the major metabolic pathways discussed in this chapter. Positron emission tomography and other imaging methods have also been applied to metabolism research and are discussed in Chapter 39. Various other methods (e.g., magnetic resonance spectroscopy, and near infra-red spectroscopy), are not discussed here but information given in references (1–4) can serve as a useful starting point.

## INDIRECT CALORIMETRY

One of the oldest, and still one of the most widely used, techniques for quantifying substrate oxidation in humans is by using indirect calorimetry (5). This technique involves measuring the $O_2$ and $CO_2$ in expired and inspired breath to determine oxygen consumption and carbon dioxide production ($VO_2$ and $VCO_2$, respectively). For example, the complete combustion of 1 mole (180 g) of glucose:

$$C_6H_{12}O_6 + 6\ O_2 \rightarrow 6\ CO_2 + 6\ H_2O$$

consumes 6 moles (134 L) of $O_2$, produces 6 moles (134 L) of $CO_2$, and has a free energy change ($\Delta G°$)

of –673 kcal. The ratio of $CO_2$ produced to $O_2$ consumed (i.e., the respiratory quotient, or RQ) is lower for a typical triglyceride, such as palmitoyl-stearyl-oleoyl glycerol, than for glucose because of the highly reduced state of lipids compared with carbohydrates:

$$C_{55}H_{104}O_6 + 78\ O_2 \rightarrow 55\ CO_2 + 55\ H_2O$$

For the same reason, even though the overall $\Delta G°$ of this reaction is much greater (–8,190 kcal), the amount of energy released per liter of $O_2$ is also lower for palmitoyl-stearyl-oleoyl glycerol (4.69 kcal/L) than for glucose (5.02 kcal/L). These differences in RQ and energy yield make it possible to estimate the overall rates of glucose oxidation, lipid oxidation, and total energy production, from the rates of $O_2$ uptake and $CO_2$ release at the mouth or across a tissue bed. In whole-body studies, the contribution of protein (amino acid) oxidation can be accounted for by measuring or estimating the rate of urinary nitrogen excretion, because urea accounts for >80% of urinary nitrogen (5). Alternatively, protein oxidation can be ignored in situations where its contribution to overall energy metabolism is known to be small (e.g., endurance exercise). Assuming that 1 g of nitrogen is excreted in the urine for every 6.25 g of protein oxidized, the final equations become:

Glucose oxidation (g/min)
  $= 4.55 \cdot VO_2 - 3.21 \cdot VCO_2 - 2.87 \cdot N$
Lipid oxidation (g/min)
  $= 1.67 \cdot VO_2 - 1.67 \cdot VCO_2 - 1.92 \cdot N$
Energy production rate (kcal/min)
  $= 3.91 \cdot VO_2 + 1.10 \cdot VCO_2 - 3.34 \cdot N$

where $VO_2$, $VCO_2$, and N are the rates of $O_2$ uptake (in L/min), $CO_2$ release (in L/min), and urinary nitrogen excretion (in g/min).

## TABLE 38–1

### Summary of Commonly Used Methods to Assess Regional and Whole-Body Substrate Metabolism

| Metabolic Event | Method | Advantage | Disadvantage |
|---|---|---|---|
| Whole-body substrate oxidation | Indirect calorimetry (inspiratory/expiratory gas exchange) | Simple, noninvasive, robust | Limited applicability during certain metabolic conditions (e.g., lipogenesis, ketogenesis, very high-intensity exercise); cannot distinguish different sources of fat/carbohydrate (e.g., plasma glucose versus glycogen). |
| Organ/tissue substrate oxidation | Organ/tissue $O_2$ and $CO_2$ balance | Specificity | Invasive, not very robust (blood gas concentration and blood flow measurements relatively variable) |
| Plasma substrate oxidation (whole body and regional) | $^{13}$C-labeled tracer method | Specificity | Requires correction for label fixation → separate infusion trial |
| Tissue substrate utilization | Biopsy | Specificity | Invasive; robustness varies (e.g., muscle TG concentration measurement difficult); only applicable when breakdown → simultaneous synthesis |
| Lipolysis | Whole-body glycerol Ra (tracer dilution method) | Relatively noninvasive | No regional information; does not include glycerol released from retroperitoneal adipose tissue |
| | Adipose tissue a-v-balance (abdominal vein catheterization) | Direct measurement, does not rely on assumptions | Invasive, technically challenging; requires simultaneous blood flow measurements; only feasible in the abdominal region |
| | Microdialysis | Relatively noninvasive; more flexible than a-v-balance with venous catheterization regarding body region | Requires several assumptions; only valid with simultaneous blood flow measurements |
| Hepatic glucose production | Whole-body glucose Ra (tracer method) | Noninvasive | Highly dependent on choice of tracer |
| | Splanchnic a-v-balance | | Invasive; net balance only (including uptake nonhepatic, splanchnic tissues) |
| | Splanchnic a-v-balance with tracer | Simultaneous assessment of uptake and release by splanchnic tissues | Invasive; not specific to liver |

## TABLE 38–1 (Continued)

### Summary of Commonly Used Methods to Assess Regional and Whole-Body Substrate Metabolism

| Metabolic Event | Method | Advantage | Disadvantage |
|---|---|---|---|
| Insulin sensitivity | Hyperinsulinemic-euglycemic clamp (no tracers) | Simple, rapid data analysis (plasma glucose concentration) | Cannot distinguish effects on endogenous glucose production and peripheral glucose uptake (only net response); time consuming if staged-insulin infusion |
| | Two-stage hyperinsulinemic-euglycemic clamp with tracers | Assessment of insulin sensitivity to endogenous glucose production and peripheral glucose uptake | Time consuming |
| Protein synthesis | Tracer incorporation into protein | Very robust; no assumptions necessary (i.e., measurement of direct incorporation of tracer); applicable to secreted proteins (e.g., albumin, pepsin) | Often invasive (tissue biopsy), no information on breakdown |
| | a-v-balance method across limb | Information on net anabolism/catabolism | Invasive, cannot determine synthesis and breakdown rates; highly variable (mostly due to blood flow measurements); contribution of tissues (e.g., skin) other than the tissue of interest (e.g., muscle); not applicable to secreted proteins |
| | a-v-balance with tracer | Gives synthesis and breakdown rates | Invasive, highly variable (mostly due to blood flow measurements); contribution of tissues (e.g., skin) other than the tissue of interest (e.g., muscle); not applicable to secreted proteins |
| Lipoprotein kinetics | Bolus tracer injection and monoexponential slope analysis | Quick, relatively short blood sampling period | Does not account for tracer recycling |
| | Bolus tracer injection and compartmental model analysis | Accounts for tracer recycling | Prolonged blood sampling required; complex analysis |

Although commercially produced "turnkey" metabolic carts are widely available, some carts may not provide accurate or precise measurements of $VO_2$ and $VCO_2$. In addition, reliable measurements require that the research participant is in a true metabolic steady-state, so that $VO_2$ and $VCO_2$ measured at the mouth accurately reflect the rates of $O_2$ consumption and $CO_2$ production at the cellular level. This is especially true for $VCO_2$, because body $CO_2$ stores are large relative to their rate of turnover. Therefore, obtaining valid and reliable estimates of cellular gas exchange by measuring respiratory gas exchange may not be possible during very high intensity exercise, when

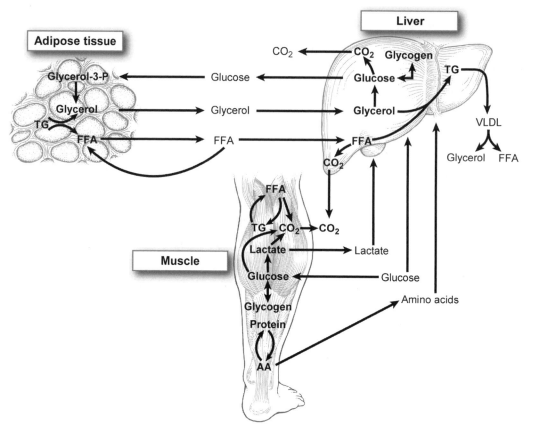

***FIGURE 38–1*** ● Summary of the major metabolic pathways that are customarily assessed by the methods described in this chapter.

hyperventilation can result in considerable non-metabolic $CO_2$ "production."

The estimation of glucose and lipid oxidation rates from $VO_2$ and $VCO_2$ values may not represent true total oxidation rates because other metabolic processes that consume $O_2$ or release $CO_2$ (e.g., lipogenesis, gluconeogenesis) will also affect the results. As a result, the estimated rates of glucose and lipid oxidation actually represent net, not gross, rates of substrate utilization (5). Therefore, correct interpretation of indirect calorimetry data, when there is significant conversion of metabolic substrates without complete oxidation (e.g., lactate or ketone body formation, lipogenesis, gluconeogenesis), requires careful consideration of the metabolic conditions at the time of the study.

## METHODS BASED ON BLOOD OR TISSUE SAMPLING

### Measurement of Blood or Plasma Substrate Concentrations

Some information about metabolism can be gained by measuring the concentration of substrates; for example, free fatty acids or glucose, in blood. However, plasma substrate concentrations are not a direct measure of substrate production or release (e.g., when concentration rises) or utilization or uptake (e.g., when concentration falls) from the circulation, because blood substrate concentration reflects the net balance between release and uptake rates. Therefore, arteriovenous balance or isotopic tracer methods must be used to assess the kinetics responsible for plasma substrate concentration.

### Arteriovenous Balance Technique

The regional kinetics of a substrate can be determined by measuring the amount of a substrate in the blood (or plasma) that enters and leaves a particular tissue or tissue bed (e.g., skeletal muscle, the splanchnic region), along with the rate of blood (or plasma) flow through that tissue. The rate of uptake or release can then be calculated by multiplying the arteriovenous (a-v) concentration difference by the flow. However, this technique can be challenging because it requires placement of arterial catheters, additional catheters into veins directly draining the organ of interest, and accurate measurements of blood flow across the tissue. The high rate of blood flow through many tissues (e.g., liver, kidney, contracting muscle) can make it difficult to accurately quantify the rate of substrate uptake or release, because even a small a-v difference in concentration can result in a large calculated rate of uptake or release when multiplied by a high flow; consequently, even very small errors in blood flow measurements can result in very large errors in the calculated uptake and release rates. Similarly, accurate detection of low rates of substrate consumption across an organ/tissue presents a challenge and heavily depends on the precision of the substrate concentration measurement; very small errors in this difference will cause large errors in calculated consumption or production.

Moreover, even when measurements are made with great precision during carefully controlled conditions, the data must be interpreted carefully. Although arterial blood sampled anywhere in the body represents arterial blood delivered to any tissue, most venous blood vessels that can be cannulated do not drain only one tissue or cell type. Therefore, a-v balance measurements reflect the metabolism of a mixture of different cells or tissues. In addition, unless an isotope-labeled tracer is used, the a-v balance technique assesses only *net* rates of substrate uptake or release; true total rates will be underestimated to the extent that there is simultaneous exchange (e.g., uptake of fatty acids by muscle and release by adipocytes as blood transits a limb).

## Tissue Biopsy

Measuring the change in the concentration or content of an intracellular substrate over time in tissue samples can also be used to determine substrate utilization. This technique has been used most commonly to measure the rate of muscle glycogen utilization during exercise by obtaining muscle biopsies before and after exercise and to measure the concentration of glycogen in those samples, but it has also been used to quantify the use of intramuscular triglyceride. Liver glycogen and triglyceride metabolism have also been studied by obtaining serial liver biopsies, but the increased risk of that procedure limits its usefulness in clinical investigation. The biopsy technique can only quantify the net rate of substrate depletion (or accretion), not total substrate metabolism. However, this potential limitation is not an issue when the rate of substrate utilization is in orders of magnitude greater than the simultaneous rate of substrate synthesis, such as when measuring muscle glycogen use during endurance exercise (6). In contrast, during exercise, changes in intramuscular triglyceride content can

underestimate the true contribution of this energy source to overall energy metabolism because of a high rate of synthesis that occurs simultaneously with breakdown (7).

Another limitation of the biopsy approach is that only a very small amount of tissue (typically 10–100 mg) is removed from the organ, which may not be representative of the tissue as a whole. This issue is particularly relevant when attempting to quantify changes in intramuscular triglyceride content, because triglycerides are heterogeneously distributed throughout muscle.

## REGIONAL ADIPOSE TISSUE METABOLISM

### Microdialysis

Microdialysis probes have been used for the last 30 years to investigate neurotransmitter activity in rat brains (8). More recently, microdialysis has been shown to be a useful tool for in situ studies of regional adipose tissue metabolism in humans (9) (Figure 38–2). The microdialysis probe consists of a double lumen catheter with a dialysis membrane glued to one end. It is implanted percutaneously into subcutaneous adipose tissue using a guide cannula with peel-away sheath. Dialysis solvent (usually Ringer's solution) is perfused through the inner cannula of the probe. The perfusion fluid equilibrates with the fluid surrounding the dialysis membrane by diffusion in both directions and exits through the outer cannula where it is collected from a side arm. Therefore, the outgoing tissue dialysate mirrors the composition of extracellular adipose tissue fluid (Figure 38–1). Assessment of adipose tissue interstitial substrate (usually glycerol) concentration, which can be used to calculate venous concentrations, in combination with arterial glycerol concentration and adipose tissue blood flow permits assessment of a-v balance across regional subcutaneous adipose tissue depots. In addition, pharmacologic agents can be delivered to the extracellular space along with the ingoing perfusate causing high local concentrations without systemic effects (10,11). Therefore, in situ pharmacological experiments can be performed without evoking confounding systemic influences.

### Abdominal Vein Catheterization

Abdominal vein catheterization, used in conjunction with arterial blood sampling and adipose tissue blood flow measurements, permits assessment of a-v balance across regional subcutaneous abdominal adipose tissue. Using the Seldinger technique, a superficial vein of the abdominal wall (superficial epigastric or superficial circumflex iliac) is cannulated in an anterograde direction by advancing a small catheter over a guide wire until the tip is positioned inferior to the inguinal ligament as judged by surface anatomy (12). Blood obtained from this catheter represents drainage from adipose tissue without any contribution from underlying muscle. In this location, muscle is completely separated from subcutaneous fat by a sheet of avascular fibrous tissue.

## Adipose Tissue Blood Flow

Measurement of adipose tissue blood flow is needed to assess regional fat metabolism using a-v balance principles. Subcutaneous adipose tissue blood flow can be determined by [133]xenon washout (13). This technique involves injection of 6–9 MBq of [133]xenon, dissolved in 0.1 mL of sterile saline, into subcutaneous adipose tissue (e.g., abdominal or gluteal adipose tissue depots). After the initial fast washout period, the disappearance of [133]xenon is continuously monitored by a detector that is coupled to a multichannel analyzer that is set to register the 81-keV [133]xenon peak. This approach gives reliable measurements of adipose tissue blood flow for at least 3 hours (14).

## ISOTOPIC TRACER METHODS

One of the most powerful methods for quantifying substrate metabolism in humans is to administer (by infusion, injection, or ingestion) very small amounts of a compound that is labeled with a radioactive or stable isotope (i.e., an isotopic tracer). Originally, this approach was used to delineate different biochemical pathways in vivo, by determining what other compounds or substances became labeled as a result of intermediary metabolism.

However, much more quantitative information can be obtained by measuring the dilution of the tracer by naturally occurring unlabeled material (i.e., the tracee), which makes it possible to calculate the tracee rate of appearance (Ra) in the bloodstream. In addition, the rate of incorporation or conversion of the tracer into another molecule (e.g., amino acid into protein or glucose to $CO_2$) can be determined, making it possible to calculate the rate of synthesis or formation of the product.

## General Tracer Theory

The major assumptions underlying the use of isotopic tracers in metabolic research are that (1) metabolism of the tracer is identical to that of the tracee; that is, no isotope effects would result in discrimination between the two in a biological system, (2) the tracer is given in truly trace amounts, so its administration does not change any metabolic processes, and (3) there is no significant recycling of the tracer within the time frame of the experiment, because this would artificially increase the tracer-to-tracee ratio (TTR) and result in an underestimation of Ra. Fortunately, these assumptions are valid in most experimental conditions. However, in some situations these assumptions are violated (15), in which case this approach is invalid.

## Radioactive and Stable Isotope Tracers

Tracers labeled with either radioactive (e.g., [14]C, [3]H) or stable (e.g., [13]C, [2]H) isotopes have been used in metabolic research. Although the general principles of using radioactive and stable isotope labeled tracers are the same, there are some differences between the two approaches, each with unique advantages and disadvantages. For example, when using a

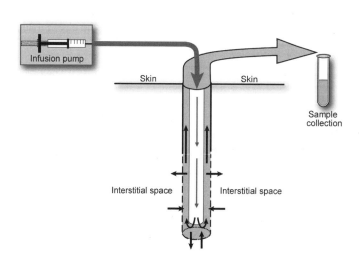

**FIGURE 38–2** ● A microdialysis probe—consisting of a double lumen catheter with a dialysis membrane glued to one end and implanted percutaneously—is perfused through the inner cannula of the probe with perfusate solution. The perfusion fluid equilibrates with the fluid surrounding the dialysis membrane by diffusion in both directions and exits through the outer cannula where it is collected from a side arm. Therefore, the outgoing tissue dialysate mirrors the composition of extracellular adipose tissue fluid.

radioactive isotope labeled tracer, the high sensitivity of liquid scintillation counting makes it possible to detect extremely small amounts of labeled material. This feature reduces the quantity that must be administered or the size of the tissue sample (e.g., blood, muscle) that is needed for analysis. It also facilitates measuring the incorporation of the label into secondarily labeled products. However, the overall sensitivity of this strategy in humans can be limited at times by the maximum acceptable radiation dose that can be given to a study participant. Also, the use of radioactive isotope labeled tracers cannot be justified in certain populations, such as children and pregnant women. In addition, measurement of the ratio of tracer to tracee (i.e., the specific radioactivity), which is needed to assess metabolic kinetics, requires separate measurements of radioactivity and concentration by different methods, which can obviously result in greater total analytical error.

Tracers labeled with stable isotopes have several advantages over radioactive tracers. The use of stable isotopes does not expose the individual to potentially hazardous ionizing radiation, so these tracers can be used safely in infants, children, and pregnant women. In addition, the TTR or the enrichment (i.e., amount of tracer relative to tracee), is measured directly by mass spectrometry, which eliminates the need for separate concentration measurements. The analysis of biological samples by using selected ion monitoring gas chromatography mass spectrometry (SIM-GCMS), also makes it possible to determine the position of a label within a molecule more easily, accurately, and precisely than when radioactive tracers are used. This greatly expands the number and type of possible measurements that can be made, because it allows simultaneous analysis of several tracers within the same substrate.

The principle disadvantage of using stable isotopic tracers is that SIM-GCMS is not as sensitive as liquid scintillation counting, which increases the amount of tracer that must be infused and the size of the tissue sample required for analysis. In appropriate situations, isotope ratio mass spectrometry (IRMS), which is a much more sensitive technique than SIM-GCMS, can be used to detect very low levels of tracer enrichment. This approach requires a larger sample size than does SIM-GCMS, and samples must be combusted or converted into a simple gas (e.g., $CO_2$, $N_2$) before analysis. GC combustion IRMS (GC-C-IRMS) uses an in-stream combustion or catalysis chamber to convert specific compounds eluted from a GC into a simple gas that can be analyzed by continuous flow IRMS. This approach makes it possible to measure lower levels of enrichment than is normally possible using GCMS and requires less sample than classical IRMS.

## MEASUREMENT OF SUBSTRATE RATE OF APPEARANCE BASED ON ISOTOPIC DILUTION

### Steady-State Conditions

Isotopic tracer studies are ideally performed when a dynamic physiological steady-state exists; that is, when the rate of appearance (Ra) and rate of disappearance (Rd) of the tracee are equal and not changing with respect to time. Measurement of substrate (e.g., glucose) Ra or Rd can provide insights into metabolic events that cannot be achieved by measuring substrate concentrations alone. For example, a decrease in plasma glucose concentration can be the result of an increase in glucose Rd or a decrease in glucose Ra, or a combination of both. During steady-state conditions, Ra can be determined by injecting a bolus of tracer into the circulation and then determining the area under the resultant specific activity- or enrichment-time curve in plasma:

$$Ra = Dose \ of \ tracer/Area \ under \ curve$$

This approach assumes that the tracee is released into and is cleared from a single, defined pool, such as the plasma compartment, and does not require any assumptions regarding the distribution of the tracer or tracee throughout the body, or about their route of entry and exit from the system. The Ra value reflects the sum total of the tracee that has had the opportunity to exchange with and "dilute" the tracer before its disposal.

Despite its apparent simplicity, there are certain limitations to the bolus injection approach. First, it can sometimes be difficult to adequately resolve the initial phases of the TTR-time curve, due to the rapid speed with which changes tend to occur and the inability to differentiate dilution of the tracer by newly formed tracee from that due to preexisting tracee (i.e., initial distribution and mixing). Second, accurately quantifying the low TTR that forms the "tail" of the curve can be challenging, particularly when stable isotope labeled tracers are used. Injecting a larger dose of tracer can minimize this latter problem, but there is a practical limit to how much can be administered before metabolism itself might be affected by the amount of tracer given. Finally, determining the area under the specific activity or enrichment-time curve following the bolus injection of tracer generally entails the use of nonlinear least-squares regression, which makes the approach mathematically complex.

A more common approach for determining Ra is to first administer the tracer as a continuous infusion until a plateau (or pseudoplateau) in plasma specific activity or TTR is reached; that is, an isotopic steady-state is achieved. Then, sequential blood samples are obtained to assess the specific activity or TTR at plateau. Ra can be calculated by dividing the tracer infusion rate by the TTR:

$$Ra = \text{Infusion rate of tracer/Plateau TTR}$$

Conceptually, this approach is exactly the same as the bolus injection technique, because the calculated Ra reflects the appearance of tracee that has "diluted" the tracer.

A potential problem of the constant infusion approach is that tracer may have to be infused for many hours before a plateau in specific activity or enrichment is achieved. Therefore, a bolus of tracer (priming dose) is often given at the start of the infusion to reduce the time required to reach equilibrium and the time required to measure Ra (Figure 38–3). The size of this priming dose is chosen based on a priori knowledge of the approximate mass and rate of turnover of tracee within the body, with the goal being that the rate of decline in the TTR resulting from the prime is perfectly matched by the rate of rise in the TTR due to the constant infusion, so a plateau is rapidly established. For example, when studying basal glucose kinetics, it would take more than 8 hours for the TTR to reach a plateau if the tracer were given as an unprimed infusion. With the use of an appropriate priming dose, however, measurement of basal glucose Ra can be performed within 3–4 hours.

## Nonsteady-State Conditions

Although theoretically isotope labeled tracer studies are best performed in a physiological steady-state, in reality, the body is always in transition from one state to another—from fed to postabsorptive to long-term fasted states. In addition, constraining the measurement of substrate kinetics to only steady-state or quasi-steady-state conditions means measurements will only be made during static situations and the dynamic regulation of metabolism cannot be assessed. Therefore, it can be important to quantify Ra during nonsteady-state conditions.

The most common approach for calculating substrate kinetics during nonsteady-state conditions is to use the Steele equation, which assumes changes in the TTR (or in tracee concentration) occur within a single, well-mixed pool that represents some fraction of the total system (16). The calculation of Ra by using this equation is:

$$Ra = (F - p{\cdot}V{\cdot}C_t{\cdot}dE/dt)/E_t$$

where F is the rate of tracer infusion, p is the pool fraction, V is the total volume of distribution of the tracee, $C_t$ is the tracee concentration at time t, and $dE/dt$ is the rate of change in the TTR, and $E_t$ is the TTR at time t. The product $p{\cdot}V{\cdot}C_t$ represents the total mass of tracee assumed to instantly mix with the tracer, which when multiplied by $dE/dt$, can be used to correct the tracer infusion rate for any "extra" tracer being added to or removed from the system. The rate of substrate disposal, Rd, which is not equal to Ra during nonsteady-state conditions, is calculated as:

$$Rd = Ra - p{\cdot}V{\cdot}dC/dt$$

Solid line: desired priming dose
Broken line: over prime
Dotted line: under prime

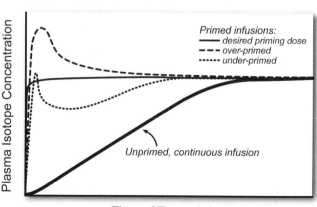

**FIGURE 38–3** ● Isotopic enrichment in plasma during constant and primed infusion of isotope-labeled tracer into the bloodstream. An optimal priming dose shortens the time necessary to achieve isotopic steady-state in plasma substrate enrichment during constant infusion of a labeled tracer.

where p and V are as defined above and $dC/dt$ is the rate of change in tracee concentration at the time of measurement.

The assumption that changes in the TTR and tracee concentration occur instantly within a single well-mixed pool is an oversimplification. Nonetheless, for substances with a small, rapidly turning over pool (e.g., glycerol or plasma free fatty acids), the Steele equation provides accurate estimates of Ra during nonsteady-state conditions. In contrast, it is impossible to obtain accurate estimates of nonsteady-state Ra for urea using the Steele equation, because urea is distributed throughout total body water within large, slowly mixing pools.

### Precursor-Product Methods

Isotope labeled tracer techniques can measure the rate of synthesis of certain compounds by determining the incorporation of a labeled precursor into the product. Specific examples of precursor-product applications are discussed next.

## MEASUREMENT OF SYNTHESIS RATES BASED ON TRACER INCORPORATION

### Gluconeogenesis

Quantifying the rate of gluconeogenesis usually involves infusing an isotope labeled precursor of glucose (e.g., $^{14}$C- or $^{13}$C-labeled lactate) and then measuring the TTR of both the precursor and glucose at isotopic steady-state. The percentage of glucose coming from that precursor can then be calculated based on the ratio of these two values. The absolute rate of gluconeogenesis can be calculated by multiplying the percentage of glucose produced by the precursor by total glucose Ra (measured by using another tracer). The use of labeled lactate underestimates the true rate of gluconeogenesis because of dilution of the label inside liver cells by other metabolic processes (17). In addition, the use of one labeled precursor for gluconeogenesis (e.g., lactate) may not measure gluconeogenesis from other precursors (e.g., glycerol), which can be significant during specific physiological conditions (e.g., when plasma glycerol concentrations are high during short-term fasting (18)).

The limitations of using a labeled lactate precursor can be partially circumvented by measuring the rate of incorporation of labeled bicarbonate into glucose (19). Gluconeogenically derived glucose can become labeled by infusing labeled bicarbonate as a result of $CO_2$ fixation by pyruvate carboxylase and subsequent randomization of the label within oxaloacetate in the tricarboxylic acid (TCA) cycle. This approach accounts for gluconeogenesis from all pyruvate-level substrates. However, this method still does not account for dilution of the label within the intrahepatic oxaloacetate pool or for gluconeogenesis from glycerol.

At present, the only method for quantifying gluconeogenesis, using isotopic tracers, that does not underestimate gluconeogenesis, is based on measuring the incorporation of $^2$H from $^2$H$_2$O into the five position of glucose (20). Gluconeogenically derived glucose becomes labeled in this position as a result of the interconversion of malate and fumarate in the mitochondria, as well as a result of the equilibration of glyceraldehyde-3-phosphate and dihydroxyacetone phosphate in the cytosol. The absolute rate of gluconeogenesis can then be calculated by multiplying the percentage of glucose produced by gluconeogenesis by total glucose Ra. This method accounts for gluconeogenesis from all possible sources. However, the methods needed to measure the low amounts of $^2$H that become bound to glucose are technically complex.

### Protein Synthesis

The synthesis rate of individual body proteins in any accessible protein pool is usually determined by using a primed constant infusion of a labeled amino acid tracer and measuring the rate of incorporation of the tracer into the protein (Figure 38–4). Proteins of interest are obtained by chemical extraction of tissue biopsy samples (e.g., myofibrillar proteins from muscle biopsy samples) or body fluid samples (e.g., albumin and apolipoproteins in plasma). The fractional synthesis rate (FSR) of proteins (i.e., the proportion of the protein pool that is newly synthesized during a specific time period) can be calculated as:

$$FSR = (\Delta E_{protein} / (E_{precursor})) \times 100$$

where $\Delta E_{protein}$ is the increment of protein tracer enrichment between two sequential samples, and $E_{precursor}$ is the average precursor enrichment during the time period. The time period for sample collection depends on the protein of interest. The collection interval needs to be short enough so sampling occurs during the linear part of the incorporation of label into product (Figure 38–4) and long enough so that changes in product labeling are large enough that they can be reliably measured. Therefore, sampling times will vary, depending on how fast proteins are synthesized and catabolized (turnover rate); a shorter interval between samples is needed for rapidly turning over proteins (e.g., very low density

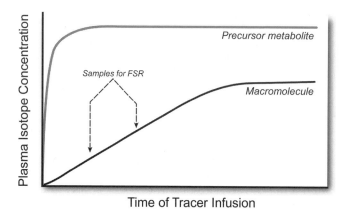

**FIGURE 38–4** ● Isotopic enrichment in precursor (e.g., muscle intracellular free amino acid) and product (e.g., muscle protein) pool during constant infusion of isotope-labeled tracer into the bloodstream. Samples for the calculation of the FSR of the macromolecule are taken during the linear part of the enrichment curve of the macromolecule, when the enrichment in the precursor pool is constant.

lipoprotein (VLDL) apolipoprotein B-100, which has a turnover rate of approximately 30% per hour) and a longer interval between samples is needed for slowly turning over proteins (e.g., muscle protein which has a turnover rate of approximately 0.05% per day). The absolute rate of protein synthesis can be estimated by multiplying the FSR by the protein pool size (e.g., muscle mass times proportion of muscle mass that is protein, which is usually approximately 18%).

To measure the true synthesis rate of macromolecules, it is imperative to know the enrichment of the appropriate precursor pool. In the case of protein synthesis, the immediate precursor is intracellular transfer RNA (tRNA), which provides the amino acids for protein synthesis. Accurate measurement of tRNA tracer enrichment, however, is technically difficult (21) and often not even possible because of the "inaccessibility" of this precursor pool (e.g., liver tRNA for hepatic proteins, which are secreted into the circulation) in human research participants. Surrogate markers of the precursor pool can be used to provide an estimate of the "true" precursor TTR. These markers include the TTR of amino acids in intracellular free water (obtained by tissue biopsy) or the keto-acid corresponding to the tracer amino acid (e.g., keto-isocaproic acid (KIC) in the case of leucine) in blood (22–24). In other cases, the plateau enrichment of a relatively fast turning over protein (e.g., VLDL apo-B100) that is produced from the same precursor amino acid pool as a slower turning over protein (e.g., albumin) can be used to represent the precursor pool enrichment (25). This approach takes advantage of the principle that the plateau enrichment of a macromolecule (here, VLDL apo-B100) must be the same as the steady-state enrichment of the precursor pool (here, tRNA-bound amino acids in hepatocytes). The extent to which

the final, plateau enrichment in the end product is lower than that in the sampled precursor pool indicates the extent to which the "true" precursor pool (in the case of hepatic proteins, tRNA amino acids in hepatocytes) is diluted compared to the sampled precursor pool (e.g., plasma amino acids).

Another approach for measuring protein synthesis rate is known as the *flooding dose technique*. This technique attempts to equilibrate the free pools, by providing so much of the labeled amino acid, that an equilibrium is forced (26–28). One of the problems with this method is that the large amount of tracer administered can influence the turnover of the macromolecule of interest (e.g., leucine is a known stimulator of muscle protein synthesis). Data from several studies (29–33) shows that the rate of human muscle protein synthesis is greater when measured with a flooding dose of an essential amino acid than a nonessential amino acid.

### Lipids and Lipoproteins

Lipoproteins are a complex structure, containing apolipoproteins, triglyceride (TG), cholesterol, and phospholipids. Very low density lipoproteins (VLDL) contain the biggest proportion of TG of all lipoprotein subclasses (except for chylomicrons containing dietary fat), are produced by the liver, and secreted into the systemic circulation, where the TG in VLDL are progressively hydrolyzed by lipoprotein lipase. Each VLDL particle contains one apolipoprotein-B100 (apo-B100) molecule so that apo-B100 kinetics usually represent the kinetics of the entire particle.

A common approach used to measure the turnover rate of VLDL-TG is to inject a bolus of tracer (e.g., labeled glycerol or palmitate) and then to determine the monoexponential slope of decline in VLDL-TG enrichment (34–37). These data can be used to calculate the fractional turnover rate (FTR) of VLDL-TG (i.e., the fraction of the VLDL-TG pool that enters or leaves the pool per unit of time). However, this approach can underestimate the true VLDL-TG turnover rate, because it does not account for tracer recycling. Recycling of the tracer can occur when plasma glycerol or palmitate is incorporated into another pool, from which it is later released and incorporated into VLDL-TG without reappearing in plasma. Therefore, compartmental modeling techniques can improve the accuracy of measuring VLDL-TG kinetics by accounting for tracer recycling (38).

Glycerol is a better tracer than palmitate because glycerol recycles to a lesser extent than fatty acids. However, not all glycerol tracers are equivalent [for details see reference (38)]. Constant infusions of glycerol or palmitate tracers have also been used to measure VLDL-TG turnover rates by fitting the data to a monoexponential rise-to-plateau model (39–41). However, this method, like the monoexponential decay method, also does not account for the considerable tracer recycling that occurs during a prolonged constant infusion protocol. Theoretically it is possible to calculate the fractional turnover rate (as described in the previous section on *Protein synthesis*), by measuring the change in VLDL-TG enrichment between two subsequent samples (with linear extrapolation between the two data points) during a constant tracer infusion and then dividing this value by the precursor enrichment (slope ÷ plateau). For this approach to be valid it is critical that it is done during the linear increase in VLDL-TG enrichment, which makes it necessary to collect frequent samples (especially shortly after the tracer bolus administration) to verify linearity; furthermore, the final value relies on the correct precursor enrichment, which is inaccessible (intrahepatic glycerol/fatty acids) and has to be substituted with the enrichment values in plasma or the experiment carried out until a plateau in the VLDL-TG enrichment is attained. The reliance on only two data points is definitely another shortcoming of this approach and will certainly increase the variability of the final results.

An alternative approach to measuring VLDL-TG turnover rates, one that relies on the tracer-dilution principle in plasma during a constant infusion of labeled VLDL (42), is difficult and often unfeasible: it requires producing endogenously labeled VLDL, via ingestion or infusion of a precursor (glycerol) tracer, plasmapheresis to collect the endogenously produced tracer VLDL, and VLDL isolation and storage before reinfusion to measure VLDL Ra.

Given these complexities, this method is not likely to be used on a regular basis.

Apolipoprotein turnover rates can be assessed via bolus injection of an amino acid tracer then fitting the enrichment data to a compartmental model, such as the one for apo-B100 originally developed by Zech et al. (43). A compartmental model is a mathematical construct of a metabolic system, which is often based on the exponential functions of the tracer decay curve after bolus injection, and an understanding of the metabolic system being modeled (also see Chapter 39). This approach makes it possible to estimate kinetics that occur in nonsampled (e.g., intracellular) compartments by fitting the experimental data to the model. Given the complexity of the lipoprotein system, this is probably the best approach; however, all the methods described above for measuring TG turnover (monoexponential decline, monoexponential rise to plateau in enrichment, the slope ÷ plateau enrichment analysis, and the constant infusion of a leucine tracer in combination with mathematical modeling) have been used to assess apo-B100 kinetics.

Once the FTR (usually in pools·h$^{-1}$) has been determined, the absolute rate of VLDL-TG production can be calculated as (1) total production rate, which represents the total amount of VLDL-TG produced by the liver (usually in $\mu$mol·min$^{-1}$ or, normalized to body weight, in $\mu$mol·kg body wt$^{-1}$·min$^{-1}$) and (2) production per unit of plasma, which represents the rate of release of VLDL-TG from the liver into the bloodstream as follows:

Total VLDL-TG $_{production\ rate}$ (in $\mu$mol·min$^{-1}$)
= (VLDL-TG FTR/60) × C$_{VLDL-TG}$ x PV

VLDL-TG $_{secretion\ into\ plasma}$ (in $\mu$mol·L plasma$^{-1}$·min$^{-1}$)
= (VLDL-TG FCR/60) × C$_{VLDL-TG}$

where C$_{VLDL-TG}$ is the concentration of VLDL-TG in plasma, and PV is plasma volume, which can be estimated based on a patient's fat-free mass (PV = 0.055 L × kg FFM) (44, 45).

It is assumed that PV is equal to the VLDL-TG volume of distribution, because VLDL is restricted to the plasma compartment and does not enter the interstitial space or the lymphatic system (46). During steady-state conditions (when plasma VLDL-TG concentration is constant), the VLDL-TG production rate is equal to the rate of VLDL-TG disappearance from plasma; therefore, the FTR equals the fractional production/synthetic rate and the fractional catabolic rate.

The rate of de novo lipogenesis of VLDL-TG fatty acids can be determined by using mass isotopomer distribution analysis to assess the incorporation of [$^{13}$C]acetate into VLDL-palmitate (47). This involves a constant infusion of [$^{13}$C]acetate and subsequent blood samples to obtain plasma VLDL-TG. The contribution of de novo synthesized fatty acids to total VLDL-TG turnover is extremely small (<10% during fed conditions and even less during fasting) (48).

## MEASUREMENT OF PLASMA SUBSTRATE OXIDATION

Plasma substrate oxidation can be assessed by infusing a $^{14}$C- or $^{13}$C-labeled tracer of the substrate and measuring the appearance of $^{14}$CO$_2$ or $^{13}$CO$_2$ in breath. Dividing the TTR of the product, that is, breath CO$_2$, by the infusion rate of the tracer/label (once steady-state in the TTR of the plasma substrate has been achieved) calculates the fractional rate of oxidation of substrate (i.e., percent uptake of substrate that was oxidized to CO$_2$). The absolute rate of oxidation (usually expressed as μmol·min$^{-1}$) can then be calculated by multiplying the Rd of substrate by the fractional oxidation rate or as (VCO$_2$ × E$_{CO2}$) / E$_{substrate}$, where E$_{CO2}$ is the enrichment of CO$_2$ in expired breath and E$_{substrate}$ the enrichment of the substrate in plasma.

As in other precursor-product methods, accurate calculation of plasma substrate oxidation requires isotopic steady-state conditions in both the precursor (substrate) and product (CO$_2$) pools. Therefore, a bolus (approximately 80 times the expected rate of $^{13}$CO$_2$ production) of labeled bicarbonate along with a bolus of the tracer (e.g., [1-$^{13}$C]leucine) is injected at the start of the experiment. This bicarbonate prime greatly speeds equilibration of the secondarily labeled bicarbonate pools, so an apparent plateau in the TTR of expired CO$_2$ can be achieved within minutes instead of hours. Some of the labeled carbons of an oxidized tracer do not appear in breath because it is incorporated into other metabolites that remain in the body. Therefore, the data for plasma substrate oxidation are usually corrected by dividing the calculated oxidation rate by the fraction of infused labeled bicarbonate that is recovered in breath CO$_2$. This bicarbonate correction factor, which is usually 0.7–0.8 in resting patients, but may approach 1.0 during exercise or during very prolonged tracer infusion, can be determined by measuring the recovery in breath of infused label bicarbonate (e.g., NaH$^{14}$CO$_3$).

The use of a bicarbonate correction factor is not adequate for specific substrates, such as fatty acids, which loses its labeled carbon during exchange reactions of the tricarboxylic acid (TCA) cycle; loss of label by these exchange reactions can lead to a significant underestimation of the true rate of substrate oxidation despite using a bicarbonate correction. Therefore, the use of an acetate correction factor has been proposed for fatty acids, based on the principle that infusing acetate labeled in the same position as the acetyl-CoA, which is produced from the substrate being studied, makes it possible to account for the amount of label that enters the TCA cycle but does not appear in breath carbon dioxide (49). This approach assumes that the only fate of acetate is oxidation and that plasma acetate is taken up and metabolized by the same tissues and in the same proportions as the acetate derived from the substrate of interest.

## EXAMPLES OF SPECIFIC APPLICATIONS

### Assessment of Insulin Action: The Euglycemic Hyperinsulinemic Clamp Technique

The euglycemic hyperinsulinemic glucose clamp technique is considered the gold standard for assessing insulin sensitivity in vivo (50,51). This procedure involves infusing insulin at a constant rate, while infusing 20% dextrose (monohydrated glucose) at a variable rate designed to "clamp" plasma glucose concentration at euglycemic levels. Plasma glucose concentration is monitored frequently (i.e., every 5–15 minutes) and the glucose infusion rate is adjusted as needed to maintain the desired glucose concentration. Eventually (i.e., after one to several hours, depending on the insulin concentration and the patient's sensitivity to insulin) a plateau in the rate of glucose infusion is achieved. This rate of glucose infusion reflects tissue glucose uptake at that prevailing insulin level. At high insulin infusion rates, this procedure provides a measure of insulin sensitivity in skeletal muscle because muscle is the major site of glucose disposal. The euglycemic hyperinsulinemic glucose clamp can be used in conjunction with isotope labeled tracer infusions and conducted in stages of low and high insulin infusion rates to assess insulin action in the liver (suppression of glucose production) and adipose tissue (suppression of lipolysis) in response to low insulin infusion rates, and in skeletal muscle (glucose uptake) in response to high insulin infusion rates.

A variation of the euglycemic hyperinsulinemic clamp is the hyperglycemic clamp, in which plasma glucose concentration is elevated and then maintained at some investigator-determined point above basal by infusing dextrose. The plasma insulin concentration that results from the increase in endogenous secretion provides an index of beta cell sensitivity and responsiveness to hyperglycemia.

## Determination of Muscle Protein Synthesis

The two most commonly used tracers for measuring muscle protein synthesis are leucine and phenylalanine, usually labeled with either $^2H$ or $^{13}C$; other amino acids that have been successfully, although only sporadically, used to measure muscle protein synthesis include valine, glycine, alanine, proline, and serine. Another useful tracer for the measurement of muscle protein FSR is α-keto-isokaproic acid (α-KIC; the corresponding keto-acid of leucine) (23,24). The use of a KIC and/or leucine tracer, offers an advantage in that it allows monitoring or confirmation of an isotopic steady-state in intracellular free leucine enrichment by measuring the enrichment of KIC in plasma. Decisions concerning the choice of label are driven predominately by the price of a specific tracer and the analysis techniques available (e.g., GC-MS, GC-C-IRMS).

Muscle protein is not a homogenous pool of protein but rather it is comprised of a variety of specific proteins that can be classified broadly into myofibrillar (contractile), sarcoplasmic (located within the cytoplasm and responsible for most metabolic functions), mitochondrial (muscle respiratory function) proteins, and collagen (the connective tissue component). Each of these classes of proteins has unique kinetic characteristics and kinetics probably vary also to some extent even within each class of proteins. Most studies of muscle protein metabolism have relied on the measurement of mixed muscle protein (i.e., crude protein extract from muscle tissue); however, numerous investigators now measure the rates of individual muscle protein subclasses to obtain more specific information. Data obtained from studies measuring either mixed or myofibrillar protein synthesis are largely comparable because the major subclasses of proteins in the muscle behave very similarly; however, myofibrillar protein synthesis rate is more sensitive than mixed muscle protein (i.e., greater changes in myofibrillar than in the rate of mixed muscle protein synthesis have been observed), while its basal rate is lower than that of sarcoplasmic and mitochondrial (52,53). Recent observations made (JA Babraj, B. Mittendorfer, and MJ Rennie unpublished) indicate that muscle collagen is not responsive to feeding (unlike myofibrillar and sarcoplasmic proteins), which suggests that it is ultimately important to measure the rates of individual protein classes or more specific proteins to further increase our knowledge base.

The major advantage of measuring dynamic changes in muscle protein kinetics, such as those enabled by using tracer infusions, is that these measurements can be made over short time periods to detect acute alterations in muscle protein metabolism, such as those that occur through the course of the day; muscle protein synthesis (and breakdown) fluctuate several-fold throughout the day depending on the body's metabolic condition, with synthesis being greater (e.g., during feeding and after exercise) than during fasting, which leads to overall maintenance (or growth or loss) of muscle mass.

Technical as well as physiologic considerations need to be taken into account when designing such studies. During basal, fasting conditions, the sensitivity of the analytical technique used to measure the extent of labeling in muscle protein, largely dictates the time of tracer infusion (between two biopsies) necessary to obtain robust results; it usually requires at least 2.5 hours of tracer infusion (but measurements have been made up to approximately 12 hour between biopsies) to reliably measure the increase in the amount of tracer between the first and second biopsy, although measurements have been made with as little as 30 minutes between biopsies (53). During conditions when muscle protein synthesis is stimulated (e.g., during feeding and after exercise), measurements can safely be made in a somewhat shorter period of time (though routinely, measurements are made between 3 and 5 hours), whereas the time between biopsies has to be prolonged when the rates of muscle protein synthesis are suppressed (e.g., during prolonged fasting).

The sensitivity of analysis can be improved by choosing, for instance, [1,2-$^{13}C$]leucine over [1-$^{13}C$]leucine as a tracer, allowing for acceptable signal resolution during shorter infusion periods or during conditions when synthesis rates are very low. Unfortunately, the cost of such studies may become prohibitively high.

As researchers learn more about muscle physiology, it is apparent that analytical issues are not the only ones to be considered when designing the study protocol. For example, it has recently been shown that muscle protein synthesis responds rapidly (within 30 minutes) to increased availability of amino acids but is then (after 2.5 to 3 hours) inhibited for at least 4 hours, despite continued amino acid availability (53). These findings suggest that there is an upper limit to the ability of muscle to build up protein that is independent of the availability of precursors (i.e., amino acids) for muscle protein synthesis. Therefore, measurements made during longer periods of increased amino acid availability likely underestimate the "true" effect of feeding.

# MEASUREMENT OF WHOLE BODY LIPID KINETICS

The breakdown of stored triglycerides (lipolysis) results in the release of fatty acids and glycerol. Fatty acids are of primary importance as energy substrates, and glycerol serves mostly as a gluconeogenic precursor. The rate of appearance of fatty acids and glycerol into the bloodstream provides an index of whole body lipolytic activity. The rate of release of fatty acids into the bloodstream is usually measured by the constant infusion of an isotope labeled fatty acid. Isotopic steady-state can usually be achieved within 30 minutes of the start of the tracer infusion because the fatty acid turnover is rapid, and the effective volume of distribution is small. Because of the small pool size and rapid turnover rate, no priming dose of fatty acid tracer is necessary. To assess glycerol kinetics, the glycerol tracer is usually administered as a primed, constant infusion (54,55). Although glycerol is distributed throughout the total volume of extracellular fluid, a steady-state can nonetheless be achieved rapidly during a constant infusion because of the rapid turnover time of the pool. Samples for the calculation of substrate kinetics are usually obtained once an isotopic steady-state in the sampled compartment (e.g., blood) is achieved ( approximately 30 to 90 minutes after the start of the tracer infusion).

In many circumstances of interest (e.g., exercise, catecholamine infusion) there is a nonsteady-state of lipolysis. Under these circumstances, fatty acid and glycerol Ra are calculated by using Steele's equation for nonsteady-state conditions (16,56). The volume of distribution for fatty acids is usually assumed to be the plasma volume [i.e., approximately 55 mL per kg FFM (44,45)] for fatty acids and 300 mL per kg body wt for glycerol (57).

# SUMMARY

- There are numerous methods used to quantify substrate metabolism in human research participants, including uptake and release of substrates into the circulation (whole-body level) and from a specific tissue/organ; oxidation of substrates at the whole-body level and in specific tissues/organs, and synthesis of macromolecules (e.g., proteins, glucose) from specific precursors (e.g., amino acids, glycerol) that use isotope labeled tracers, especially those labeled with stable isotopes.
- The use of stable isotope labeled tracers is probably the most flexible and powerful of all the methods described (see also Table 38–1) and those not included here (e.g., magnetic resonance imaging, near infrared spectroscopy).

- Each method, however, is based on different principles, and therefore each has its own unique advantages and disadvantages (Table 38–1).

# REFERENCES

1. Perseghin G. Petersen KF, Shulman GI. Cellular mechanism of insulin resistance: potential links with inflammation. Int J Obes Relat Metab Disord 2003;27:S6–S11.
2. Roden M, Petersen KF, Shulman GI. Nuclear magnetic resonance studies of hepatic glucose metabolism in humans. Recent Prog Horm Res 2001;56:219–237.
3. Shulman RG, Rothman DL. 13C NMR of intermediary metabolism: implications for systemic physiology. Annu Rev Physiol 2001;63:15–48.
4. Cerretelli P, Binzoni T. The contribution of NMR, NIRS and their combination to the functional assessment of human muscle. Int J Sports Med 1997:4:S270–S279.
5. Frayn KN. Calculation of substrate oxidation rates in vivo from gaseous exchange. J Appl Physiol 1983; 55:628–634.
6. Azevedo JJ Jr, Linderman JK, Lehman, SL et al. Training decreases muscle glycogen turnover during exercise. Eur J Appl Physiol Occup Physiol 1998;78:479–486.
7. Guo Z, Burguera B, Jensen M. Kinetics of intramuscular triglyceride fatty acids in exercising humans. J Appl Physiol 2000;89:2057–2064.
8. Ungerstedt U. Measurement of neurotransmitter release by intracranial dialysis In: Measurements of neurotransmitter Release in Vivo. Marsden. CA, (Ed.), New York: John Wiley and Sons 1984:81–105.
9. Arner P, Bolinder J, Eliasson A et al. Microdialysis of adipose tissue and blood for in vivo lipolysis studies. Am J Physiol 1988;255:E737–E742.
10. Arner P, Kriegholm E, Engfeldt P et al. Adrenergic regulation of lipolysis in situ at rest and during exercise. J Clin Invest 1990; 85:893–898.
11. Arner P, Kriegholm E, Engfeldt P. In situ studies of catecholamine-induced lipolysis in human adipose tissue using microdialysis. J Pharmacol Exp Ther 1990;254:284–288.
12. Frayn KN, Coppack SW, Humphreys SM et al. Metabolic characteristics of human adipose tissue in vivo. Clin Sci (Land), 1989;76:509–516.
13. Larsen O, Lassen N, Quaade F. Blood flow through human adipose tissue determined with radioactive xenon. Acta Physiol Scand 1966;66:337–345.
14. Bulow J, Astrup A, Christensen NJ et al. Blood flow in skin, subcutaneous adipose tissue and skeletal muscle in the forearm of normal man during an oral glucose load. Acta Physiol Scand 1987; 130:657–661.
15. Zello GA, Marai L, Iung AS et al. Plasma and urine enrichments following infusion of L-[1-13C]phenylalanine and L-[ring-2H5]phenylalanine in humans: evidence for an isotope effect in renal tubular reabsorption. Metabolism 1994; 43:487–491.
16. Steele R. Influences of glucose loading and of injected insulin on hepatic glucose output. Ann NY Acad Sci 1959;82:420–430.
17. Coggan AR, Raguso CA, Williams BD et al. Glucose kinetics during high-intensity exercise in endurance-trained and untrained humans. J Appl Physiol 1995; 78:1203–1207.
18. Baba H, Zhang X, Wolfe R. Glycerol gluconeogenesis in fasting humans. Nutrition 1995;11:149–153.
19. Coggan A, Swanson S, Mendenhall L et al. Effect of endurance training on hepatic glycogenolysis and

gluconeogenesis during prolonged exercise in men. Am J Physiol Endocrinol Metab 1995; 268:E375–E383.

20. Landau B. Quantifying the contribution of gluconeogenesis to glucose production in fasted human subjects using stable isotopes. Proc Nutr Soc 1999;58:963–972.

21. Watt PW, Lindsay Y, Scrimgeour CM et al. Isolation of aminoacyl-tRNA and its labeling with stable-isotope tracers: use in studies of human tissue protein synthesis. Proc Natl Acad Sci USA 1991;88:5892–5896.

22. Nakshabendi IM, Obeidet W, Russell RI et al. Gut mucosal protein synthesis measured using intravenous and intragastric delivery of stable tracer amino acids. Am J Physiol 1995;269:E996–E999.

23. Chinkes D, Klein S, Zhang XJ et al. Infusion of labeled KIC is more accurate than labeled leucine to determine human muscle protein synthesis. Am J Physiol 1996; 270:E67–71.

24. Bennet WM, O'Keefe SJ, Haymond MW. Comparison of precursor pools with leucine, alpha-ketoisocaproate, and phenylalanine tracers used to measure splanchnic protein synthesis in man. Metabolism 1993;42:691–695.

25. De Feo P, Volpi E, Lucidi P et al. Ethanol impairs postprandial hepatic protein metabolism. J Clin Invest 1995; 95:1472–1479.

26. Chinkes DL, Rosenblatt J, Wolfe RR. Assessment of the mathematical issues involved in measuring the fractional synthesis rate of protein using the flooding dose technique. Clin Sci (Lond) 1993;84:177–183.

27. Garlick PJ, Wernerman J, McNurlan MA et al. Measurement of the rate of protein synthesis in muscle of postabsorptive young men by injection of a "flooding dose" of [1-13C]leucine. Clin Sci (Lond) 1989;77:329–336.

28. Garlick PJ, McNurlan MA. Measurement of protein synthesis in human tissues by the flooding method. Curr Opin Clin Nutr Metab Care 1998;1:455–460.

29. Smith K, Barua JM, Watt PW et al. Flooding with L-[1-13C]leucine stimulates human muscle protein incorporation of continuously infused L-[1-13C]valine. Am J Physiol 1992;262: E372–E376.

30. Smith K, Downie S, Watt P et al. Increased incorporation of [$^{13}$C]valine into plasma albumin as a result of a flooding dose of leucine in man. Clin Nutr 1992b;11:77 (Abstract).

31. Smith K, Essen P, McNurlan MA et al. A multi-tracer investigation of the effect of a flooding dose administered during the constant infusion of tracer amino acid on the rate of tracer incorporation into human muscle protein. Proc Nutr Soc 1992; 59:109A (Abstract).

32. Smith K, Downie S, Barua JM et al. Effect of a flooding dose of leucine in stimulating incorporation of constantly infused valine into albumin. Am J Physiol 1994; 266:E640–E644.

33. Smith K, Reynolds N, Downie S et al. Effects of flooding amino acids on incorporation of labeled amino acids into human muscle protein. Am J Physiol 1998; 275:E73–E78.

34. Farquhar JW, Gross RC, Wagner RM et al. Validation of an incompletely coupled two-compartment nonrecycling catenary model for turnover of liver and plasma triglyceride in man. J Lipid Res 1965;79:119–134.

35. Reaven GM, Hill DB, Gross RC et al. Kinetics of triglyceride turnover of very low density lipoproteins of human plasma. J Clin Invest 1965;44:1826–1833.

36. Sane T, Nikkila EA. Very low density lipoprotein triglyceride metabolism in relatives of hypertriglyceridemic probands. Evidence for genetic control of triglyceride removal. Arteriosclerosis 1988;8:217–226.

37. Nikkila EA, Kekki M. Polymorphism of plasma triglyceride kinetics in normal human adult subjects. Acta Med Scand 1971;190:49–59.

38. Patterson BW, Mittendorfer B, Elias N et al. Use of stable isotopically labeled tracers to measure very low

density lipoprotein-triglyceride turnover. J Lipid Res 2002;43:223–233.

39. Siler SQ, Neese RA, Parks EJ et al. VLDL-triglyceride production after alcohol ingestion, studied using [2-$^{13}$C$_1$] glycerol. J Lipid Res 1998;39:2319–2328.

40. Parks EJ, Krauss RM, Christiansen MP et al. Effects of a low-fat, high-carbohydrate diet on VLDL-triglyceride assembly, production, and clearance. J Clin Invest 1999;104:1087–1096.

41. Wang W, Basinger A, Neese RA et al. Effect of nicotinic acid administration on hepatic very low density lipoprotein-triglyceride production. Am J Physiol Endocrinol Metab 2001; 280:E540–E547.

42. Sidossis LS, Mittendorfer B, Walser E et al. Hyperglycemia-induced inhibition of splanchnic fatty acid oxidation increases hepatic triacylglycerol secretion. Am J Physiol 1998;275:E798–E805.

43. Zech LA, Grundy SM, Skinberg D et al. Kinetic model for production and metabolism of very low density lipoprotein triglycerides: evidence for a slow production pathway and results for normolipidemic subjects. J Clin Invest 1979; 63:1262–1273.

44. Boer P. Estimated lean body mass as an index for normalization of body fluid volumes in humans. Am J Physiol 1984;247:F632–F636.

45. Egusa G, Beltz WF, Grundy SM et al. Influence of obesity on the metabolism of apolipoprotein B in humans. J Clin Invest 1985; 76:596–603.

46. Reichl D. Lipoproteins of human peripheral lymph. Eur Heart J 1990;11 Suppl E:230–236.

47. Hellerstein MK, Christiansen M, Kaempfer S et al. Measurement of de novo hepatic lipogenesis in humans using stable isotopes. J Clin Invest 1991;87:1841–1852.

48. Aarsland A, Chinkes D, Wolfe RR. Contributions of de novo synthesis of fatty acids to total VLDL-triglyceride secretion during prolonged hyperglycemia/hyperinsulinemia in normal man. J Clin Invest 1996;98:2008–2017.

49. Sidossis LS, Coggan AR, Gastaldelli A et al. A new correction factor for use in tracer estimations of plasma fatty acid oxidation. Am J Physiol 1995;269:E649–E656.

50. DeFronzo R, Tobin J, Andres R. Glucose clamp technique: a method for quantifying insulin secretion and resistance. Am J Physiol 1979;237:E214–E223.

51. Finegood D, Bergman R, Vranic M. Estimation of endogenous glucose production during hyperinsulinemic-euglycemic glucose clamps. Comparison of unlabeled and labeled exogenous glucose infusates. Diabetes 1987;36:914–924.

52. Bates PC, Millward DJ. Myofibrillar protein turnover. Synthesis rates of myofibrillar and sarcoplasmic protein fractions in different muscles and the changes observed during postnatal development and in response to feeding and starvation. Biochem J 1983;214:587–592.

53. Bohe J, Low JF, Wolfe RR et al. Latency and duration of stimulation of human muscle protein synthesis during continuous infusion of amino acids. J Physiol 2001;532:575–579.

54. Mittendorfer B, Horowitz JF, Klein S. Gender differences in lipid and glucose kinetics during short-term fasting. Am J Physiol 2001;281:E1333–E1339.

55. van Hall G, Sacchetti M, Rådegran G et al. Human skeletal muscle fatty acid and glycerol metabolism during rest, exercise and recovery. J Physiol 2002;543:1047–1058.

56. Gastaldelli A, Coggan AR, Wolfe RR. Assessment of methods for improving tracer estimation of non-steady-state rate of appearance. J Appl Physiol 1999; 87: 1813–1822.

57. Beylot M, Martin C, Beaufrire B et al. Determination of steady state and nonsteady-state glycerol kinetics in humans using deuterium-labeled tracer. J Lipid Res 1987;28:414–422.

# CHAPTER 39

# Medical Images as Scientific Data

William J. Powers, Tom O. Videen

The fields of genetics and genomics are not the only areas that have experienced enormous growth in new knowledge in recent years. The past 30 years have also witnessed an explosion in the field of medical imaging, beginning with the development of x-ray computed tomography (CT) in the early 1970s, followed by positron emission tomography (PET) and single photon emission computed tomography (SPECT) in the late 1970s, and then magnetic resonance imaging (MRI) in the 1980s. These techniques and others (including ultrasonography) are central to the modern practice of medicine and all physicians are familiar with their use to aid in the diagnosis of disease and the management of patients. They can substitute for direct visualization at surgery or autopsy, or replace more invasive studies requiring selective catheterization or biopsy. The value of individual medical imaging techniques for clinical practice ultimately depends on their ability to provide information that will lead to an improvement in patient outcome (1). These same advances in medical imaging are also revolutionizing translational research and experimental medicine.

Medical imaging can provide both structural and physiological information about the human body. Structural imaging provides information about the physical structure of organs. X-ray, ultrasound, and magnetic resonance imaging (MRI) all employ the differing physical properties of various tissues to produce these structural images. Physiological imaging uses the data provided by the imaging device to measure a biological process such as cardiac ejection fraction or brain metabolism. By their very nature, both structural and physiological imaging provide spatial information. They generate measurements that are derived from a specific location within the body, usually an organ or a part of an organ. Furthermore, most imaging systems have a restricted field of view that encompasses only part of the body. Finally, for physiological imaging, differences in organ physiology often require developing techniques that are organ specific. As a consequence, medical imaging techniques are particularly suited to studies of the physiology and pathology of individual organs (such as brain, lung, or heart) rather than for studies of whole body processes.

The role of medical imaging techniques in translational research and experimental medicine is very different than its role in medical diagnosis and treatment. Medical imaging can be used to generate measurements to test biological hypotheses in the same way that more familiar techniques such as serum assays are used. These studies can be either observational or interventional. Observational studies (Chapter 7) using medical imaging generally fall into two general designs. Between-group designs consist of a diseased group and control group or consist of groups with different disease severities. One or more medical imaging measurements are made in all patients; the hypothesis is that there will be a difference in the measurements among the groups. Within-group designs consist of one group, usually with a disease. One or more medical imaging measurements are made in all patients; the hypothesis is that there will be an association or correlation between different medical imaging measurements or between some medical imaging measurement and another clinical variable such as disease severity.

An example of an observational study with a between-group design is the measurement of blood-to-brain glucose transport by PET in poorly controlled diabetics and in normal patients, testing the hypothesis that transport is reduced in diabetics (2).

An example of an observational study with a within-group design is the measurement of cerebral oxygen extraction fraction by PET in patients with symptomatic carotid artery occlusion, testing the hypothesis that increased oxygen extraction fraction is associated with an increased risk of subsequent stroke (3).

Interventional studies include an intervention as part of the experiment. The endpoint or outcome of the study is the effect of the intervention on the medical imaging measurement. These studies can have either a between-group or within-group design format (Chapter 8). An example of between-group design with medical imaging is the measurement of cerebral infarct size by CT in patients with acute ischemic stroke, randomized to receive tissue plasminogen activator, or placebo, testing the hypothesis that tissue plasminogen activator reduces infarct size (4). An example of a study with a within-group design is the measurement of regional cerebral blood flow in patients with acute intracerebral hemorrhage before and after pharmacological blood pressure reduction to test the hypothesis that induced hypotension decreases blood flow in the area around the hemorrhage (5). While these four basic designs have proven to be extremely useful for clinical research using medical images as scientific data, they have many variations and other designs may be more suitable to the specific hypothesis to be tested.

The use of medical imaging to produce accurate quantitative data for scientific investigation of physiological or pathological processes in vivo requires a very different approach to imaging than normally used in clinical medicine and a degree of rigor that is not familiar to most practicing clinicians. In the remainder of this chapter, we address the requirements necessary for application of these technologies to translational research and experimental medicine.

## PRINCIPLES OF QUANTITATIVE IMAGING

### Signal and Noise

Medical imaging devices record signals that are derived from some physical or chemical property of the tissue under study. These signals have a magnitude (amplitude or intensity) and a location. Many medical imaging devices generate data in the form of individual quantitative values derived from contiguous, discreet adjacent volumes of tissue ("voxels"). Each voxel in the dataset has a numerical value that is the same for the entire voxel. The precision of the measurement of the numerical value within each voxel depends on the amount of relevant signal that is acquired by the device for that voxel. This principle is easily demonstrated by radionuclide imaging. In radionuclide imaging, the number of radioactive decay events that take place inside the body are measured by external radiation detectors. Radioactive decay is a random process. Thus, the number of decays will vary somewhat within successive time intervals even when the number of nuclei at risk for decay remains relatively constant (i.e., the total measurement time is very short compared to the decay rate). This variability has a standard deviation equal to the square root of the total number of decays measured (6). Thus, the measurement precision (expressed as the standard deviation/the number of decays) will be 10% in a voxel with 100 measured decay events whereas it will be 3% in a voxel with 1,000 measured decay events. Similar considerations apply to CT, MRI, and other medical imaging modalities although the mathematic expressions are more complicated. Measurements based on small amounts of signal will be less precise and more variable than measurements based on larger amounts of signal. Because the amount of signal acquired by the device is usually proportional to the acquisition time, longer acquisition times usually produce more precise regional measurements. In addition to the magnitude of the true signal, the amount of "noise" will affect measurement precision (Chapter 3). The term *noise* refers to effects on the signal that are recorded by the imaging device but do not derive from the biological process under study. These effects can be due to other processes (e.g., radioactivity from another source outside the structure under study) or arise from the electronic components and computational processes of the imaging device. The effect of noise on the precision of a measurement depends on its magnitude relative to the true signal. The signal to noise ratio must be high or the variability introduced by fluctuations in the noise will make it impossible to measure the signal accurately.

An important source of noise in medical imaging is motion of the object under study during data acquisition. The signal recorded in a single voxel of the imaging device will no longer be derived from a single region in the object. For clinical research, motion of the person is a persistent problem. Various restraining devices are used to reduce motion, particularly for studies of the head. Sedative drugs may be employed, but they may affect the measurement being made (e.g., measurements of cerebral blood flow and metabolism) and pose some risk to the participant. Reducing the acquisition time reduces the chance that movement occurs. However, because the amount of signal acquired by the device is usually proportional to the acquisition time, shorter acquisition times usually produce less precise regional measurements. A different problem arises from normal physiological motion of organs such as the heart or lungs. In these cases, to obtain accurate regional imaging data, image acquisition must be synchronized with the organ's movement (for example, by using an electrocardiogram or respiratory monitor). Very short image acquisitions are collected at the same point in the cardiac or respiratory cycle and then the images are summed. This is known as cardiac or respiratory gating.

## Spatial Resolution

Each medical imaging device has an intrinsic spatial resolution that is determined by the size of the object that can be measured accurately and separately from the surrounding tissue. High spatial resolution devices provide accurate measurements of small volumes or structures, while low resolution devices only provide accurate measurements of larger volumes. Spatial resolution is measured by imaging objects of various sizes and known signal magnitudes to determine how small an object can be and still have its magnitude measured accurately. It is important that the spatial resolution of the imaging device is adequate for the size of the structure under study. Because all imaging devices have a finite spatial resolution, the voxels at the border between two structures of different signal magnitude will contain some signal contribution from both structures. This results in an image that shows a gradual transition of values between two structures even when such a transition doesn't exist (Figure 39–1). The lower the spatial resolution, the more pronounced is this *partial volume effect*. In certain specific circumstances, when there are additional data about the underlying signal distribution, a correction for the partial volume effect can be applied to the image (7,8).

The spatial resolution of the image itself is not always the same as, although it is obviously related

to, the spatial resolution of the device. The resolution of the image is determined by the size of the individual picture elements ("pixels") that are used to create the image. Although it would seem logical that these would be the same size as the actual data voxels generated by the imaging device, this is not necessarily so. Because smaller pixels produce more visually pleasing images, mathematical interpolation sometimes is used to create smaller pixels for image display. In this case, the original pixels are subdivided and the values of the new, smaller pixels are calculated as a weighted average of the original pixel value and the values from surrounding pixels. Creating smaller pixels by interpolation does not improve the quantitative accuracy with which small objects are measured because the device resolution remains the same; it simply produces more visually appealing pictures. Alternatively, image resolution may be lower than the device's resolution. Combining smaller pixels into larger pixels improves the precision of the measurement in each new larger pixel by increasing the amount of signal. However, measurements of small objects made from these larger pixel images will be less accurate unless the new pixel size is still small compared to the object size.

For CT and MRI, device resolution is often expressed as the dimension of the voxels and image resolution as the dimension of the pixels. For SPECT and PET measurements, radioactivity from a given region in the object is redistributed or smeared over a larger area. For a point source of radioactivity, this redistribution approximates the form of a Gaussian (bell-shaped) curve with the maximum value occurring at the original point. As a consequence of this redistribution of radioactivity, the radioactivity measured in the voxels in a given region, regardless of their size, contain only a portion of the radioactivity actually within that region in the original structure. The remainder has been redistributed into surrounding voxels. Similarly, some

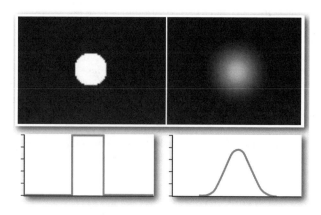

**FIGURE 39–1** ● Partial volume effect in a medical image. An object with an abrupt increase in intensity at its edges (upper left) shows a more gradual transition in signal when imaged with a medical imaging device (upper right). Corresponding profiles of intensity drawn through the center of the object (lower left) and image (lower right) are shown beneath.

radioactivity originally in these surrounding voxels has been redistributed into the region of interest. Thus, the regional radioactivity measurements made with PET or SPECT represent some portion of the radioactivity actually within that region as well as a contribution from radioactivity in surrounding regions. The resolution of PET or SPECT images is expressed as the measured width of the image of a very small object at one-half its maximum intensity—the so-called "full width at half maximum" (FWHM). This is the distance that two objects of the same size and intensity must be apart to be distinguished as separate (Figure 39–2). Additionally, an object must be at least twice the FWHM in size for its radioactivity to be measured accurately. For objects just twice the FWHM in size, only the magnitude of the pixel in the center provides the true radioactivity measurement (Figure 39–3).

## Spatial Uniformity

Clinical interpretation of medical images depends heavily on recognition of abnormal areas of increased or decreased signal within a familiar background pattern. Thus, an area of increased density within the normally dark lung fields in a chest radiograph is easily recognized as an abnormality by the trained observer. Variations in the overall intensity of the film due to differences in body habitus or shadows produced by overlying structures have little effect on the accuracy of this pattern recognition. The trained interpreter can easily compensate for these variations and still identify the abnormal area as distinct from the normal background pattern of

low x-ray density in the lung fields. However, if the signal magnitude (x-ray density) is to be used as a valid measurement for a research study (for example, of lung water content), then a much more rigorous standard for image quality must be met: the *sensitivity*, which is the quantitative relationship between the signal magnitude recorded by the image (in this case x-ray density), and the *magnitude* of the physical quantity of interest (in this case, lung water content) must be uniform across the entire image. In the example of a chest radiograph, this requirement for *spatial uniformity of sensitivity* may be violated if the energy of the x-ray beam is not the same everywhere within the entire the field of view. In areas with higher beam energy, lung regions with the same water content will appear darker than in regions with lower beam strength. Spatial uniformity of sensitivity for an imaging device may be tested by analyzing the image produced by a large test object with uniform composition (uniform phantom). With tomographic imaging processes (x-ray CT, SPECT, PET and MRI), spatial uniformity of sensitivity must be guaranteed not only within each slice (transverse) but across all slices as well (transaxial).

A particular difficulty occurs when characteristics of the object of interest itself affect the relationship between the intensity of the image and physical quantity. This phenomenon is easily observed in the anterior-posterior chest radiograph where the interposition of the heart between the x-ray beam and the film make it impossible to determine the x-ray density of the retrocardiac lung tissue. Because the disruption of the relationship between signal (image)

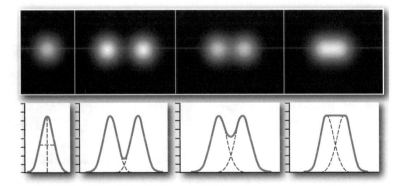

**FIGURE 39–2** ● Effect of image resolution on the ability to distinguish separate objects in PET and SPECT images. Image resolution in PET and SPECT images is expressed as the measured width of the image of a very small object at one-half its maximum intensity—full-width half-maximum (FWHM) (Far left, top image, bottom intensity profile through the center of the image with the maximum height marked by a vertical line and the width at one-half the maximum height marked by a horizontal line.) When two objects are close together, their intensity profiles are superimposed on each other but they can still be distinguished as separate if the centers are more that two FWHM apart (near left and near right, top and bottom). When the centers are less than or equal to two FWHM apart, their intensity profiles are superimposed such that they cannot be distinguished as separate objects (far right, top and bottom).

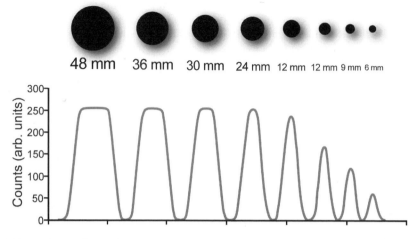

**FIGURE 39–3** ● Effect of image resolution on the ability to accurately measure radioactivity in objects in PET and SPECT images. The objects in the top row have different diameters but all contain the same concentration of radioactivity. The bottom row shows intensity profiles through the center of each object as they would be appear in an image with a resolution of 12 mm FWHM. For objects greater than or equal to twice the FWHM, the peak intensity is an accurate measure of the radioactivity in the object. As the size of the object becomes less than twice the FWHM, the peak intensity will progressively underestimate the radioactivity in the object. Adapted from Cherry SR, Sorenson JA, Phelps ME. Physics in Nuclear Medicine. 3rd Ed. Philadelphia: WB Saunders, 2003, Figure 17–16.

and the physical quantity depends on the individual body characteristics of the person, correcting this problem must be based on some individually measured quantity as well. The simple individual solution of obtaining a lateral chest radiograph only partially solves the problem because of variations in the x-ray absorption by overlying extrapulmonary tissue in other locations. Even x-ray computed tomography (CT), with multiple different projections from different angles, does not always solve this problem due to the effect of dense bone on the x-ray beam. The resultant distortions must be adjusted for when using x-ray CT to obtain quantitative measurements of x-ray density.

A similar problem occurs with imaging of radioactive molecules within the body. A variable fraction of the particles emitted by radioactive decay is absorbed by the surrounding tissue depending on the particle energy and mass, tissue composition, and path length. Thus, radioactive sources of the same strength at different places in the body may cause different intensities of radioactivity to be recorded by external radiation detectors. Similarly, external radiation detectors will record different intensities from the same source depending on their placement. Furthermore, the radioactivity from overlapping superficial and deep structures is superimposed and cannot be distinguished by an overlying external radiation detectors. Although application of CT technology can deal with the issue of overlapping structures, cor-

rection for the attenuation of the radioactive signal by tissue absorption must be performed separately if the radioactivity of the tissue region is to be measured accurately. Single photon emission computed tomography (SPECT) uses a calculated attenuation correction whereas positron emission tomography (PET) employs the physical properties of positron decay to accurately measure the correction for each individual (9) (Figure 39–4).

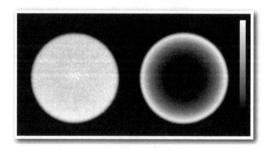

**FIGURE 39–4** ● **Effect of attenuation correction on a PET image.** PET images of a large object filled with a radioactive solution of water with (left) and without (right) attenuation correction for the fraction of the particles emitted by radioactive decay absorbed by the water. The corrected image shows uniform intensity throughout. The uncorrected image shows progressively lower intensity as the distance from the surface of the object increases, reflecting the greater distance that the deeper particles have to travel through the water and thus the greater likelihood that they will be absorbed.

Spatial nonuniformity can also be a problem in research studies when imaging is used to measure the size of anatomic structures or pathological lesions. The relationships between the linear dimensions or volumes measured on the image and the actual dimensions of the object may vary across the image. Imaging a three-dimensional grid of a known size can provide the necessary information to determine the accuracy of such approaches. Spatial image distortion can be a particular problem with magnetic resonance imaging due to inhomogeneities of the magnetic field. Unfortunately, these inhomogeneities may vary depending on the actual object under study (such as those produced by air-bone interfaces), making accurate length and volume measurements very difficult.

## Temporal Uniformity

When the experimental design calls for a comparison to be made among images acquired at different times with the same equipment, the equipment must be tested to ensure that sensitivity remains the same over time. Because most clinical image interpretation is based on detecting an abnormal signal (lesion) against a known background, some change from day to day in sensitivity has little impact on clinical utility as long as the lesion and background are affected more or less the same. Such "drift" can be catastrophic when an accurate quantitative measurement is necessary. Temporal uniformity of the sensitivity of medical imaging devices should not be assumed. It can be confirmed by imaging an object of known signal strength over time or prior to each research scan. In cases where sensitivity varies unpredictably from scan to scan, a standard of known signal can be placed in the field of view and imaged at the same time as the research object. An appropriate correction to the signal from the structure of interest can then be made based on any change in the signal from the standard as long as spatial uniformity is established.

An alternative strategy to deal with temporal nonuniformity is to use the ratio of the measurement in the structure of interest to some other reference region within the tissue. Commonly used ratios are structure to whole organ or structure to some part of the organ. The measurement of the structure of interest is often said to be "normalized" to the reference region. Such ratios or normalization strategies almost always reduce the variability of measurements across different patients or within the same patients studied more than once. However, this strategy also has some significant disadvantages. First, it produces only dimensionless data because the measurement units of the structure of interest are divided by the same measurement units of the reference region.

Second, any biological changes that occur in the reference region will produce inaccuracy in the measurement of the structure of interest. Thus, this technique is best used when previous studies have documented that no change occurs in the reference region under the given experimental circumstances (10). If this criterion has not been met, it is important to remember that any change in the ratio is only relative. Thus, an increase in the structure to reference ratio could be caused by an increase, decease, or no change in the actual measurement in the structure. In some cases, determining relative change is an appropriate experimental goal and provides valuable information. However, the interpretation of the results must always be tempered by acknowledging that the actual measurement changes may be different.

## Linearity

Because the signal magnitude recorded by the medical imaging device is used to measure the magnitude of the physical quantity of interest, it is important to thoroughly understand the quantitative relationship between the two. In ideal circumstances, this relationship (the sensitivity) is constant across a wide range in magnitude of the physical quantity. When graphed, a straight line with 0 intercept results and the sensitivity is said to exhibit *linearity*. Under conditions of linearity, changes in the magnitude of the physical quantity always produces proportional changes in the signal. This, however, is not always the case. The sensitivity may vary with the magnitude of the physical quantity. Under these circumstances, the use of the medical imaging device as a measurement instrument must be restricted to its linear range or corrections for nonlinearity must be applied.

Radiation detection devices always exhibit some degree of nonlinearity. The signals produced by a radiation detector have a finite duration. At some critical rate of radioactive decay, the decay particles will hit the radiation detection system so fast that signals will overlap and not be recorded as separate. These decay particles are called *dead time losses*. Below the critical rate, the device response is linear, but above this critical rate the sensitivity decreases as the radioactivity increases (Figure 39–5). PET and SPECT scanners incorporate corrections for dead time losses, but these corrections may become inaccurate at higher rates of radioactive decay (11).

Another commonly encountered situation in which nonlinearity occurs is the use of magnetic resonance contrast agents to measure cerebral hemodynamics. The relationship between the signal change produced by these paramagnetic compounds and the tissue concentration of the contrast agent is

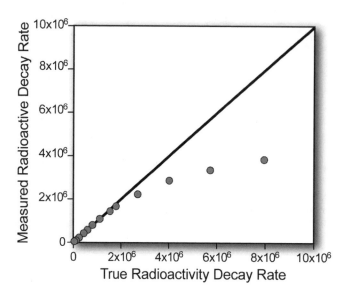

**FIGURE 39–5**  ●  Variation in sensitivity of a radiation detector with radioactive decay rate. The relationship between the rate of radioactive decay measured by the radiation detector is linear at actual decay rates below $2 \times 10^6$, but becomes nonlinear at higher rates. The solid line is the line of identity.

not linear but logarithmic (12). Techniques that use these agents incorporate this relationship into their mathematical computations.

Linearity of a medical imaging device should never be assumed; it must be established empirically for the experimental conditions. Linearity can be checked by imaging a series of objects with known concentrations of the quantity of interest to determine whether the sensitivity is constant. With PET and SPECT, a single radioactive object can be imaged over time to determine if the half-life of the signal decay corresponds to the known half-life of the radionuclide decay.

## Standardization of Different Imaging Devices for Longitudinal or Multicenter Studies

Sometimes, research studies may necessitate imaging on different imaging devices. This can happen with single center studies when a single device is not always available or when the original device is replaced. Multicenter studies almost always require imaging with multiple imaging devices. The challenges presented by this requirement are formidable. Each device has it own signal to noise characteristics, sensitivity, resolution and other characteristics that determine precision and accuracy. Therefore, measurements made on different devices are not necessarily equivalent and may not be directly comparable. Several strategies can be used to deal with this issue. The most rigorous is to design a test object called a phantom that mimics the images that will be acquired for the study and to collect images of the phantom from each different device. Appropriate corrections to the image

data can then be calculated. Similarly, the same human volunteers can be studied on different imaging devices and the results can be used to calculate appropriate corrections. This second approach is less accurate because of biological variability and is most suitable for single center studies with only two devices. A less rigorous approach that has been used with success in PET studies involves selecting an image resolution for all scans that is equal to or lower than the device resolution of the lowest resolution device. The image data are then expressed as a ratio of measurements of the target to a suitable reference region; for example, an affected side of the brain versus the opposite side (13). This approach minimizes the effects of different device resolutions and sensitivities. It still requires spatial uniformity and an adequate signal to noise for measurement precision (e.g., collecting adequate radioactive decay events in a PET image). This approach is being used in the Carotid Occlusion Surgery Study, a multicenter clinical trial to determine whether extracranial-intracranial bypass surgery can reduce the risk of subsequent stroke in patients with symptomatic carotid artery occlusion who are identified to be at high risk because of increased cerebral oxygen extraction measured by PET (http://www.cosstrial.org).

## Multimodality Imaging

Combining data from different imaging modalities is a particularly effective means of studying human physiology and pathophysiology. The most common combinations involve structural images (x-ray CT or proton MRI) with physiological images

(PET, SPECT or MRI). Alternatively, multiple different physiological images may be used. This approach provides accurate anatomic localization of the regional physiological data (e.g., cerebral glucose metabolism in the caudate nucleus) and also allows correlation of different physiological measurements in the same region (e.g., metabolism of glucose, oxygen, and fatty acids in the left ventricle). Multimodality imaging requires that all the individual images be aligned to each other so that the anatomic regions in each image correspond to one another. If the images are acquired sequentially on the same device without the subject moving, this is automatic. Such is the case for multiple sequential PET images or x-ray CT and PET images on the new generations of combined PET-CT devices. If the images are acquired at different times, then they must be aligned subsequently off line. There are a variety of strategies for doing this: (1) Rigid frames may be affixed to the subject and then fastened to each different device in a specified location. (2) External landmarks, called fiducial markers, can be affixed to the human volunteer and detected by each different imaging device. The fiducial markers in the separate images are then aligned to one another. (3) A variety of algorithms have been developed to use the data in the images themselves for alignment. These off-line alignment strategies only work well when the organs under study don't change shape or position with changes in body position. Thus, they work well for the brain but not so well for the heart, lungs, or abdominal contents.

A second issue that arises with multimodality imaging is the effect of differing device resolution. Generally, the resolution of the structural images is better than that of the physiological images. Defining an anatomic structure on a high-resolution image and then obtaining data from corresponding pixels in a lower resolution image will still yield a low-resolution measurement. Often, composite images are created that combine high-resolution anatomy with lower resolution physiology. These can give the impression that the resolution of the physiological image is better than it actually is. It is also important to consider the effect of differing resolutions when comparing physiological data from different images. The corresponding pixels in images of different resolution that have been aligned did not acquire their signal from the same anatomic location. The signal in pixels in the low-resolution image are more affected by surrounding structures. Thus, to accurately compare the values, the two images should have the same resolution. This usually requires selecting an image resolution for all images that is equal to or below the device resolution of the lowest resolution device.

## IMAGE DATA AS BIOLOGIC MEASUREMENTS

### Relation of Image Signal to Biology

Thus far, we have discussed many important issues involved in obtaining accurate and precise quantitative data from medical images. These raw data are in the form of signals that arise from the physical or chemical properties of the tissue under study. Physical properties of tissue used for creating medical images include the absorption of radiation (conventional radiography and x-ray CT), the reflection of ultrasound waves at tissue interfaces (ultrasonography), radioactive decay (SPECT and PET), and the behavior of molecules placed in a magnetic field (MRI and MR spectroscopy). In some cases, the images generated from these physical properties provide direct physical measurements of the tissue structure that can be used for research purposes, such as the diameter of the aorta measured by ultrasonography or the size of brain structures measured by MRI. In other cases, the physical property of the tissue is the measurement of biological interest. A recent example of this is the apparent diffusion coefficient (ADC) measured by magnetic resonance imaging. The ADC is a measure of the rate at which molecules diffuse through a medium (air or soft tissue) and may be altered by a variety of pathological processes (14).

Much more commonly, it is not a physical or chemical property but a biological process that is of scientific interest. In most cases, the signal is not equivalent to the physiological process but is affected by it as well as by other factors. *A thorough understanding of the relationship between the signal recorded by the imaging device and the biological process under study is the single most important requirement for using medical imaging in biologic research.* Such a thorough understanding is not necessary for most *clinical* imaging applications and, in fact, often does not exist. Interpretation of clinical images is based on prior empiric observations of the relationships between image signals and pathology. Knowledge of the accuracy of these interpretations is also derived from prior studies of false-positive and false-negative findings. There is no requirement to understand the biological basis for these empiric relationships. These different requirements for understanding the biological basis of the medical image underscore the fundamental difference between the use of image data for biologic research and for the practice of clinical medicine.

## Tracers and Indicators

Because the signal recorded by the imaging device is not equivalent to a biological process, the initial-raw image must be processed in some manner to produce physiological data. These data are often represented in image format as well, where each pixel has a value equivalent to the physiological measurement for its location. Much of this image processing is based on the principles of tracer kinetics. A tracer is a particle introduced into a physical or biological system that is used to study the properties of the system by measuring the amount and location of the tracer, usually as a function of time. By definition, a tracer is present in such small quantities that its presence does not alter the properties of the system. The term *indicator* is used to refer to both tracers and substances used for the same purpose but present in larger quantities. Because these larger quantities may alter the system by their presence, interpretation of such studies is more difficult.

Application of tracer kinetics to the interpretation of medical images requires three components: a tracer, a device for measuring the tracer, and a mathematical model that relates the measurement of the tracer to the process under study. There are many different methods for measuring the amount and location of the tracer including direct sampling of body fluids such as blood and urine. In this chapter, we restrict this discussion to tracer methods in humans that use some sort of external imaging device to measure the amount and location of the tracer. (Some examples of nonimaging applications of tracer kinetics are given in Chapter 38.) The most commonly used tracers are exogenous substances that are administered internally. These are often radioactive molecules (radiotracers) such as $^{99m}$Tc-sestamibi for SPECT or $^{18}$F-fluorodeoxyglucose for PET. Nonradioactive substances can be used as well. Examples include iodinated contrast for arteriography and x-ray CT, gadolinium-based contrast for MRI, $^{13}$C-glucose for MR spectroscopy, and microbubbles for cardiac ultrasound. Indicators can be endogenous as well, either naturally occurring substances such as $^{23}$Na for sodium MR imaging or substances created endogenously such as magnetization of intravascular water molecules for MRI or oxygenation of hemoglobin for near infrared spectroscopy.

## Temporal Sampling

Some of the important issues regarding imaging devices and measurement accuracy have already been discussed. When imaging devices are used to measure the amount and location of indicators as a function of time, an additional important issue must be considered—temporal sampling. The rate at which the individual image measurements are obtained must be faster than the rate at which the biological process occurs. For example, the normal mean transit time for radioactive red blood cells through the cerebral circulation is 4–7 sec (15). When individual images of the fraction of injected red bloods cells residing in the cerebral vasculature are acquired every 0.1 sec, the transit time can be calculated accurately. Individual images acquired every 5 sec would clearly be inadequate, and it would be difficult to detect small differences in the transit time between groups if images were acquired every 1 sec.

Two factors limit the rate of temporal sampling. The first is the design of the imaging device. Each device has a minimum time interval during which it can acquire data as separate and discrete measurements. The second factor is the trade-off between temporal sampling rate and measurement precision. As noted previously, measurements based on small amounts of signal will be less precise and more variable than measurements based on larger amounts of signal. Because the amount of signal acquired by the device is proportional to image acquisition time, longer acquisition times produce more precise measurements. Therefore, although the scanning device may permit rapid temporal sampling, the shorter these acquisition intervals are, the less precise the measurements will be during each interval. Increasing the amount of indicator to increase the amount of signal acquired per unit time is one obvious strategy to permit more precise, shorter individual acquisition times, but this approach has practical limitations. If endogenous, the amount of tracer is limited by its natural abundance. If exogenous, the amount of tracer is limited by its effect on the process under study or by toxic effects. Toxic effects may be delayed or occur in different organs or systems. Delayed toxic effects are a particular problem with radiotracers and limit the amount of tracer that may be used safely. Design of devices with improved sensitivity can help this problem, but sometimes it is just not possible to obtain adequate precision and adequate temporal sampling with available imaging devices.

## Tracer Kinetic Models

Tracer kinetic models that relate measurements of the indicator to the biologic process under study employ a wide variety of mathematical techniques. Tracer kinetic models must take into account a variety of factors, including delivery of the tracer to the tissue, distribution and metabolism of the tracer within the tissue, egress of tracer and tracer metabolites from the tissue, recirculation of tracer and metabolites, and the amount of tracer and tracer metabolites remaining in the blood. This topic is far beyond the scope of this chapter and the interested reader is referred to specialty articles (16–19). We will, however, illustrate some of the concepts involved by considering three fundamental tracer kinetic principles: the Fick principle, the central volume principle, and the compartmental principle.

The *Fick principle* states that the change in the quantity (q) of a substance in an organ is equal to the arterial blood flow F times the arterial concentration $C_A$ minus the venous blood flow times venous concentration $C_V$. Because arterial blood flow equals venous blood flow:

$$\frac{dq(t)}{dt} = F[C_A(t) - C_V(t)] \qquad (1)$$

The total amount of tracer taken up by the organ at time T, q(T), can be obtained by integration. Rearranged,

$$F = \frac{q(T)}{\int_0^T (C_A(t) - C_V(t))\, dt} \qquad (2)$$

With this equation, three quantities must be known to compute organ blood flow: q(T), $C_A(t)$, and $C_V(t)$. Alternatively, if organ blood flow is known, the Fick principle can be used to determine substrate metabolism,

$$MR = F\,(C_A - C_V) \qquad (3)$$

where MR (metabolic rate) is the steady-state rate of substrate utilization by the organ, F is the blood flow in volume of blood per unit time, and $C_A$–$C_V$ is the steady state difference in concentration of the substance in arterial and venous blood. Medical imaging is particularly suited to measure q(T) for organs or regions of an organ. Tracer kinetic models based on the Fick principle are commonly used to measure organ blood flow with medical imaging.

*The central volume principle* is based on the concept of transit time. If a bolus of a tracer is introduced into arterial blood flowing into a tissue, the tracer particles will flow through the tissue and then exit via the venous drainage (15). Because all particles will not take the same path, they will take different times to transit the tissue. The mean transit time, $\bar{t}$, for the particles is determined by the volume in which the tracer is distributed $V_d$ and the flow F through the tissue:

$$\bar{t} = \frac{V_d}{F} \qquad (4)$$

The mean transit time can be determined by measuring the total amount of tracer injected $q_o$ and the residual amount that remains in the tissue as a function of time q(t),

$$\bar{t} = \frac{\int_0^\infty q(t)\,dt}{q_0} \qquad (5)$$

Medical imaging devices are particularly suited to measure q(t). With radioactive tracers, this residual amount (residue function) in an organ can be measured with external radiation detection devices. However, external radiation detection devices don't measure all the radioactivity emitted; some is absorbed by the tissue and some exits at angles not covered by the detector crystals. The efficiency of detection $\varepsilon$ is dependent on the particular external radiation detection device, the structure under study, and the position of the device relative to the structure. If the volume of the tracer injection is small enough, the injection is fast enough, and the temporal sampling rate is rapid enough, all the tracer going to the tissue region under study will still be in the tissue during the initial acquisition period and will thus be measured by the external detector as the initial portion of the residue curve. Thus, the initial height will be equal to $q_0$. Both the initial height and the remainder of the residue curve will be measured at the same efficiency, so $\bar{t}$ can be measured accurately. In this case,

$$\bar{t} = \frac{\varepsilon \int_0^\infty q(t)\,dt}{\varepsilon\, q_0} = \frac{\text{Area}}{\text{Height}} = \frac{V_d}{F} \qquad (6)$$

The area and initial height of the residue curve are determined by the medical imaging device. If the volume of distribution of the tracer in the organ is known from previous in vitro experiments, F can be determined (20).

Methods based on the *compartmental principle* differ from those based on the Fick and central volume principles because they make certain assumptions about the behavior of the tracer in the tissue. Compartmental models consist of a finite number of homogenous, well-mixed pools (i.e., compartments) that interact by the exchange of material. A fundamental assumption of compartmental models is that the concentration of the tracer in a compartment is instantaneously the same everywhere once it is introduced into the compartment. Compartment models are reasonable approximations of the behavior of freely diffusible tracers in some organs. (Another example of compartment models was described in Chapter 20 on pharmacokinetics.) Compartmental models, however, do not accurately describe all biologic systems. The behavior of tracers confined to the intravascular blood pool, for instance, does not conform to compartmental principles.

The change in quantity of tracer in each compartment is expressed in terms of the fraction of the quantity in one compartment that moves to the other compartment in a given time period, for example per minute (1/min or $min^{-1}$). For a simple two-compartment model with exchange in both directions (Figure 39–6):

$$\frac{dq_1(t)}{dt} = k_{12}q_2 - k_{21}q_1 \qquad (7)$$

$$\frac{dq_2(t)}{dt} = k_{21}q_1 - k_{12}q_2 \qquad (8)$$

where $q_1$ and $q_2$ are the quantities of tracer in compartments 1 and 2 respectively, $k_{12}$ is the rate constant for movement of tracer from compartment 2 to 1, and $k_{21}$ is the rate constant for movement from compartment 1 to 2. Integration of these differential equations provides equations that express the amount of tracer in each compartment as a function of time. The sum of the quantities in all compartments represents the total amount of tracer in the system. With the exception of measurements of blood, it is usually not possible to measure separately the amount of tracer in each compartment with medical imaging devices because these compartments may not be actual physical entities and, if they are, may be completely spatially interdigitated with each other. Thus, most physiological image processing that relies on compartmental models uses image measurements of the overall sum of the tracer in all compartments to calculate the tracer quantities and rate constants for the individual compartments.

Calculation of rate constants by compartmental modeling often employs parameter estimation. Parameter estimation is a mathematical technique in which various different combinations of values for the rate constants are used to predict how much total tracer should be in the system as a function of time. Each prediction is checked against the actual measured total amount of tracer in the system over time. When the technique works, there is a unique combination of values for the rate constants that results in a prediction that very closely matches the real data (Figure 39–7). These values are then assumed to represent the properties of the system and used to calculate biologically relevant measurement values, such as blood-to-organ transport or organ metabolism. However, just because the model produces a prediction that fits the actual data uniquely and well does not mean that the values of the rate constants are equivalent to actual biological quantities. All models must be validated for biological accuracy.

## Validation of Tracer Kinetic Models

No matter how comprehensive tracer kinetic models may be, fundamentally, they are all simplifications of extremely complex biological systems. As simplifications, all models are inaccurate to some degree and rely on certain implicit and explicit assumptions that may or may not be true, or may be true only in certain cases. *Therefore, it is necessary to validate the accuracy of the model-based method under the conditions it will be used.* Such validations are often technically difficult, time consuming, and don't produce any new scientific knowledge, but they are the necessary foundation for any research using the method.

The ideal means to validate a model-based method is to compare values obtained with the method to values obtained simultaneously by a reference standard (often called a gold standard) for a wide range of values under variety of different conditions. These reference standards are often invasive or otherwise inappropriate for use in humans. Thus, a common strategy is to validate the model-based method in a relevant animal model with the assumption that such validations will apply to the use of the noninvasive imaging method in humans.

An excellent example is the validation in nonhuman primates of a PET imaging method to measure the cerebral oxygen extraction fraction (OEF) by comparison with a direct measurement of OEF (21, 22). This method was developed to be used under a wide variety of physiologic and pathologic conditions. In the validation studies, OEF, the cerebral metabolic rate of oxygen, and cerebral blood flow were varied over a wide range by manipulating $P_aCO_2$ and by intravenous methohexital and sodium cyanide infusions. The results are presented both in the form of a graph and a regression equation: OEF (PET) = 1.03 OEF (reference) + 0.01, r = .94 (Figure 39–8A). The graph provides the data to determine whether there is a systematic difference at different

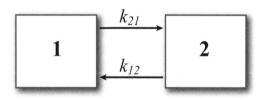

**FIGURE 39–6** ● Diagram of a **two-compartment model.** Diagram of a two-compartment tracer kinetic model. $k_{12}$ is the rate constant for movement of tracer from compartment 2 to 1 and $k_{21}$ is the rate constant for movement from compartment 1 to 2.

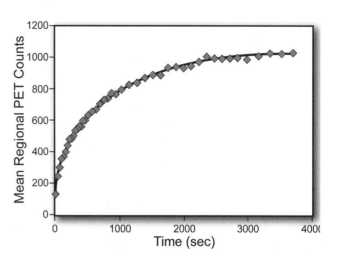

**FIGURE 39–7** ● **Parameter estimation curve.** The diamonds represent brain radioactivity measurements made with PET at different times after intravenous administration of 178 microcuries on $^{11}$C-glucose to newborn infant. The solid line shows the final estimated regional time-radioactivity curve based on the combination of parameters that provide the curve that fits the measured data best. Adapted from Powers WJ, Rosenbaum JL, Dence CS et al. Cerebral glucose transport and metabolism in preterm infants. J Cereb Blood Flow Metab 1998; 18:632–638, Figure 2.

OEF values. The value of r > .90 indicates the excellent correlation between the two methods, but is not sufficient to demonstrate the validity of a new method, unless the slope is close to one and the intercept close to zero. In this case, the slope of 1.03 and the intercept of 0.01 along with the r value of .94 demonstrates that the PET method produces essentially identical values to the reference method. Another way of displaying the data is by the method of Bland and Altman (Figure 39–8B) (Chapter 3) (23).

Validation studies do not always show such close agreement between methods, but can still provide important information. For instance, Figure 39–9 shows a comparison of a PET method for measurement of cerebral blood flow (CBF) to a reference standard in nonhuman primates. The PET method is accurate at CBF levels of 15–40 ml $100g^{-1}$ $min^{-1}$ but underestimates higher values (24). Thus, this method should not be used when accurate measurements of CBF > 40 ml $100g^{-1}$ $min^{-1}$ are required.

Sometimes it is not feasible or possible to perform this type of rigorous validation. There may be no reference standard for a new measurement, or there may be no way to manipulate the values in a controlled manner to the extent necessary to encompass the range of values expected under the experimental conditions. Under these circumstances, some degree of validation can be obtained by determining whether the measurement changes in direction and magnitude as expected under known conditions or if it produces values that are plausible when compared to those obtained in other species or circumstances.

In addition to an empiric validation, a rigorous error analysis of the method, as revealed by computer simulations, can be valuable. Such analyses determine how errors arising from different sources affect the final measurement. For example, a researcher might want to determine how inaccurate

the final measurement of organ blood flow would be if there was a 10% underestimation in the measurement of blood tracer concentration. Errors may affect the final measurement by more or less magnitude than the original error. These error analyses serve two purposes. They indicate the degree of quality control necessary for each component of the method to produce a final measurement of the required precision and accuracy. They also provide some indication of what conditions may render the method sufficiently inaccurate to preclude its use. However, even error analysis cannot test the validity of the underlying assumptions of the model and their effect on measurement accuracy under different conditions. For methods that have not been rigorously validated under the identical conditions in which they will be used, the likelihood that these assumptions are violated and the effect of violations on the accuracy of the final measurement should be carefully analyzed for each experiment.

## A Special Problem in the Statistical Analysis of Image Data

The majority of statistical analyses in translational research and experimental medicine involve detecting differences between groups of measurements or associations among pairs of measurements. These analyses are, by and large, based on the concept that the individual measurements or measurement pairs are independent observations, not influenced by one another. The number of independent measurements or measurement pairs determines the degrees of freedom of the statistical analysis, which in turn determines the probability that the magnitude of the observed difference between groups or the observed association between pairs could have occurred by chance if the groups are actually not different or if no association exists (Chapters 24

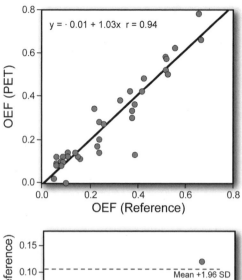

$y = \cdot 0.01 + 1.03x \quad r = 0.94$

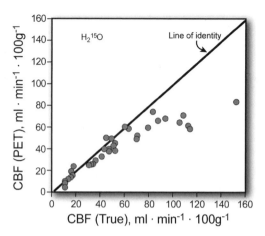

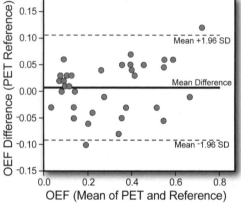

**FIGURE 39–9** ● Validation plot of PET versus reference measurement of cerebral blood flow. The PET method is accurate at CBF levels of 15–40 ml $100g^{-1}$ $min^{-1}$ but underestimates higher values. Adapted from Raichle ME, Martin WRW, Herscovitch P et al. Brain blood flow measured with intravenous $H_2{}^{15}O$. II. Implementation and validation. J Nucl Med 1983;24:790–798, Figure 3.

**FIGURE 39–8** ● Validation plots of PET versus reference measurements of cerebral oxygen extraction fraction. **A.** (upper) XY plot **B.** (lower) Bland-Altman plot. Data from Mintun MA, Raichle ME, Martin WRW et al. Brain oxygen utilization measured with O-15 radiotracers and positron emission tomography. J Nucl Med 1984;25:177–187 and Altman DI, Lich LL, Powers WJ. Brief inhalation method to measure cerebral oxygen extraction fraction with PET: accuracy determination under pathologic conditions. J Nucl Med 1991;32:1738–1741.

and 25). The higher the degrees of freedom, the smaller is the magnitude of the difference or association that is necessary to reach a given probability. Because a 5% probability threshold ($p < 0.05$) is conventionally accepted as the criterion for statistical significance, the interpretation of the results of a study can be highly dependent on the number of measurements entered into the analysis.

The special problem posed by image data is the correct choice for the degrees of freedom for each analysis. Each medical image contains thousand of pixels, each with its own numeric value. The values in each pixel are not independent of the immediately adjacent pixels, so treating individual pixel values as independent measures for statistical analysis is

clearly incorrect. However, as pixels or groups of pixels get further from each other, the measurements do become more independent but are still related because they are derived from the same person. Exactly how to deal with these issues is the subject of research and debate (25,26). The most conservative approach is to perform analyses in which the number of measurements is equal to the number of research participants. Because these are truly independent measurements, the results will be statistically valid.

## SUMMARY

- The use of medical images to produce quantitative data for scientific investigation requires a degree of rigor that is not necessary for most clinical applications. Four basic requirements provide a foundation for applying imaging technologies to translational research and experimental medicine.
- Strict quality control measures to establish and ensure the quantitative accuracy of the image data.
- A thorough understanding of the properties of the imaging device and how these properties may affect the experimental results.
- A thorough understanding of the relationship between the signal recorded by the imaging device and the biological process under study.
- Validation of the accuracy of any model-based method under the conditions it will be used.

## REFERENCES

1. Jaeschke R, Guyatt GH, Sackett DL. Users' guides to the medical literature. III. How to use an article about a diagnostic test. B. What are the results and will they help me in caring for my patients? JAMA 1994;271:703–707.
2. Fanelli CG, Dence CS, Markham J et al. Blood-to-brain glucose transport and cerebral glucose metabolism are not reduced in poorly controlled type I diabetes mellitus. Diabetes 1998;47:1444–1450.
3. Grubb Jr RL, Derdeyn CP, Fritsch SM et al. The importance of hemodynamic factors in the prognosis of symptomatic carotid occlusion. JAMA 1998;280:1055–1060.
4. The NINDS rt-PA Stroke Study Group. Effect of intravenous recombinant tissue plasminogen activator on ischemic stroke lesion size measured by computed tomography. Stroke 2000;31:2912–2919.
5. Powers WJ, Zazulia AR, Videen TO et al. Autoregulation of cerebral blood flow surrounding acute (6–22 hours) intracerebral hemorrhage. Neurology 2001;57:18–24.
6. Cherry SR, Sorenson JA, Phelps ME. Physics in Nuclear Medicine. 3rd Ed. Philadelphia: Saunders, 2003:32–135.
7. Videen TO, Dunford-Shore JE, Diringer MN et al. Correction for partial volume effects in regional blood flow measurements adjacent to hematomas in humans with intracerebral hemorrhage: implementation and validation. J Comput Assist Tomogr 1999;23:248–256.
8. Zazulia AR, Diringer MN, Videen TO et al. Hypoperfusion without ischemia surrounding acute intracerebral hemorrhage. J Cereb Blood Flow Metab 2001;21:804–810.
9. Powers WJ. Positron Emission Tomography. In: Aminoff MJ, Daroff RB, eds. Encyclopedia of the Neurological Sciences. San Diego: Academic Press, 2003;4:34–38.
10. Fox PT, Raichle ME. Stimulus rate dependence of regional cerebral blood flow in human striate cortex, demonstrated by positron emission tomography. J Neurosphys 1984;51:1109–1120.
11. Cherry SR, Sorenson JA, Phelps ME. Physics in Nuclear Medicine. 3rd Ed. Philadelphia: Saunders, 2003:178–182.
12. Rosen BR, Belliveau JW, Vevea JM et al. Perfusion imaging with NMR contrast agents. Magn Reson Med 1990; 14:249–265.
13. Derdeyn CP, Videen TO, Simmons NR et al. Count-based PET method for predicting ischemic stroke in patients with symptomatic carotid arterial occlusion. Radiology 1999;212:499–506.
14. Roberts TLP, Rowley HA. Diffusion weighted magnetic resonance imaging in stroke. Eur J Radiol 2003; 45:185–194.
15. Phelps ME, Eichling JO. A quick method for calculation of the vascular mean transit time. J Nucl Med 1974;15:814–817.
16. Peters AM. Fundamentals of tracer kinetics for radiologists. Br J Radiol 1998;71:1116–1129.
17. Zierler KL. Equations for measuring blood flow by external monitoring of radioisotopes. Circ Res 1965; 16:309–321.
18. Weisskoff RM, Chesler D, Boxerman JL et al. Pitfalls in MR measurement of tissue blood flow with intravascular tracers: which mean transit time? Magn Reson Med 1993;29:553–558.
19. Larson KB, Markham J, Raichle ME. Tracer-kinetic models for measuring cerebral blood flow using externally detected radiotracers. J Cereb Blood Flow Metab 1987;7:443–463.
20. Hoedt-Rasmussen K, Sveinsdottir E, Lassen NA. Regional cerebral blood flow in man determined by intra-arterial injection of radioactive inert gas. Circ Res 1966;18:237–247.
21. Mintun MA, Raichle ME, Martin WRW et al. Brain oxygen utilization measured with O-15 radiotracers and positron emission tomography. J Nucl Med 1984; 25:177–187.
22. Altman DI, Lich LL, Powers WJ. Brief inhalation method to measure cerebral oxygen extraction fraction with PET: accuracy determination under pathologic conditions. J Nucl Med 1991;32:1738–1741.
23. Bland JM, Altman DG. Measuring agreement in method comparison studies. Stat Methods Med Res 1999;8:135–160.
24. Raichle ME, Martin WRW, Herscovitch P et al. Brain blood flow measured with intravenous $H_2^{15}O$. II. Implementation and validation. J Nucl Med 1983;24:790–798.
25. Petersson KM, Nichols TE, Poline JB et al. Statistical limitations in functional neuroimaging. I. Non-inferential methods and statistical models. Philos Trans R Soc Lond B Biol Sci 1999;354:1239–1260.
26. Petersson KM, Nichols TE, Poline JB et al. Statistical limitations in functional neuroimaging. II. Signal detection and statistical inference. Philos Trans R Soc Lond B Biol Sci 1999;354:1261–1281.

# INDEX

Page numbers followed by "f" indicate figures; those followed by "t" indicate tables.